Comprehensive Neurosurgery Board Review

Second Edition

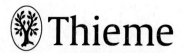

Comprehensive Neurosurgery Board Review
Second Edition

Jonathan S. Citow, MD
Private Practice
Libertyville, Illinois

R. Loch Macdonald, MD, PhD
Keenan Endowed Chair in Surgery
Head, Division of Neurosurgery, St. Michael's Hospital
Professor of Surgery, University of Toronto
Toronto, Ontario, Canada

Daniel Refai, MD
Chief Resident in Neurosurgery
Washington University School of Medicine
Barnes Jewish Hospital
St. Louis, Missouri

Thieme
New York • Stuttgart

Thieme Medical Publishers, Inc.
333 Seventh Avenue
New York, NY 10001

Editorial Director: Michael Wachinger
Executive Editor: Kay D. Conerly
Editorial Assistant: Dominik Pucek
Vice President, Production and Electronic Publishing: Anne T. Vinnicombe
Production Editors: Martha L. Wetherill, Donald Whitehead
Vice President, International Marketing and Sales: Cornelia Schulze
Chief Financial Officer: Peter Van Woerden
President: Brian D. Scanlan
Compositor: MPS Content Services
Printer: Everbest Printing Company
Cover illustrations by Markus Voll and Karl Wesker

Library of Congress Cataloging-in-Publication Data

Comprehensive neurosurgery board review / [edited by] Jonathan S. Citow, R. Loch Macdonald, Daniel Refai.—2nd ed.
      p. ; cm.
     Includes bibliographical references and index.
     ISBN 978-1-60406-031-7
     1. Nervous system—Surgery—Examinations, questions, etc.   I. Citow, Jonathan Stuart.   II. Macdonald, R. Loch (Robert Loch)
III. Refai, Daniel.
     [DNLM: 1. Nervous System Diseases—surgery—Examination Questions.   2. Neurosurgical Procedures—methods—Examination Questions.
WL 18.2 C7365   2009]
    RD593.C5966 2009
    617.4'80076—dc22
                                                                                                                     2009008432

Important note: Medical knowledge is ever-changing. As new research and clinical experience broaden our knowledge, changes in treatment and drug therapy may be required. The authors and editors of the material herein have consulted sources believed to be reliable in their efforts to provide information that is complete and in accord with the standards accepted at the time of publication. However, in view of the possibility of human error by the authors, editors, or publisher of the work herein, or changes in medical knowledge, neither the authors, editors, or publisher, nor any other party who has been involved in the preparation of this work, warrants that the information contained herein is in every respect accurate or complete, and they are not responsible for any errors or omissions or for the results obtained from use of such information. Readers are encouraged to confirm the information contained herein with other sources. For example, readers are advised to check the product information sheet included in the package of each drug they plan to administer to be certain that the information contained in this publication is accurate and that changes have not been made in the recommended dose or in the contraindications for administration. This recommendation is of particular importance in connection with new or infrequently used drugs. Some of the product names, patents, and registered designs referred to in this book are in fact registered trademarks or proprietary names even though specific reference to this fact is not always made in the text. Therefore, the appearance of a name without designation as proprietary is not to be construed as a representation by the publisher that it is in the public domain.

Printed in China

5 4 3 2 1

ISBN 978-1-60406-031-7

To Benjamin, Emma, and Harrison—thank you yet again for your patience. Less books and surgeries, more swinging and dancing. To my wife Karen—the ultimate rock, and yet so soft. Need I say more? To my mother Phyllis—still so supportive despite being almost 120 years old. Thanks as always.

Jonathan S. Citow, MD

To Sheilah, my love for almost 30 years. I pray for more than another 30. You make it all worth it. To Iain, Robyn, and Erin. I hope you can find your lives as fulfilling as I do mine. To my parents, Neil and Lea. I am proud to think you inspired me to do this work in service to humanity.

R. Loch Macdonald, MD, PhD

I wish to dedicate this book to my parents, Hamid and Ana Refai, for their tireless love and support of my education; to my wife, Anushka, for her unending love and support of my endeavors; to my brother and sister, Dean and Nily, for encouraging me to pursue my aspirations in life; and to my educators at Washington University in Saint Louis for teaching me first to be a physician and second, a neurosurgeon.

Daniel Refai, MD

To all those who dedicate their lives to learning and teaching the knowledge and skill of this profession so that those afflicted with neurosurgical illnesses may be cared for to the best of our abilities.

Scellig Stone, MD

To my loved ones...

Demitre Serletis, MD

Contents

Preface

With the expert help of my coauthors in the Division of Neurosurgery residency at the University of Toronto, we have revised *Comprehensive Neurosurgery Board Review* extensively. We have added material to cover gaps identified by readers of the first edition and updated chapters to include the latest information on the neurosciences, including such areas as molecular biology. We have removed redundancy within and between chapters as much as possible and reformatted the text to promote quick review and memory retention.

The *Comprehensive Neurosurgery Board Review, Second Edition* provides summary information for the senior resident and practicing neurosurgeon preparing for the boards. However, it is more than a "board review" book. For those of us who have been in practice for years and want to keep up with the residents, the book provides a refresher course on such neurosurgical topics as neuro-anatomy and trauma. It also serves as a quick reference for the neurosurgeon whose daily practice does not typically involve the full breadth of the field.

Acknowledgments

I am grateful to the editors and staff at Thieme for such expert help. I worked with and appreciate the help of Birgitta Brandenberg, Ivy Ip, and Kay Conerly. Thanks for another professional text that I hope will be valuable to a generation of neurosurgeons. Dominik Pucek managed the manuscript with precision and kept me on schedule. I also acknowledge Brian Scanlan. He has made Thieme a leader in neurosurgical publishing and inspired me to help edit this and other books that will live up to his standards.

Contributors

Editors

Jonathan S. Citow, MD
Private Practice
Libertyville, Illinois

R. Loch Macdonald, MD, PhD
Keenan Endowed Chair in Surgery
Head, Division of Neurosurgery, St. Michael's Hospital
Professor of Surgery, University of Toronto
Toronto, Ontario, Canada

Daniel Refai, MD
Chief Resident in Neurosurgery
Washington University School of Medicine
Barnes Jewish Hospital
St. Louis, Missouri

Assistant Editors

Greg Hawryluk, MD
Neurosurgery Resident
University of Toronto
Toronto, Ontario, Canada

Betty Kim, MD
Neurosurgery Resident
University of Toronto
Toronto, Ontario, Canada

Charles Matouk, MD
Neurosurgery Resident
University of Toronto
Toronto, Ontario, Canada

Carlo Santaguida, MD
Neurosurgery Resident
University of Toronto
Toronto, Ontario, Canada

Demitre Serletis, MD
Neurosurgery Resident
University of Toronto
Toronto, Ontario, Canada

Scellig Stone, MD
Neurosurgery Resident
University of Toronto
Toronto, Ontario, Canada

1 Anatomy

Associate Editor, **Betty Kim**

I. Meninges

A. Meningeal layers

Layer	Description

Dura	Tough layer of connective tissue
	Composed of two layers
	    External periosteal layer — adheres to the periosteum of the calvaria within the cranial cavity, does not extend beyond foramen magnum (thus, spinal dura has only one layer)
	    Inner meningeal layer — extends beyond foramen magnum and forms the spinal dura, which ends at S2

Leptomeninges Arachnoid	Translucent middle layer between the dura and pia, contains tight junctions Composed of fibroblasts, collagen fibers, and some elastic fibers Subarachnoid space = cerebrospinal fluid (CSF) + cerebral arteries + superficial cerebral veins

Pia	Directly lines the cerebrum and its fissures, lacks tight junctions
	Composed of two layers:
	    Intimal layer — avascular, receives nutrients from CSF and neural tissues
	    Epipial layer — continous with arachnoid trabeculae, absent over the convexities
	The outer layer is covered by simple squamous epithelium.
	Dentate ligament — formed by pia, stretches from midpoint between dorsal and ventral roots on the lateral spinal cord surface to attach to the arachnoid and dura
	Filum terminale — extension of epipia which condenses and continues from S2 and ends as the coccygeal ligament.

B. Virchow–Robin spaces — a perivascular potential space, between blood vessels and the surrounding sheath of leptomeninges entering the nervous tissue (brain and spinal cord)

C. Cisterns — regions where the meningeal layers (pia and arachnoid) are widely separated

    1. Surrounding the midbrain — interpeduncular, crural, ambient (contains the vein of Galen, posterior cerebral [PCAs] and superior cerebellar arteries [SCAs]), and quadrigeminal cisterns; also, cerebello-medullary (cisterna magna), pontine, chiasmatic, sylvian, and lumbar (maximal at L2) cisterns

D. Meningeal blood supply, innervation, and embryological origins

Blood Supply	Neural Innervation	Embryologic Origin
Anterior meningeal artery (ophthalmic artery)	Supratentorial dura:	Ectoderm:
	V_1: Anterior fossa	Leptomeninges
Middle meningeal artery (maxillary branch)	V_2: Middle fossa	Ependyma
Posterior meningeal artery (occipital and vertebral arteries)	V_3: Posterior fossa, mastoid air cells	Neural parenchyma
		Glia
Blood supply to the tentorium:		
Cavernous internal carotid artery	Infratentorial dura:	Mesoderm:
Superior cerebellar artery	Upper cervical roots (C2, C3)	Dura
Proximal posterior cerebral artery	Cranial nerve X	Blood vessels
	Spine:	
	Recurrent branches of the spine (via interventricular foramina)	

II. Cerebrospinal Fluid

A. Function: waste removal, carry nutrition to the brain, cushioning of the brain and regulating various brain functions via neurotransmitters, paracrine and endocrine effects. Hypothalamic hormones are secreted into the cerebrospinal fluid (CSF) and transported by the ependymal cells to the hypophyseal portal system.

B. CSF constituents

Components	Values	Additional Comments
Ions and biochemistry	Comparison with plasma:	β-transferrin: found exclusively in the CSF, used to assess CSF leak
	↑ in CSF: Cl^-	Froin's syndrome: CSF xanthochromia and clotting (due to the presence of fibrinogen) occur when CSF is loculated, usually in the lumbar thecal sac. CSF protein is increased (up to 1000 mg/L).
	↓ in CSF: K^+, Ca^{2+}, uric acid, and glucose	
	Same: Na^+, osmolarity	
	Normal values in CSF:	
	Glucose = 45–80 mg/dL (⅔ of serum value)	CSF Specific gravity: 1.007
	Protein ≤45 mg/dL	CSF pH: 7.33–7.35
Cellular	Lymphocytes: <5	Traumatic tap = 700 RBCs per 1 WBC
	PMNs and RBCs: none	

Abbreviations: CSF, cerebrospinal fluid; PMNs, polymorphonuclear neutrophils; RBCs, red blood cells; WBC, white blood cell

C. CSF production

1. Active process — Na^+ is actively secreted into the subarachnoid space via Na^+/K^+ adenosine triphosphate (ATP) pump with H_2O from vessels following the Na^+ ions

2. Sites of CSF production
   a. 70% Choroid plexus
   b. 18% Ultrafiltrate
   c. 12% Metabolic H_2O production

3. Control of CSF production
   a. Raphe nuclei send axons (serotonin) to the periependymal vessels.

b. Decreased production
    (1) Carbonic anhydrase inhibitors (acetazolamide)
    (2) Norepinephrine (NE)
c. Increased production
    (1) Volatile anesthetics and CO_2

4. CSF volumes in a 70 kg man
  a. 450 mL = CSF production each day. CSF production is 0.3–0.37 mL/minute, 20 mL/h
  b. 150 mL = total volume
  c. 25 mL = within ventricles

5. Choroid plexus — a single layer of cuboidal epithelial cells surrounding blood vessels, involved in CSF production. Primarily located in
  a. Roof of the fourth ventricle
  b. Inferior medullary velum and lateral recess to the foramen of Luschka
  c. Posterior roof of the third ventricle
  d. Floors of the bodies and roofs of the temporal horns of the lateral ventricles (LVs) (**Fig. 1.1**)

D. CSF absorption

1. Passive process — absorption by arachnoid granulation cells that transmit CSF in giant cytoplasmic vacuoles via bulk flow into the venous sinuses

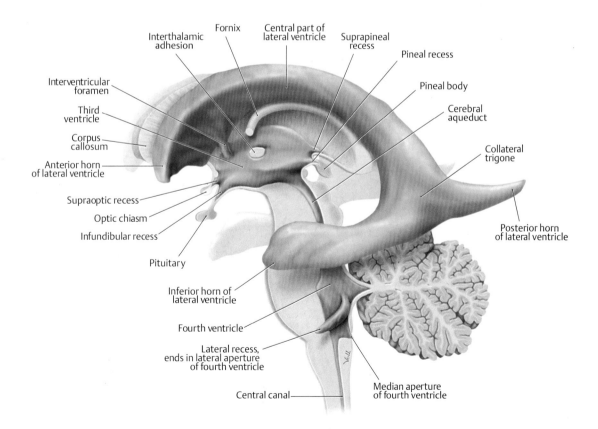

Fig. 1.1 Overview of the ventricular system and important neighboring structures. Left lateral view. The ventricular system is an expanded and convoluted tube that is the upper extension of the central spinal canal into the brain. (From THIEME Atlas of Anatomy, Head and Neuroanatomy, © Thieme 2007, Illustration by Markus Voll.)

2. Control of CSF absorption — pressure-dependent

3. Arachnoid granulations
    a. Most abundant at the superior sagittal sinus, contains arachnoid villi
    b. A pressure-dependent one-way valve, with collapsing tubules that transmit CSF when intracranial pressure (ICP) is 3–6 cm H_2O greater than the venous pressure

E. Intracranial pressure

1. Monro–Kellie doctrine — the closed skull has a fixed/constant volume with
    a. 1500 mL brain tissue
    b. 150 mL blood (arteries + veins)
    c. 150 mL CSF (total volume)
    d. Any added volume (brain swelling due to edema, increased blood volume, increased CSF, tumor, hemorrhage, etc.) forces removal of normal inhabitants of the cranial cavity.

2. Normal ICP values
    a. <10–15 mm Hg — adults and older children
    b. 3–8 mm Hg — younger children
    c. 1.5–6 mm Hg — infants

III. Brain Barriers

A. Blood–brain barrier (BBB) formed by

1. Capillary endothelial tight junctions (mainly)

2. Pinocytic activity in endothelial cells

3. Astrocytic foot processes

B. Molecular movement across the BBB

1. Diffusion

2. Carrier-mediated transport (D-glucose, amino acids)

3. Active transport

C. Permeability across the BBB

1. Highly permeable — H_2O, CO_2, O_2, lipid-soluble (ethanol, barbiturates, heroin, and anesthetics)

2. Slightly permeable — ions (Na^+, Cl^-, and K^+)

3. Impermeable — plasma proteins, protein-bound molecules, large organic molecules, and L-glucose

D. Blood–CSF barrier is formed by the tight junctions of choroid cuboidal epithelium (although blood vessels have fenestrated capillaries).

E. Circumventricular organs are midline ventricular system structures of specialized tissues with absent BBB due to fenestrated capillaries.

1. Circumventricular organs (from rostral to caudal)

Organ	Feature
Organum vasculosum (lamina terminalis)	Outlet for hypothalamic peptides Detect peptides, amino acids, and proteins in blood
Neurohypophysis	Outlet for hypothalamic hormones (vasopressin and oxytocin)
Median eminence of the hypothalamus	Release hypothalamic-releasing factors
Subfornical organ	May be involved in body fluid regulation Located between the foramina of Monro Connected to the choroid plexus
Subcommissural organ	Function: unknown, located under the posterior commissure The only circumventricular organ with an intact BBB
Pineal gland	Melatonin production Role in circadian rhythm
Area postrema	A chemoreceptor that induces emesis when stimulated by digitalis or apomorphine Located on the floor of the fourth ventricle The only paired circumventricular organ

IV. Blood Supply to the Brain

A. General – The brain constitutes only 2% of body weight (1500 g) but receives 17% of the cardiac output and uses 20% of the body's oxygen.

B. Cerebral blood flow

Cerebral Blood Flow	Flow Rate (mL/100 g of Brain Tissue per Minute)
Normal	50
Ischemic penumbra (reversible)	8–23
Irreversible neuronal death	< 8

C. Origins of great vessels

1. Brachiocephalic (innominate) — bifurcates into the right common carotid artery and left subclavian artery → vertebral artery → internal mammary artery → thyrocervical trunk → costocervical trunk

2. Left common carotid artery

3. Left subclavian artery gives off vertebral, thyrocervical, and costocervical trunks.
   a. Vertebral artery dominance
      (1) Left side = 50%
      (2) Right side = 25%
      (3) Nondominance = 25%
   b. The left vertebral artery arises from the aorta in 5% of cases; 40% of the population has a hypoplastic vertebral artery.

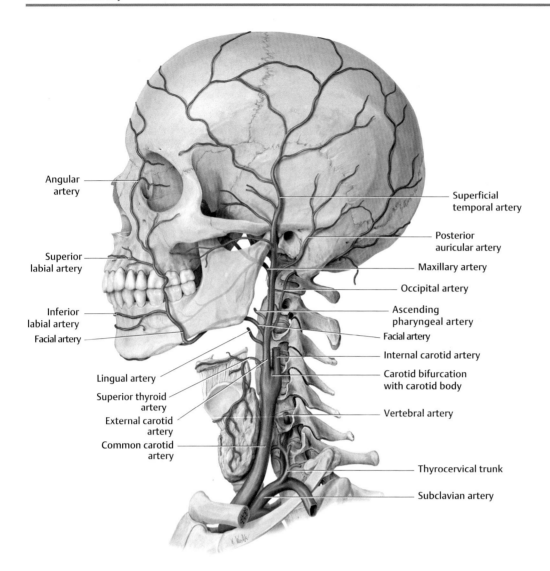

Angular artery
Superior labial artery
Inferior labial artery
Facial artery
Lingual artery
Superior thyroid artery
External carotid artery
Common carotid artery

Superficial temporal artery
Posterior auricular artery
Maxillary artery
Occipital artery
Ascending pharyngeal artery
Facial artery
Internal carotid artery
Carotid bifurcation with carotid body
Vertebral artery
Thyrocervical trunk
Subclavian artery

Fig. 1.2 Overview of arteries of the head. Left lateral view. The common carotid artery divides into internal and external carotid arteries at the carotid bifurcation, which is usually at the level of the fourth cervical vertebra. There are eight branches of the external and none of the cervical internal carotid artery. (From THIEME Atlas of Anatomy, Head and Neuroanatomy, © Thieme 2007, Illustration by Karl Wesker.)

D. External carotid artery (ECA) — vascular supply to the brain can be variable depending on several leptomeningeal anastomoses, many of which are from the external carotid circulation. The ECA is anteromedial and smaller than the internal carotid artery (ICA) and has eight major branches (mnemonic: **SALFOPS max**) (**Fig. 1.2**).

E. ECA branches

Branches	Vascular Supply and Anastomoses
Superior thyroid artery (A)	Larynx and upper thyroid Thyrocervical trunk (branch of the subclavian artery) supplies the inferior thyroid and isthmus.
Ascending pharyngeal artery (M)	Nasopharynx, oropharynx, and middle ear CNs IX, X, and XI Meninges Anastomoses with the vertebral artery branches
Lingual artery (A)	Tongue and the floor of the mouth
Facial artery (A)	Face, palate, and lips Angular branch of the facial artery anastomoses with the orbital branch of the ophthalmic artery.
Occipital artery (P)	Posterior scalp, upper cervical musculature Posterior fossa and meninges Anastomoses with the vertebral artery
Posterior auricular artery (P)	Pinna, external auditory canal, and scalp
Superficial temporal artery	Scalp and ear
Internal **max**illary artery	Deep face Gives off the middle meningeal artery (MMA) and accessory meningeal arteries Anastomoses with inferior lateral cavernous sinus trunk and ophthalmic artery through ethmoidal branches

Branch direction from the ECA (A) = anteriorly, (M) = medially, (P) = posteriorly.

F. Internal carotid artery (ICA)

   1. ICA segments
      a. Cervical segment (C1) — no branches, originates from the common carotid artery (CCA) at C3–C4 or C4–C5 level. It is the larger of the two terminal CCA branches. ICA initially lies posterolateral to the ECA then becomes medial to the ECA to enter the carotid canal just anteromedial to the internal jugular vein (IJV), separated from it by CNs IX–XII.
      b. Petrosal/intraosseous segment (C2) — enters the carotid canal in the petrous temporal bone anterior to the IJV/jugular fossa and lies behind the eustachian tube. This segment is variable and may provide collateral blood flow from ECA during ICA occlusion.
         (1) Intraosseous segment of the ICA:
            (a) Vertical segment — 10 mm in length, begins where the ICA turns anteromedially to the tympanic cavity and cochlea and anterior to IJV
            (b) Genu – slightly inferior and anterior to the cochlea and tympanic cavity
            (c) Horizontal segment – almost 20 mm in length, exits the canal at petrous apex *superior* to the cartilage-filled foramen lacerum
         (2) Intraosseous branches of the ICA:
            (a) Caroticotympanic artery — embryonic hyoid artery remnant, rises near the genu to pass superiorly to supply the middle and inner ear. Aberrant course can cause a retrotympanic pulsatile mass (differential diagnosis [DDx] = glomus tympanicum tumors). Anastomoses with inferior tympanic artery (ascending pharyngeal artery branch).

(b) Vidian artery (artery of the pterygoid canal) — typically from ECA, but can also originate from the horizontal petrous segment of ICA. Vidian artery travels through the vidian canal and foramen lacerum (anteroinferiorly). Anastomoses with ECA

(c) Periosteal arterial branches: Persistent arteries of the petrosal/intraosseous segment:

Anomalous Artery	Feature
Persistent stapedial artery	Embryonic stapedial artery that fails to involute (primitive hyoid branch of the internal carotid artery) Course: from the vertical segment, it exits through a bony canal on the cochlear promontory and traverses the footplate of stapes to terminate as the middle meningeal artery If persistent stapedial artery is present, foramen spinosum is either small or absent with enlarged geniculate fossa (Y-shaped)
Persistent otic artery	Primitive otic artery that fails to involute Embryonic carotid–basilar anastomoses Connects petrous internal carotid artery to embryonic dorsal longitudinal neural arteries; very rare

c. Intracavernous segment (**Fig. 1.3**) — extends from the ICA at exit from the carotid canal and terminates at the entrance into the subarachnoid space adjacent to the anterior clinoid. It travels in the cavernous sinus and is covered by the trigeminal ganglion. CN VI lies inferolaterally, CN III, IV, V_1, and V_2 are lateral (within the lateral dural wall).

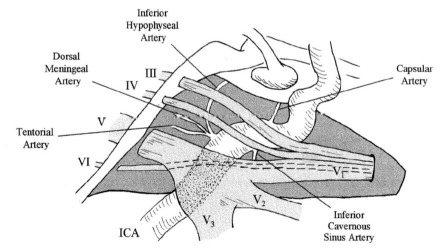

Fig. 1.3 Branches of the cavernous segment of the internal carotid artery (ICA).

(1) Intracavernous segment of ICA (proximal → distal):
   (a) C5: ascending portion — entrance into the cranium to the genu
   (b) C4: posterior genu — between C5 and C3 segments
   (c) C3: horizontal portion — between the genu
   (d) C2: anterior genu
   (e) C1 — remainder of the ICA segment

(2) Intracavernous branches of ICA:
  (a) Meningohypophyseal trunk (posterior trunk) has three branches:
      (i) Tentorial artery (of Bernasconi and Cassinari) — tentorium
      (ii) Inferior hypophyseal artery— neurohypophysis
      (iii) Dorsal meningeal artery (clival branch) — CN VI and part of the clivus
  (b) Inferolateral trunk (artery of the inferior cavernous sinus) travels to
      (i) Inferolateral cavernous sinus wall
      (ii) Tentorium (via tentorial branch)
      (iii) Foramen ovale and spinosum to supply CN III, IV, VI, and gasserian ganglion
      (iv) The most important anastomoses include
          • Maxillary artery (via artery of the foramen rotundum)
          • MMA and ophthalmic artery
  (d) Medial trunk (McConnell's capsular arteries) — supplies the anterior and inferior pituitary gland, present only in 28% of the population, the most distal branch from the C3 and C2 segment
      (i) Anterior capsular artery — courses medially over the sellar roof
      (ii) Inferior capsular artery — courses inferomedially, supplies the sella floor
(3) Persistent arteries of the intracavernous segment

Anomalous Artery	Feature
Persistent trigeminal artery	Most common primitive internal carotid artery–basilar anastomosis 0.02–0.06% of all cerebral angiograms Associated with higher incidence of vascular abnormalities (25%), aneurysms most common
Intracavernous anastomoses	Internal carotid artery aplasia; very uncommon

d. Intradural segment/supraclinoid ICA (**Fig. 1.4** and **Fig. 1.5**) — Branches of the extracavernous intradural segment include the ophthalmic, superior hypophyseal, posterior communicating, anterior choroidal branches, and branches to the hypothalamus, optic nerve, and chiasm.
  (1) Ophthalmic artery (OA) — supplies the orbit (additional minor contributions from the infraorbital branch of the maxillary artery that anastomoses with OA) (**Fig. 1.6**)
    (a) Usually the first intracranial ICA branch (intradural origin in 93%)
    (b) Course — arises superomedial or anteromedial to the ICA and under the anterior clinoid process (rarely OA originates within the cavernous sinus). OA initially lies inferolateral to CN II, and medial to CN III and VI. It crosses between CN II and the superior rectus muscle to the medial orbital wall between the medial rectus and superior oblique muscles.
    (c) In 0.5% of cases, OA arises from the MMA (with risk of blindness after embolization of the MMA if not detected).
    (d) Aneurysms arise from the superior wall of the ICA distal to the origin of the ophthalmic artery and point upward against the optic nerve.
    (e) OA branches:
      (i) Ocular branch — includes central retinal artery and ciliary artery, to supply the retina, choroid of the eye, and portions of the ON

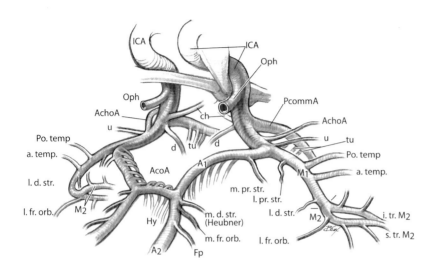

Fig. 1.4 View of the anterior circle of Willis as it would be seen from a right pterional approach.

(ii) Orbital branches:
- Lacrimal artery — supplies lacrimal gland and conjunctiva. The most significant branch of the lacrimal artery is the recurrent meningeal artery, which turns backward through the superior orbital fissure to anastomose with the MMA.
- Muscular artery — supplies extraocular muscles and the orbital periosteum

(iii) Extraorbital branches—include supraorbital, anterior and posterior ethmoidals, dorsal nasal, medial frontal, palpebral, and supratrochlear arteries. These branches possess extensive anastomoses with the ECA (via ethmoidal and anterior falcine artery) for collateral intracranial flow during proximal ICA occlusion.

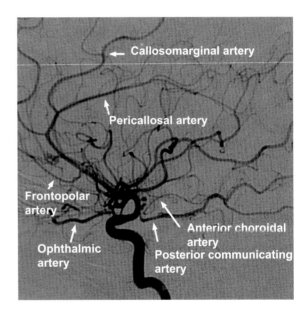

Fig. 1.5 Lateral internal carotid artery catheter angiogram.

(2) Superior hypophyseal arteries — several small arteries arising from the posteromedial portion of the intradural ICA
   (a) They course beneath the optic nerve to supply:
      (i) Pituitary (anterior pituitary lobe, pituitary stalk) and tuber cinereum
      (ii) Optic nerve and chiasm (inferior surface)
   (b) These arteries anastomose with the arteries of the contralateral as well as the inferior hypophyseal arteries to form the *hypophyseal portal system*.
   (c) Aneurysms arising from this region point inferiorly and medially.

(3) Posterior communicating artery (PcommA) — arises from the posterior aspect of the intradural ICA, courses posterolaterally above CN III to join the horizontal PCA segment (P1). The PcommA is typically smaller than the PCA and ICA.

    (a) Perforators — ~ Seven perforators evenly distributed along the PcommA course superomedially to supply the posterior hypothalamus, anterior thalamus, subthalamic nucleus, and posterior limb of the internal capsule (IC). The largest perforator (anterior thalamoperforating artery) terminates between the mamillary bodies and optic tracts.

    (b) PcommA variants are observed in 50% of cases, including absent or hypoplastic (30%), fetal origin (20%), duplicated or triplicated:

        (i) Fetal origin of the PCA ("fetal PCA") — when PcommA diameter is the same as PCA. Failed regression of fetal PCA leads to dominant blood supply of occipital lobes from ICA (via fetal PCA) rather than from the vertebrobasilar system (20% unilateral and 8% bilateral).

        (ii) Infundibulum — a funnel-shaped dilatation observed at the junction between PcommA's origin and ICA. Dilatation is usually <2 mm in diameter with wide base at the ICA origin (DDx = ICA–PcommA aneurysm); seen in 10% of PcommAs (**Fig. 1.7**).

    (c) Aneurysms usually arise from the posterior wall of the carotid artery just distal to the PcommA's origin and point posteriorly toward CN III. The PcommA is on the inferomedial side of the aneurysm. The anterior choroidal artery (ChA) is superior/superolateral to the aneurysm.

(4) Anterior choroidal artery — arises from the posteromedial surface of the ICA, 2–4 mm distal to the PcommA's origin. Aneurysms tend to be located superior or superolaterally to the origin of the anterior ChA. It anastomoses with the lateral posterior ChAs and has two segments:

    (a) Cisternal segment — courses posteromedially within the suprasellar cistern beneath (inferior and lateral) the optic tract, then turns posteromedially around the uncus

    (b) Intraventricular segment — continues from the cisternal segment. Prior to reaching the lateral geniculate body, it turns posterolaterally through the crural and ambient cisterns to enter the choroidal fissure (plexal point) of the temporal horn. Perforators (3–10) supply:

        (i) Visual system — inferior optic chiasm, posterior portion of the optic tract, optic radiation, lateral geniculate body

        (ii) Temporal lobe — uncus, parahippocampal gyrus, amygdala

        (iii) Choroid plexus in the temporal horn and atrium

        (iv) Basal ganglia — globus pallidus medius, tail of caudate, internal capsule (genu)

        (v) Diencephalon — subthalamus, lateral ventroanterior (VA) and ventrolateral (VL) thalamic nuclei

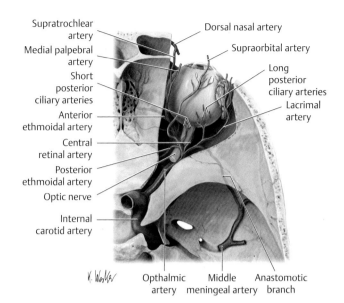

Fig. 1.6 Branches of the ophthalmic artery. Right orbit, superior view after opening of the optic canal and orbital roof. The ophthalmic artery is a branch of the internal carotid artery. It runs below the optic nerve through the optic canal to the orbit and supplies the intraorbital structures, including the eyeball. (From THIEME Atlas of Anatomy, Head and Neuroanatomy, © Thieme 2007, Illustration by Karl Wesker.)

(vi) Midbrain — middle third of the cerebral peduncle, upper red nucleus, substantia nigra

(5) Dural artery — a small branch that arises from the ICA 3–5 mm proximal to the bifurcation; courses anteriorly to supply the dura of the anterior clinoid process

(6) Carotid siphon — intracavernous and supraclinoid segments of the ICA

G. Anterior cerebral artery (ACA) (**Fig. 1.8**)

  1. ACA segments
    a. A1 — horizontal/precommunicating segment
    b. A2 — vertical/postcommunicating segment
    c. A3 — distal ACA and cortical branches
    d. Anterior communicating — connects right and left ACAs at level of A1–A2 junction

  2. Precommunicating segment (A1) — 1–12 perforating arteries called the medial lenticulostriate arteries (medial proximal striate arteries)
    a. Course posterosuperiorly through the anterior perforated substance to supply:
      (1) Optic nerve (superior surface) and optic chiasm
      (2) Anterior hypothalamus
      (3) Septum pellucidum
      (4) Anterior commissure
      (5) Pillars of the fornix and the anteroinferior striatum
    b. Note: Medial *distal* striate artery = recurrent artery of Heubner (RAH)

  3. Anterior communicating artery (AcommA) — located in the cistern of the lamina terminalis
    a. Two or more perforators arise from the AcommA that supply:
      (1) Infundibulum
      (2) Optic chiasm

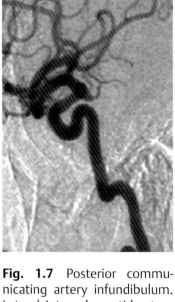

Fig. 1.7 Posterior communicating artery infundibulum. Lateral internal carotid artery angiogram demonstrates the artery arising from the tip of a pyramidal dilation.

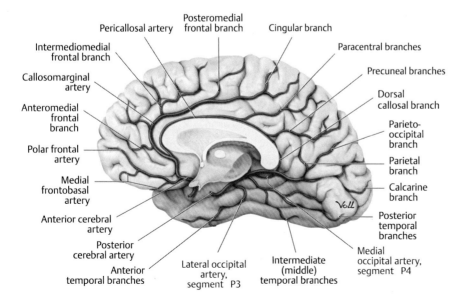

Fig. 1.8 Anterior cerebral artery. The major branches are the orbitofrontal (medial frontobasal), frontopolar (polar frontal), anterior internal frontal (anteromedial frontal), callosomarginal, middle internal frontal (intermedial frontal), posterior internal frontal (posteromedial frontal), paracentral (cingular), superior parietal (paracentral), and inferior parietal (precuneal). (From THIEME Atlas of Anatomy, Head and Neuroanatomy, © Thieme 2007, Illustration by Markus Voll.)

(3) Subcallosal area

(4) Preoptic hypothalamus

b. Perforators include the subcallosal artery and medial artery of the corpus callosum.

c. Aneurysms usually arise at the point where the dominant A1 bifurcates at the AcommA and point toward the opposite side.

4. Postcommunicating segment (A2)

A2	Feature

Recurrent artery of Heubner (medial distal striate artery)	Arises just proximal or more commonly, distal to the anterior communicating artery and courses back toward the proximal A1, hence the term recurrent
	It enters the anterior perforating substance.
	Vascular territory:
	    Head of the caudate
	    Anterior limb of the internal capsule
	    Anterior putamen and globus pallidus
	    Septal nuclei
	    Inferior frontal lobe

Orbitofrontal artery	Gyrus rectus, medial orbital gyri Olfactory bulb and tract
Frontopolar artery	Medial frontal lobe Lateral surface of the superior frontal gyrus
Anterior internal frontal artery	Anterior medial frontal lobe

5. Distal segment (A3) — distal to the pericallosal–callosomarginal junction

A3	Feature
Callosomarginal artery	Cingulate gyrus and paracentral lobule Second most common site for anterior cerebral artery aneurysms (junction of the pericallosal artery) Aneurysms usually point distally.
Pericallosal artery	Medial parietal cortex and the precuneus
Middle internal frontal artery	Medial frontal cortex
Posterior internal frontal artery	Medial posterior frontal cortex
Paracentral artery	Medial cortex around the central sulcus
Superior parietal artery	Medial superior parietal lobe
Inferior parietal artery	Medial inferior parietal lobe

H. Middle cerebral artery (MCA) (**Fig. 1.9**)

    1. MCA segments

        a. M1 — horizontal segment extends horizontal and lateral beneath the anterior perforated substance, proximal to the bifurcation (50%) or trifurcation (25%)

        b. M2 — insular segment extends from the bifurcation to the genu which courses around the island of Reil and heads posterosuperiorly into the sylvian fissure

        c. M3 — opercular segment, opercular branches emerging from the sylvian fissure, a continuation of M2 branches

        d. M4 — cortical segments

    2. M1 segment

M1	Feature
Uncal artery	More frequently arises from the distal internal carotid artery (compared with proximal M1) Supply: uncus and underlying white matter
Temporopolar artery	Supply: anterior pole of the superior, middle, and inferior temporal gyri
Anterior temporal artery	Supply: anterior pole of the superior, middle, and inferior temporal gyri

Lateral lenticulostriate arteries	Perforators (2–15) from superior surface of M1
	 Vascular territory:
	     Substantia innominata
	     Anterior commissure (lateral portion)
	     Putamen (majority)
	     Globus pallidus (lateral segment)
	     Internal capsule (superior half)
	     Head and body of the caudate (except anteroinferior portion)

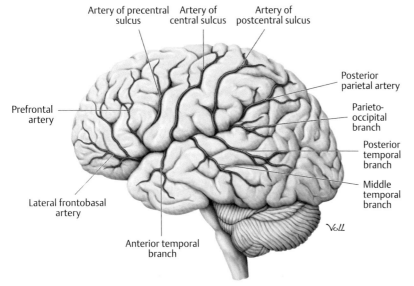

Fig. 1.9 Middle cerebral artery. The major terminal branches are the orbital frontal (lateral frontobasal), prefrontal, precentral (artery of the precentral sulcus), central (artery of the central sulcus), anterior parietal (artery of the postcentral sulcus), posterior parietal, angular (parietooccipital branch), posterior temporal, middle temporal, anterior temporal, and temporopolar arteries. (From THIEME Atlas of Anatomy, Head and Neuroanatomy, © Thieme 2007, Illustration by Markus Voll.)

3. M2 segment

M2	Feature
Superior trunk	
Orbitofrontal branch	Supply: orbital portion of the middle and inferior frontal gyri and the inferior pars orbitalis
Prefrontal branch	Supply: superior pars orbitalis, pars triangularis, anterior pars opercularis, and most of the middle frontal gyrus
Precentral branch	Supply: posterior pars opercularis, middle frontal gyrus, and inferior and middle portions of the precentral gyrus
Central branch	Supply: superior postcentral gyrus, upper central sulcus, anterior part of the inferior parietal lobule, and the anteroinferior region of the superior parietal lobule
Anterior parietal branch	Supply: superior parietal lobule
Inferior trunk	
Posterior parietal branch	Supply: posterosuperior and inferior parietal lobule and inferior supramarginal gyrus Occlusion: cortical sensory loss and hemianopsia
Angular branch	Supply: posterior aspect of the superior temporal gyrus, portions of the supramarginal and angular gyri, and superior aspect of the lateral occipital gyrus The largest cortical branch of the middle cerebral artery
Temporooccipital branch	Supply: posterior half of the superior temporal gyrus, posterior extreme of the middle and inferior temporal gyri, and the inferior lateral occipital gyrus
Posterotemporal branch	Supply: middle and posterior portion of the superior temporal gyrus, posterior ⅓ of middle temporal gyrus, and posterior extreme of the inferior temporal gyrus Occlusion: Wernicke's aphasia and hemianopsia
Middle temporal branch	Supply: superior temporal gyrus near the level of pars triangularis and pars opercularis, central part of the middle temporal gyrus, and middle and posterior parts of the inferior temporal gyrus

I. Posterior cerebral artery (PCA) (**Fig. 1.10**)

    1. PCA segments
        a. P1 — precommunicating segment, extends from the tip of the basilar artery to PcommA origin, within the interpeduncular cistern
        b. P2 — ambient segment, extends from the PcommA to the dorsal aspect of the midbrain (P2A and P2P, anterior and posterior, respectively)
        c. P3 — quadrigeminal segment, extends from the lateral portion of the quadrigeminal cistern (origin of the posterior temporal artery) to the anterior limit of the calcarine fissure
        d. P4 — terminal cortical branches

    2. Vascular territory — parietooccipital sulcus (medial) and inferior temporal sulcus (lateral)

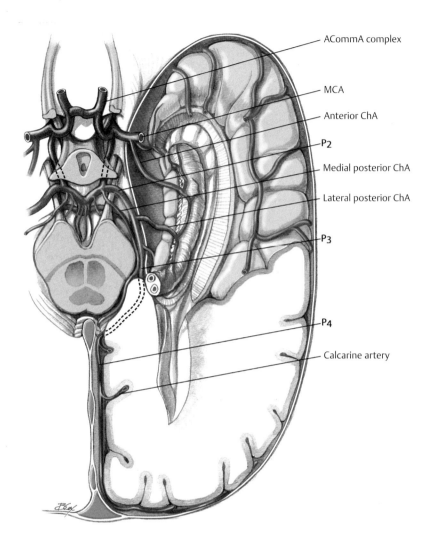

ACommA complex

MCA

Anterior ChA

P$_2$

Medial posterior ChA

Lateral posterior ChA

P$_3$

P$_4$

Calcarine artery

Fig. 1.10   Posterior cerebral artery. View of inferior surface of brain.

3. P1 segment

P1 Segment	Feature
Posterior thalamoperforator arteries	From the basilar artery and P1, travels through the posterior perforated substance behind the mamillary bodies Supply: thalamus, hypothalamus, subthalamus, and midbrain (cranial nerves III and IV)
Medial posterior choroidal arteries	Travels anteromedially along the roof of the third ventricle Supply: midbrain tectum, posterior thalamus, pineal gland, and tela choroidea of the third ventricle
Meningeal branches	Supply: tentorium and the falx

4. P2 segment

P2 Segment	Feature
Lateral posterior choroidal artery	Main branch of P2, courses over the pulvinar and through the choroidal fissure Supply: posterior portion of the thalamus and choroid plexus (temporal horn and atrium)
Thalamogeniculate arteries	Medial geniculate body, lateral geniculate body, pulvinar, superior colliculus, and crus cerebri
Cortical branches	Inferior temporal artery group Supply: inferior portion of the temporal lobe

5. P3 segment

P3 Segment	Feature
Posterior temporal artery	Posterior temporal lobe, occipitotemporal and lingual gyri Anterior temporal artery branch travels to the inferior temporal lobe to supply the inferior cortex. Anastomoses with middle cerebral artery
Internal occipital artery	
Parietooccipital artery	Located in the parietooccipital sulcus Supply: posterior ⅓ of the medial hemispheres, cuneus, precuneus, superior occipital gyrus, and precentral and superior parietal lobules Anastomoses with anterior cerebral artery
Calcarine artery	Located in the calcarine sulcus Supply: occipital pole and the visual cortex Anastomoses with middle cerebral artery
Posterior pericallosal artery	Supply: splenium of the corpus callosum Anastomoses with anterior cerebral artery

J. Choroidal arteries (ChAs)

Choroidal Arteries	Feature
Anterior ChAs	Arise from the ICA
	Course: goes through the choroidal fissure → temporal horn of LV
	Vascular territory:
	Choroid of the LVs (especially in the lateral horn)
	Hippocampus, amygdala, uncus
	Globus pallidus, caudate tail, putamen
	Thalamus (VL)
	IC (posterior limb and retrolenticular)
	Optic tract, lateral geniculate nucleus, optic radiation
	Historically, this artery was sacrificed to treat Parkinson's disease: decreased tremor likely due to decreased blood supply to VL thalamus.
Posterior ChAs (medial and lateral)	Arise from the PCA
	Medial branches supply pineal gland, tectum, thalamus, choroid of the third ventricle
	Lateral branches enter the choroidal fissure and anastomose with the anterior choroidal arteries forming variable anastomotic network

Abbreviations: ChAs, choroidal arteries; IC, internal capsule; ICA, internal carotid artery; LV, lateral ventricles; PCA, posterior cerebral artery; VL, ventrolateral

K. Circle of Willis (**Fig. 1.11**)

    1. Arteries that form a polygon encircling the ventral surface of the diencephalon (adjacent to the optic chiasm, mamillary bodies, and infundibulum), located in the interpeduncular fossa, suprasellar and adjacent cisterns. The carotid and vertebrobasilar systems are connected via the circle of Willis. Complete in 25% of individuals, 50% have posterior circulation variations. Consists of the "anterior and posterior circulation":

        a. Anterior circulation — AcommA, A1, ICA

        b. Posterior circulation — PcommA, P1, basilar tip

    2. Penetrating arteries of the circle of Willis

Arteries	Feature
Anteromedial arteries	Arise from ACA and AcommA, including RAH
	Enter the anterior perforated substance
	Supply: anterior hypothalamus, preoptic nucleus, and supraoptic nucleus
Posteromedial arteries	Arise from proximal PCA and PcommA
	Supply: hypophysis, infundibulum, and tuberal hypothalamus
	Thalamoperforating arteries supply: mamillary bodies, subthalamus, and midbrain
Anterolateral arteries	Striate arteries from proximal MCA and RAH
	Enter the anterior perforated substance
	Supply: head of caudate, lateral globus pallidus, putamen, claustrum internal capsule, and the external capsule
Posterolateral arteries	Arise from PCA (thalamogeniculate arteries)
	Supply: caudal thalamus (geniculate bodies, pulvinar, lateral nucleus, and lateral ventral nucleus)

Abbreviations: ACA, anterior cerebral artery; AcommA, anterior communicating arteries; MCA. middle cerebral artery; PCA, posterior cerebral artery; PcommA, posterior communicating artery; RAH, recurrent artery of Heubner

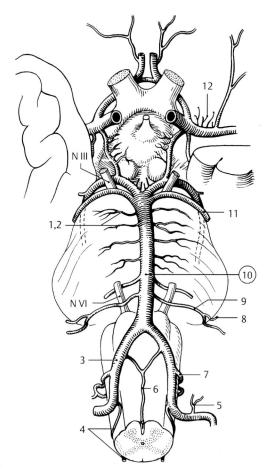

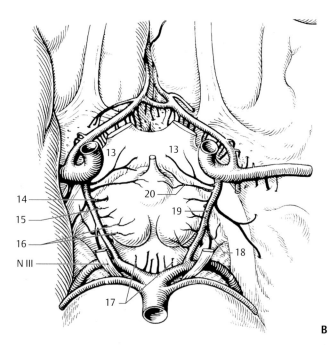

Fig. 1.11 The circle of Willis with the arteries including main perforating arteries of the brain (A) viewed from inferior and left in situ showing posterior circulation and (B) close-up view of circle of Willis itself. 1. Pontine arteries. 2. Circumferential pontine arteries. 3. Vertebral artery. 4. Posterior spinal artery. 5. Meningeal branches of vertebral artery. 6. Anterior spinal artery. 7. Posterior inferior cerebellar artery. 8. Labyrinthine artery. 9. Anterior inferior cerebellar artery. 10. Basilar artery. 11. Superior cerebellar artery. 12. Mesencephalic arteries. 13. Arteries to optic chiasm. 14. Thalamotuberal artery. 15. Hypothalamic branch. 16. Mammillary arteries. 17. Posterior thalamoperforating arteries. 18. Branch to oculomotor nerve. 19. Posterior communicating artery. 20. Artery of tuber cinereum. (From Dauber W. Pocket Atlas of Human Anatomy. Stuttgart, Germany: Thieme; 2007. Reprinted by permission.)

L. Vertebral artery

  1. Course — arises from the subclavian artery, enters the foramina transversarium at C6 in 90%, turns lateral at C2, travels posteriorly along the atlas, entering the skull via foramen magnum

  2. Anastomoses — ECA, thyrocervical and costocervical trunks

  3. Supply — pyramids inferior olivary nucleus, CNs X and XII, and the reticular formation

4. Vertebral artery branches

Branches	Feature
Extracranial	Three branches: 1. Segmental spinal branches 2. Muscular branch anastomoses with muscular branch of ECA (ascending pharyngeal, thyrocervical, and costocervical) 3. Meningeal branch Anterior meningeal branch → dura around the foramen magnum Posterior meningeal branch → falx and posterior fossa dura Blood supply to the falx cerebelli = posterior meningeal branches, occipital, ascending pharyngeal and PICA arteries
Posterior spinal artery	Supply: gracile and cuneate fasciculi and the inferior cerebellar peduncle
Anterior spinal artery	Supply: pyramid, medial lemniscus, medial longitudinal fasciculus, olive and vagal and hypoglossal nuclei
PICA	Occasionally arises extracranially, 1–25% of vertebral arteries terminate in the PICA Supply: choroid of fourth ventricle, posterior lateral medulla, tonsils, vermis, and posteroinferior cerebellar hemispheres Five segments: 1. Anterior medullary segment 2. Lateral medullary segment — supply CNs IX, X, and XI 3. Tonsillomedullary segment — forms a large loop 4. Telovelotonsillar segment — between tela choroidea and inferior medullary velum rostrally superior pole of the tonsils caudally 5. Hemispheric branches Occlusion = lateral medullary syndrome (Wallenberg's)

Abbreviations: CN, cranial nerve; ECA, external carotid artery; PICA, posterior inferior cerebellar artery

M. Basilar artery

1. Union of two vertebral arteries near the pontomedullary junction, extends along the ventral pons and terminates as paired PCAs (within the interpeduncular cistern)

2. Basilar artery branches

Branches	Feature
Anterior inferior cerebellar artery	Course: crosses cranial nerve (CN) VI and the cerebellopontine angle cistern to the internal auditory canal and passes anterior and inferior to CNs VII and VIII Supply: CNs VII and VIII, inferolateral pons, middle cerebellar peduncle, flocculus, and anterolateral hemispheres Branches: internal auditory artery, recurrent perforating artery, and subarcuate artery
Labyrinthine artery	Internal auditory artery Supply: structures of the labyrinth
Paramedian artery	Supply: ventral pons and midbrain
Pontine arteries	Long and short circumferential pontine arteries Supply: ventral pons
Superior cerebellar artery	Course: travels posterolateral around the pontomesencephalic junction below the tentorium, CNs III and IV Supply: superior vermis and cerebellar hemispheres, deep cerebellar white matter, and dentate nuclei
Posterior cerebral arteries	Refer to above

N. Regional blood supply

Structures	Vascular Supply
Striatum	Mainly: MCA (lenticulostriate arteries) Rostrally: RAH Caudally: anterior ChA
Internal capsule	Anterior limb: ACA (RAH, MCA lateral [lenticulostriate arteries]) Genu: ICA perforators, MCA lateral (lenticulostriate arteries) Posterior limb: anterior ChA and PcommA
Thalamus	PCA by way of posterior thalamoperforators, thalamogeniculate arteries, and the medial posterior ChAs Rostrally from PcommA (anterior thalamoperforating arteries) and basilar bifurcation perforators (posterior thalamoperforating arteries)
Medulla	Anterior and posterior spinal arteries PICA and vertebral arteries
Pons	Basilar paramedian branches Short and long circumferential branches of the basilar artery that anastomose with AICA at the middle cerebellar peduncle SCA

Midbrain	Basilar artery, PCA, SCA, PcommA, and anterior ChA
	Stroke syndromes include:
	  Weber's syndrome: CN III palsy with contralateral hemiplegia
	  Benedikt's syndrome: Weber's + red nucleus lesion (coarse intentional tremor, hyperkinesias, and ataxia of the upper limb)

Cerebellum	PICA: inferior cerebellar peduncle, vermis, tonsils, and choroid of the fourth ventricle AICA: middle cerebellar peduncle, choroid of the fourth ventricle, and anterior cerebellum SCA: superior cerebellar peduncle, choroid of the fourth ventricle and the deep nuclei

Abbreviations: ACA, anterior cerebral artery; AICA, anterior inferior cerebellar artery; ChA, choroidal artery; CN, cranial nerve; ICA, internal carotid artery; MCA, middle cerebral artery; PCommA, posterior communicating artery; PCA, posterior cerebral artery; PICA, posterior inferior cerebellar artery; RAH, recurrent artery of Heubner; SCA, superior cerebellar artery

O. Supratentorial venous drainage (**Fig. 1.12** and **Fig. 1.13**)

    1. Diploic veins — communicate with the scalp, meningeal veins, and dural sinuses

    2. Meningeal veins — epidural vessels of the dura, which follow meningeal arteries. Drainage into dural sinuses or into extracranial pterygoid vertebral plexus

    3. Dural sinuses — no valves, communicates with emissary veins

    4. Cerebral veins — superficial veins and deep cerebral veins

    5. Dural sinuses

Dural Sinus	Feature
Superior sagittal sinus	Extends from foramen cecum (near crista galli) to the internal occipital protuberance (becomes transverse sinus) Drains predominantly (60%) into the right transverse sinus
Inferior sagittal sinus	Cortical veins from the medial hemisphere join to form the ISS to join great cerebral vein of Galen to form the straight sinus Drains into → straight sinus → torcula → drains predominantly into the left transverse sinus
Transverse sinus	From the confluence, courses laterally then curves down the occipitopetrosal junction to become the sigmoid sinus
Sigmoid sinus	Courses along the posterior aspect of the temporal bone (petromastoid) to become the superior jugular bulb at the jugular foramen and then the IJV Receives blood from the inferior petrosal sinus
Confluence of sinuses (torcula Herophili)	Dilatation at the internal occipital protuberance that communicates with superior sagittal, straight, transverse, and occipital sinuses
Petrosal sinuses	Superior petrosal sinus — receives veins from the pons, medulla, cerebellum, and inner ear Inferior petrosal sinus — receives veins from the cerebellum and labyrinthine veins
Straight sinus	Courses posteroinferiorly along the falx to the tentorium and terminates at the TS Formed by the vein of Galen and ISS

Cavernous sinus	Drains into:
	    Superior petrosal sinus → transverse/sigmoid sinus junction
	    Inferior petrosal sinus → IJV
	Communicates with the basilar sinus, pterygoid and pharyngeal venous plexus

Abbreviations: ISS, inferior sagittal sinus; IJV, internal jugular vein; TS, transverse sinus

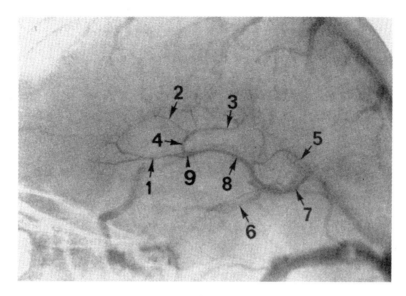

Fig. 1.12 Venous anatomy on lateral catheter angiogram. 1. Septal vein. 2. Anterior caudatevein. 3. Terminal vein. 4. Thalamostriate vein. 5. Atrial vein. 6. Basal vein of Rosenthal. 7. Vein of Galen. 8. Internal cerebral vein. 9. Venous angle. (From Alleyne Jr. CH. Neurosurgery Board Review. New York, NY: Thieme;1997. Reprinted by permission.)

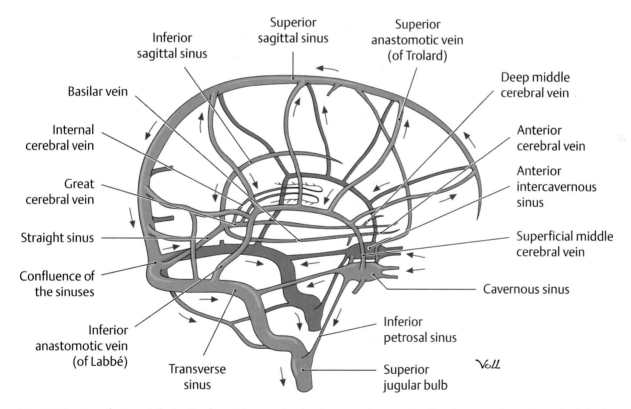

Fig. 1.13 Dural sinus tributaries from the cerebral veins (after Rauber and Kopsch). Right lateral view. Venous blood collected deep within the brain drains to the dural sinuses through superficial and deep cerebral veins. The red arrows in the diagram show the principle directions of venous blood flow in the major sinuses. (From THIEME Atlas of Anatomy, Head and Neuroanatomy, © Thieme 2007, Illustration by Markus Voll.)

6. Cerebral veins

Cerebral Veins	Feature
Superficial veins	
Superficial middle cerebral veins	Course along the sylvian fissure Drain into the cavernous sinus Drain into the vein of Trolard → superior sagittal sinus Drain into vein of Labbé → transverse sinus Mnemonic: **T**rolard = **T**op, **L**abbé = **L**ower
Superior anastomotic vein	Vein of Trolard, drains from the sylvian fissure → superior sagittal sinus
Inferior anastomotic vein	Vein of Labbé, drains from the sylvian fissure → transverse sinus
Deep veins	
Internal cerebral veins	Course: located in the tela choroidea of the roof of the third ventricle (velum interpositum), extend from the interventricular foramen, travel over the thalamus and posteriorly to the quadrigeminal cistern, where they join to contribute to the vein of Galen Formed by the union of the thalamostriate, choroidal, septal, epithalamic, and lateral ventricular veins
Basal vein of Rosenthal	Drains the anterior and medial temporal lobe Course: passes posterosuperiorly through the ambient cistern, joins the internal cerebral vein to form the vein of Galen
Vein of Galen	Receives both internal cerebral veins, basal veins of Rosenthal, occipital veins, and posterior callosal vein Travels under the splenium and merges with the inferior sagittal sinus to form the straight sinus

V. Blood Supply to the Spinal Cord

A. Summary of spinal cord blood supply (**Fig. 1.14** and **Fig. 1.15**)

Artery	Vascular Territory
Vertebral arteries	
Posterior spinal artery	Supplies posterior ⅓ of the spinal cord
Anterior spinal artery	Supplies anterior ⅔ of the spinal cord Two anterior spinal arteries join at the medulla to enter the anterior median fissure as a single artery (to become the anterior median spinal artery)
Radicular arteries	

Anterior radicular arteries	Comprised of 2–17 arteries:
	  Cervical 6, thoracic 2–4, lumbar 1–2 arteries
	Artery of Adamkiewicz:
	  A major anterior radicular artery originating at the lower thoracic or upper lumbar spine (the largest); travels with the spinal roots
	  Most frequent on the left side (75% of population)
	  Joins the anterior spinal artery

Posterior radicular arteries	Comprised of 10–23 arteries Divide at the posterolateral spinal cord surface and joins the paired posterior spinal arteries

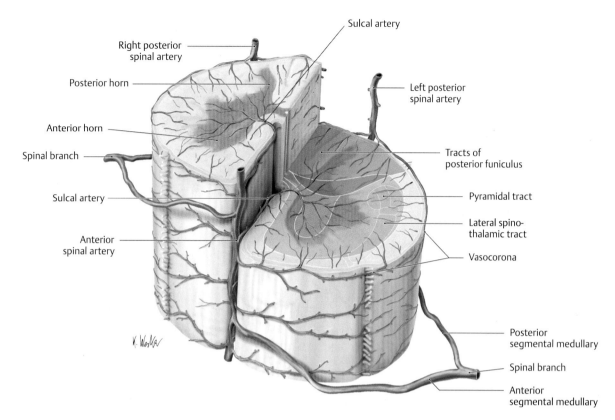

Fig. 1.14 Blood supply to the spinal cord segments. In each spinal cord segment, the anterior spinal artery gives off several (5–9) sulcal arteries that course posteriorly in the anterior median fissure. Typically, each sulcal artery enters one half of the spinal cord, supplying the anterior horn, base of the posterior horn, and anterior and lateral funiculi (approximately ⅔ of the total area) in that half; the sulcal arteries tend to alternate direction (left or right) to supply both halves of the spinal cord segment. The paired posterior spinal arteries provide the blood supply to the posterior third of the cord, including the posterior horn and funiculus. All three spinal arteries contribute numerous delicate anastomosing vasocorona on the pial surface of the spinal cord, which in turn send branches into the periphery of the cord. The sulcal arteries are end arteries within the spinal cord and their occlusion may produce clinical symptoms. (From THIEME Atlas of Anatomy, Head and Neuroanatomy, © Thieme 2007, Illustration by Karl Wesker.)

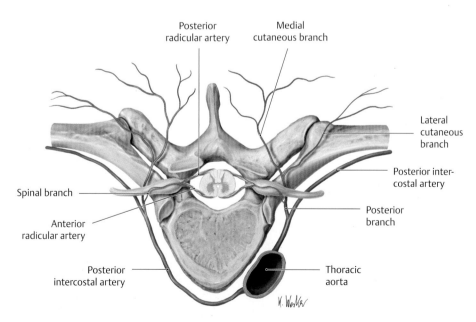

Fig. 1.15 Blood vessels supplying the spinal cord. Thoracic vertebra viewed from above. The spinal branches arise from the posterior branches of segmental arteries and divide into an anterior and posterior radicular artery. The radicular arteries supply the dorsal and ventral roots, and peripheral portions of the dorsal and ventral horns. They also communicate with the vasocorona. These arteries have a better developed connection with the anterior spinal artery at some levels and with the posterior spinal artery at other levels. (From THIEME Atlas of Anatomy, Head and Neuroanatomy, © Thieme 2007, Illustration by Karl Wesker.)

1. Radicular arteries
    a. Derived from segmental vessels from the aorta, which includes the ascending cervical, deep cervical, intercostals, lumbar, and sacral arteries
    b. Passes through the intervertebral foramina to divide into the anterior and posterior radicular arteries to supply the thoracic, lumbar, sacral, and coccygeal spinal segments
    c. The anterior ramus of the segmental artery supplies the cord while the posterior ramus branches in the foramen supply the dorsal root ganglion (DRG) and nerve roots via anterior and posterior radicular branches
    d. A single thoracic radicular artery (artery of Adamkiewicz) arises from the aorta at T7 (most vulnerable to low flow); 75% arise from T9–T12; 80% arise from the left

2. Posterior arterial system
    a. Paired posterior spinal arteries form a leptomeningeal perimedullary network that anastomoses with the anterior system, most prominently at the level of the conus where the anastomotic loop is located.
    b. Blood from the posterior medullary arteries flows centripetally in the perforating branches from the leptomeningeal system of the spinal cord surface to the posterior columns and posterior horns.

3. Anterior arterial system
    a. Single midline artery that feeds into the anterior medullary artery in the anterior median fissure
    b. Flows centrifugally via penetrating branches to the anterior and intermediate gray and via pial radial network to the white matter of the anterior and lateral funiculi

B. Regional arterial supply of the spinal cord

Level	Arterial Supply
Cervical	Vertebral artery (proximal portion of the subclavian artery) Posterior inferior cerebellar artery Ascending cervical artery (from the thyrocervical trunk) Deep cervical artery (from the costocervical trunk)
Thoracic	Thyrocervical and costocervical trunk Intercostal artery (aorta: T3–T11) Subcostal artery (aorta: T12)
Lumbar	Lumbar artery (aorta L4–L5)
Sacrum	Lateral sacral artery (internal iliac artery) supplies sacral neural elements. Middle sacral artery The aorta and iliac arteries send branches to the thoracolumbar spine.

C. Intraspinal arteries

    1. Segmental arteries → spinal branches (lies ventral to the root) pass through the intervertebral foramina → anterior or posterior radicular arteries → anterior or posterior spinal arteries.

D. Spinal cord ischemia

    1. Most vulnerable at transitional regions where the arterial supply is derived from >1 source

    2. Border zone region is especially vulnerable at T1–T4 and L1 (e.g., with an intercostal artery occlusion or an aortic dissection) anterior aspect of the spinal cord. Also vulnerable are areas between the anterior and posterior medullary arteries (between the intermediate and dorsal horns and lateral and posterior fasciculi).

E. Venous drainage of the spinal cord — highly variable, typically follows the arterial system

    1. Both anterior spinal veins (located in the anterior sulcus) and the posterior spinal veins lie adjacent to the spinal arteries, which eventually drain into the intervertebral veins exiting the spinal canal via intervertebral foramina.

    2. Anterior and posterior radicular veins

VI. Intracranial–Extracranial Anastomoses

A. Occipital artery ↔ vertebral (C1 and C2)

B. Ascending pharyngeal artery ↔ vertebral

C. Ascending pharyngeal artery ↔ ICA via petrous and cavernous branches

D. Facial artery (angular branch) ↔ ICA via angular branch of the facial artery to the orbital branch of the ophthalmic artery

E. Posterior auricular artery ↔ ICA via stylomastoid artery

F. Maxillary artery branch ↔ ICA via

    1. MMA ↔ ethmoidal branch of the ophthalmic artery

    2. Artery of foramen rotundum ↔ inferior lateral trunk

    3. Accessory meningeal artery ↔ inferior lateral trunk

    4. Vidian artery ↔ petrous ICA

    5. Pharyngeal artery ↔ cavernous ICA

    6. Temporal branches ↔ ophthalmic artery

    7. Infraorbital artery ↔ ophthalmic artery

VII. Persistent Fetal Carotid–Basilar and Carotid–Vertebral Anastomoses (Fig. 1.16)

Anastomoses	Feature

Primitive trigeminal	Most frequent persistent fetal circulation* (besides fetal PcommA)
	Present in 0.1 to 0.5% of angiograms
	Connects cavernous ICA with embryonic dorsal longitudinal neural arteries. Typically associated with hypoplastic PcommA and basilar and vertebral arteries proximal to the anastomosis. Increased frequency of aneurysms and AVMs (**Fig. 1.17**)
	Arises from:
	  ICA just proximal to the cavernous sinus
	  Meningohypophyseal trunk
	Curves medially to join basilar artery between SCA and AICA

Persistent otic/acoustic	Extremely rare, first to disappear Connects petrous ICA via internal auditory meatus to the basilar artery Connects petrous ICA with embryonic dorsal longitudinal neural arteries
Primitive hypoglossal	Second most frequent persistent fetal circulation, but much less common than the primitive trigeminal artery Present in 0.02–0.3% of angiograms Connects cervical ICA with embryonic dorsal longitudinal neural arteries: arises from the cervical ICA and connects to the basilar artery through the hypoglossal canal Typically bilateral hypoplastic vertebral arteries (thus, this primitive artery may be the main supply to the brainstem and cerebellum)
Proatlantal intersegmental	Connects ECA or cervical ICA with embryonic dorsal longitudinal neural arteries Suboccipital anastomoses between cervical ICA and vertebral artery Courses between the arch of C1 and the occiput

Abbreviations: AICA, anterior inferior cerebellar artery; AVMs, arteriovenous malformations; ECA, external carotid artery; ICA, internal carotid artery; PcommA, posterior communicating artery; SCA, superior cerebellar artery.

*Stages of regression during embryogenesis (14 mm stage) — otic → hypoglossal → trigeminal (thus, most common)

VIII. Cortical Anatomy

A. General anatomy (**Fig. 1.18, Fig. 1.19, Fig. 1.20, Fig. 1.21**)

1. Contains 14 billion cortical neurons

2. Cells that develop later pass more superficially from the germinal zone and form connections with the cells they pass.

3. Cell types — stellate, fusiform, pyramidal (source of main output)

4. Neurotransmitters
   a. Excitatory — glutamate and aspartate
   b. Inhibitory — gamma-aminobutyric acid (GABA; stays in the cortex, augmented by barbiturates and anticonvulsants)

5. Neocortex — six layers, distinguished by cell density, type, and their arrangement of cells Allocortex — three layers, located in the olfactory cortex, hippocampus, and dentate gyrus

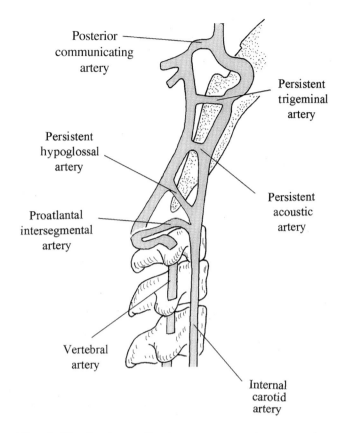

Fig. 1.16 Persistent fetal anastomoses between the anterior and posterior circulations.

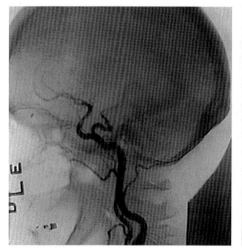 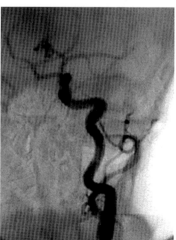 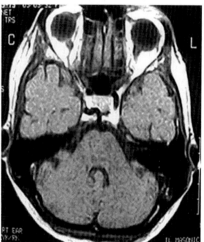

A–C

Fig. 1.17 (**A**) Lateral and (**B**) anteroposterior catheter angiograms, and (**C**) axial T1-weighted magnetic resonance image of a persistent trigeminal artery.

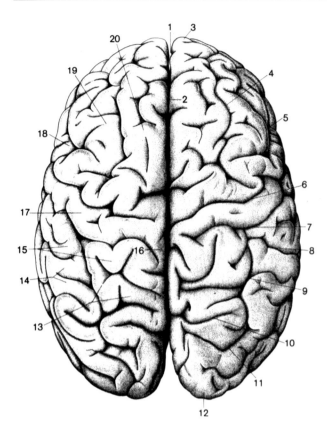

Fig. 1.18 Brain surface anatomy, superior view. 1. Longitudinal fissure of cerebrum. 2. Superior margin of cerebrum. 3. Frontal pole. 4. Superior frontal sulcus. 5. Inferior frontal sulcus. 6. Precentral sulcus. 7. Central sulcus. 8. Postcentral sulcus. 9. Intraparietal sulcus. 10. Parietooccipital sulcus. 11. Transverse occipital sulcus. 12. Occipital pole. 13. Superior parietal lobule. 14. Inferior parietal lobule. 15. Postcentral gyrus. 16. Paracentral lobule. 17. Precentral gyrus. 18. Inferior frontal gyrus. 19. Middle frontal gyrus. 20. Superior frontal gyrus. (From Frick H, Leonhardt H, Starck D. Human Anatomy 2. New York, NY: Thieme, 1991. Reprinted by permission.)

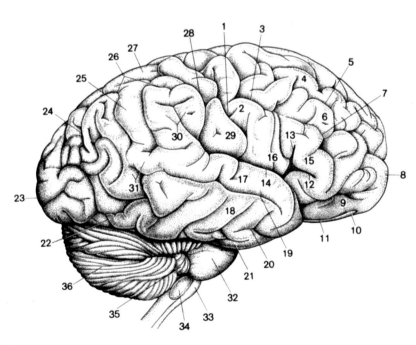

Fig. 1.19 Brain surface anatomy, right lateral view. 1. Central sulcus. 2. Precentral gyrus. 3. Precentral sulcus. 4. Superior frontal gyrus. 5. Superior frontal sulcus. 6. Middle frontal gyrus. 7. Middle frontal sulcus. 8. Frontal pole. 9. Orbital gyri. 10. Olfactory bulb. 11. Olfactory tract. 12–14. Lateral sulcus. 12. Anterior ramus. 13. Ascending ramus. 14. Posterior ramus. 15. Frontal operculum. 16. Frontoparietal operculum. 17. Superior temporal gyrus. 18. Middle temporal gyrus. 19. Superior temporal sulcus. 20. Inferior temporal sulcus. 21. Inferior temporal gyrus. 22. Preoccipital notch. 23. Occipital pole. 24. Transverse occipital sulcus. 25. Inferior parietal lobule. 26. Intraparietal sulcus. 27. Superior parietal lobule. 28. Postcentral sulcus. 29. Postcentral gyrus. 30. Supramarginal gyrus. 31. Angular gyrus. 32. Pons. 33. Pyramid (medulla oblongata). 34. Olive. 35. Flocculus. 36. Cerebellar hemisphere. (From Frick H, Leonhardt H, Starck D. Human Anatomy 2. New York, NY: Thieme;1991. Reprinted by permission.)

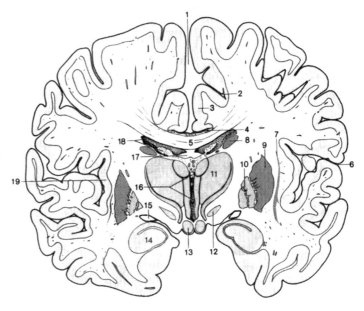

Fig. 1.20 Coronal section through the brain. 1. Longitudinal fissure of cerebrum. 2. Cingulate sulcus. 3. Cingulate gyrus. 4. Sulcus of corpus callosum. 5. Corpus callosum. 6. Lateral sulcus. 7. Claustrum. 8–9. Corpus striatum. 8. Caudate nucleus. 9. Putamen. 9–10. Lentiform nucleus. 10. Globus pallidus. 11. Thalamus. 12. Subthalamic nucleus. 13. Mamillary body. 14. Amygdala. 15. Optic tract. 16. Third ventricle and choroid plexus. 17. Body of fornix. 18. Lateral ventricle and choroid plexus. 19. Cortex of insula. (From Frick H, Leonhardt H, Starck D. Human Anatomy 2. New York, NY: Thieme; 1991. Reprinted by permission.)

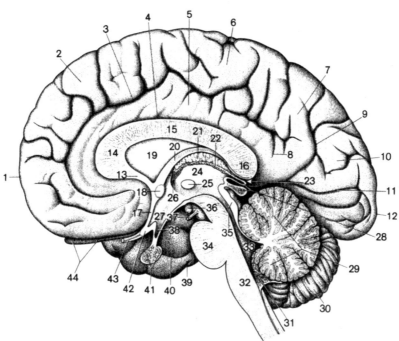

Fig. 1.21 Brain surface anatomy, view of medial surface of right hemisphere. 1. Frontal pole of frontal lobe. 2. Medial frontal gyrus. 3. Cingulate sulcus. 4. Sulcus of corpus callosum. 5. Cingulate gyrus. 6. Paracentral lobule. 7. Precuneus. 8. Subparietal sulcus. 9. Parietooccipital sulcus. 10. Cuneus. 11. Calcarine fissure. 12. Occipital pole of occipital lobe. 13–16. Corpus callosum (cut surface). 13. Rostrum. 14. Genu. 15. Body. 16. Splenium. 17. Lamina terminalis (cut surface). 18. Anterior commissure (cut surface). 19. Septum pellucidum. 20. Fornix. 21. Tela choroidea of third ventricle. 22. Choroid plexus of third ventricle (cut edge). 23. Transverse cerebral fissure. 24. Thalamus. 25. Interthalamic adhesion (cut surface). 26. Interventricular foramen of Monro. 27. Hypothalamus. 28. Suprapineal recess and pineal body (cut surface). 29. Vermis of cerebellum (cut surface). 30. Cerebellar hemisphere. 31. Choroid plexus of fourth ventricle. 32. Medulla oblongata (cut surface). 33. Fourth ventricle. 34. Pons (cut surface). 35. Tectal lamina (cut surface) and mesencephalic aqueduct of Sylvius. 36. Mamillary body. 37. Oculomotor nerve. 38. Infundibular recess. 39. Temporal lobe lateral occipitotemporal gyrus. 40. Rhinal fissure. 41. Hypophysis (cut surface) with adenohypophysis (anterior lobe) and neurohypophysis (posterior lobe) of pituitary gland. 42. Optic chiasm (cut surface). 43. Optic nerve. 44. Olfactory bulb and tract. (From Frick H, Leonhardt H, Starck D. Human Anatomy 2. New York, NY: Thieme; 1991. Reprinted by permission.)

B. Neocortical layers (**Fig. 1.22**)

Layer		Feature	Fibers and Projections
Molecular	I	Most superficial layer Contains horizontal axons, Golgi type II cells, terminal dendritic processes	Receives diffuse afferent fibers from the lower brain to control the excitability of the region
External granular	II	Contains closely packed granule cells Poorly myelinated	
External pyramidal	III	Contains pyramidal neurons, granule cells, and Martinotti cells	Commissural fibers to connect the two hemispheres Ipsilateral cortico-cortico association fibers
Internal granular	IV	Contains closely packed stellate cells Dense horizontal myelinated plexus forms the external band of Baillarger	Main sensory input Enlarged in the sensory cortex
Internal pyramidal	V	Contains the largest cells (Betz cells) Contains pyramidal neurons, granule cells, and Martinotti cells Dense myelinated plexus forms the internal band of Baillarger	Main efferents to the brain stem and spinal cord Enlarged in the motor cortex
Multiform	VI	Contains spindle-shaped cells	Efferent fibers to the thalamus

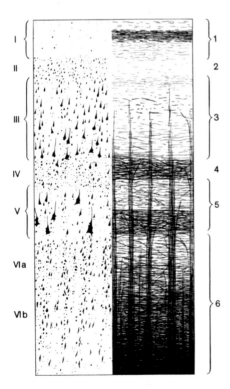

Fig. 1.22 Isocortex layers. 1. Molecular layer. 2. External granular layer. 3. External pyramidal layer. 4. Internal granular layer. 5. Internal pyramidal layer. 6. Multiform layer. 1–3. External principle zone. 4–6. Internal principle zone. (From Frick H, Leonhardt H, Starck D. Human Anatomy 2. New York, NY: Thieme; 1991.)

C. Brodmann's areas (**Fig. 1.23**)

Area	Functional Area	Location	Function
1, 2, 3	1° somatosensory cortex	Postcentral gyrus	Touch
4	1° motor cortex	Precentral gyrus	Voluntary motor control
5	3° somatosensory cortex, posterior parietal association	Superior parietal lobule	Stereognosis
6	Supplementary motor control, supplementary eye field, premotor adjacent cortex	Precentral gyrus and rostral adjacent cortex	Limb and eye movement planning
	Supplementary eye field, premotor adjacent cortex Cortex; frontal eye fields		
7	Posterior parietal association	Superior parietal lobule	Visuomotor control, perception
8	Frontal eye fields	Superior, middle frontal Gyri, medial frontal lobe	Saccadic eye movements
9, 10, 11, 12	Prefrontal association cortex	Superior, middle frontal	Thought, cognition
	Frontal eye fields	Gyri, medial frontal lobe	Movement planning
13, 14, 15, 16		Insular cortex	
17	Primary visual cortex	Banks of calcarine fissure	Vision
18	Secondary visual cortex	Medial and lateral Occipital gyri	Vision, depth
19	Tertiary visual cortex, middle	Medial and lateral	Vision, color, motion
	Temporal visual area	Occipital gyri	Depth
20	Visual inferotemporal area	Inferior temporal gyrus	Form vision
21	Visual inferotemporal area	Middle temporal gyrus	Form vision
22	Higher order auditory cortex	Superior temporal gyrus	Hearing, speech
23, 24, 25, 26, 27	Limbic association cortex	Cingulate gyrus, subcallosal area, retrosplenial area, parahippocampal gyrus	Emotions
28	Primary olfactory cortex, limbic association cortex	Parahippocampal gyrus	Smell, emotions
29, 30, 31, 32, 33	Limbic association cortex	Cingulate gyrus and limbic association cortex	Emotions
34, 35, 36	Primary olfactory cortex; limbic association cortex	Parahippocampal gyrus	Smell, emotions

(Continued on page 34)

C. Brodmann's areas (**Fig. 1.23**) (*Continued from page 33*)

Area	Functional Area	Location	Function
37	Parietal-temporal-occipital association cortex, middle temporal visual area	Middle and inferior temporal gyri at temporo-occipital junction	Perception, vision, reading, speech
38	Primary olfactory cortex, limbic association cortex	Temporal pole	Smell, emotions
39	Parietal-temporal-occipital association cortex	Inferior parietal lobule (angular gyrus)	Perception, vision, reading, speech
40	Parietal-temporal-occipital association cortex	Inferior parietal lobule (supramarginal gyrus)	Perception, vision, reading, speech
41	Primary auditory cortex	Heschl's gyri and superior temporal gyrus	Hearing
42	Secondary auditory cortex	Heschl's gyri and superior temporal gyrus	Hearing
43	Gustatory cortex	Insular cortex, fronto parietal operculum	Taste
44	Broca's area, lateral premotor cortex	Inferior frontal gyrus (frontal operculum)	Speech, movement planning
45	Prefrontal association Cortex	Inferior frontal gyrus (frontal operculum)	Thought, cognition, planning behavior
46	Prefrontal association cortex (dorsolateral prefrontal cortex)	Middle frontal gyrus	Thought, cognition, planning behavior, eye movement
47	Prefrontal association cortex	Inferior frontal gyrus (frontal operculum)	Thought, cognition, planning behavior

° = standard abbreviation for primary.

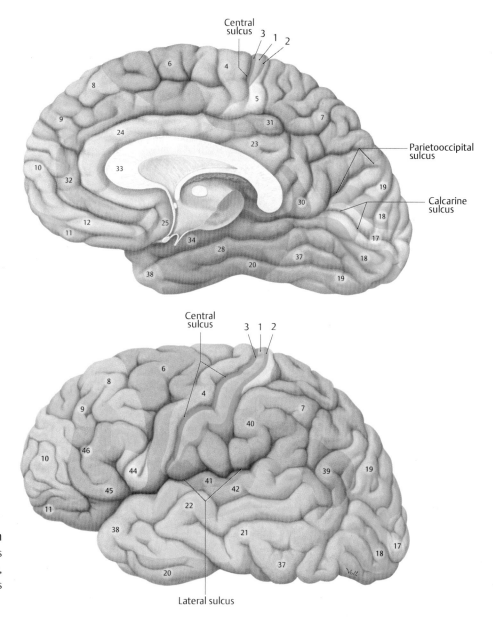

Fig. 1.23 Brodmann areas in the neocortex. (From THIEME Atlas of Anatomy, Head and Neuroanatomy, © Thieme 2007, Illustration by Markus Voll.)

D. Sensory cortices

1. Main sensory areas — somatosensory area (areas 3, 1, 2), visual area (area 17), auditory area (areas 41, 42), gustatory area (area 43), and olfactory area (multiple Brodmann areas, not distinctly localized)

2. Sensory cortex

Sensory Area	Feature
Primary somatosensory area (S1)	Postcentral gyrus (areas 3,1,2) Input: VPLc and VPM thalamic nuclei (medial lemniscus, spinothalamic, and trigeminothalamic tracts) Input for area 3a: muscle spindles Input for area 3b: cutaneous (skin) Input for area 1: muscle spindles and skin Input for area 2: deep (joint) receptors Course: ML/STT → VPLc/VPM → S1 Face and tongue have bilateral representation (**Fig. 1.24**).
Secondary somatosensory area (S1)	Located on the superior bank of the lateral sulcus Input: ipsilateral VPLc and VPM thalamic nuclei Input: bilateral S1 Output: ipsilateral S1 and motor cortex Information is bilateral and the homunculus is inverted (face rostral), processing of the thalamic tracts but not medial lemniscus
Somatosensory association area	Superior parietal lobule (areas 5, 7) Integrates sensory data; lesion causes tactile agnosias or astereognosis
Primary visual cortex (V1; area 17)	Located in the walls and floors of the calcarine sulcus, extends around the occipital pole Input: LGB → geniculocalcarine fibers pass close to the outer wall of the lateral ventricles (external sagittal stratum) → calcarine sulcus Output: internal sagittal stratum → corticofugal fibers → superior colliculus and LGB Macula → posterior ⅓ of the calcarine cortex (occipital pole) Vertical meridian has commissural fibers for bilateral representation. Ganglion cell receptive field — a region of the retina that affects the firing of one retinal ganglion cell. It is either "on-center and off-surround" or "off-center and on-surround." These cells fire at a constant steady rate. LGB also has "on and off" areas that contribute to visual processing. The cortex no longer has concentric receptive fields. The ocular dominance columns have alternating right and left stripes. Orientation columns each represent 180 degrees. Band of Baillarger in the striate cortex is the stripe of Gennari visible to the naked eye; are collaterals of the primary visual cortical axons (the recognizable layer IVb on myelin-stained sections due to dense plexus of myelinated axons)
Secondary visual cortex (V2, V3; areas 18, 19)	Input: LGB and pulvinar V2 = area 18, V3 = area 19 (more lateral) Lesion causes visual agnosia

Primary auditory cortex (area 41)	Transverse gyri of Heschl located in the superior temporal gyrus, buried in the temporal operculum of the sylvian fissure; the first cortical structure for auditory information processing
	The association area 42 surrounds area 41.
	Input: MGB with fibers that pass through the sublenticular IC
	    Ventral MGB has tonotopic organization (high frequencies medial).
	    Dorsal and medial MGB → ipsilateral area 41
	    Isofrequency cell columns are present in the cortex.
	    Each cochlea projects bilaterally but more to the contralateral side.
	    Trapezoid body — the only auditory commissure needed for sound localization
	Unilateral lesion — bilateral partial deafness, but mostly contralateral
	Area 22 lesion (dominant hemisphere): word deafness or sensory aphasia with normal hearing

Gustatory area (area 43)	In the postcentral operculum adjacent to the tongue sensory area Input: ipsilateral nucleus solitarius → VPMpc → area 43
Vestibular cortex	Located in the inferior parietal lobule near S1 (head) Bilateral representation, slightly more contralateral

Abbreviations: IC, internal capsule; LGB, lateral geniculate body; MGB, medial geniculate body; ML, medial lemniscus; STT, spinothalamic tract; VPLc, ventroposterolateral pars caudalis; VPM, ventroposteromedial; VPMpc, ventroposteromedial pars compacta

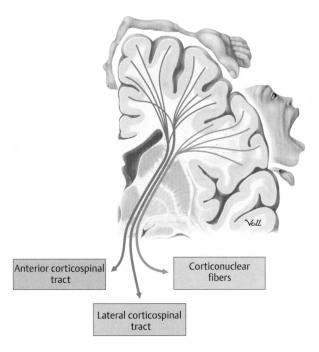

Fig. 1.24 Motor homunculus. Coronal section anterior view of the left hemisphere. Axons for the head area are the corticonuclear fibers and the corticospinal fibers split into lateral and anterior corticospinal tracts below the diencephalon. (From THIEME Atlas of Anatomy, Head and Neuroanatomy, © Thieme 2007, Illustration by Markus Voll.)

E. Motor cortex

1. Main motor areas — primary motor (area 4), premotor (area 6a), supplemental motor (areas 6a), frontal eye fields (area 8)

2. Motor cortex

Motor Cortex	Feature

Primary motor cortex M1 (area 4)	Precentral gyrus, involved in voluntary motor control, the thickest cortex
	Pyramidal cells of Betz (layer V) make up 3% of the corticospinal fibers.
	Output includes corticobulbar and corticospinal fibers:
	  From area 4 (31%), area 6 (29%), and parietal cortex 40%
	  Not somatotopic
	  Unilateral projection, except bilateral to the eye, face, tongue
	  Columns may be present (like those of the visual and somatosensory cortex)
	Neurotransmitters — glutamate and aspartate (±)

Premotor cortex (area 6a)	Voluntary motor control for responses dependent on sensory input Located on the lateral aspect of the cortex, anterior to area 4 Input: cortical, VL and VA thalamic nuclei Unilateral lesion: no deficit
Supplemental motor cortex M2 (area 6a)	Programming, planning, and initiating of motor movements Somatotopic organization of neurons Located on the medial aspect of the hemisphere anterior to area 4, medial superior frontal gyrus Input: bilateral Output: ipsilateral areas 4, 6, 5, and 7, contralateral M2, bilateral spinal cord, caudate, putamen, and thalamus Lesion — hemiparesis/plegia, diminished spontaneous speech, may have volitional movement with effort

Frontal eye fields (area 8)	Rostral to the premotor area (caudal middle frontal gyrus)
	Initiate saccades — stimulation causes contralateral eye deviation
	Occipital eye center (area 17) controls ipsilateral pursuit.
	Eye fields do not reach CNs III, IV, and VI nuclei directly, but goes to:
	  Rostral interstitial nucleus of the MLF
	  Interstitial nucleus of Cajal
	  Paramedian pontine reticular formation
	  Superior colliculus
	Lesion causes impaired saccades, especially in the dominant hemisphere.

Abbreviations: CN, cranial nerve; MLF, medial longitudinal fasciculus; VA, ventroanterior; VL, ventrolateral

F. Input to the motor area

1. Ipsilateral thalamic VL and ventrolateral pars oralis (VLo) → M1

2. Contralateral cerebellum → M1

3. Medial globus pallidus (GP) → ipsilateral thalamic ventroanterior pars compacta (VApc), VLo, centromedial (CM) → M2 and premotor cortex (not M1)

4. S1 (all but area 3) to all of the motor cortex

5. M2 → M1 and premotor cortex

6. Motor cortex has reciprocal fibers with the thalamus (except for thalamic reticular nuclei, which receives afferent fibers from the entire cortex but does not send them back.

G. Cerebral dominance

Dominant Hemisphere	Nondominant Hemisphere
Usually left hemisphere	Usually right hemisphere
Language, math, analytical thought Sign language mainly left hemisphere	Spatial analysis, face recognition, music, emotion Pictures may communicate language to the nondominant hemisphere, but letters require the dominant hemisphere for analysis.
Lesions in the dominant angular and supramarginal gyri: Gerstmann's syndrome: Right/left dissociation, finger agnosia, acalculia, Fail to appreciate the existence of hemiparesis agraphia	Lesion in the nondominant inferior parietal lobule: Failure to recognize a side of the body (neglect) Fail to appreciate the existence of hemiparesis
Handedness: Right-handed individuals are nearly always left-brain language dominant. Left-handed individuals are usually left-brain language dominant: 85%: left hemisphere dominance, 15%: bilaterally dominant Rare: right hemisphere dominance Men are more frequently left-handed, dyslexic, and prone to stutter. Handedness may be determined by testosterone during brain development.	

H. Cerebral topography

Fissure	Surface marking
Sylvian fissure	Localization: 1. Mark a point ¾ of the way on a line over the superior sagittal sinus from the nasion to the inion. 2. Mark the frontozygomatic point: 2.5 cm up along the orbital rim above the zygomatic arch. The sylvian fissure extends along the line connecting the 75% point and the frontozygomatic point. Pterion is located 3 cm behind the frontozygomatic point along the sylvian line. Angiographic localization: Sylvian point — the most posterior branch of the middle cerebral artery leaving the sylvian fissure, should be 5 cm from midline on an anteroposterior film, correspond to the top of the insula.
Rolandic fissure	Location: 1. Mark the upper Rolandic point: 2 cm posterior to the halfway point along the midline nasion/inion line. Also measured as 2.5 cm behind the pterion along the sylvian line. 2. Mark the lower Rolandic point: junction between the line from the upper Rolandic point to the midzygomatic arch and the sylvian fissure line. The Rolandic fissure lies between these two points. The motor strip is usually 4–5 cm behind the coronal suture.

IX. Diencephalon

A. General information (**Fig. 1.25**)

Components of the Diencephalon	Anatomical Border
Thalamus	Extends from the posterior commissure to the foramen of Monro
Epithalamus	Lateral border — IC, tail of caudate, stria terminalis
Habenular trigone	Inferior aspect contains epithalamic subcomponents.
Pineal gland	Note: diencephalons + telencephalon = cerebrum
Stria medullaris	
Roof of the third ventricle	
Hypothalamus	
Subthalamus (see Section X. Basal Ganglia)	
Metathalamus (MGB and LGB)	

Abbreviations: IC, internal capsule; LGB, lateral geniculate body; MGB, medial geniculate body

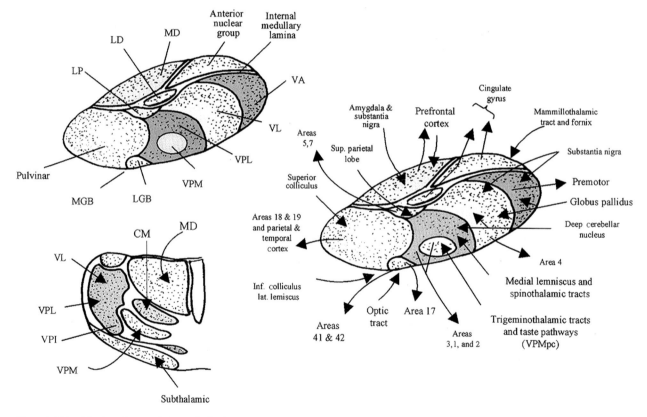

Fig. 1.25 Thalamic nuclei and their projections. CM, centromedial; Inf, inferior; lat., lateral; LD, lateral dorsal; LGB, lateral geniculate body; LP, lateral posterior; MD, mediodorsal; MGB, medial geniculate body; Sup., Superior; VA, ventroanterior; VL, ventrolateral; VPI, ventral posterior inferior; VPL, ventroposterolateral; VPM, ventroposteromedial; VPMpc, ventroposteromedial pars mammillothalamic.

B. Thalamus (**Fig. 1.26** and **Fig. 1.27**)

    1. Thalamic function

        a. Integrate, correlate, and relay motor, sensory, visual, limbic, and conscious systems

        b. Interpretation and conscious perception of pain

        c. Enhance cortical areas (focusing attention)

    2. Classification of thalamic nuclei

        a. Specific groups of nuclei — anterior, medial, ventrolateral, and dorsal nuclei

        b. Important relay station to the primary motor and sensory cortices

        c. Nonspecific groups of nuclei — intralaminar nuclei

        d. Reciprocal connections with association cortices

        e. Midline and intralaminar nuclei — input = reticular formation, output = diencephalon

        f. Reticular nucleus — modifies collateral inputs from thalamocortical and corticothalamic fibers

    3. Thalamic medullary laminae divide the nuclei

        a. Internal medullary lamina (IML) — between the medial and ventrolateral thalamic nuclei

        b. External medullary lamina (EML) — between the lateral and reticular nuclei

    4. Thalamic nuclei

Nuclei	Feature

Anterior nuclear group:
  Anteroventral
  Anterodorsal
  Anteromedial
	Input: mammillothalamic tract and fornix
	Output: cingulate gyrus via anterior limb of the IC
	Involved in the regulation of visceral function

Mediodorsal nuclear group	Between IML and periventricular gray Integrates somatic and visceral activities and controls affective behavior; disconnected during prefrontal lobotomies MD lesion — Korsakoff's psychosis Input: amygdala, orbitofrontal, and temporal cortex Output: frontal association cortex or prefrontal area Reciprocal connections with the frontal eye fields

Intralaminar nuclear
  group:
  Centromedial
  Parafascicular nuclei
  Rostral intralaminar
	Enclosed by the IML, input = RAS, output = diffuse cortex
	CM: input = area 4, output = putamen
	Parafascicular nucleus: input = area 6, output = caudate
	Rostral intralaminar nucleus: input = reticular formation, output = diffuse cortical areas
	A thalamic pacemaker for controlling electrical activities and wakefulness

Midline nuclei	Periventricular gray and the massa intermedia Output: amygdala and cingulate gyrus
Lateral nuclear group Dorsal tier:	LD: output = cingulum and supralimbic parietal lobe LP: input = parietal lobe, output = areas 5 and 7

LD, LP, pulvinar	Pulvinar: input = superior colliculus, reciprocal connections with occipital cortex, temporal and parietal lobes
	Extrageniculate visual pathways → secondary visual areas
	The three visuotopic thalamocortical pathways include
	  1. LGB → area 17
	  2. Inferior pulvinar → area 18
	  3. Lateral pulvinar → area 19
	Medial pulvinar may connect with the superior temporal gyrus.

(Continued on page 42)

4. Thalamic nuclei (*Continued from page 41*)

Nuclei	Feature

Lateral nuclear group
Ventral tier:
    VA, VL, VP (VPLo,
      VPLc, VPM, VPI)
Metathalamus (medial
    and lateral
    geniculate bodies)
	All are relay nuclei.
	Caudal portion carries specific sensory information.
	Rostral portion has input from the striatum, cerebellum, and SN.
	
	VA recruits cortical response, programming of movements from BG.
	Mammillothalamic tract passes through the VA.
	Input: GP, SN, and areas 6 and 8
	Output: frontal cortex and intralaminar nuclei
	
	VLo: Input = GP
	        Output = premotor and supplementary motor cortex
	VLc: Input = contralateral deep cerebellar nuclei and the red nuclei; reciprocal
	        connections with area 4
	
	VPLo: Input = contralateral deep cerebellar nuclei
	        Output = motor cortex
	VPLc: Input = medial lemniscus
	        Output = sensory cortex (limbs are lateral, back is dorsal)
	VPM: Input = contralateral spinal, principal sensory nuclei of CN V and ipsilateral dorsal
	        trigeminal tract
	        Output = sensory cortex to
	            Face, has bilateral VPM representation
	            Taste fibers from the nucleus solitarius → central tegmental tract uncrossed to
	                the VPMpc → parietal operculum area 43
	VPI: Output = ipsilateral S2 (S2 also receive bilateral input from S1 areas)
	
	Medial geniculate body:
	    The auditory relay nucleus
	    Located in the caudal ventral thalamus
	    Input: inferior colliculus via inferior brachium
	    Reciprocal connections — primary auditory cortex, spatial representation of tonal
	        frequency. Tonotopic, high-frequency sounds lie medially.
	Heschl's gyrus is located in the superior temporal convolution (area 41), where higher
	        frequencies remain medial.
	
	Lateral geniculate body:
	The visual relay nucleus, located rostral and lateral to MGB and ventral to pulvinar.
	        Composed of six layers:
	    Layers 1,2: magnocellular
	    Layers 3–6: parvicellular
	    Input: retinal ganglion cells
	    Retina → LGB (crossed/uncrossed fibers of the optic tract)
	    Crossed fibers from contralateral eye → 1, 4, 6 layers
	    Uncrossed fibers → 2, 3, 5 layers
	    Reciprocal connections — calcarine cortex (area 17) and pulvinar
	    No binocular fusion since fibers from different eyes end in different layers
	    Mnemonic: Lower retina → **L**ateral geniculate → **L**ower calcarine cortex

Posterior thalamic nuclear complex	Input: spinothalamic tract, ML, and S1 Output: retroinsular cortex and posterior auditory cortex
Thalamic reticular nuclei	Forms a shell over the dorsal thalamus Migrated derivative of the ventral thalamus Located between the IC and external medullary lamina It samples passing fibers and gates the activity of the thalamus but has no cortical projections.

Abbreviations: BG, basal ganglia; CN, cranial nerve; GP, globus pallidus; IC, internal capsule; IML, internal medullary lamina; LD , lateral dorsal; LGB, lateral geniculate body; LP, lateral posterior; MGB, medial geniculate body; ML, medial lemniscus; RAS, reticular activating system; SN, substantia nigra; VA, ventroanterior; VL, ventrolateral; VP, ventroposterior; VPLo, ventroposterolateral pars oralis; VPLc, ventroposterolateral pars caudalis; VPM, ventroposteromedial; VPI; ventral posterior inferior; VPMpc, ventroposteromedial pars compacta

5. Neurotransmitters
    a. Input: excitatory (aspartate and glutamate) from the deep cerebellar nuclei and cortex
    b. Output: GABA

6. Thalamic radiations — portions of the IC with reciprocal connections between the thalamus and cortex. There are four thalamic peduncles:
    a. Anterior: fibers from the medial and anterior thalamic nuclei → frontal lobe
    b. Superior: connections → sensorimotor to precentral and postcentral gyri
    c. Posterior: connections → visual to calcarine cortex
    d. Inferior: connections → auditory to Heschl's gyri

C. Epithalamus

1. Habenulum — involved in pathways of smell and basic emotions that influence visceral responses. Habenular nucleus and commissure = convergence of the limbic pathways. The nucleus is located in the habenular trigone.
    a. Input:
        (1) GP → lateral habenulum
        (2) Septal nuclei, lateral preoptic region, and anterior thalamic nuclei → medial habenulum (via stria medullaris)
        (3) Other inputs include lateral hypothalamus, substantia innominata, midbrain raphe nuclei, ventral tegmentum, and superior cervical ganglia

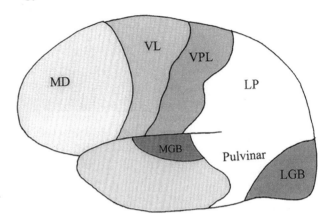

Fig. 1.26 Thalamocortical projections. LGB, lateral geniculate body; LP, lateral posterior; MD, mediodorsal; MGB, medial geniculate body; VL, ventrolateral; VPL, ventroposterolateral.

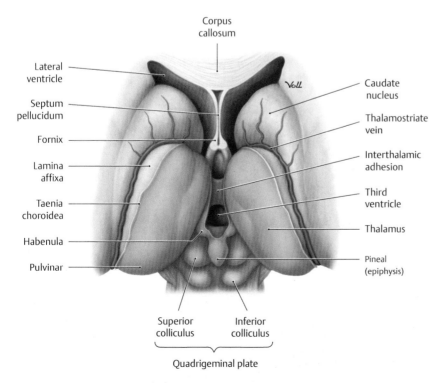

Corpus callosum

Lateral ventricle

Septum pellucidum

Fornix

Lamina affixa

Taenia choroidea

Habenula

Pulvinar

Caudate nucleus

Thalamostriate vein

Interthalamic adhesion

Third ventricle

Thalamus

Pineal (epiphysis)

Superior colliculus   Inferior colliculus

Quadrigeminal plate

Fig. 1.27 Arrangement of the diencephalon around the third ventricle. Posterior view of an oblique transverse section through the telencephalon with the corpus callosum, fornix, and choroid plexus removed. Removal of the choroid plexus leaves behind its line of attachment, the taenia choroidea. The thin wall of the third ventricle has been removed with the choroid plexus to expose the thalamic surface medial to the boundary line of the taenia choroidea. This thin layer of telencephalon, called the lamina affixa, is colored brown in the drawing and covers the thalamus (part of the diencephalon), shown in blue. Because the thalamostriate vein marks this boundary between the diencephalon and telencephalon, it is featured prominently in the drawing. Lateral to the vein is the caudate nucleus, which is part of the telencephalon. (From THIEME Atlas of Anatomy, Head and Neuroanatomy, © Thieme 2007, Illustration by Markus Voll.)

b. Output:
   (1) Fasciculus retroflexus → interpeduncular nuclei and the midbrain raphe nuclei → reticular nuclei, hypothalamic nuclei, and preganglionic autonomic nuclei
   (2) Note: fasciculus retroflexus = habenulointerpeduncular or Meynert's fasciculus

2. Pineal gland (epiphysis)

Pineal Gland	Feature
Borders	Attached to the roof of the third ventricle by Ventral commissure (posterior commissure) Dorsal commissure (habenular commissure)
Components	Glia and pinealocytes
Functions	Neurosensory photoreceptors Secretion of Serotonin (5-hydroxytryptamine [5-HT]) — from pinealocytes Norepinephrine — from terminating sympathetic neurons Thyroid-releasing hormone, luteinizing hormone-releasing hormone, and somatostatin (which inhibits growth hormone) Melatonin, made from 5-HT Daily levels fluctuate with diurnal light (maximal secretion in dark). Oversecreting pineal gland delays puberty. Hypofunctioning pineal gland causes precocious puberty. Sympathetic innervation inhibits the pineal gland: light contacting the retina → suprachiasmatic nucleus of hypothalamus → dorsal longitudinal fasciculus → upper intermediolateral cell column of superior colliculi → pineal inhibited
Lesions	Bilateral lesions of the hypothalamic suprachiasmatic nuclei (which relays retinal input to the pineal gland), abolishes circadian rhythms of eating and drinking; affects the estrous cycle.

D. Internal capsule (IC) (**Fig. 1.28** and **Fig. 1.29**)

1. IC contains fibers from thalamic radiations, corticospinal, bulbar, reticular, and pontine tracts.

2. IC components

Components	Fibers	Blood Supply: Branches
Anterior limb	Anterior thalamic radiation Prefrontal corticopontine tract	ACA: recurrent artery of Heubner (caudal) MCA: lenticulostriates (lateral and rostral)
Genu	Corticobulbar tract Corticoreticular tract	MCA: lenticulostriates ICA: perforators
Posterior limb	Superior thalamic radiation Frontopontine tract Corticospinal/tectal/rubral/reticular tracts Note: Motor fibers are anterior to the sensory. Rostral to caudal: cervical, thoracic, lumbar, sacral	MCA: lenticulostriates (lateral and rostral) Anterior ChA (caudal) Anterior ChA PcommA (caudal)
Retrolenticular portion	Posterior thalamic radiation (visual information) Parietal and occipital corticopontine fibers	Anterior ChA
Sublenticular portion	Inferior thalamic radiation (auditory information) Temporal and parietooccipital corticopontine fibers	Anterior ChA

Abbreviations: ACA, anterior cerebral artery; ChA, choroidal artery; ICA, internal carotid artery; MCA, middle cerebral artery; PCommA, posterior communicating artery

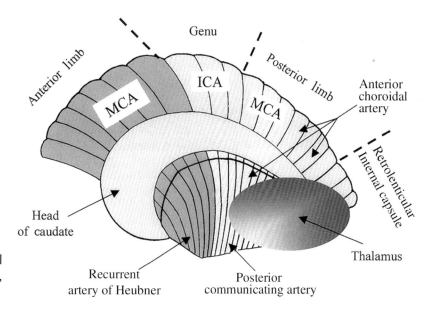

Fig. 1.28 Blood supply to the internal capsule. ICA, internal carotid artery; MCA, middle cerebral artery.

X. Basal Ganglia

A. Basal ganglia includes (**Fig. 1.30**)

   1. Corpus striatum = neostriatum + paleostriatum

   2. Amygdala

   3. Subthalamic nuclei

   4. Substantia nigra (SN)

B. Definitions

   1. Neostriatum (or striatum) = caudate + putamen

   2. Paleostriatum = GP

   3. Corpus striatum = neostriatum + paleostriatum (caudate, putamen, GP)

   4. Archistriatum = amygdala.

   5. Lentiform nuclei = putamen + GP

   6. Diencephalic = paleostriatum, subthalamic nucleus

   7. Telencephalic = neostriatum, archistriatum

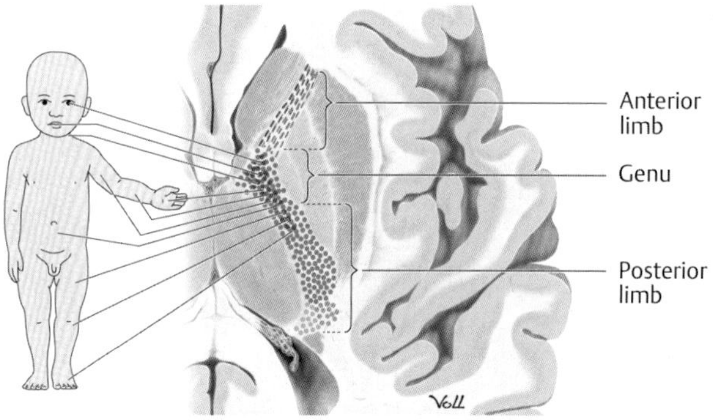

C. Caudate subcomponents

   1. Head — contiguous with the anterior perforated substance

   2. Body — separated from the thalamus by the stria terminalis and the terminal vein

   3. Tail — in the roof of the temporal horn near the amygdala

   4. Nucleus accumbens septi — located where the caudate and putamen meet anteriorly

Fig. 1.29 Somatotopic organization of the internal capsule. Transverse section shows both ascending and descending projection fibers that pass through the internal capsule. The figure of the child shows sites where pyramidal tract fibers pass. Anterior limb contains frontopontine (red dashes) and anterior thalamic peduncle (blue dashes) fibers, genu contains corticonuclear fibers (red dots) and posterior limb contains corticospinal fibers (red dots), posterior thalamic peduncle fibers (blue dots), temporopontine tract (orange dots), and the posterior thalamic peduncle (light blue dots). (From THIEME Atlas of Anatomy, Head and Neuroanatomy, © Thieme 2007, Illustration by Markus Voll.)

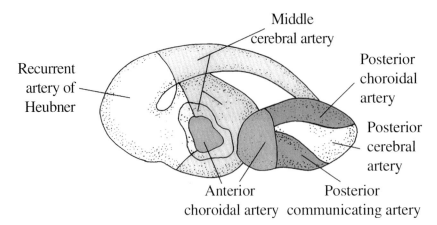

Fig. 1.30 Blood supply to the thalamus and striatum.

D. Striatum

    1. Striatal input — cortex, thalamic CM and parafascicular nuclei, SN, midbrain dorsal raphe nucleus, and the lateral amygdala. These fibers include

        a. Corticostriate fibers (most important input) which travel from

            (1) Area 4 → bilateral putamen

            (2) Premotor cortex → ipsilateral caudate and putamen

            (3) Prefrontal cortex → caudate

        b. Amygdalostriate fibers:

            (1) Amygdala → caudate and putamen

        c. Thalamostriate fibers, which travel from

            (1) Intralaminar CM nucleus (the largest intralaminar nucleus) → putamen

            (2) Parafascicular nucleus (PF) → caudate

        d. Nigrostriatal fibers, which travel from

            (1) SN → caudate and putamen (inhibitory dopamine)

        e. Raphe nucleus sends inhibitory fibers (serotonin)

    2. Striatal output

        a. Striatonigral fibers: head of caudate → substantia nigra pars reticulata (SNpr)

        b. Striatopallidal fibers: caudate/putamen → globus pallidus interna (GPi; inhibitory, GABA)

        c. Nigrothalamic fibers — terminate in VA, VLm, MD (GABA)

E. Medullary lamina

    1. Lateral medullary lamina — between putamen and GP

    2. Medial medullary lamina — divides medial and lateral GP (MGP, LGP)

    3. Accessory medullary lamina — divides MGP into inner and outer segments

F. Globus pallidus (GP)

    1. GP input

        a. Striatum (GABA and enkephalin) → LGP

        b. Striatum (substance P) → MGP

        c. Lateral part of subthalamus has reciprocal fibers (glutamate) → LGP, and the medial part connects to the MGP

        d. Note: Huntington's disease has decreased substance P and enkephalin in GP and SN.

2. GP output (four bundles)
   a. Ansa lenticularis (main output tract) — from MGP, passes around the IC → Forel's field H1 (FFH1), the prerubral field
   b. Lenticular fasciculus (FFH2 fibers) — from MGP, passes through the IC to join ansa lenticularis in Forel's field and enters the thalamic fasciculus
   c. Thalamic fasciculus (FFH1 fibers) — composed of the joined ansa lenticularis, lenticular fasciculus, and cerebellothalamic tract (fibers from the contralateral deep cerebellar nuclei) → thalamic VA and VL. The pallidotegmental fibers are from the MGP → Forel H fibers → pedunculopontine nucleus
   d. Pallidosubthalamic fibers
      (1) LGP → subthalamus (ST)
      (2) MGP → stria medullaris → lateral habenulum
      (3) GP → VA, VL, and CM

G. Subthalamus (ST) — located posterolateral to the hypothalamus, ventral to the thalamus, and medial to the IC. Lesion causes contralateral hemiballismus.

  1. ST contains
     a. Subthalamic nuclei (of Luys), lens-shaped, located over the rostral SN
     b. Zona incerta, gray matter between the thalamic and lenticular fasciculi. Laterally it is continuous with the thalamic reticular nucleus. Input: motor cortex
     c. Sensory fasciculi (medial lemniscus, spinothalamic and trigeminothalamic tract → VP thalamus)
     d. Cerebellar and globus pallidus fibers → thalamus

  2. Subthalamic fasciculus contains
     a. Dentatothalamic fibers traverse the red nucleus to the field of Forel H1 to enter VL.
     b. Ansa lenticularis bands sharply around the medial edge of the IC to enter VL.
     c. Lenticular fascicularis crosses at the internal capsule, goes to the ST to form the field of Forel H2.

  3. General pathway — LGP → ST → MGP and LGP, which passes through the peduncular IC

  4. ST input— LGP, prefrontal, premotor, and motor cortex, CM and PF thalamic nuclei and pedunculopontine nucleus

  5. Output: LGP (mainly), MGP, and SN

  6. Neurotransmitter used — glutamate

H. Claustrum

  1. Input: lateral hypothalamus, thalamic CM nucleus, and locus ceruleus

  2. Reciprocal connections with area 6

I. Substantia nigra (SN)

  1. SN input: striatum → SNpr (pigmented neurons), GP, ST, pedunculopontine nucleus, and dorsal raphe nucleus

  2. SN output (Note: SN does not have output to the GP)
     a. SNpc → striatum
     b. SNpr → thalamus and pedunculopontine nucleus

J. Corpus striatum — output inhibitory to MGP and SNpr that inhibits the thalamic output to the premotor and supplementary motor cortex, but not to area 4.

K. BG circuits

    1. Putamen circuit — involved in discrete motor movements

        a. Fibers from motor and somatosensory cortex → putamen → GP → thalamus → supplementary motor cortex

    2. Caudate circuit — involved with cognitive function

        a. Fibers from cortical association areas → caudate → GP → thalamus → supplementary motor cortex

L. Summary of BG pathways

    1. Striatum – reciprocal connections with SN (to the SNpr and from the SNpc)

    2. GP — reciprocal connections with ST

    3. LGP → ST

    4. MGP → thalamus (VL, VA, and CM)

    5. There are no afferent fibers from the cortex or thalamus to the GP.

    6. SNpc inhibits the putamen, which inhibits GP, which in turn inhibits the thalamus.

O. Neurotransmitters

    1. Glutamate — cortex → striatum fibers

    2. GABA — putamen → GP fibers

XI. Hypothalamus

A. Hypothalamus — controls visceral, autonomic, endocrine, and emotional function (**Fig. 1.31**). It extends from the anterior perforated substance and optic chiasm to the optic tracts and the mamillary bodies. It has an anterior and posterior part, median and lateral eminences, and an infundibulum.

    1. Hypothalamic structures (**Fig. 1.31**)

Structures	Feature
Preoptic area	Periventricular gray of the most rostral third ventricle portion; contains medial and lateral preoptic nuclei
Medial hypothalamic area	Continuous with the periaqueductal gray Contains the supraoptic, tuberal, and mamillary regions (anterior, middle, and posterior regions, respectively). Supraoptic region (anterior) — contains paraventricular and supraoptic nuclei (secretes vasopressin and oxytocin), *anterior* hypothalamic nucleus, and suprachiasmatic nucleus (which acts as a biologic clock with bilateral afferent input from the retinas) Tuberal region — region where the fornix separates the hypothalamus into *medial* and *lateral* portions Mamillary region — contains the mamillary bodies and *posterior* hypothalamic nuclei
Lateral hypothalamic area	Contains the lateral hypothalamic nucleus
Median eminence	Region where the central nervous system interacts with the pituitary, funnel-like extension of the tuber cinereum

Note: Rostral and lateral is the basal olfactory region, whereas medial is the septal region with the medial and lateral septal nuclei and the nucleus accumbens septi.

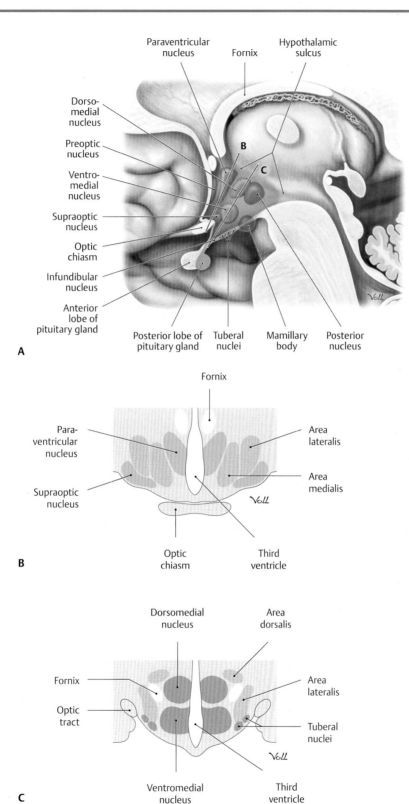

Fig. 1.31   Nuclei in the right hypothalamus. (**A**) Midsagittal section of the right hemisphere viewed from the medial side. (**B, C**) Coronal sections. The hypothalamus is a small nuclear complex located ventral to the thalamus and separated from it by the hypothalamic sulcus. (From THIEME Atlas of Anatomy, Head and Neuroanatomy, © Thieme 2007, Illustration by Markus Voll.)

2. Hypothalamic input

Fibers	Feature
General	Main inputs come from the two oldest cortical areas: Pyriform cortex → amygdala → stria terminalis → hypothalamus, and hippocampus → fornix → septum, etc. A closed loop is formed from the cingulate gyrus → entorhinal cortex → hippocampus → hypothalamus → anterior thalamic nucleus back to the cingulate gyrus.
Medial forebrain bundle	From basal olfactory areas, septal nuclei, periamygdala, and subiculum → lateral preoptic and lateral hypothalamic areas Information related to basic emotional drives and smell
Fornix	Hippocampus → mamillary bodies
Stria terminalis	Travels within the terminal sulcus (between the thalamus and caudate). Amygdala → hypothalamus (anterior and preoptic nuclei) Information related to emotional drives and smell
Mamillary peduncle	Brainstem reticular formation → lateral mamillary nucleus
Dorsal longitudinal fasciculus	Midbrain's central gray → periventricular hypothalamus
Retinohypothalamic tract	Retinal ganglion cells → both suprachiasmatic nuclei and various hypothalamic nuclei (circadian rhythms)
Nucleus solitarius (NSol)	NSol rostral segment (taste) → medial hypothalamus NSol caudal segment (visceral) → lateral hypothalamus
Other inputs	Midbrain raphe nucleus, pons parabrachial nucleus, locus ceruleus, lateral geniculate body, and the thalamus (thalamohypothalamic)

3. Hypothalamic output

Output	Feature
Mammillothalamic tract	"Hypothalamic–thalamic tract of Vicq d'Azyr" Mamillary bodies → anterior thalamic nucleus; major tract
Dorsal longitudinal fasciculus (major tract)	Mamillary bodies → midbrain tegmentum and central gray
Medial forebrain bundle	Lateral hypothalamus → hippocampus
Stria terminalis	Hypothalamus → amygdala
Mammillotegmental tract	Mamillary bodies → midbrain ventral and dorsal tegmentum
Descending autonomic projections	Paraventricular, lateral hypothalamus, and posterior hypothalamus → dorsal motor nucleus X, nucleus solitarius, nucleus ambiguous, medulla, and spinal intermediolateral cell column
Supraoptichypophyseal tract	Supraoptic and paraventricular nuclei → posterior pituitary gland (releases oxytocin, vasopressin, cholecystokinin, enkephalins, glucagon, dynorphin, and angiotensin)
Tuberohypophyseal tract	Arcuate nucleus of the tuber region → median eminence and the infundibular stem. Releasing hormones are secreted into the fenestrated capillaries that form the hypophyseal portal system draining into the anterior pituitary gland.

4. Hypothalamic controls
   a. Parasympathetic — anterior and medial (ventromedial) hypothalamic nuclei
   b. Sympathetic — posterior and lateral hypothalamic nuclei
   c. Decreases body temperature — anterior hypothalamic nucleus
   d. Increases body temperature — posterior hypothalamic nucleus
   e. Satiety center — medial hypothalamic nucleus
   f. Feeding center — lateral hypothalamic nucleus
   g. Arousal center — posterior hypothalamic nucleus

B. Pituitary gland is located within the sella turcica of the sphenoid bone.

1. Anterior and posterior pituitary lobe

Adenohypophysis	Neurohypophysis
75% of the gland	25% of the gland
Ectodermal origin from roof of the stomodeum	Diencephalic origin
Three components:	Three components:
1. Pars tuberalis includes	1. Pars nervosa (posterior lobe)
Portion of the infundibular stalk	2. Infundibulum
Median eminence of hypothalamus	3. Nuclei (supraoptic and paraventricular)
2. Pars intermedia	
3. Pars distalis: majority of the gland, has no direct arterial supply	

C. Hypophyseal portal system is formed by the superior hypophyseal arteries (supraclinoid ICA) and the inferior hypophyseal arteries (branch of cavernous ICA meningohypophyseal trunk). These arteries join in and around the pituitary stalk and form sinusoids that feed the infundibulum and the anterior pituitary gland. The superior hypophyseal artery supplies the infundibulum and the median eminence. The inferior hypophyseal artery supplies the posterior pituitary lobe.

XII. Olfactory System (Also See Section XV)

A. Olfactory sense — the only sensory system without a thalamic relay. It functions to help find food and mates, and to avoid predators.

B. Rhinencephalon — composed of the olfactory bulbs, tracts, tubercles, striae, and the anterior olfactory nucleus and pyriform cortex. It is a paleopallium (archipallium is part of the hippocampus, dentate gyrus, fasciolar gyrus, and indusium griseum).

1. Rhinencephalon

Components	Feature
Olfactory receptors	Located in the upper posterior nasal cavity Epithelium with primary bipolar cells with kinocilium
Olfactory nerve	Consists of a group of unmyelinated fibers extending through the cribriform plate to synapse with mitral cells (second neurons) in the olfactory bulb Mitral and tufted cells gather to form the glomeruli. Granule cells have no axons in the olfactory nerve. Neurotransmitters used — glutamate and aspartate
Olfactory bulb	Connects to the olfactory tract → lateral olfactory stria and gyrus Connects to the olfactory tract → medial olfactory stria and gyrus Lateral olfactory tract = axons of the mitral and tufted cells
Lateral olfactory stria	Output: Anterior olfactory nucleus; some fibers cross in the anterior commissure to the contralateral anterior nucleus and olfactory bulb to the internal granule cells Olfactory tubercle Amygdala Pyriform cortex → entorhinal cortex → hippocampus, insula, and frontal lobe via uncinate fasciculus Pyriform cortex → amygdala, lateral preoptic hypothalamus, and nucleus of the diagonal band Pyriform cortex → MD thalamic nucleus → orbitofrontal cortex
Medial olfactory stria	Output: Subcallosal area Septal area (paraterminal gyrus)
Olfactory cortex	Two components: 1. Primary olfactory cortex = pyriform cortex + periamygdaloid cortex. 2. Secondary olfactory cortex = entorhinal area of the anterior parahippocampus (area 28), which is posterior to the primary cortex. Note: Pyriform cortex is the lateral olfactory gyrus from the lateral olfactory stria to the amygdala.
Anterior perforated substance	Transmits perforating arteries Located in front of the optic tract, behind the olfactory trigone, anteromedially continuous with the subcallosal gyrus and bounded laterally by the lateral stria (olfactory tract and uncus)
Septal area	Composed of the subcallosal area and the parateriminal gyrus Medial and lateral septal nuclei Located rostral to the anterior commissure and preoptic area Medial septal nucleus becomes continuous with the nucleus and tract of the diagonal band of Broca, which extends to the amygdala. Septal input: fornix and the mamillary peduncle Septal output: Stria medullaris → medial habenular nucleus Medial forebrain bundle → lateral hypothalamus, midbrain, and the tegmentum Fornix → hippocampus
Anterior commissure	Anterior portion of the AC connects the two olfactory bulbs. Posterior portion of the AC connects the two GP, putamen, external capsules, claustrums, and inferior and middle frontal gyri.

Abbreviations: AC, anterior commissure; GP, globus pallidus; MD, mediodorsal

XIII. Hippocampal Formation (Fig. 1.32, Fig. 1.33, Fig. 1.34)

A. Limbic system — controls behavior and emotion. Components include

1. Limbic cortex (parahippocampal gyrus, hippocampal formation and dentate gyrus, cingulate gyrus, insula and orbitofrontal cortex)

2. Subcortical limbic structures (amygdala, hypothalamus, septal nuclei, habenular nuclei, anterior and dorsomedial thalamic nuclei, and the indusium griseum)

3. Fibers (mammillothalamic tract, fornix, stria medullaris thalami, and stria terminalis) (**Fig. 1.34**)

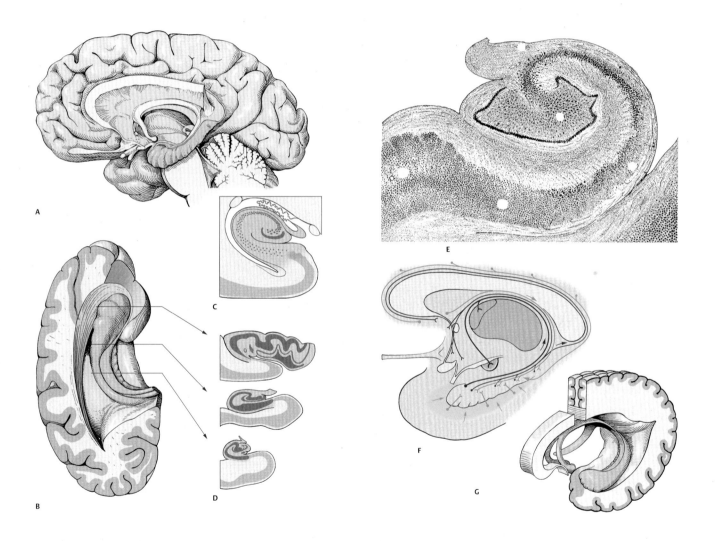

Fig. 1.32 Hippocampus. (**A**) After removal of the remainder of the left hemisphere (after Ludwig and Klinger). (**B**) View from above (after Sobotta). (**C**) Frontal section through the hippocampus and Ammon's horn (schematic). (**D**) Ammon's horn, sections at different levels. (**E**) Ammon's horn, frontal section through the hippocampus. (**F**) Fiber connections of the hippocampus. (**G**) Hippocampus and fornix (after Feneis). (From Kahle W, Frotscher M. Color Atlas of Human Anatomy. Volume 3: Nervous System and Sensory Organs. New York, NY: Thieme; 2003. Reprinted by permission.)

Fig. 1.33 Normal hippocampus (hematoxylin and eosin).

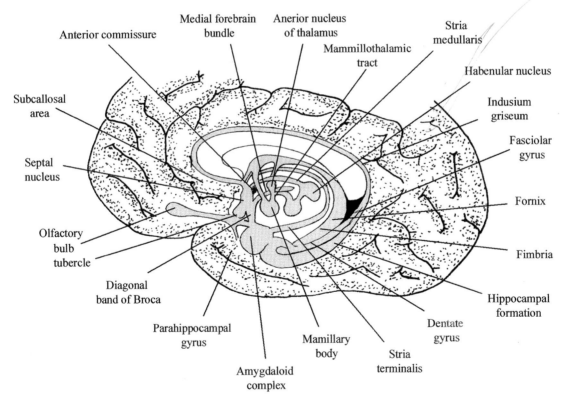

Fig. 1.34 Limbic structures and connections.

B. The hippocampal formation — composed of the presubiculum, subiculum, prosubiculum, hippocampus, and dentate gyrus. All are archipallium with three layers (molecular, pyramidal, and polymorphic layer). The inferior parahippocampus is isocortex with the six layers. Divided into four cornu ammonis (CA) zones

C. Indusium griseum — composed of the supracallosal gyrus and medial and lateral longitudinal striae. They are the remnants of the hippocampus that course over the dorsal surface of the corpus callosum. Connects septal area with hippocampus

D. Hippocampal input

    1. Entorhinal cortex (area 28) → hippocampus and dentate gyrus

    2. Medial septal nucleus → fimbria

    3. Cingulate gyrus → cingulum → presubiculum/entorhinal cortex → hippocampus

E. Hippocampal output (via fornix)

    1. Fornix components: fimbriae → crura → body → columns. Fibers include
        a. Precommissural fornix (minority) — fibers are located anterior to interventricular foramen, and rostral to anterior commissure. Hippocampus → precommissural fornix → caudal septal nucleus
        b. Postcommissural fornix (majority), cingulate gyrus — Fibers are located anterior to the interventricular foramen and caudal to the anterior commissure.
        c. Subiculum → postcommissural fornix (larger) to either
            (1) Medial nucleus of the mamillary body
            (2) Anterior thalamic nucleus
            (3) Lateral septal area of the rostral hypothalamus
            (4) Medial frontal cortex
            (5) Cingulate and parahippocampal gyri

    2. Dentate fibers do not leave the hippocampus. The subiculum may serve as the main output for the hippocampus and dentate gyrus. It is the sole direct cortical projector.
        a. Output:
            (1) Hippocampus and subicular cortex (presubiculum, subiculum, and postsubiculum) → alveus → fimbria → two forniceal crura → forniceal commissure → body of the fornix under the corpus callosum → separation at the rostral thalamus into anterior columns
            (2) CA1 pyramidal cell axons → subiculum and fornix
            (3) CA3 pyramidal cell axons → CA1 and fornix

F. Function: involved with recent memory (not remote memory) and consolidation of short-term memory into long-term memory. Unilateral injury to the mamillary body and the fornix does not seem to impair memory. The hippocampus has no olfactory function. Stimulation or lesioning causes psychomotor seizures.

G. Circuit of Papez — suggested involvement with emotion, combining the subjective/autonomic/ somatic elements. Bidirectional connection from the subiculum → mamillary bodies → mammillothalamic tract → anterior thalamic nucleus → entorhinal cortex → subiculum

H. Amygdala — merges caudally with the uncus of the parahippocampal gyrus

    1. Inputs: lateral olfactory tract, pyriform cortex, hypothalamus, paraventricular thalamus and the nucleus of the solitary tract → lateral parabrachial nucleus → amygdala. Also inputs from
        a. Locus ceruleus (noradrenergic fibers)
        b. SN and ventral tegmentum (dopaminergic fibers)

       c. Substantia innominata (SI) and the lateral olfactory area (cholinergic fibers)

       d. Raphe nucleus (serotonergic fibers)

  2. Outputs:

       a. Stria terminalis — mainly to the nucleus of the stria terminalis (at the caudate/thalamic junction) → hypothalamus

       b. Ventral amygdalofugal tract — amygdala and pyriform area → lateral preoptic area, septal area, nucleus of the diagonal band, substantia innominata (SI), hippocampus, and brainstem nuclei to regulate autonomic functions (with fear or stress)

       c. Amygdalocortical

       d. Amygdalostriate → nucleus accumbens

  3. Amygdala stimulation — arousal and arrest reaction with the initial reaction of flight, fear, rage with pupillary dilation and growling

       a. Stria terminalis injury — does not change the response

       b. Stria terminalis stimulation — increases the respiratory rate

       c. Ventral amygdalofugal fiber injury — does not produce any responses upon stimulation.

  4. Function: Amygdala serves as an interface between the cortex and the autonomic functions controlled by the hypothalamus and the brainstem. It dictates the emotions and behaviors for a specific situation. Significant reciprocal cortical input/output exists.

I. Substantia innominata (nucleus basalis of Meynert) — located in the basal forebrain, extends from the olfactory tubercle to the hypothalamus

  1. Input: amygdala, temporal lobe, pyriform cortex, and entorhinal cortex

  2. Output: cortex (diffuse)

  3. Subcommissural region contains

       a. Diagonal band of Broca

       b. Anterior commissure

       c. Median forebrain bundle (MFB)

       d. Ansa lenticularis, ansa peduncularis

       e. Inferior thalamic peduncle

  4. Contains high concentration of cholinergic neurons and is the single major source of cholinergic (ACh) fibers to the cortex. Cells degenerate here in Alzheimer's disease.

  5. Cholinergic areas of the central nervous system (CNS)

       a. Substantia innominata

       b. Pedunculopontine nucleus

       c. Lateral dorsal tegmental nucleus

       d. Medial habenular nucleus

J. C-shaped structures — limbic association areas, hippocampus and fornix, amygdala and stria terminalis, caudate nucleus, and the lateral ventricles

XIV. Cerebellum (Fig. 1.35, Fig. 1.36, Fig. 1.37)

A. General

Cerebellum	Description
Function	Controls muscle tone, coordination, and equilibrium
Gross anatomy	Divided into the cortex, medullary substance, intrinsic nuclei, hemisphere, and vermis. Contains many convolutions called folia. Composed of: Three lobes: anterior, posterior, and flocculonodular Nine lobules of the vermis: lingula, centralis, culmen, declive, folium, tuber, pyramis, uvula, and nodulus
Phylogenic classification	Archicerebellum: The oldest component: flocculus and nodulus Involved with vestibular function Paleocerebellum: Anterior lobe, rostral to the primary fissure (lingula, centralis, and culmen), controls muscle tone with inputs from the stretch receptors Neocerebellum: The newest component: posterior lobe between the primary fissure and the lateral fissures (declive, folium, tuber, pyramis, and uvula) Controls coordination with inputs from the contralateral cortex (via pontine relay nuclei)
Cerebellar cortical layers	There are three cerebellar cortical layers (superficial to deep): 1. Molecular layer: Contains basket cells (–) and outer stellate cells (–). Axons from each basket cell touch 10 Purkinje cells. 2. Purkinje cell layer: Contains Purkinje cells (–, GABA). The myelinated axons synapse with the deep nuclei and the lateral vestibular nucleus and send collateral fibers to excite Golgi type 2 cells. 3. Granular layer: Contains granule cells (+, glutamate) and Golgi type 2 cells (–). Granule cells supply 4–5 dendrites to form a glomerulus. It sends unmyelinated axons up to the molecular layer, bifurcating into parallel fibers that contact Purkinje cell dendrites. Golgi type 2 cells have axons that synapse in the glomeruli of the granular layer and dendrites that extend to the molecular layer, where they synapse with parallel fibers.
Afferent fibers to the cerebellar cortex	Arrives via cerebellar peduncles (superior, middle, and inferior) Input: spinocerebellar, cuneocerebellar, olivocerebellar, vestibulocerebellar, and pontocerebellar tracts These fibers lose their myelin in the cortex, end as mossy/climbing fibers. All cerebellar cells are inhibitory except granule cells, climbing fibers, and mossy fibers.

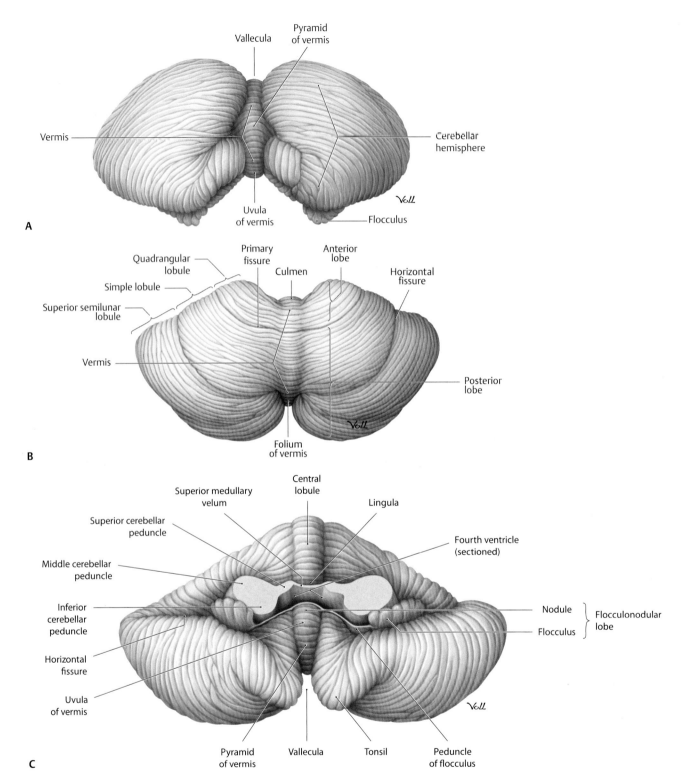

Fig. 1.35 Cerebellum (**A**) Inferior view. (**B**) Superior view. (**C**) Anterior view. The cerebellum has been removed from the posterior fossa and detached from the brainstem at the cerebellar peduncles. (**B**) The primary fissure separates the anterior from the posterior lobe. (**B**) The posterolateral fissure separates the posterior from the flocculonodular lobe. (From THIEME Atlas of Anatomy, Head and Neuroanatomy, © Thieme 2007, Illustration by Markus Voll.)

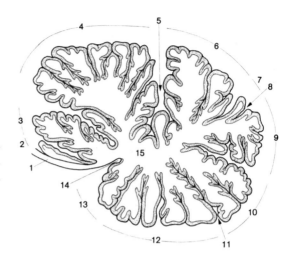

Fig. 1.36 View of medial side of right cerebellum sectioned in sagittal plane, showing parts of the cerebellar vermis. 1. Superior medullary velum. 2. Lingula. 3. Central lobule. 4. Culmen. 5. Primary fissure. 6. Declive. 7. Folium of vermis. 8. Horizontal fissure. 9. Tuber of vermis. 10. Pyramid of vermis. 11. Secondary fissure. 12. Uvula, separated from the nodulus by the dorsolateral fissure. 13. Nodulus. 14. Fastigium. 15. Corpus medullare. (From Frick H, Leonhardt H, Starck D. Human Anatomy 2. New York, NY: Thieme;1991. Reprinted by permission.)

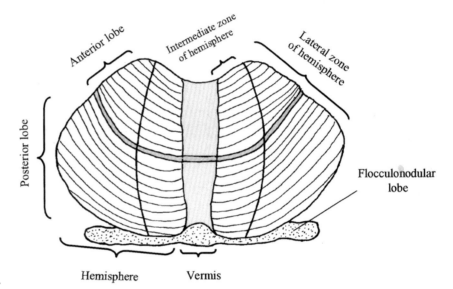

Fig. 1.37 Cerebellar functional zones.

B. Spinocerebellar tracts

1. Dorsal spinocerebellar tract
   a. Uncrossed; conveys proprioception from the joints, muscle spindles, and Golgi tendon organs of the ipsilateral lower extremities and upper trunk to Clarke's nucleus in lamina VII of the intermediate zone in the spinal cord. Fibers then enter the inferior cerebellar peduncle to the cerebellar vermis and intermediate zone of the cerebellum as well as the fastigial and interposed nuclei.

2. Ventral spinocerebellar tract
   a. Crossed; conveys efferent copies of motor commands that reach the α motor neurons and exteroceptive and proprioceptive information for the lower extremities
   b. The initial cell bodies are "spinal border cells" in the anterior and intermediate horns. The tract ascends bilaterally, crosses within the spinal cord, enters the superior cerebellar peduncle, and crosses partly again in the cerebellum but remains mainly contralateral.

3. Cuneocerebellar tract
   a. Conveys proprioception of the upper extremities in the fasciculus cuneatus but synapses in the accessory cuneate nucleus in the caudal medulla above the cuneate nucleus and then enters the inferior cerebellar peduncle ipsilaterally
   b. The upper extremity equivalent to the dorsal spinocerebellar tract

4. Rostral spinocerebellar tract
   a. It provides internal feedback, ipsilateral, and enters the inferior cerebellar peduncle.
   b. The upper extremity equivalent to the ventral spinocerebellar tract

5. Trigeminocerebellar tract
   a. Conveys mesencephalic nucleus of V → middle cerebellar peduncle → dentate and emboliform Conveys chief sensory nucleus of V → quadrangular lobe and tonsil. Conveys spinal nucleus of V (uncrossed and crossed) → tonsil

6. Vestibulocerebellar tract
   a. Monitors head position, eye movement, and equilibrium
   b. Conveys CN VIII fibers → inferior cerebellar peduncle → ipsilateral flocculonodular
   c. Conveys inferior and medial vestibular nuclei → juxtarestiform body → bilateral flocculonodular lobe and fastigial nuclei

7. Tectocerebellar tract
   a. Conveys information from the tectum (auditory and visual reflexes) → anterior medullary velum → superior cerebellar peduncle → anterior and posterior lobes

8. Reticulocerebellar tract
   a. Modulates circuit from the cerebral cortex to the cerebellum
   b. Conveys information from
      (1) Medulla → inferior cerebellar peduncle → vermis
      (2) Pons (reticulotegmental nucleus) → middle cerebellar peduncle → vermis

C. Afferent to the cortex

1. Mossy fibers (+) from spinocerebellar, pontocerebellar, and vestibulocerebellar tracts to the granular layer to form the center of a glomerulus with mossy fiber rosette (up to 44 connections per fiber). The mossy fiber stimulates granule cells, whereas Golgi type 2 cells inhibit them for feedback. The glomerulus contains
   a. One mossy fiber rosette (+)
   b. Up to 20 dendrites of granule cells
   c. Golgi type 2 cell's axons and dendrites

2. Climbing fibers (+, glutamate) from the contralateral inferior olivary complex to the molecular layer, where they synapse on Purkinje's cell dendrites, granule cell parallel fibers (stimulates Purkinje's cells), and other inhibitory cells such as basket and stellate cells (to silence the background). Climbing fibers may synapse with more than one cell. If the fiber discharges, so does the Purkinje cell (all or none response).

D. Corticonuclear projections, bidirectional and unilateral

1. Vermis-fastigial nucleus

2. Paravermian zone-interposed nucleus

3. Hemisphere-dentate nucleus

E. Deep nuclei — contain neurons that release excitatory neurotransmitters (aspartate and glutamate). The deep nuclei project to the granular layer.

    1. There are four paired nuclei.

        a. Fastigial nucleus — in the midline roof of the fourth ventricle, sends fibers to the vestibular system bilaterally

        b. Globose nucleus — involved with tone

        c. Emboliform nucleus — involved with tone

        d. Dentate nucleus — the largest, shaped like a bag that is open medially toward the superior cerebellar peduncle; involved with coordination

    2. Note: nucleus interpositus = globus + emboliform nucleus

F. Extracerebellar inputs to the deep nuclei can overcome the tonic inhibition from the cortex. The red nucleus sends crossed fibers to the nucleus interpositus. Stimulation from

    1. Pons — sends crossed and uncrossed fibers to the dentate nuclei

    2. Inferior olivary nucleus

        a. Principal olivary nucleus → dentate nucleus (crossed)

        b. Medial and dorsal accessory olivary nuclei → interposed nucleus (crossed)

        c. Medial accessory olive → fastigial nucleus (crossed)

    3. Trigeminal sensory nucleus

    4. Reticulotegmental tract

    5. Locus ceruleus

    6. Raphe nucleus via climbing and mossy fibers

G. Cerebellar afferent fibers

Cerebellar Peduncles	Feature
Inferior cerebellar peduncle	Restiform body — contains only afferent fibers from the inferior olivary complex, pons and dorsal spinocerebellar tract Juxtarestiform body — contains afferent and efferent fibers from the vestibular system → uvula, nodulus, and fastigial nucleus; located medial to the restiform body
Middle cerebellar peduncle	Contains only afferent fibers Cerebral cortex → ipsilateral pons → contralateral cerebellar hemisphere (corticopontine fibers) and bilaterally to the vermis (mossy fibers) Nodulus is the only part of the cerebellum without pontine input.
Superior cerebellar peduncle	Receives afferent fibers from the ventral spinocerebellar tract Also contains efferent fibers

H. Efferent cerebellar fibers (mainly from the deep nuclei

Cerebellar Peduncles	Feature
Inferior cerebellar peduncle (via juxtarestiform body)	Fastigial nucleus → contralateral reticular nucleus, pons, spinal cord, and bilaterally to the lateral and inferior vestibular nuclei Vermian cortex and flocculonodular lobe (through Purkinje fibers that bypass the deep nuclei) to the ipsilateral vestibular nuclei Flocculus → superior and medial vestibular nuclei Nodulus/uvula → superior, medial, and inferior vestibular nuclei Fastigial nuclei → vestibular nuclei Vestibulocerebellar feedback: uvula and flocculonodular lobes
Superior cerebellar peduncle (main)	Dentate nucleus → contralateral thalamic VL, VPLo, and centrolateral nucleus → cortex, controls coordination Ipsilateral cerebellar lesion — ipsilateral dyscoordination because it controls the contralateral cerebral cortex. Nucleus interpositus → contralateral red nucleus (some to the thalamus VL and VA), crossing back to the ipsilateral spinal cord; controls ipsilateral tone control Dentate nucleus sends crossed fibers → principal olive Emboliform nucleus → dorsal accessory olive Globose nucleus → medial accessory olive

Abbreviations: VA, ventroanterior, VL, ventrolateral; VPLo, ventroposterolateral pars oralis

I. Somatotopic organization

  1. Touch — ipsilateral in the anterior lobe and bilateral in the posterior lobe

  2. Audiovisual information lies midline

J. Cerebellar organization

  1. Vermian zone
       a. Purkinje fibers — inhibits the vestibular nuclei to decrease extensor muscle tone
       b. Fastigial nucleus receives ipsilateral inhibition from the vermis but gives bilateral stimulation to the vestibular nuclei, pons, medulla, thalamus, and cervical motor neurons. Controls posture, tone, equilibrium, and locomotion.

  3. Paramedian zone — sends fibers to the nucleus interpositus → thalamus and red nucleus. Controls ipsilateral flexor tone.

  4. Lateral zone — the hemispheres represent the largest efferent pathway, fibers to:
       a. Dentate nucleus → thalamic VL
       b. VPLo → motor cortex area 4 for ipsilateral coordination. This is the largest efferent pathway.

K. Functional considerations

Cerebellar Lesions	Feature
General	Ipsilateral deficits that gradually attenuate with time Injuries to the superior cerebellar peduncle and dentate nucleus result in the most severe and persistent deficits.
Neocerebellar lesions (posterior lobe)	Hypotonia, fatigability, pendular and sluggish deep tendon reflexes, asynergia with decreased coordination, dysmetria, dysdiadokinesis, rebound with the upper limb hitting the chest when dropped, decomposition of movement breaking a task into multiple acts, intention tremor (mainly proximal), ataxia of axial muscles, nystagmus when looking to the side of the lesion, and slow dysarthric speech.
Paleocerebellar lesions (anterior lobe)	Transient increased extensor tone Anterior lobe normally inhibits the lateral vestibular nucleus. Reticular formation tonically decreases extensor tone. Stimulation of nucleus interpositus to the red nucleus elicits ipsilateral limb flexion.
Archicerebellar (posterior vermis and flocculus)	Truncal ataxia and equilibrium disorders

XV. Cranial Nerves

A. General information

1. Cranial nerves carry fibers of six different modalities
    a. General somatic efferent (GSE) — CNs III, IV, VI, XII
    b. General visceral efferent (GVE) — CNs III, VII, IX, X
    c. Special visceral efferent (GVE) — CNs V, VII, IX, X, X, muscles from branchial arches
    d. General somatic afferent (GSA) — CNs V, VII, IX, X, transmit visceral information, but not pain
    e. General visceral afferent (GVA) — CNs IX, X
    f. Sensory afferent (SA) — CNs I, II, VII, VIII, IX

2. Ganglia associated with cranial nerves

Cranial Nerves	Sensory Ganglia*	Autonomic Ganglia*
Oculomotor nerve (CN III)		Ciliary ganglion
Trigeminal nerve (CN V)	Trigeminal ganglion	
Facial nerve (CN VII)	Geniculate ganglion	Pterygopalatine ganglion Submandibular ganglion
Vestibulocochlear nerve (CN VIII)	Spiral ganglion Vestibular ganglion	
Glossopharyngeal nerve (CN IX)	Superior ganglion Inferior (petrosal) ganglion	Otic ganglion
Vagus nerve (CN X)	Superior (jugular) ganglion Inferior (nodose) ganglion	Prevertebral and intramural ganglia

Source: From Schuenke M, Schulte E, Schumacher U. Atlas of Anatomy, Head and Neuroanatomy. Stuttgart, Germany: Thieme; 2007. Reprinted by permission.

*There are sensory, motor, and autonomic ganglia. Sensory ganglia are analogous to spinal ganglia in the dorsal roots of the spinal cord. They contain cell bodies of pseudounipolar primary afferent neurons. The autonomic ganglia in the head are parasympathetic and contain cell bodies of multipolar neurons.

B. Cranial nerve I (olfactory nerve)

    1. Sensory afferent — Primary neurons in the olfactory epithelium function simultaneously as neurosecretory cells and as sensory receptors (other types SA have separate receptors). Primary neurons send 20 bundles of axons (olfactory nerves proper) across the cribriform plate (ethmoid bone) to synapse with secondary neurons (mitral and tufted cells) within the olfactory bulbs.

        a. Mitral cells → lateral olfactory area

        b. Tufted cells → anterior olfactory nucleus, lateral, intermediate, and medial olfactory areas

        c. Olfactory tract carries these secondary neuron axons to three areas.

            (1) Primary (lateral) olfactory area (via lateral olfactory stria), composed of

                (a) Uncus

                (b) Entorhinal area (anterior portion of the hippocampal gyrus)

                (c) Limen insula (insular and frontal lobe junction)

                (d) Part of the amygdala

            (2) Anterior perforated substance (or intermediate olfactory area) via intermediate olfactory stria between the olfactory trigone and the optic tract

            (3) Medial olfactory area (septal area), via medial olfactory stria, in the subcallosal region of the medial frontal lobe. This region mediates emotional response to odors with its limbic connections.

    2. Miscellaneous

        a. Diagonal band of Broca connects all three olfactory areas.

        b. Pyriform cortex — pear-shaped area, which contains the uncus, entorhinal area, and limen insula of the primary olfactory area

    3. Efferent fibers from the olfactory areas travel in

        a. Medial forebrain bundle from all three olfactory areas → hypothalamus

        b. Stria medullaris thalami from olfactory areas → habenular nucleus

        c. Stria terminalis from amygdala → anterior hypothalamus and preoptic area

    4. The hypothalamus sends olfactory information to

        a. Reticular formation

        b. Salivatory nuclei

        c. Dorsal motor nucleus of X — responsible for nausea, accelerated peristalsis, and enhanced gastric secretion

    5. Anterior olfactory nucleus is located between the olfactory bulb and olfactory tract.

        a. Input: receives fibers from tufted cells

        b. Output:

            (1) Anterior commissure → contralateral olfactory bulb

            (2) Ipsilateral olfactory cortical areas

C. Cranial nerve II (optic nerve) (**Fig. 1.38**)

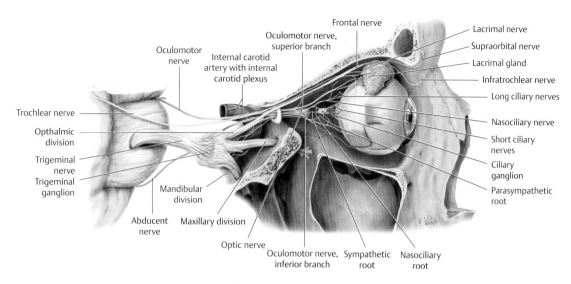

Fig. 1.38 Innervation of the orbit. Right orbit, lateral view with the temporal bony wall removed. The orbit receives motor, sensory, and autonomic innervation from four cranial nerves: the oculomotor nerve (CN III), the trochlear nerve (CN IV), the abducent nerve (CN VI) and the ophthalmic division of the trigeminal nerve (CN V1). The oculomotor nerve also conveys presynaptic parasympathetic fibers to the ciliary ganglion. The postsynaptic sympathetic fibers pass into the orbit by way of the internal carotid plexus and ophthalmic plexus. (From THIEME Atlas of Anatomy, Head and Neuroanatomy, © Thieme 2007, Illustration by Karl Wesker.)

1. Sensory afferent — Bipolar cells of the retina (primary sensory neurons) connect to ganglion cells (secondary neurons). The three types of retinal ganglion cells include

Cell Type	Response Type	Transmission Rate	Cell Body
X cells	Tonic response to: Pretectum, lateral geniculate body	Slow	Largest
Y cells	Phasic response to: Lateral geniculate body, superior colliculus	Rapid	
W cells	Tonic and phasic response to: Superior colliculus, pretectum	Very slow	Smallest

2. Course: ganglion cells send axons to the optic nerve (1 million fibers) → optic canal → optic chiasm → optic tract → to either
   a. Thalamic LGB for conscious vision
      (1) LGB has tertiary neurons that form the optic radiations → primary visual cortex (surrounds the calcarine fissure)
   b. Pretectal area — light reflex
   c. Superior colliculus — eye movement reflexes
   d. Suprachiasmatic nuclei — neuroendocrine function

3. Meyer's loop courses anteriorly toward the temporal pole before turning posteriorly. It carries fibers from the contralateral superior visual quadrant.

4. Von Willebrand's knee — contains fibers from the contralateral optic nerve that travel across a short distance into the other optic nerve before continuing through the optic tract. Visual lesions are discussed in Chapter 4.

5. Visual images are inverted by the lens.

6. Fibers from the right visual field cross to the left retina and terminate in the left cortex. These fibers from the right eye cross to the left optic tract in the chiasm, and fibers from the left eye stay on the left side traveling through the left optic nerve and tract.

D. Cranial nerve III (oculomotor nerve) (**Fig. 1.38**)

1. General somatic efferent — oculomotor nuclear complex is located at the level of the superior colliculus with three subnuclei that supply individual muscles of the ocular region.

Subnuclei	Muscle Innervation
Lateral	Ipsilateral inferior rectus, inferior oblique, and medial rectus
Medial	Contralateral superior rectus
Central	Levator palpebrae superioris (bilateral) innervation

a. Course of GSE CN III
   (1) Lower motor nerve (LMN) axons travel through the tegmentum (midbrain) → red nucleus (midbrain) → medial aspect of cerebral peduncles → interpeduncular cistern at the midbrain/pons junction
   (2) CN III passes between the PCA and SCA → oculomotor trigone in the posterior roof of the cavernous sinus → superior orbital fissure → anulus of Zinn → orbit
   (3) Within the orbit, the nerve divides into:
      (a) Superior division — supply superior rectus and levator palpebrae superioris muscles. It ascends lateral to the optic nerve.
      (b) Inferior division — supply inferior rectus, inferior oblique, and medial rectus muscles. Parasympathetic fibers travel with the inferior division and may branch off directly or from the nerve to the inferior oblique muscles to enter the ciliary ganglion (see below).

2. General visceral efferent — Edinger-Westphal nucleus is located in the midbrain (superior to the oculomotor complex).
   a. Course of GVE CN III
      (1) Parasympathetic fibers travel with CN III (dorsal and superficial aspect) until they branch from the inferior oblique branch in the orbit and terminate in the ciliary ganglion near the apex of the cone of the extraocular muscles.
      (2) Postganglionic fibers form 6–10 short ciliary nerves, which travel with branches of V1 to gain entry into the rear of the orbit (near the optic nerve) and travel anteriorly between the choroid and sclera to terminate in the ciliary body and iris.
      (3) Controls
         (a) Pupillary constrictor muscles = pupillary constriction
         (b) Ciliary muscles = lens bending for accommodation

E. Cranial nerve IV (trochlear nerve) (**Fig. 1.38**)

1. General somatic efferent — Trochlear nucleus is located at the level of the inferior colliculus. It gives rise to the trochlear nerve, which crosses in the superior medullary velum of the midbrain (behind the aqueduct), exits the contralateral side just below the inferior colliculus, and courses around the peduncles, emerging between the PCA and SCA with CN III. It then travels in the lateral wall of the cavernous sinus,

through the superior orbital fissure, into the orbit above the anulus of Zinn, crosses medially near the roof of the orbit over the levator palpebrae and superior rectus muscles to innervate the contralateral superior oblique muscle. It causes inward and downward rotation (intortion).

2. **Mnemonic:** SO_4 = **S**uperior **O**blique CN 4, LR_6 = **L**ateral **R**ectus, the rest CN III

3. Unique properties of the trochlear nerve
    a. The only cranial nerve to exit from the dorsum of the brainstem
    b. The smallest cranial nerve
    c. The longest intracranial course
    d. The only nerve in which all LMN axons decussate
    e. The only nerve to decussate outside the CNS

F. Cranial nerve V (trigeminal nerve) (**Figs. 1.38** and **1.39**)

1. General — nucleus of V is located in the dorsolateral brainstem extending from the midbrain to upper cervical segments composed of
    a. Motor nucleus
    b. Sensory nuclei with three subnuclei:
        (1) Mesencephalic nucleus — conveys proprioceptor information from the muscles of mastication. Note: cell bodies in the nucleus are first order.
        (2) Chief sensory nucleus — conveys light touch from face
        (3) Spinal nucleus — conveys pain, temperature, and deep pressure information

2. The trigeminal nerve leaves the midlateral surface of the pons as a large sensory root (portio major) and a smaller motor root (portio minor).

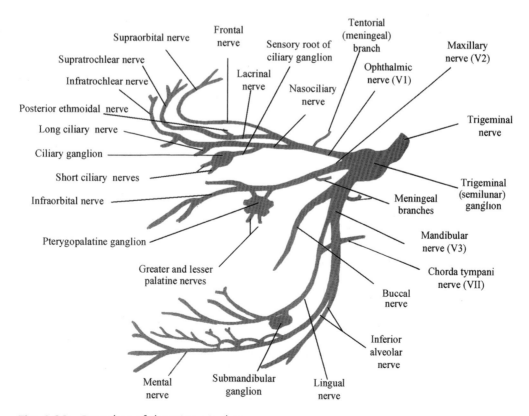

Fig. 1.39   Branches of the trigeminal nerve.

3. The sensory ganglion (semilunar, gasserian, or trigeminal ganglion) lies in Meckel's cave on the floor of the middle fossa.
    a. Three nerve divisions, ophthalmic (V_1), maxillary (V_2), and mandibular (V_3) exit the skull via superior orbital fissure, foramen rotundum, and foramen ovale, respectively. V_1 fibers lie ventral whereas V_3 fibers lie dorsal in the trigeminal nerve. Medial rotation of the nerve occurs after the ganglion.
    b. Sensory branches

V_1	V_2	V_3
Lacrimal	Zygomatic	Buccal
Frontal	Infraorbital (with superior alveolar	Auriculotemporal
Nasociliary (with long and short	nerves)	Lingual
ciliary nerves)	Pterygopalatine	Inferior alveolar
Meningeal branch (dura of the	Meningeal branch (dura to the	Motor branches
anterior and middle cranial fossa)	anterior and middle fossa)	Meningeal branch (dura to the
		anterior and middle fossa)

    c. Sympathetic fibers to the orbit travel with the ICA and then with long and short ciliary nerves from V_1 to the eye.
    d. Parasympathetic fibers from the ciliary ganglion travel with the short ciliary nerves (passes through the ciliary ganglion without synapsing) to the eye.

4. Special visceral efferent — motor nucleus of V sends fibers to V_3 branch to supply the muscles of
    a. Mastication (masseter, temporalis, medial and lateral pterygoids)
    b. Mylohyoid
    c. Anterior belly of the digastric muscle (Note: posterior belly = CN VII)
    d. Tensor tympani
    e. Tensor veli palatini
        (1) Note: The branches to the tensor veli palatini and the tensor tympani pass through the otic ganglion without synapsing.

5. General somatic afferent — sensation to the face, forehead, nose, mouth, teeth, and dura of anterior and middle fossae
    a. Course of GSA CN V
        (1) Fibers from V_1, V_2, and $V_3 \rightarrow$ trigeminal ganglion $\rightarrow$ spinal trigeminal tract $\rightarrow$ spinal trigeminal nucleus $\rightarrow$ ventral (crossed) and dorsal (uncrossed, mainly V_3) trigeminothalamic tracts $\rightarrow$ thalamic VPM
    b. Function:
        (1) Spinal trigeminal nucleus — pain, temperature, and some touch
        (2) Principal sensory nucleus of CN V — touch and pressure
        (3) Mesencephalic nucleus of CN V — proprioception of the jaw and eyes
        (4) Ventral trigeminothalamic tract — pain, touch, and pressure are crossed
        (5) Dorsal trigeminothalamic tract — touch and pressure are uncrossed
    c. Spinal trigeminal nucleus — extends from the pons to C2
        (1) Rostral — merges with the primary sensory nucleus of CN V
        (2) Caudal — merges with the substantial gelatinosa at C2
        (3) Input: CNs VII, IX, and X
        (4) Spinal trigeminal nucleus subcomponents:

(a) Pars oralis — extends from pons to hypoglossal nucleus, subserves the nose and mouth
(b) Pars interpolaris — extends down to the obex, subserves the face
(c) Pars caudalis — extends down to C2, subserves the forehead, jaw, and cheek
d. Mesencephalic nucleus of CN V contains primary sensory neurons. Fibers travel with the motor root (portio minor).

6. Trigeminal reflexes
   a. Bilateral blinking — corneal from CN V_1 → VII
   b. Elevation of the eyes (Bell's phenomenon) — CN III
   c. Tearing — V_1 → superior salivatory nucleus
   d. Salivation — CN V → inferior salivatory nucleus
   e. Sneezing — CN V → nucleus ambiguous → respiratory center of the reticular formation → phrenic nerves → intercostal muscles
   f. Vomiting — CN V → X
   g. Jaw jerk (masseter) — mesencephalic nucleus → LMN of temporalis and masseter

G. Cranial nerve VI (abducens nerve) (**Fig. 1.38**)

1. General somatic efferent — abducens nucleus is ventral to the fourth ventricle in the pontine tegmentum. Axons course ventrally and emerge at the pontomedullary junction just lateral to the pyramid. The nerve travels in the subarachnoid space of the posterior fossa then bends over the petrous apex to enter the cavernous sinus via Dorello's canal. In the cavernous sinus, it travels just lateral to the ICA and enters the orbit at the medial end of the superior orbital fissure, goes through the anulus of Zinn (tendinous ring) to innervate lateral rectus muscle.
   a. Nucleus — associated with a horizontal gaze center with
      (1) Motor fibers → ipsilateral lateral rectus muscle
      (2) Interneurons → medial longitudinal fasciculus (MLF) to the contralateral medial rectus muscle
      (3) Note: vertical gaze center is located in the rostral interstitial nucleus of the MLF (between the midbrain and diencephalon). Parapontine reticular formation (PPRF) connects horizontal and vertical gaze centers.
   b. Input:
      (1) Medial vestibular nucleus, PPRF, reticular formation, and nucleus prepositus
   c. CN VI lesions — most frequently injured CN due to its long intracranial course
      (1) A lesion of the nerve causes impaired ipsilateral lateral gaze.
      (2) A lesion of the nucleus impairs ipsilateral gaze of both eyes.

H. Cranial nerve VII (facial nerve) (**Fig. 1.40**)

1. Special visceral efferent — the facial motor nucleus in the pontine tegmentum sends axons dorsally toward the fourth ventricle that loop around the CN VI nucleus (forming the facial colliculus), and then travel ventrally to emerge from the pontomedullary junction between CNs VI and VIII.
   a. Nervus intermedius is lateral to the motor facial branch at the brainstem. Facial nerve then travels with CN VIII through the internal acoustic meatus to the petrous temporal bone. Axons travel in the facial canal between the cochlea and vestibular organs and then turn laterally and caudally.
   b. Nerve to the stapedius arises 6 mm above the stylomastoid foramen. It is the first muscle branch. The branchial motor fibers then exit the facial canal at the stylomastoid foramen and immediately innervate the stylohyoid, posterior belly of the digastric and occipitalis muscles. Remaining fibers travel in the substance of the parotid gland to innervate the muscles of facial expression, platysma, and the buccinator.

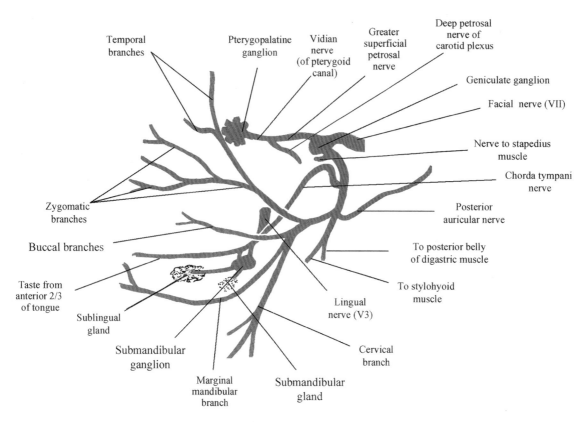

Fig. 1.40   Branches of the facial nerve.

2. GVE, GSA, and SVA fibers travel in the nervus intermedius, which exits the brainstem between the motor branches of CNs VII and VIII.
   a. General visceral efferent — superior salivatory nucleus sends axons to the nervus intermedius to
      (1) Greater superficial petrosal nerve → pterygopalatine ganglion → lacrimal gland (lacrimation) and the mucosa of the nose and mouth (secretion)
         (a) Course in detail — Great superficial petrosal nerve exits the petrous temporal bone via greater petrosal foramen to the middle fossa, passing deep to the trigeminal ganglion and down the foramen lacerum to the pterygoid canal (vidian canal), where it joins the deep petrosal nerve (sympathetic fibers from the plexus that surrounds ICA) to form the nerve of the pterygoid canal. This nerve goes to the pterygopalatine fossa where the pterygopalatine ganglion is suspended from the V_2 nerve. Fibers from this ganglia travel with V_2 → lacrimal gland and the mucosa of the nose and mouth.
      (2) Chorda tympani joins lingual nerve (V_3) → submandibular ganglion → submandibular and sublingual glands for salivation.
         (a) Note: Both olfactory areas and the limbic system send input to the hypothalamus, which influences the superior salivatory nucleus via dorsal longitudinal fasciculus.
         (b) Course in detail — Chorda tympani nerve exits petrotympanic fissure to join the lingual branch of V_3 ~1 cm below the foramen ovale to the submandibular gland (suspended from the lingual nerve).
   b. General somatic afferent — sensation of the external auditory meatus and the back of the ear → the geniculate ganglion (at the facial genu in petrous bone) → spinal trigeminal tract

c. Special visceral afferent — taste to the anterior ⅔ of the tongue, travels in the chorda tympani → geniculate ganglion → rostral nucleus solitarius

3. Branches of the facial nerve (proximal to distal)
    a. Greater superficial petrosal nerve (just before the geniculate ganglion)
    b. Nerve to the stapedius
    c. Chorda tympani
    d. Motor branches: **T**emporal, **Z**ygomatic, **B**uccal, **M**andibular, **C**ervical branches (**Mnemonic:** "Ten Zebras Bit My Clock").

4. CN VII Lesions
    a. Upper motor neuron (UMN) — Upper half of face is bilateral innervation. Therefore, an UMN lesion affects only the contralateral lower face.
    b. Lower motor nerve — LMN lesion affects the entire ipsilateral face, decreased sensation and taste, impaired salivation and lacrimation, and hyperacusis depending on exactly where the lesion is in relation to branches of the nerve (Bell's palsy — CN VII dysfunction).
    c. Mimetic or emotional innervation — Involuntary contraction of the face can occur with emotion even after a corticobulbar fiber lesion.

I. Cranial nerve VIII (vestibulocochlear nerve) (**Fig. 1.41**)

1. Special somatic afferent — Hearing is detected in the organ of Corti, which sends fibers to the spiral ganglion (first neuron, at the modiolus in the center of the cochlea) → cochlear nerve → cochlear nuclei (second neuron) including ventral nuclei (crossed and uncrossed) and dorsal nuclei (uncrossed) → ventral (trapezoid body), intermediate and dorsal acoustic striae (mostly crossed) → lateral lemniscus → inferior colliculus (third neuron) → MGB (fourth neuron) → temporal lobe Heschl's convolutions (fifth neuron).

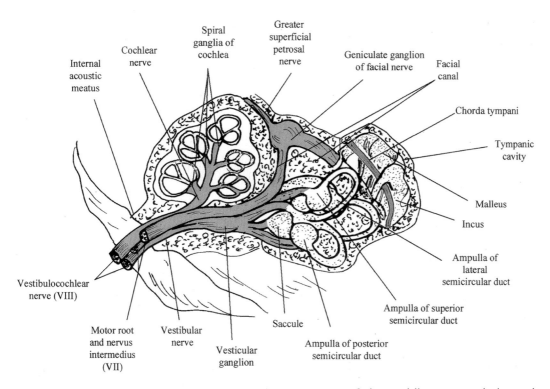

Fig. 1.41 The vestibulocochlear nerve and components of the middle ear, vestibula, and cochlea.

a. Ventral cochlear nucleus also sends fibers to the reticular formation, trapezoid body (en route to the superior olivary complex), lateral lemniscus and its nucleus. Involved with low frequencies (while dorsal cochlear nucleus is involved with high frequencies).

2. Olivocochlear bundle involved in suppression of auditory input
   a. Acoustic reflexes — superior olivary complex to
      (1) Both motor CN VII nuclei → stapedius muscles. Decrease amplitude of sound waves by decreasing the movement of ossicles.
      (2) Both motor CN V nuclei → tensor tympani muscles. Decrease the sensitivity of tympanic membrane by pulling it taut.

3. Special somatic afferent — semicircular canals, utricle, and saccule → superior and inferior ganglia to CN VIII to the superior, inferior, medial, and lateral vestibular nuclei to:
   a. Uncrossed fibers via juxtarestiform body → vestibulocerebellum
   b. Vestibulospinal tract → LMNs (facilitates extensors)
   c. MLF → nuclei of CN III, IV, VI, PPRF, superior colliculus, and interstitial nucleus of Cajal
   d. Hair cells (feedback modification)

4. Vestibular nuclei
   a. Lateral vestibular nucleus (Dieter's nucleus) → ipsilateral lateral vestibulospinal tract → innervate antigravity extensors
   b. Medial, superior, inferior vestibular nuclei give rise to the medial vestibulospinal tract, which descends bilaterally to the cervical segments of the spinal cord.
   c. Medial and inferior vestibular nuclei have reciprocal connections with the cerebellum.

5. All nuclei contribute to the MLF.
   a. Descending MLF continues as the medial vestibulospinal tract → cervical LMNs
   b. Utricle sends fibers → superior vestibular ganglion → lateral vestibular nucleus
   c. Saccule sends fibers → inferior vestibular ganglion → inferior vestibular nucleus
   d. Superior vestibular nucleus (uncrossed) → coordinates head/eye movements
   e. Medial vestibular nucleus (crossed) → coordinates eye with head movements

6. Lesions
   a. Lateral lemniscus lesion — contralateral deafness (although true unilateral deafness is generally due to CN VIII or more distal lesion)
   b. Vestibular damage — decreased equilibrium, vertigo, and nystagmus
   c. MLF (unilateral damage) rostral to the CN VI nucleus — weakness of the ipsilateral lateral rectus, contralateral nystagmus, and normal convergence
   d. MLF (bilateral damage) — internuclear ophthalmoplegia (INO) damage, no eye adduction

J. Cranial nerve IX (glossopharyngeal nerve) (**Fig. 1.42**)

1. Glossopharyngeal nerve leaves the medulla between the olive and inferior cerebellar peduncle. The most rostral 3–4 rootlets between the olive and the inferior cerebellar peduncle will join to form a single nerve. The nerve sends off a tympanic branch before exiting the skull via jugular foramen, where it lies anterior to CNs X and XI. The nerve perforates the dura and arachnoid to form the superior and inferior (petrosal) glossopharyngeal ganglia.

2. General somatic afferent sensation to
   a. Back of the ear
   b. Inner surface of the tympanic membrane

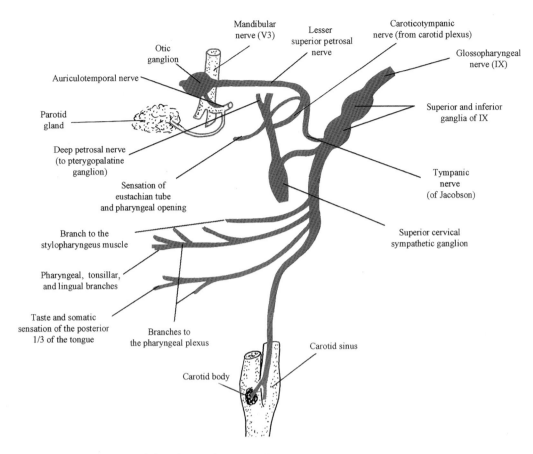

Fig. 1.42 Branches of the glossopharyngeal nerve.

     c. Posterior ⅓ of the tongue
     d. Upper pharynx → superior ganglion → spinal trigeminal nucleus

  3. General visceral afferent and special visceral afferent:
     a. Carotid body and sinus, taste buds of the posterior ⅓ of the tongue, posterior pharynx, and eustachian tube → inferior ganglion (petrosal ganglion) → caudal nucleus solitarius → reticular formation and hypothalamus → reflex control of heart rate, respiratory rate, and blood pressure
       (1) Taste — rostral nucleus solitarius sends taste fibers that ascend in the central tegmental tract → contralateral thalamic VPM
       (2) Carotid sinus reflex — Baroreceptors at the carotid bifurcation sense increases in blood pressure → CN IX → nucleus solitarius → dorsal X nucleus → decrease in blood pressure and heart rate.
       (3) Carotid body — a chemoreceptor that detects blood O_2 and CO_2
     b. Similar pathway as the carotid sinus
     c. Note: Hering's nerve is a branch of CN IX from the carotid body and sinus.

  4. General visceral efferent — Parotid salivation is controlled by fibers from the inferior salivatory nucleus to CN IX, to the tympanic nerve (Jacobson's nerve) that leaves CN IX before exiting the jugular foramen, goes through the inferior ganglion (the sensory fibers supply sensation to the tympanic cavity, eustachian tube, and mastoid air cells), through the tympanic plexus to the lesser petrosal nerve, then through a small canal lateral to the canal for the greater superficial petrosal nerve back into the cranium, through the foramen ovale, to synapse in the otic ganglion (below foramen ovale and surrounding a branch of V3) and travels with the auriculotemporal nerve (V3) to the parotid gland.

5. Special visceral efferent — Rostral nucleus ambiguous innervates stylopharyngeus muscle and part of the superior pharyngeal constrictor.

6. CN IX injury
   a. CN IX injury — decreased gag reflex, sinus reflex, and taste. In isolation, a unilateral injury is difficult to detect.
   b. Glossopharyngeal neuralgia — pain behind the ear or in the mouth, often precipitated by swallowing or coughing.

K. Cranial nerve X (vagus nerve)

1. Vagus nerve leaves the medulla between the olive and inferior cerebellar peduncle as 8–10 rootlets that converge into a single nerve to exit the skull via the jugular foramen. The superior (jugular) and inferior (nodose) ganglia are just beneath the jugular foramen. The inferior ganglion contains important sensory fibers of CN X.

2. General somatic afferent
   a. Sensation from the ear, external auditory meatus, and external surface of the tympanic membrane travels in the auricular branch (Arnold's nerve)
   b. Sensation from the posterior fossa dura travels in meningeal branches → superior ganglion of CN X → spinal trigeminal tract
   c. Fibers from larynx and pharynx regions → inferior ganglion of CN X → trigeminal spinal nucleus and tract
      (1) Recurrent laryngeal nerve supplies the vocal cords and subglottis.
      (2) Inferior laryngeal nerve supplies the larynx above the vocal folds. It pierces the thyrohyoid membrane and unites with the external laryngeal nerve to form the superior laryngeal nerve.

3. General visceral afferent and special visceral afferent — sensation of the pharynx, larynx, trachea, lungs, heart, esophagus, stomach, and thoracoabdominal viscera down to the splenic flexure, aortic arch baroreceptors, aortic body (chemoreceptor), and taste sensation in the epiglottis → inferior ganglion of CN X → tractus solitarius
   a. Rostral portion of the nucleus SVA (gustatory) input from CN VII, IX
   b. Caudal portion of the nucleus (mainly GVA) from CN X
   c. Commissural nucleus at the obex where both solitary nuclei merge
   d. Efferent fibers from the nucleus → thalamic VPM, salivary nucleus, dorsal motor nucleus of CN X, nucleus ambiguous, parabranchial nucleus, hypoglossal nucleus, phrenic nerve nuclei, and thoracic LMN.
   e. Medullary respiratory center — nucleus ambiguous, nucleus solitarius, and reticular formation. Responds to vagal input and CO_2 accumulation. The medullary vasomotor center is less well defined.

4. General visceral efferent — Parasympathetic inputs arise from the dorsal motor nucleus of CN X → vagus nerve → thorax and abdomen, which branches into the right and left gastric nerves to innervate abdominal viscera up to the splenic flexure. Input to the dorsal motor nucleus of CN X from the hypothalamus, olfactory system, reticular formation, and solitary nucleus.

5. Special visceral afferent — nucleus ambiguous → LMNs → pharynx constrictor muscles and internal muscles of the larynx. Nucleus ambiguous → stylopharyngeus muscle (CN IX), trapezius and sternocleidomastoid muscles (CN XI). Rostrally it joins dorsal X and caudally to form the CN XI nucleus.

6. Branches of CN X (neck)
    a. Pharyngeal branch of CN X supplies all muscles of the pharynx and soft palate except: stylopharyngeus (CN IX) and tensor veli palatini (CN V). Muscles of the pharynx and soft palate include
        (1) Superior, middle, and inferior constrictors, levator palati, salpingo- and palatopharyngeus, one tongue muscle (palatoglossus)
    b. Laryngeal nerve
        (1) Superior laryngeal nerve divides into the internal and external laryngeal nerves. The external branch supplies the inferior constrictor, cricothyroid, pharyngeal plexus, and superior cardiac nerve.
        (2) Recurrent laryngeal nerve supplies the intrinsic laryngeal muscles except the cricothyroid.
    c. Cervical cardiac branches
        (1) Right-sided branches travel behind the subclavian artery → deep cardiac plexus
        (2) Left-sided branches travel with the trachea (upper nerve) → deep cardiac plexus. Also travel across the arch of the aorta → superficial cardiac plexus.

7. CN X injury

Unilateral CN X Injury	Bilateral CN X Injury
Hoarseness	Asphyxia
Dysphagia	Dysphagia
Dyspnea	Dysarthria
Uvular deviation to the normal side	Paralysis of the esophagus and stomach with pain and emesis
Ipsilateral decreased cough reflex (decreased sensation)	Tachycardia
Ipsilateral decreased carotid sinus reflex	

L. Cranial nerve XI (spinal accessory nerve)
    1. Special visceral efferent
        a. Cranial portion from the nucleus ambiguous (CNs IX, X, and XI) to join with CN X and form the recurrent laryngeal nerve
        b. Motor cortex fibers → posterior limb of the internal capsule → pyramid decussation → lateral corticospinal tract → accessory nucleus → the spinal portion from C1–6 exits between the ventral and dorsal roots as rootlets → ascends posterior to the dentate ligament to enter the foramen magnum (posterior to the vertebral artery → joins with CN X to exit jugular foramen → jugular foramen → sternocleidomastoid and upper trapezius muscles. Note: Similar to CN X, CN IX has two ganglia; fibers from CN IX form a single compact root (unlike the fibers from CN X that are more spread out).

M. Cranial nerve XII (hypoglossal nerve)
    1. General somatic efferent — the nucleus lies near the floor of the fourth ventricle beneath the hypoglossal trigone. The nerve exits the medulla between the inferior olive and the pyramid. It travels through the hypoglossal foramen and innervates
        a. All intrinsic muscles of the tongue
        b. All but one of the extrinsic muscles of the tongue (genioglossus, styloglossus, and hypoglossus). Note: Palatoglossus is innervated by CN X.

XVI. Brainstem (Figs. 1.43, 1.44, 1.45, 1.46, 1.47, 1.48, 1.49, 1.50, 1.51)

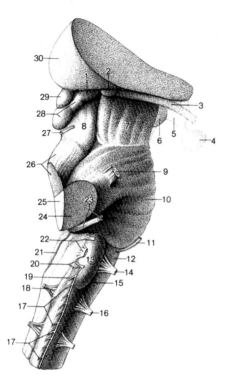

Fig. 1.43 Lateral view of the brainstem. 1. Medial geniculate body. 2. Lateral geniculate body. 3. Optic tract. 4. Hypophysis. 5. Infundibulum. 6. Mamillary body. 7, 8. Cerebral peduncle. 7. Ventral part (crus cerebri). 8. Dorsal part (mesencephalic tegmentum). 9. Trigeminal nerve. 10. Pons. 11. Abducens nerve. 12. Pyramid (medulla oblongata). 13. Olive. 14. Hypoglossal nerve. 15. Ventrolateral sulcus. 16. Ventral root of the first cervical nerve. 17. Spinal roots of accessory nerve. 18. Dorsal root of first cervical nerve (retracted). 19. Dorsolateral sulcus (medulla oblongata). 20. Cranial roots of accessory and vagus nerve. 21. Tenia of fourth ventricle. 22. Glossopharyngeal and vagus nerves. 23. Facial nerve with nervus intermedius and vestibulocochlear nerve. 24. Middle cerebellar peduncle. 25. Inferior cerebellar peduncle. 26. Superior cerebellar peduncle. 27. Trochlear nerve. 28. Inferior colliculus and brachium of inferior colliculus. 29. Superior colliculus. 30. Pulvinar. (From Frick H, Leonhardt H, Starck D. Human Anatomy 2. New York, NY: Thieme; 1991. Reprinted by permission.)

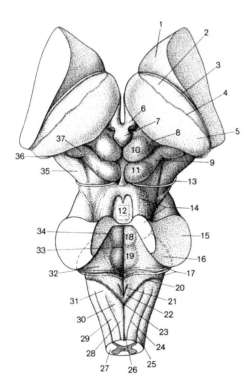

Fig. 1.44 Dorsal view of brainstem with cerebellum removed. 1. Caudate nucleus. 2. Lamina affixa. 3. Terminal stria and superior thalamostriate vein in terminal sulcus. 4. Tenia choroidea. 5. Pulvinar. 6. Habenular trigone. 7. Pineal body. 8–11. Mesencephalon. 8. Brachium of superior colliculus. 9. Brachium of inferior colliculus. 10, 11. Tectum. 10. Superior colliculus. 11. Inferior colliculus. 12. Superior medullary velum. 13. Trochlear nerve. 14. Superior cerebellar peduncle. 15. Middle cerebellar peduncle. 16. Inferior cerebellar peduncle, 17. Stria medullares (fourth ventricle) and lateral recess of fourth ventricle. 18. Median eminence. 19. Facial colliculus. 20. Tenia of fourth ventricle. 21. Trigone of hypoglossal nerve. 22. Trigone of vagus nerve (ala cinerea). 23. Obex. 24. Dorsal intermediate sulcus. 25. Dorsolateral sulcus. 26. Dorsal median sulcus. 27. Lateral funiculus. 28. Fasciculus gracilis. 29. Fasciculus cuneatus. 30. Tuberculum gracile. 31. Tuberculum cuneatum. 32. Vestibular area. 33. Median sulcus. 34. Sulcus limitans. 35. Cerebral peduncle. 36. Lateral geniculate body. 37. Medial geniculate body. (From Frick H, Leonhardt H, Starck D. Human Anatomy 2. New York, NY: Thieme;1991. Reprinted by permission.)

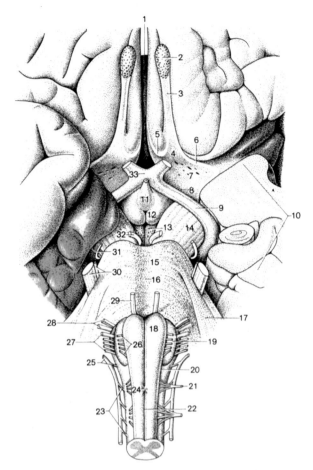

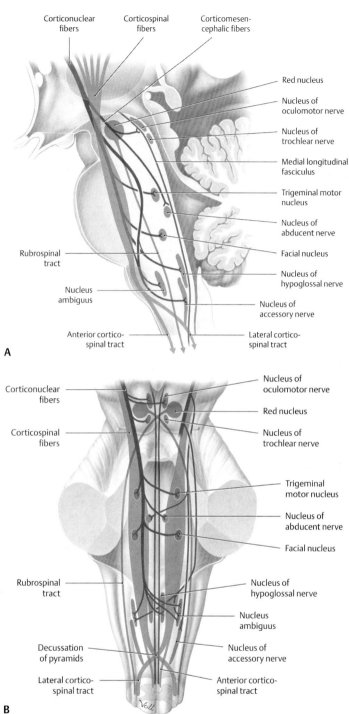

Fig. 1.45 Ventral view of brainstem. 1. Corpus callosum in depths of anterior interhemispheric or longitudinal cerebral fissure. 2. Olfactory bulb. 3. Olfactory tract. 4. Olfactory trigone. 5. Medial olfactory stria. 6. Lateral olfactory stria. 7. Anterior perforated substance. 8. Diagonal band of Broca. 9. Optic tract. 10. Cut surface of left temporal lobe. 11. Infundibulum with hypophyseal stalk. 12. Mamillary body. 13. Interpeduncular fossa with interpeduncular perforated substance. 14. Ventral part of cerebral peduncle. 15. Pons. 16. Basilar sulcus. 17. Middle cerebellar peduncle. 18. Pyramid (medulla oblongata). 19. Olive. 20. Ventrolateral sulcus. 21. Ventral root of first cervical nerve. 22. Ventral median fissure. 23. Spinal roots of accessory nerve. 24. Decussation of pyramids. 25. Accessory nerve and cranial roots. 26. Hypoglossal nerve. 27. Glossopharyngeal and vagus nerve. 28. Facial nerve with nervus intermedius and vestibulocochlear nerve. 29. Abducens nerve. 30. Motor and sensory roots of trigeminal nerve. 31. Trochlear nerve. 32. Oculomotor nerve. 33. Optic chiasm. (From Frick H, Leonhardt H, Starck D. Human Anatomy 2. New York, NY: Thieme;1991. Reprinted by permission.)

Fig. 1.46 Descending tracts in the brainstem. (**A**) Midsagittal section viewed from the left side. (**B**) Posterior view with the cerebellum removed. The descending tracts shown here begin in the telencephalon and terminate partly in the brainstem, but mostly in the spinal cord. Corticonuclear fibers of the corticospinal tract terminate in the brainstem and corticospinal fibers terminate in the spinal cord. (From THIEME Atlas of Anatomy, Head and Neuroanatomy, © Thieme 2007, Illustration by Markus Voll.)

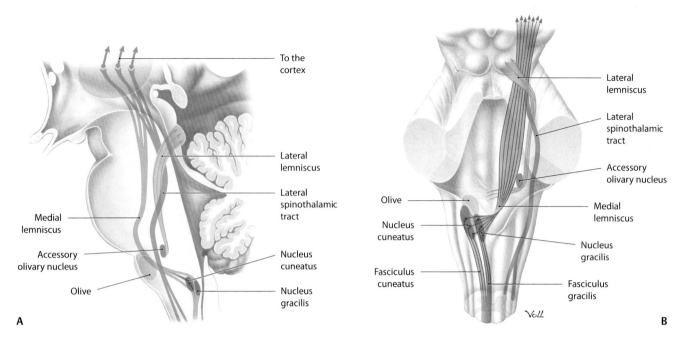

Fig. 1.47   Ascending tracts in the brainstem. (**A**) Left lateral view. (**B**) Posterior view. Two major ascending fiber bundles, the posterior funiculus (violet) and the lateral spinothalamic tract (dark blue), carry sensory information from the spinal cord to the brainstem. The posterior funiculus consists of the medial fasciculus gracilis and the lateral fasciculus cuneatus. (From THIEME Atlas of Anatomy, Head and Neuroanatomy, © Thieme 2007, Illustration by Markus Voll.)

A. The midbrain (MB) consists of the tectum, tegmentum, and crus cerebri.

   1. Midbrain at the level of the superior colliculus (**Fig. 1.48**) — contains the superior colliculus, oculomotor nucleus, red nucleus, superior cerebellar peduncle, and SN
      a. Superior colliculus — laminated with alternating gray and white zones
      b. Superficial layers — connected to the visual system
      c. Deep layers — connected to the muscles for head and eye movements
         (1) Superior colliculus

Superior Colliculus Input	Superior Colliculus Output
All fibers enter via brachium of the superior colliculus.	Parabigeminal nucleus
Retina — mainly contralateral, unlike the equal representation in LGB, cortex	Pulvinar
	LGB
Cortex — frontal, parietal, temporal, occipital	PPRF
Brainstem nuclei — parabigeminal nucleus, inferior colliculus, SN, nucleus cuneatus	Rostral interstitial nucleus of the MLF (RiMLF)
	Reticular formation
Spinal cord	Spinal cord

Abbreviations: LGB, lateral geniculate body; MLF, medial longitudinal fasciculus; PPRF, paramedian pontine reticular formation; RiMLF, rostral interstitial nucleus of the MLF; SN, substantia nigra

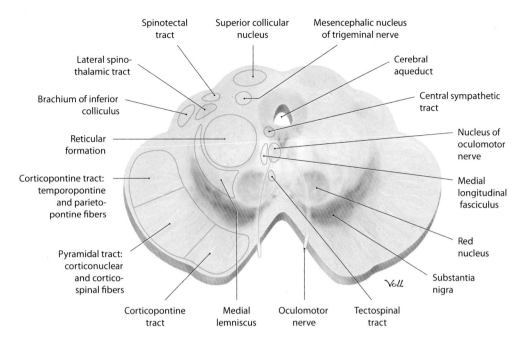

Fig. 1.48 Transverse section through the midbrain at the level of the superior colliculus and oculomotor nerve nucleus. (From THIEME Atlas of Anatomy, Head and Neuroanatomy, © Thieme 2007, Illustration by Markus Voll.)

(2) Unilateral damage of the superior colliculus — contralateral visual field neglect, impaired tracking, but no deficit with eye movements

(3) Stimulation — contralateral conjugate deviation (although there are no direct projections to the extraocular muscles) by

    (a) Stimulating rostral interstitial nucleus of the MLF (RiMLF) to excite the ipsilateral CN III

    (b) Stimulating PPRF to excite the contralateral CN VI and RiMLF

d. Oculomotor nucleus

    (1) Oculomotor nuclear

Nuclear Component	Feature

Lateral part	Composed of cell columns (all ipsilateral) for:
	  Inferior rectus muscle (dorsal)
	  Inferior oblique muscle (intermediate)
	  Medial rectus muscle (ventral)

Medial part	Cell column (contralateral) for: Superior rectus muscle

Central part	Cell columns for:
	  Levator palpebrae superioris muscles
	  Edinger-Westphal nuclei

(2) Oculomotor rootlets — pass through the red nucleus to enter the interpeduncular fossa. The oculomotor complex has no direct cortical or superior colliculus connections; all goes through the reticular formation neurons.

(3) Direct input of the oculomotor nucleus:
   (a) Bilateral medial and ipsilateral superior vestibular nuclei (via MLF)
   (b) Nucleus of Cajal
   (c) Contralateral abducens nucleus
   (d) Perihypoglossal nucleus
   (e) RiMLF
   (f) Pretectal olivary nucleus
   (g) Flocculus → nucleus prepositus → ipsilateral oculomotor nucleus (vertical eye movements)

(4) PPRF projects directly to the main conjugate horizontal gaze center (abducens nucleus) and the main conjugate vertical gaze center (RiMLF).

(5) Direct light reflex — retinal ganglion cells → optic nerve → optic tract → brachium of superior colliculus → pretectal area → posterior commissure → both oculomotor nuclei → Edinger-Westphal subnucleus → ciliary ganglion → pupillary sphincter muscle

e. Rostral interstitial nucleus of the MLF — located above the oculomotor nucleus in the MLF at the junction of the midbrain/diencephalon. It is the main center for vertical eye movements (especially downward). It reacts to vestibular and visual stimulation.
   (1) Input: superior vestibular nucleus and PPRF
   (2) Output: mainly to the oculomotor complex (inferior rectus portion)

f. Accessory oculomotor nuclei

Accessory Nuclei	Feature

Interstitial nucleus of Cajal	Located along the MLF in the rostral midbrain
	Input: superior and medial vestibular nuclei, pretectum, frontal eye fields, and the fastigial nuclei
	Output:
	  Ipsilateral medial vestibular nucleus and spinal cord
	  Both trochlear nuclei
	  Contralateral oculomotor nuclei (cross in the posterior commissure), not to the medial rectus part
	Function: vertical eye movements, pursuit, head movements, and posture

Darkshevich's nucleus	Located dorsolateral to the oculomotor nucleus Output: nucleus of the posterior commissure
Nucleus of the posterior commissure	Connections with the pretectal area and the posterior thalamic nuclei

g. Pretectal region — located rostral to the superior colliculus at the posterior commissure. Nuclei are involved in the pupillary light reflexes.

h. Posterior commissure — posterior to the aqueduct, at the junction of the midbrain/diencephalon. Involved with the light reflex. Contains fibers from the pretectal nuclei, nucleus of the posterior commissure, interstitial nuclei, and Darkshevich's nucleus.

i. Subcommissural organs — modified ependymal cells in the aqueduct below the posterior commissure. It has no BBB.

2. Midbrain at the level of the inferior colliculus — the inferior colliculus is responsible for the tonotopic organization of auditory information and projects via brachium of the inferior colliculus to the MGB.
   a. Parabigeminal area
      (1) Located ventrolateral to the inferior colliculus
      (2) Connections to the superior colliculus (involved with the visual system)
   b. Trochlear nucleus roots cross in the superior medullary velum, emerge on the contralateral side under the inferior colliculus, traveling between the PCA and SCA with the oculomotor nerve to enter the cavernous sinus.
   c. Periaqueductal gray

Periaqueductal Gray	Feature
Components	Contains: Mesencephalic nucleus of V Locus ceruleus Ventral and dorsal tegmental nuclei Dorsal nucleus of the raphe sends: $\quad$ 5-HT + CCK → SN and putamen Median nucleus of the raphe (forms mesolimbic system with outputs to the brainstem reticular formation hypothalamus, septal area, entorhinal cortex, hippocampus, cerebellum, locus ceruleus, and raphe nucleus of the pons and medulla)
Function	Central analgesia, vocalization, control of reproductive behavior, aggressive behavior, and upward gaze
Connections	Hypothalamus, reticular formation, spinal cord, locus ceruleus, and raphe nucleus

Abbreviations: 5-HT, 5-hydroxytryptamine (serotonin); CCK, cholecystokinin; SN, substantia nigra

   d. Interpeduncular nucleus
      (1) Located just dorsal to the interpeduncular fossa
      (2) Input: habenular nucleus via fasciculus retroflexus
      (3) Output: diffuse cholinergic fibers to various parts of the CNS

3. Midbrain tegmentum
   a. The ventral surface of the midbrain, containing reticular formation and tracts, periaqueductal gray (surrounding the cerebral aqueduct), substantia nigra (sensorimotor), red nucleus, and the oculomotor and trochlear nuclei. (Note: Tectum is the dorsal surface, or the "roof" of the midbrain, containing the inferior colliculi and the superior colliculi.)
      (1) Red nucleus — located in the reticular formation
         (a) Fibers of the oculomotor nerve and superior cerebellar peduncle pass through it.
         (b) Input:
            (i) Deep cerebellar nuclei:
               • Rostral ⅓ from the dentate nuclei
               • Caudal ⅔ from the interposed nuclei
               • Fibers exit the cerebellum via superior peduncle and cross to the contralateral side in the midbrain to reach the red nucleus.
            (ii) Cerebral cortex—from the precentral, premotor, supplementary motor, and motor cortices

(c) Output:

  (i) Contralateral cervical and lumbar spine via rubrospinal tract

  (ii) Contralateral nucleus interpositus, facial nucleus, medulla, and spinal cord via crossed ventral tegmental tract

  (iii) Ipsilateral inferior olivary nucleus via uncrossed central tegmental tract

(d) There are no direct connections to the thalamus.

  (i) Red nucleus stimulation — increased tone in the contralateral flexors and decreased in the contralateral extensors. Maintains flexor muscle tone.

  (ii) Interposed nucleus stimulation — increased ipsilateral flexion

(2) Midbrain reticular formation

(3) Pedunculopontine nucleus

  (a) Located in the lateral tegmentum ventral to the inferior colliculus

  (b) Input: cortex, mGP, and SNpr

  (c) Output: thalamus and SNpc; a major source of ACh output

  (d) Stimulation — causes walking movements; controls locomotion

4. Substantia nigra — located between the crus cerebri and midbrain tegmentum

SN	Feature
SNpc	Contains large cells Neurotransmitters — dopamine and CCK
SNpr	Contains fewer cells Ventral to the SNpc, thus closer to crus cerebri Neurotransmitters: GABA and 5-HT
Input	Caudate, putamen and lateral GP to the SNpr [GABA], subthalamus, dorsal raphe nucleus (5-HT and CCK), and pedunculopontine nucleus (ACh). There is also input with enkephalin and substance P (the highest concentration in the brain).
Output	(1) SNpc (dopamine) → striatum, a closed loop (2) SNpr → VA and MD thalamus (3) SNpr → superior colliculus (initiates eye movements) and pedunculopontine nucleus

Abbreviations: 5-HT, 5-hydroxytryptamine (serotonin); ACh, acetylcholine; CCK, cholecystokinin; GABA, gamma-aminobutyric acid; GP, globus pallidus; MD, mediodorsal; SNpc, substantia nigra pars compacta; SNpr, substantia nigra pars reticulata; VA, ventroanterior

5. Crus cerebri

  a. Corticospinal and corticobulbar tracts — middle ⅔ of the crus cerebri (lower extremities located laterally)

  b. Corticopontine tracts — extreme medial and lateral ends of crus cerebri (frontopontine medially and parieto-temporo-occipitopontine located laterally)

B. Pons (**Fig. 1.49**)

1. Reticular formation involved with wakefulness (central tegmental tract), muscle tone (reticulospinal tract), respiration, blood pressure regulation, sensory transmission. Located in the pons and medulla, stimulation induces reflexes and cortically induced movements. Contains four zones:

  a. Reticular formation zones

Zones	Feature
Median zone	Contains raphe nuclei Dorsal and median raphe nuclei send ventral tegmental tract → median forebrain bundle → hypothalamus, striatum, thalamus, amygdala, hippocampus, cortex, and olfactory bulb
Paramedian zone	Input: cortex Output: cerebellum
Medial zone	The effector zone with ascending and descending fibers
Lateral zone	The sensory zone with output to the effector zone

b. Pontine reticular formation
   (1) Sends crossed reticulospinal fibers (muscle tone) → spinal cord LMN
   (2) Fibers to central tegmental tract (wakefulness) → thalamic intralaminar nuclei (for arousal)
c. Bulbar pressor area — the main control and the depressor area located in the rostral medulla/caudal pons
d. Ascending reticular activating system (ARAS) — involved with cortical arousal. The main ascending pathway is the central tegmental tract to intralaminar thalamic nuclei.

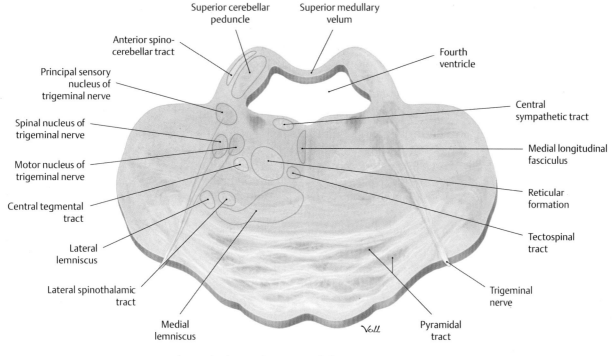

Fig. 1.49   Transverse section through the midportion of the pons. (From THIEME Atlas of Anatomy, Head and Neuroanatomy, © Thieme 2007, Illustration by Markus Voll.)

2. Isthmus rhombencephali — located between the cerebellum and midbrain, has the superior medullary velum with the decussating trochlear nerves over the roof of the fourth ventricle. The parabrachial nuclei are adjacent to the superior cerebellar peduncles.

3. Locus ceruleus
   a. Pigmented (melanin)
   b. Neurotransmitter – NE with wide projections
   c. Function: controls cortical activation and paradoxical (rapid eye movement [REM]) sleep.

C. Medulla

  1. Medulla at the level of the olivary nuclei (**Fig. 1.50**)

Component	Feature

Floor of the fourth ventricle	Three eminences (medial to lateral):
	  1. Hypoglossal eminence over CN XII nucleus
	  2. Intermediate eminence over dorsal motor nucleus of CN X
	     Dorsal motor nucleus of CN X lies medially.
	     Solitary nucleus lies laterally.
	  3. Lateral eminence over the area vestibularis
	Sulcus limitans — separates efferent and afferent (lateral) fibers
	Note: Roof of the fourth ventricle — tela choroidea and the choroid plexus lie in the inferior medullary velum.

Inferior olivary complex	Principal olivary nucleus sends efferent fibers → cerebellum (hemispheres) Medial and dorsal accessory olivary nuclei send fibers → vermis Olivocerebellar fibers cross to the inferior cerebellar peduncles (these fibers make up most of the peduncle) to become climbing fibers and reach Purkinje cells. The complex also has descending fibers.

Medullary reticular formation	Afferent fibers from cortex, deep cerebellar nuclei, and cranial nerves
	Output: gigantocellular reticular nucleus →
	  Central tegmental tract crossed to the intralaminar thalamic nuclei for arousal and from the midbrain to the olive
	  Reticulospinal tract:
	    Rostral fibers stimulate LMNs
	    Caudal fibers inhibit LMNs

Raphe nuclei	Extends from the midbrain to medulla
	Neurotransmitters — serotonin, CCK, and enkephalin:
	  Provides endogenous analgesia via substantia gelatinosa
	  Controls deep sleep, mood, and aggression
	Nucleus magnus projects to layers I and II of the spinal cord to inhibit pain.
	  Less firing of the nucleus magnus = less arousal
	  Destruction of nucleus magnus = insomnia.

Tracts	Medial lemniscus (ML) Spinothalamic tracts Anterior and lateral tracts merge and branch to the reticular formation. Dorsal spinocerebellar tract → inferior peduncle Ventral spinocerebellar tract → superior cerebellar peduncle, MLF, rubrospinal, rubrobulbar, and vestibulospinal tracts
Inferior cerebellar peduncles	Carries fibers from the spinal cord + medulla → cerebellum Crossed olivocerebellar fibers (the majority) Uncrossed dorsal spinocerebellar fibers and fibers from the lateral vestibular nuclei, paramedian reticular nuclei, accessory cuneate nuclei, arcuate nuclei, and perihypoglossal nuclei

Abbreviations: CCK, cholecystokinin; CN, cranial nerve; LMN, lower motor neuron; MLF, medial longitudinal fasciculus

D. Spinomedullary junction

  1. Spinomedullary junction (**Fig. 1.51**)
    a. Decussation of the pyramids
    b. Termination of the fasciculi gracilis and cuneatus

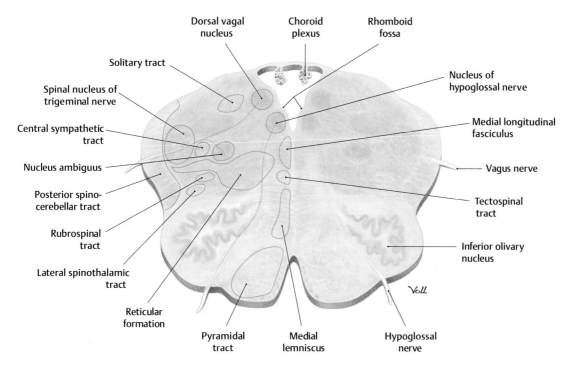

Fig. 1.50 Transverse section just above the middle of the medulla oblongata. (From THIEME Atlas of Anatomy, Head and Neuroanatomy, © Thieme 2007, Illustration by Markus Voll.)

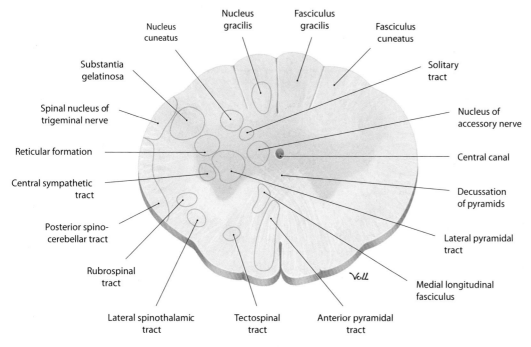

Fig. 1.51 Transverse section through the lower portion of the medulla oblongata. (From THIEME Atlas of Anatomy, Head and Neuroanatomy, © Thieme 2007, Illustration by Markus Voll.)

    c. Replacement of Lissauer's zone by the spinal trigeminal tract

    d. Replacement of the spinal gray by the reticular formation and cranial nerve nuclei

2. Internal changes at the spinomedullary junction

Internal Changes	Feature
Corticospinal decussation	Anterior corticospinal tract travels in the anterior fasciculus, uncrossed. Lateral corticospinal tract travels in the dorsolateral fasciculus, crossed.
Medial lemniscus decussation	DRG → posterior column fibers → nucleus gracilis (medial, lower extremities) or nucleus cuneatus (upper extremities) cross as the internal arcuate fibers → medial lemniscus → VPL → sensory cortex There is somatotopic organization with touch and kinesthetic fibers intermingled. Accessory cuneate nucleus — lateral and rostral to the cuneate nucleus. Functions similar to Clarke's column in the thorax to send fibers that are the upper limb equivalent of the posterior spinocerebellar tract. Upper limb muscle spindles, Golgi tendon organs, and cutaneous afferent fibers → primary spinal ganglion → second neurons in the accessory cuneate nucleus → cuneocerebellar fibers → inferior cerebellar peduncle
Spinal trigeminal tract and nucleus	Input from CNs V, VII, IX, and X
Reticular formation	Fibers from the red nucleus and spinothalamic tract → reticular nuclei → inferior cerebellar peduncles and up as mossy fibers. The cortex → arcuate nuclei (anterior to the pyramids) → stria medullaris (floor of the fourth ventricle) → cerebellum
Area postrema	In the floor of the fourth ventricle above the obex It is a chemoreceptor, sensitive to apomorphine and digitalis with afferent fibers from the spinal cord and nucleus solitarius.

Abbreviations: CNs, cranial nerves; DRG, dorsal root ganglion; VPL, ventroposterolateral

3. Associations

Brainstem	Artery	Cranial Nerves	Cerebellar Penduncle	Cerebellar Surface
Midbrain	SCA	Under CNs III and IV and above CN V	Superior	Tentorial
Pons	AICA	Passes CNs VI, VII, and VIII	Middle	Petrosal
Medulla	PICA	Passes CNs XII, IX, X, and XI	Inferior	Suboccipital

Abbreviations: AICA, anterior inferior cerebellar artery; CNs, cranial nerves; PICA, posterior inferior cerebellar artery; SCA, superior cerebellar artery

XVII. Spine and Spinal Cord

A. General information (**Fig. 1.52**)

1. Spinal cord extends from the foramen magnum to L1–L2 in the adult. The cervical and lumbar enlargements contain LMNs for the upper and lower limbs, respectively.

    a. The spinal cord tapers to a distal end called the conus medullaris.

    b. The long nerve roots extending past the conus medullaris form the cauda equina.

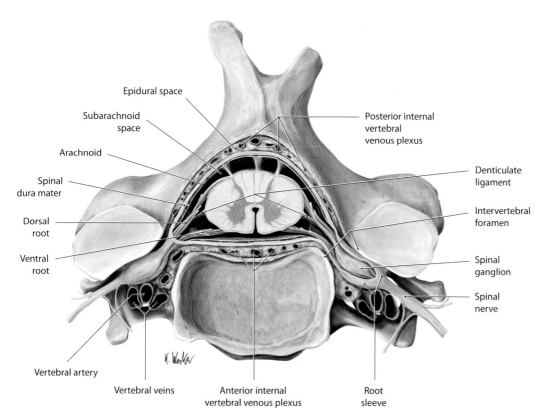

Fig. 1.52 Spinal cord and spinal nerve in the vertebral canal at the level of the C4 vertebra. Transverse section viewed from above. The spinal cord occupies the center of the vertebral foramen and is anchored within the subarachnoid space to the spinal dura mater by the denticulate ligament. The root sleeve, an outpouching of the dura mater in the intravertebral foramen, contains the spinal ganglion and the dorsal and ventral roots of the spinal nerve. The spinal dura mater is bounded externally by the epidural space, which contains venous plexuses, fat, and connective tissue. The epidural space extends upward as far as the foramen magnum where the dura becomes fused with the cranial periosteum. (From THIEME Atlas of Anatomy, Head and Neuroanatomy, © Thieme 2007, Illustration by Karl Wesker.)

    c. Filum terminale consists of pia from the conus medullaris, the rest of ependymal cells, glia, and fat that extends through the thecal sac to its end at S2. Together with the dura it forms the coccygeal ligament that attaches to the posterior coccyx.

2. There are 31 pairs of spinal nerves and spinal segments that have paired ventral and dorsal roots (8 cervical, 12 thoracic, 5 lumbar, 5 sacral, and 1 coccygeal) (**Fig. 1.53**).
    a. At 3 months' gestation, spinal cord extends to the end of the spinal canal.
    b. At birth the conus lies at L3.
    c. In adults the conus lies at L1–L2.

3. Nerve roots exit through the intervertebral foramen.
    a. C1 root exits between the occiput and the atlas.
    b. Cervical roots exit above their respective pedicles, except for the C8 root, which exits between C7 and T1. All of the other roots exit under their respective pedicles.
    c. There is no dorsal root for C1 (thus, no C1 sensory dermatome).

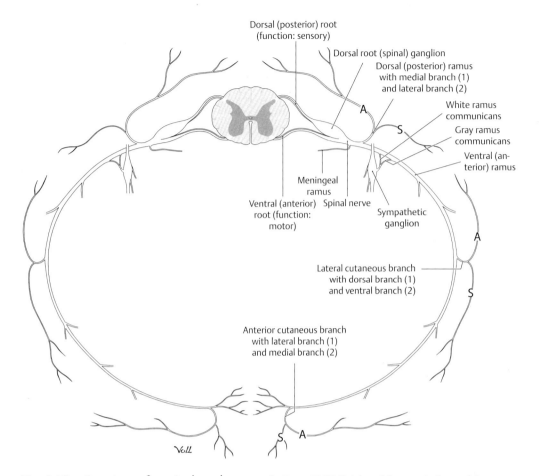

Dorsal (posterior) root
(function: sensory)

Dorsal root (spinal) ganglion

Dorsal (posterior) ramus
with medial branch (1)
and lateral branch (2)

White ramus
communicans

Gray ramus
communicans

Ventral (an-
terior) ramus

Meningeal
ramus

Ventral (anterior)   Spinal nerve
root (function:
motor)

Sympathetic
ganglion

Lateral cutaneous branch
with dorsal branch (1)
and ventral branch (2)

Anterior cutaneous branch
with lateral branch (1)
and medial branch (2)

Fig. 1.53   Structure of a spinal cord segment. (From THIEME Atlas of Anatomy, General Anatomy and Musculoskeletal System, © Thieme 2005, Illustration by Markus Voll.)

    d. In the posterior nerve roots:
      (1) Pain and temperature fibers are lateral.
      (2) Posterior column proprioceptive fibers are medial.

4. Anterior median fissure extends deeply to near the gray commissure.
    a. Posterior median sulcus extends down to the posterior median septum.
    b. Posterolateral sulci (there are two) are located near the dorsal root entry zones (DREZ).
    c. Posterior intermediate sulci separate the fasciculus gracilis from the fasciculus cuneatus.

5. Three paired funiculi
    a. Anterior funiculus — extends from the anterior median fissure to the ventral root. Contains ascending fibers from the spinal gray matter and contains descending fibers from the brainstem and cortex.
    b. Lateral funiculus — between the ventral roots and dorsal roots
      (1) Contains ascending fibers from the spinal gray
      (2) Contains descending fibers from the brainstem and cortex

c. Posterior funiculus — extends from the posterior horn to the posterior median septum. It is divided in the upper thoracic and cervical cord by a posterior intermediate septum. It is the largest funiculus, mainly composed of ascending fibers from the DRG.

6. Central gray — butterfly shaped
   a. The posterior horns extend almost to the surface (in contrast, the anterior horns only extend out a short distance). The gray commissure is around the central canal.

7. Regional spinal cord features

Region	Feature
Cervical cord	Oval shaped, wider than tall In the posterior funiculi Fasciculus gracilis (medial), fasciculus cuneatus (lateral)
Thoracic cord	Contains less gray matter There is no fasciculus cuneatus at lower levels. Lateral horn contains intermediolateral cell column. Dorsal nucleus of Clarke is located at the base of the dorsal horn and extends throughout the thoracic cord (especially large at T10–L2).
Lumbar cord	Nearly circular, contains substantial gray matter and less white matter than in the cervical cord. The sacral cord is similar to the lumbar cord.

B. Rexed's laminae

1. Ten layers determined by Rexed (Note: Between T4–L2, there is no layer VI.) (**Fig. 1.54** and **Fig. 1.55**)

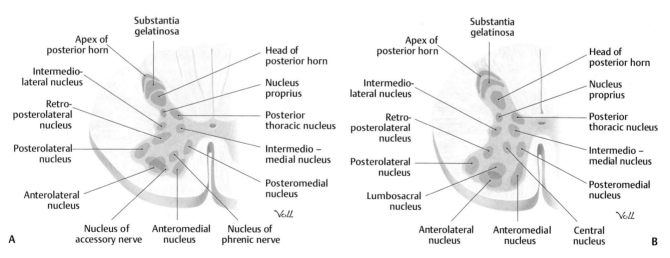

Fig. 1.54   Cell groups in the gray matter of the spinal cord. (**A**) Cervical cord, (**B**) lumbar cord. Besides the somatotopic organization of the anterior horn, the gray matter contains a particular pattern of neuron clustering. The larger anterior (ventral) horn contains the motor nuclei (red) and is the source of the ventral (motor) root of the spinal nerve, whereas the more slender posterior (dorsal) horn contains the cell bodies of secondary sensory neurons (blue) and receives the dorsal (sensory) root. The sensory neurons of the posterior horn receive synapses from entering processes of spinal (dorsal root) ganglion cells, and in turn send their axons to other, mostly cranial, levels. (From THIEME Atlas of Anatomy, Head and Neuroanatomy, © Thieme 2007, Illustration by Markus Voll.)

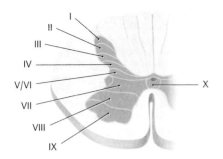 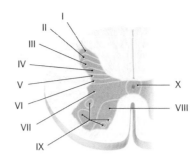 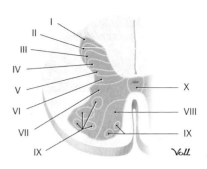

Fig. 1.55 Synaptic layers in the gray matter. (**A**) Cervical cord. (**B**) Thoracic cord. (**C**) Lumbar cord. Motor neurons are shown in red and sensory neurons in blue. The gray matter can also be divided into layers of axon termination, based on cytological criteria. This was first done by Swedish neuroanatomist Bror Rexed (1914–2002), who divided the gray matter into laminae I–X. This laminar architecture is especially well defined in the posterior (dorsal) horn, where primary sensory axons make synapses in specific layers. (From THIEME Atlas of Anatomy, Head and Neuroanatomy, © Thieme 2007, Illustration by Markus Voll.)

Layer	Feature
I	Posteromarginal nucleus (marginal zone) caps the surface of the dorsal horn. Input: DRG and layer II DRG axons ascend or descend over layer I in Lissauer's tract before synapsing. Mainly pain and temperature (fast pain, Aδ) that travel in the contralateral spinothalamic tract Neurotransmitters — substance P, enkephalin, 5-HT, and somatostatin

II	Also called the substantia gelatinosa
	Input: posterior columns, dorsolateral, and lateral funiculi with C fibers (slow pain)
	Modulates sensation via layers III and IV, but there are no ascending pathways.
	Neurotransmitter — substance P
	Note: Layers I and II possess large amounts of substance P and opiate receptors.
	    Layers I and II output:
	        Ventral and lateral horns — reflexes
	        Rostral — sensory transmission

III/IV	Also called the nucleus proprius Contains interneurons that convey low intensity stimuli to the thalamus
V	Unknown function
VI	Input: Group 1 muscle afferents → medial zone Descending spinal pathways → lateral zone

VII	Also called the zona intermedia
	Located between the anterior and posterior horns, includes the lateral horns
	Dorsal nucleus of Clarke extends from C8–L2:
	    Sends fibers to the ipsilateral dorsal spinocerebellar tract (Note: Contralateral ventral spinocerebellar
	        tract arrives from layers V and VI.)
	Central cervical nucleus extends from C1–C4:
	    Sends crossed fibers to the cerebellum and inferior vestibular nucleus
	Intermediolateral cell column
	    Medial part of layer VII, extends the entire length of cord with visceral input
	    Sends sympathetic fibers along with the ventral roots via white rami communicantes
	Note: Parasympathetic fibers arise from pelvic nerves in sacral area (S2–S4).

VIII	Located at the base of the anterior horn
IX	Contains α and gamma motor neurons Medial nuclear group — controls the axial muscles Lateral nuclear group — controls the limb's appendicular muscles Ventral group — controls extensors Dorsal group — controls flexors
X	Unknown function

Abbreviations: Aδ, delta; 5-HT, 5-hydroxytryptamine (serotonin); DRG, dorsal root ganglion

2. Dorsal root afferents
    a. Medial bundle — large myelinated fibers to the posterior columns or medial posterior horn from the encapsulated receptors such as the Golgi tendon organs, muscle spindles, Pacinian corpuscles, and Meissner's corpuscles
    b. Lateral bundle — thin nonmyelinated fibers that convey crude touch, pain, and temperature from free nerve endings. Collateral fibers present for reflexes. The thick fibers pass through or around layer II to end in layers III and IV (or they may end in Clarke's column).
    c. Main neurotransmitter (spinal and cranial sensory ganglia) — glutamate

C. Spinal cord tracts — ascending/descending/flexor and extensor tracts (**Fig. 1.56** and **Fig. 1.57**)

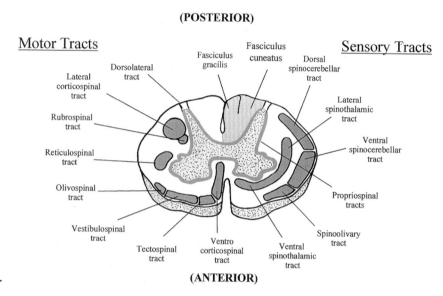

Fig. 1.56 Spinal cord pathways.

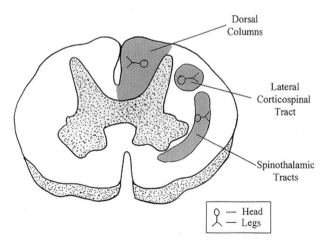

Fig. 1.57 Somatotopic organization of pathways in the spinal cord.

1. Ascending tracts

Ascending Tracts	Feature
Posterior columns	Convey fine touch, vibration, and proprioception Posterior intermediate septum starts at T6, divides the fasciculi gracilis and cuneatus Most lower limb group I afferent fibers go to Clarke's column and the dorsal spinocerebellar tract, not the fasciculus gracilis and posterior columns. Lower limb fibers are medial. Note: group Ia (muscle spindles), Ib (Golgi tendon organs) Descending fibers in the posterior column go to layer VI.
Anterior spinothalamic tract	Convey mainly light touch Fibers originate from layers I, IV, and V; most cross in the anterior commissure (but 10% remain ipsilateral). Fibers terminate in the reticular formation, periaqueductal gray, intralaminar thalamic nuclei, and thalamic VPL. The lower limb fibers are lateral.
Lateral spinothalamic tract	Convey pain and temperature. Fibers originate from layers I, IV, and V, cross the contralateral lateral spinothalamic tract, and ascend to the reticular formation and thalamic VPL.
Spinotectal tract	May convey pain stimuli Fibers originate from layers I and V, cross to the anterolateral spinal cord, ascend to the superior colliculi and periaqueductal gray.
Dorsal spinocerebellar tract	Convey touch, pressure, and proprioception from lower limbs. Type Ia, Ib, and II fibers from the Golgi tendon organs and muscle spindles go to Clarke's nucleus (C8–L3) → ipsilateral dorsal spinocerebellar tract in the posterolateral spinal cord → inferior cerebellar peduncle → cerebellar vermis
Ventral spinocerebellar tract	Convey lower limb posture and coordination information Type Ib fibers from the Golgi tendon organs go to layers V, VI, and VII to a nucleus (LI–coccyx) and samples efferent copies of the motor command reaching the α motor neurons. Fibers are bilateral but mainly crossed to the contralateral ventral spinocerebellar tract → superior cerebellar peduncle and cross again to the anterior vermis; mostly contralateral. There is no loss of touch or proprioception with disruption (since there is no conscious processing of this information).
Cuneocerebellar tract	Conveys touch, pressure, and proprioception from the upper limbs (the upper limb equivalent of the dorsal spinocerebellar tract) Ia and Ib fibers travel in the fasciculus cuneatus → accessory cuneate nucleus in the medulla → cuneocerebellar tract → inferior peduncle → lobule 5 of the cerebellum
Rostral spinocerebellar tract	Provides efferent copies, enters the inferior peduncle (the upper limb equivalent of the ventral spinocerebellar tract) Ipsilateral
Spinoolivary tract	Conveys cutaneous and group Ib receptor impulses from DRG→ posterior columns → nuclei cuneatus and gracilis → accessory olivary nucleus and crosses to the contralateral anterior lobe of the cerebellum. There are also fibers from the DRG that cross and travel in the anterior spinal cord → dorsal and medial accessory olivary nucleus.

Spinoreticular tract	Modulates motor, sensory, behavior, and awareness
	Impulses travel in the anterolateral spinal cord:
	    Ipsilateral — reticular formation in the medulla
	    Bilateral — pons and midbrain

Abbreviations: DRG, dorsal root ganglion; VPL, ventroposterolateral

2. Descending tracts

Descending Tracts	Feature

Corticospinal tract	Conveys voluntary skilled movements
	Fibers originate from:
	  Betz cells: 3% of fibers in layer 5 of the motor cortex
	  Area 4: 30% of fibers
	  Premotor area 6: 30% of fibers
	  Postcentral areas 3, 1, and 2 and parietal (area 5) cortex, 40% of these fibers from the parietal lobe
	Fibers go through the pyramid (60% myelinated) to the spinomedullary junction:
	  Lateral corticospinal tract — 90% of the fibers, almost all are crossed, travel in the posterolateral funiculus, and enter the intermediate gray to laminas IV, V, VI, and VII. A few go to anterior horns in lamina IX.
	  Anterior corticospinal tract — 10% of the fibers, ipsilateral but cross in the anterior white commissure to enter lamina VII.
	  Anterolateral corticospinal tract — ipsilateral, to the posterior horn and intermediate gray
	Neurotransmitters — glutamate and aspartate

Tectospinal tract	Conveys reflex posture movements in response to visual and possibly auditory stimuli Fibers from the superior colliculi cross in the midbrain to join the medial longitudinal fasciculus (MLF) at the medulla and travel in the anterior funiculus to the cervical levels C1–C4 to synapse in laminas VI, VII, and VIII. Fibers have more direct connections to the anterior motor neurons than the corticospinal tracts.
Rubrospinal tract	Involved in the maintenance of flexor tone Fibers from red nucleus cross in the ventral tegmentum, travel anteriorly, and partially intermingle with the corticospinal tract to descend to laminas V, VI, and VII over the entire length of the cord. Red nucleus input — both cerebral cortices and the contralateral cerebellar nucleus interpositus via superior peduncle, with somatotopic organization from cortex to the spinal cord Red nucleus stimulation — contralateral flexion and inhibition of extension
Vestibulospinal tract	Involved in the maintenance of extensor tone Fibers from lateral vestibular nucleus travel ipsilaterally within the entire length of the cord in the anterior part of the lateral funiculus laminas VII, VIII, and IX and directly to the α and gamma motor neurons and interneurons, with somatotopic organization. Stimulation causes extension.
Pontine reticulospinal tract	Involved in the maintenance of extensor tone (antigravity muscles) Axial (especially the neck muscles) limb muscles Fibers from medial pons travel ipsilaterally in the medial anterior funiculus near the MLF and go to the entire length of the cord to laminas VII and VIII. Fibers are not somatotopic.
Medullary reticulospinal tract	Involved in inhibition of extensor tone Fibers from the medial reticular formation of the medulla (especially the nucleus reticularis gigantocellularis) travel bilaterally in the anterior part of the lateral funiculus and go to the entire the length of the cord to lamina VII. Fibers are not somatotopic. Lateral tegmental system conveys impulses from the reticular formation to the spinal cord for sympathetic control. This system has substantial cortical input to influence voluntary movement, muscle tone, respiration, pressor/depressor function, and regulation of sensory impulses. Nucleus raphe magnus sends fibers bilaterally in the dorsolateral funiculus to laminas I, II, and V in the cervical enlargement.
Medial longitudinal fasciculus (MLF)	Involved in head, neck, and eye movements Fibers travel in the posterior part of the anterior funiculus with input from the medial and inferior vestibular nuclei, pontine reticular formation, superior colliculus, and interstitial nucleus of Cajal mainly to the cervical segments in laminas VII and VIII.
Descending autonomic pathways	Travels from the hypothalamus, Edinger-Westphal nucleus, locus ceruleus, solitary nucleus → lateral funiculus → intermediolateral cell column (thoracic, lumbar, and sacral spine) for sympathetic and parasympathetic control

3. Flexor tracts
   a. Lateral reticulospinal (medullary) tract
   b. Rubrospinal tract (to upper limbs only)

4. Extensor tracts
   a. Medial and lateral vestibulospinal tracts
   b. Medial (pontine) reticulospinal tract

5. Damage to the anterior lobe of the cerebellum removes tonic inhibition of the lateral vestibular nucleus resulting in increased extension.

D. Spinal canal diameters

Level	Normal Anteroposterior Spine Diameters
C1–C2	15 mm
C3–T12	12 mm
L1–L5	15–20 mm

E. Spinal ligaments and joints (**Fig. 1.58**)

Ligaments/Joints	Feature
Uncovertebral joints	Extends between the lateral uncinate processes of the cervical vertebral bodies
Zygapophyseal joints	From the facets, innervated by the fibers of the posterior spinal nerve rami (medial branch). Medially, the facet joints have no capsules and are covered only by ligamentum flavum.
Hemifacets	Hemifacets of the synovial costovertebral joints are above, below, and at the tranverse processes of T1–T10.
Anterior longitudinal ligament	Extends from the basiocciput to S1. Adherent to the vertebral bodies. The segment between C1 and the anterior basion is also called anterior atlantooccipital membrane.
Posterior longitudinal ligament	Extends from C1 to S1. PLL merges rostrally with the dura. It is thinner at the midline and not adherent to the vertebral bodies (only to the anulus). Fat and veins lie between the PLL and vertebral bodies. The tectorial membrane is the rostral extension of PLL connected to the posterior basion.
Transverse atlantal ligament	Extends between the tubercles of the lateral masses of the atlas and holds the dens against the anterior arch. The superior and inferior cruciate ligaments emerge from the transverse ligament. Superior CL — connects transverse ligament to the posterior basion Inferior CL — connects transverse ligament to the posterior body of axis
Apical ligament	Extends from the tip of the dens to the basion
Alar ligaments	The two alar ligaments extend from the dens to the lateral margins of foramen magnum.
Dentate ligaments	Extensions of pia connecting the lateral midlines of spinal cord to dura

Abbreviations: ALL, anterior longitudinal ligament; CL, cruciate ligament; PLL, posterior longitudinal ligament

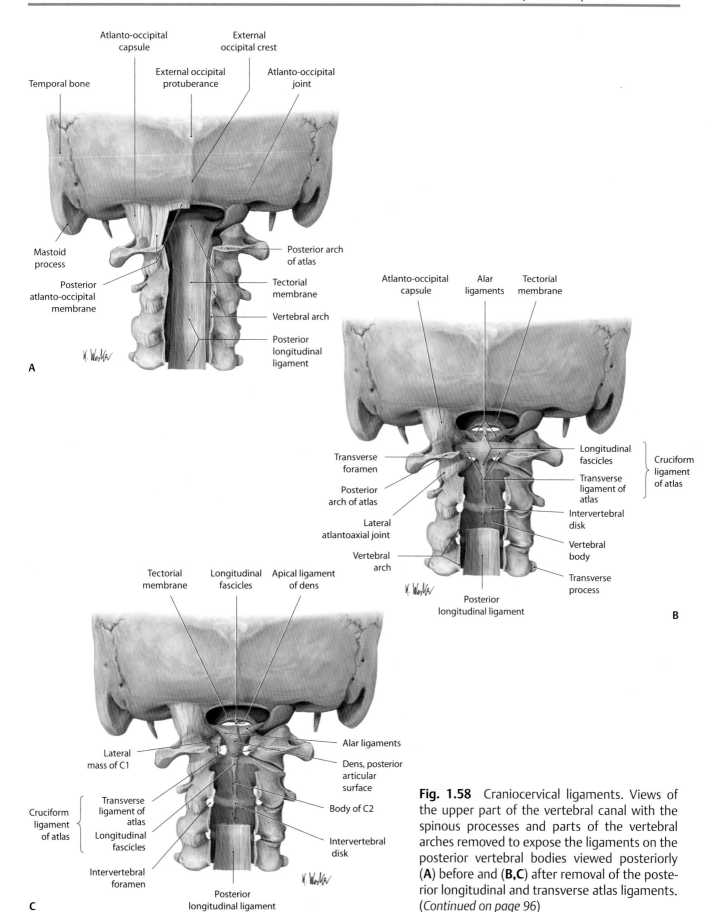

Fig. 1.58 Craniocervical ligaments. Views of the upper part of the vertebral canal with the spinous processes and parts of the vertebral arches removed to expose the ligaments on the posterior vertebral bodies viewed posteriorly (**A**) before and (**B,C**) after removal of the posterior longitudinal and transverse atlas ligaments. (*Continued on page 96*)

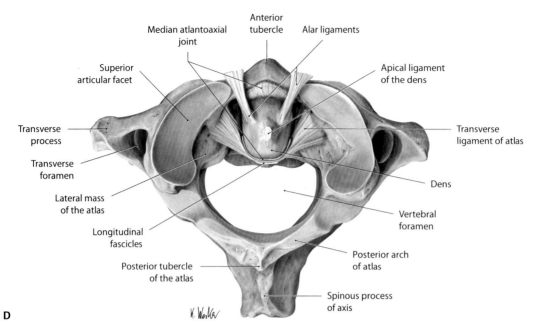

Median atlantoaxial
joint

Anterior
tubercle

Alar ligaments

Superior
articular facet

Apical ligament
of the dens

Transverse
process

Transverse
ligament of atlas

Transverse
foramen

Lateral mass
of the atlas

Dens

Longitudinal
fascicles

Vertebral
foramen

Posterior tubercle
of the atlas

Posterior arch
of atlas

Spinous process
of axis

D

Fig. 1.58 Craniocervical ligaments. (*Continued from page 95*) (**D**) The ligaments of the median atlantoaxial joint are shown from a superior view. (From THIEME Atlas of Anatomy, General Anatomy and Musculoskeletal System, © Thieme 2005, Illustration by Karl Wesker.)

XVIII. Cranial Foramina and Miscellaneous Structures

A. Cranial foramina and contents (**Fig. 1.59**)

Cranial Foramina	Structures within the Foramina	
Cribriform plate	Olfactory nerves Ethmoidal nerves Ethmoidal arteries	
Optic canal	CN II Ophthalmic artery	
Superior orbital fissure	CN III, IV, VI CN V$_1$ — all three branches (nasociliary, frontal, lacrimal) Sympathetic fibers from ICA plexus Middle meningeal artery (orbital branch) Lacrimal artery (recurrent meningeal branch) Superior ophthalmic vein	
Inferior orbital fissure	CN V$_2$ Zygomatic nerve Maxillary nerve (pterygopalatine branch) Infraorbital artery and vein Inferior ophthalmic vein	
Foramen rotundum	CN V$_2$ (**mnemonic:** CN ro**two**ndum)	
Foramen ovale	CN V$_3$ (**mnemonic:** ova**lee** = CN **three**) Lesser superficial petrosal nerve	
Foramen spinosum	Middle meningeal artery and veins	
Foramen lacerum	Usually nothing, 30% with vidian artery ICA traverses upper portion	
Carotid canal	Sympathetic nerves ICA	
Internal acoustic meatus	CN VII, VIII Labyrinthine vessels	
Stylomastoid foramen	CN VII Stylomastoid artery	
Jugular foramen	Pars nervosa: anteromedial CN IX Jacobson's nerve	Pars venosa: posterolateral CN X, XI Arnold's nerve Internal jugular vein Inferior petrosal sinus Posterior meningeal artery
Hypoglossal canal	CN XII Posterior meningeal artery	
Foramen magnum	Spinal cord and spinal roots of CN XI Vertebral arteries Anterior and posterior spinal arteries	
Foramen cecum	Emissary veins (SSS → frontal sinus and nose) Anterior falcine artery Located between the frontal crest and crista galli	
Supraorbital foramen	CN V$_1$: supraorbital vessels and nerve	
Infraorbital foramen	CN V$_2$: infraorbital vessels and nerve	

(Continued on page 98)

(Continued from page 97)

Cranial Foramina	Structures within the Foramina
Mandibular foramen	CN V$_3$ inferior alveolar nerve
Incisive foramen	CN V$_2$: nasopalatine nerve Vessels to anterior hard palate
Mental foramen	CN V$_3$: mental nerve (leaves mandible through this foramen)
Dorello's canal	CN VI: not a true foramen
Greater palatine foramen	Greater palatine nerves Vessels to the hard palate and gingiva Located medial to the third molar
Lesser palatine foramen	Lesser palatine nerves Vessels to the soft palate
Pterygopalatine fossa	CN V$_2$: maxillary artery Pterygopalatine ganglion Vidian nerve
Infratemporal fossa	CN V$_3$ Chorda tympani nerve Otic ganglion, inferior Inferior alveolar nerve Lingual nerve Buccal nerve Muscles: temporalis, medial, and lateral pterygoids Maxillary artery Pterygoid venous plexus

Vidian canal (pterygoid canal)	Vidian nerve = nerve of the pterygoid canal
	The union between the following two nerves:
	    Greater superficial petrosal nerve (parasympathetic) and
	    Deep petrosal nerve (sympathetic)
	Located at the base of medial pterygoid plate (sphenoid bone)
	Connects foramen lacerum to the pterygopalatine fossa

Petrotympanic fissure	Transmits chorda tympani
Greater petrosal foramen	Greater superficial petrosal nerve
Lesser petrosal foramen	Lesser superficial petrosal nerve

Abbreviations: CN, cranial nerve; ICA, internal carotid artery; SSS, superior sagittal sinus

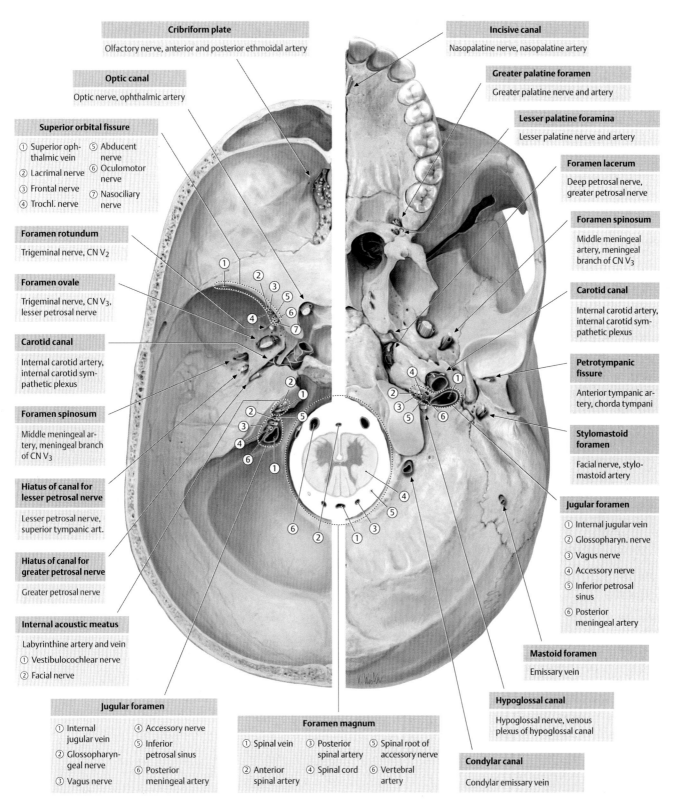

Cribriform plate

Olfactory nerve, anterior and posterior ethmoidal artery

Optic canal

Optic nerve, ophthalmic artery

Superior orbital fissure

① Superior oph-   ⑤ Abducent
thalmic vein   nerve
② Lacrimal nerve ⑥ Oculomotor
③ Frontal nerve   nerve
④ Trochl. nerve   ⑦ Nasociliary
                             nerve

Foramen rotundum

Trigeminal nerve, CN V$_2$

Foramen ovale

Trigeminal nerve, CN V$_3$, lesser petrosal nerve

Carotid canal

Internal carotid artery, internal carotid sympathetic plexus

Foramen spinosum

Middle meningeal artery, meningeal branch of CN V$_3$

Hiatus of canal for lesser petrosal nerve

Lesser petrosal nerve, superior tympanic art.

Hiatus of canal for greater petrosal nerve

Greater petrosal nerve

Internal acoustic meatus

Labyrinthine artery and vein
① Vestibulocochlear nerve
② Facial nerve

Incisive canal

Nasopalatine nerve, nasopalatine artery

Greater palatine foramen

Greater palatine nerve and artery

Lesser palatine foramina

Lesser palatine nerve and artery

Foramen lacerum

Deep petrosal nerve, greater petrosal nerve

Foramen spinosum

Middle meningeal artery, meningeal branch of CN V$_3$

Carotid canal

Internal carotid artery, internal carotid sympathetic plexus

Petrotympanic fissure

Anterior tympanic artery, chorda tympani

Stylomastoid foramen

Facial nerve, stylomastoid artery

Jugular foramen

① Internal jugular vein
② Glossopharyn. nerve
③ Vagus nerve
④ Accessory nerve
⑤ Inferior petrosal sinus
⑥ Posterior meningeal artery

Mastoid foramen

Emissary vein

Hypoglossal canal

Hypoglossal nerve, venous plexus of hypoglossal canal

Condylar canal

Condylar emissary vein

Jugular foramen

① Internal   ④ Accessory nerve
jugular vein   ⑤ Inferior
② Glossopharyn-   petrosal sinus
geal nerve   ⑥ Posterior
③ Vagus nerve   meningeal artery

Foramen magnum

① Spinal vein   ③ Posterior   ⑤ Spinal root of
                        spinal artery   accessory nerve
② Anterior   ④ Spinal cord   ⑥ Vertebral
spinal artery   artery

Fig. 1.59 Sites where nerves and blood vessels pass through the skull base. Left half of drawing: internal view of the base of the skull. Right half of drawing: external view of the base of the skull. Because the opening into the cranium is not identical to the site of emergence on the external aspect of the base of the skull for some neurovascular structures, the site of entry into the cranium is shown on the left side and the site of emergence is shown on the right side. (From THIEME Atlas of Anatomy, Head and Neuroanatomy, © Thieme 2007, Illustration by Karl Wesker.)

B. Skull anatomy

Structures	Description
Optic strut	Bone between the optic foramen and superior orbital fissure
Transverse crest	Bone in the internal auditory canal (porus acusticus) Above the acoustic and inferior vestibular nerve (to saccule) Below the facial and superior vestibular nerve (to utricle and semicircular canals)
Bill's bar	Bony bar extending from the transverse crest to the roof of the porus acusticus Separates facial nerve from the superior vestibular nerve
Falciform ligament	Dura extending between anterior clinoid and planum sphenoidale, covering the optic nerve
Liliequist's membrane	Two sleeves of arachnoid connecting the posteroinferior wall of the ICA cistern and the superior aspect of the interpeduncular cistern: Attached to the medial temporal lobes laterally Attached to the hypothalamus superiorly Separates basilar artery (posterior fossa) from suprasellar cistern
ICA dural rings	Proximal dural ring: Just distal to the exit from the cavernous sinus Composed of a reticular layer between the oculomotor nerve and the lateral aspect of internal carotid artery
Glasscock's triangle	Bone overlying the petrous internal carotid artery bordered by the foramen spinosum, arcuate eminence, dorsal aspect of V_3, and the groove of the greater superficial petrosal nerve

C. Craniometric points

External Landmarks	Feature
Nasion	Midline frontonasal suture
Glabella	Most forward point on the midline supraorbital ridge
Asterion	Junction between the frontal, parietal, temporal, and greater wing of sphenoid bones
	Located two fingerbreadths above the zygomatic arch and a thumb's breadth behind the frontal process of the zygomatic bone
Lambda	Junction between lambdoid and sagittal sutures
Bregma	Junction between coronal and sagittal sutures
Inion	Indentation under the external occipital protuberance that overlies the torcula
Opisthion	Posterior margin of the foramen magnum in the midline

XIX. Orbit and Tendinous Ring (Anulus of Zinn) (Fig. 1.60 and Fig. 1.61)

A. Tendinous ring — where the origins of extraocular muscles (all except inferior oblique) fuse to the dura/periosteum. The following structures from the superior orbital fissure pass above or through the tendinous ring to enter the orbit.

Right Orbit

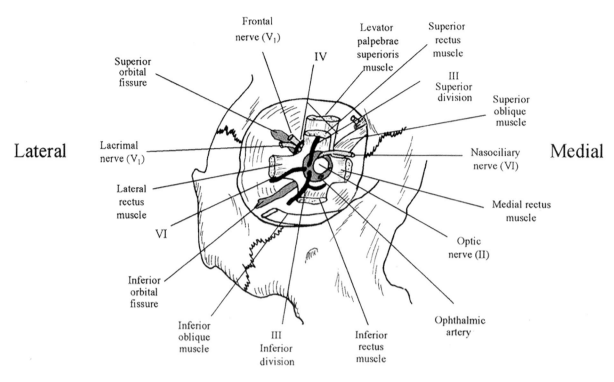

Frontal nerve (V₁)

Levator palpebrae superioris muscle

Superior rectus muscle

IV

III Superior division

Superior oblique muscle

Superior orbital fissure

Lateral

Lacrimal nerve (V₁)

Nasociliary nerve (VI)

Medial

Lateral rectus muscle

Medial rectus muscle

VI

Optic nerve (II)

Inferior orbital fissure

Inferior oblique muscle

III Inferior division

Inferior rectus muscle

Ophthalmic artery

Fig. 1.60   Tendinous ring.

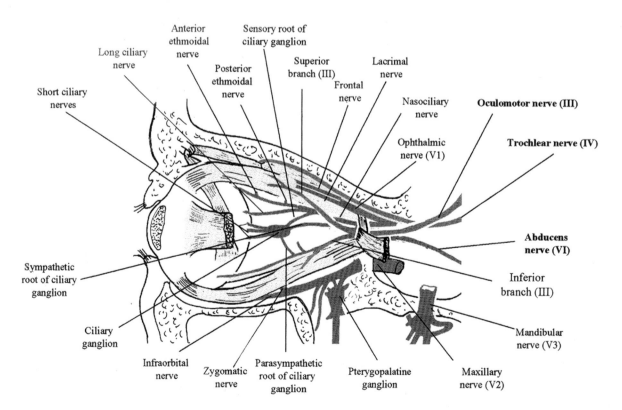

Anterior ethmoidal nerve

Sensory root of ciliary ganglion

Long ciliary nerve

Posterior ethmoidal nerve

Superior branch (III)

Lacrimal nerve

Short ciliary nerves

Frontal nerve

Nasociliary nerve

Oculomotor nerve (III)

Ophthalmic nerve (V1)

Trochlear nerve (IV)

Abducens nerve (VI)

Sympathetic root of ciliary ganglion

Inferior branch (III)

Ciliary ganglion

Mandibular nerve (V3)

Infraorbital nerve

Zygomatic nerve

Parasympathetic root of ciliary ganglion

Pterygopalatine ganglion

Maxillary nerve (V2)

Fig. 1.61   Nerves and ganglia in and around the orbit.

Above the Anulus	Through the Anulus	Mnemonic
CN V$_1$: lacrimal nerve	CN III: superior division	**L**uscious → **L**acrimal
CN V$_1$: frontal nerve	CN III: inferior division	**F**rench → **F**rontal
CN IV	CN V$_1$: nasociliary nerve	**T**arts → **T**rochlear
	CN VI	**S**tand → **S**uperior division III
		Naked → **N**asociliary
		In → **I**nferior division III
		Anticipation → **A**bducens

B. Optic nerve and ophthalmic artery — enter orbit through the optic canal and pass through the anulus of Zinn

C. Superior and inferior ophthalmic veins — pass through the superior and inferior orbital fissures, respectively. Do not pass through the anulus of Zinn.

D. Ophthalmic artery lies under CN II intracranially. The central retinal artery branches 15 mm proximal to the globe and supplies the deeper layers of the retina. The ophthalmic artery pial plexus supplies CN II. The short posterior ciliary arteries supply the sclera and outer retinal layers including the rods and cones. The ophthalmic artery crosses over laterally to the top of CN II, and the long posterior ciliary branches supply the ciliary body and iris. The two dural layers split at the optic canal with one layer over the optic nerve and one layer becoming the periosteum of the orbit. The subarachnoid space usually extends to the globe.

XX. Innervation and Muscles of the Head and Neck

A. Muscles of the head and their innervation

Region	Innervation
Eye	CN III superior division: levator palpebrae superioris and superior rectus CN III inferior division: inferior rectus, medial rectus, and inferior oblique CN IV: superior oblique CN VI: lateral rectus Müller's muscle (eyelid retractor, sympathetic)
Tympanic cavity	CN V: tensor tympani CN VII: stapedius
Face and scalp	CN VII: all areas
Mastication	CN V: temporalis, masseter, medial pterygoid, lateral pterygoid (the only one to open mouth)
Tongue	CN XII: all intrinsics and extrinsics (genioglossus, hyoglossus, and styloglossus), except the palatoglossus (innervated by CN X)
Palate	CN V: tensor veli palatini CN X: levator veli palatini, palatoglossus, and palatopharyngeus
Pharynx	CN IX: stylopharyngeus CN X: salpingopharyngeus, superior, middle, inferior pharyngeal constrictors
Larynx	CN X: all, cricothyroid by the external branch of the superior laryngeal nerve All others by the recurrent laryngeal nerve

B. Muscles of the neck and their innervation

Regions	Innervation
Cervical	CN VII: platysma CN XI, C2: sternocleidomastoid
Suprahyoid	CN V: anterior belly of the digastric CN VII: posterior belly of the digastric, stylohyoid, mylohyoid C1 by way of CN XII: geniohyoid
Infrahyoid	C1 by way of CN XII: thyrohyoid Ansa cervicalis (C1–C3): sternohyoid, sternothyroid, and omohyoid
Anterior vertebral	C1, C2: rectus capitus anterior, rectus capitus lateralis C1–C4: longus capitus C2–C8: longus coli
Lateral vertebral	C3,4: middle scalene C3–C8: posterior scalene C5–C8: anterior scalene
Suboccipital	All from the posterior rami C1: rectus capitus posterior major and minor, obliquus capitus superior C1, C2: obliquus capitus inferior

XXI. Peripheral Nerve Plexi

A. Cervical plexus organization from C1–C5 (**Fig. 1.62**)

Branches	Root	Innervation
Sensory branch	C2, C3	Lesser occipital nerve — sensation of posterolateral scalp and around ear. (Note: the greater occipital nerve (C2) does not form a plexus because it arises from the dorsal ramus)
	C2, C3	Greater auricular nerve — sensation around the ear
	C2, C3	Transverse cutaneous nerve — sensation to the anterior neck
	C3, C4	Supraclavicular nerve — sensation to the lower neck
Motor branch	C1, C3 ansa cervicalis	Omohyoid, sternothyroid, and sternohyoid Note: Superior root or descendens hypoglossi is from C1. Inferior root or descendens cervicalis is from C2, C3.
	C1 via XII	Geniohyoid and thyrohyoid
	C1, C2	Rectus capitis lateralis, longus capitis, and rectus capitis anterior
	C2–C4	Longus capitis and longus colli
	C3–C4	Scalene muscles and levator scapulae
	C3–C5	Phrenic nerve to diaphragm

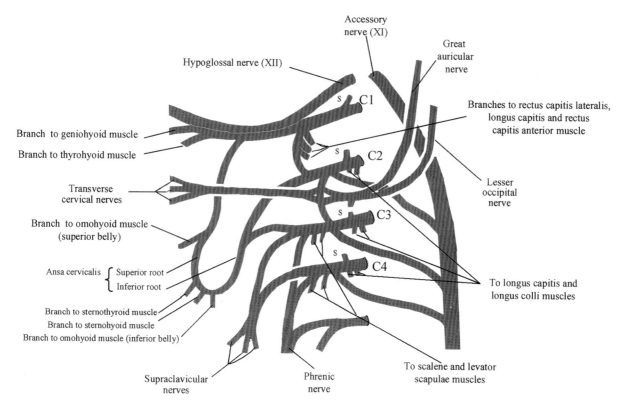

Fig. 1.62   Cervical plexus.

B. Brachial plexus — formed by the ventral rami (Note: Dorsal rami innervate paraspinal muscles.) (**Fig. 1.63**)

1. Brachial plexus organization

Subdivision	Level	Innervation
Roots C5–T1 (ventral rami)	C5–C8	Longus colli and scalene muscles
	C5	Dorsal scapular nerve → rhomboids and levator scapula
	C5–C7	Long thoracic nerve → serratus anterior
Trunks	Upper	Suprascapular nerve → supra- and infraspinatus Nerve to the subclavius muscle Note: partially covered by the anterior scalene
	Middle	No branches Note: under the anterior scalene
	Lower	No branches Note: behind the subclavian artery
Divisions	No branches	
Cords (reference: in relation to the axillary artery)	Lateral	Lateral pectoral nerve → pectoral muscles Terminates as musculocutaneous and median nerves
	Posterior	Upper/lower subscapular nerves → teres major, subscapularis Thoracodorsal nerve → latissimus dorsi Terminates as the axillary and radial nerves
	Medial	Medial pectoral nerve → pectoral muscles Medial brachial cutaneus nerve → arm Medial antebrachial cutaneous nerve → forearm Terminates as median cutaneous and ulnar nerve
Nerves	Musculocutaneous	Coracobrachialis, biceps, and brachialis
	Axillary	Deltoid and teres minor
	Radial	Triceps, brachioradialis, extensor carpi radialis longus and brevis; continues as the posterior interosseus nerve (C7, C8) → supinator, extensor carpi ulnaris, extensor digitorum, extensor digiti minimi, abductor pollicis longus, extensor pollicis longus and brevis, and extensor indicis
	Median	Forearm pronators and flexors — pronator teres, flexor carpi radialis, palmaris longus, flexor digitorum superficialis Hand — lumbricales 1, 2, opponens pollicis, abductor pollicis brevis, and flexor pollicis brevis (also by ulnar nerve) (**mnemonic: loaf** — muscles of the hand) The anterior interosseus nerve (median nerve branch) supplies flexor digitorum profundus 1 and 2, flexor pollicis longus, and pronator quadratus
	Ulnar	Forearm — flexor carpi ulnaris, flexor digitorum profundus 3 and 4 Hand — abductor, opponens, flexor digiti minimi, lumbricales 3 and 4, dorsal and palmar interosseus, flexor pollicis brevis (also by median nerve), and adductor pollicis

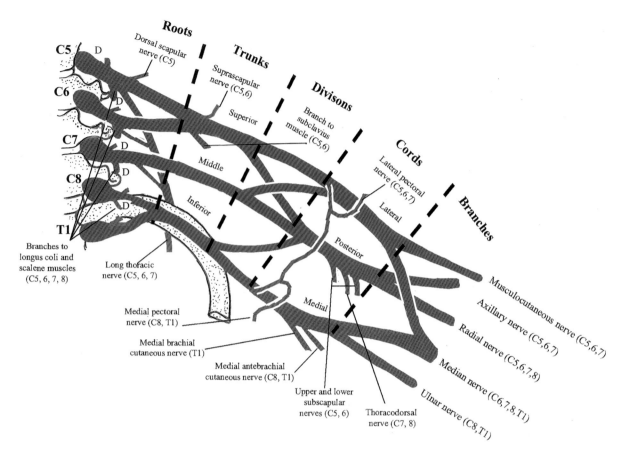

Fig. 1.63   Brachial plexus.

C. Lumbosacral plexus (**Fig. 1.64**)

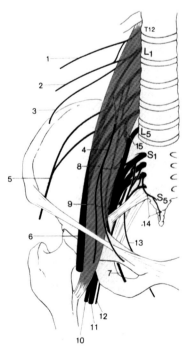

Fig. 1.64   Lumbosacral plexus. 1. Subcostal nerve. 2–7. Lumbar plexus. 2. Iliohypogastric nerve. 3. Ilioinguinal nerve. 4. Genitofemoral nerve. 5. Lateral femoral cutaneous nerve. 6. Femoral nerve. 7. Obturator nerve. 8–13. Sacral plexus. 8. Superior gluteal nerve. 9. Inferior gluteal nerve. 10, 11. Sciatic nerve. 10. Peroneal portion. 11. Tibial portion. 12. Posterior femoral cutaneous nerve. 13. Pudendal nerve. 14. Coccygeal plexus. 15. Lumbosacral trunk. (From Frick H, Leonhardt H, Starck D. Human Anatomy 2. New York, NY: Thieme; with permission 1991.)

1. Subdivisions include ventral primary rami of L1–L4 and S1–S4 spinal nerves.
    a. L4 and L5 roots join medial to the psoas muscle to form the lumbosacral trunk.
    b. S1–S4 roots join in front of the pyriformis muscle to join lumbosacral trunk to form sacral plexus.

2. Lumbosacral plexus organization

Nerve	Roots	Innervation
Superior gluteal nerve	L4–S1	Gluteus medius and minimus, and tensor fascia lata
Inferior gluteal nerve	L5–S2	Gluteus maximus
Femoral nerve	L2–L4	Iliacus, psoas, quadriceps femoris (rectus femoris, and vastus lateralis, intermedius, and medialis), and sartorius Anterior femoral cutaneous nerve (sensory) → knee Saphenous nerve medially from the knee (sensory) → foot
Obturator nerve	L2–L4	Anterior division — adductor brevis, adductor longus, gracilis, and pectineus Posterior division — obturator externus and adductor magnus (supplied also by sciatic nerve)
Sciatic nerve (exits through the greater sciatic foramen)	L4–S3	Semimembranosus, semitendinosus, biceps femoris, and adductor magnus (also by obturator nerve): Tibial nerve — gastrocnemius, soleus, tibialis posterior, flexor hallucis longus, and flexor digitorum longus Medial plantar nerve — abductor hallucis, flexor digitorum brevis, and flexor hallucis brevis Lateral plantar nerve — abductor digiti minimi, flexor digiti minimi, adductor hallucis, and interosseus muscles Common peroneal nerve: Superficial peroneal nerve — peroneus longus and brevis Deep peroneal nerve — tibialis anterior, extensor digitorum longus, extensor hallucis longus, peroneus tertius, and extensor digitorum brevis Sensory from posterior femoral cutaneous nerve: Tibial nerve — majority of the lower leg and sole of the foot Sural nerve — a patch of the lateral foot
Lateral femoral cutaneus nerve	L2, L3	Sensory to the anterior and lateral thigh
Pudendal nerve	S2–S4	Sensory to the perineum and external genitalia Motor to the external anal and urethral sphincters (from the nucleus of Onufrowicz in the anterior horn of S2–S4)
Pelvic nerves	S2–S4	Parasympathetic for bowel, bladder, and sexual function

XXII. Structures to Memorize

A. Fascicles and commissures

Fascicles and Commissures	Features
Medial longitudinal fasciculus	Eye movements with vestibular input
Dorsal longitudinal fasciculus	Periventricular hypothalamus and mamillary bodies to midbrain central gray
Medial lemniscus	Posterior column continuation to the thalamus
Lateral lemniscus	Part of the auditory pathway
Commissure of Probst	Connects the nuclei of the lateral lemniscus
Central tegmental tract	Connects: Gustatory nucleus (rostral nucleus solitarius) → medial thalamic VPM (wakefulness) Red nucleus → inferior olive
Medial forebrain bundle	Connects septal area, hypothalamus, basal olfactory areas, hippocampus/subiculum → midbrain, pons, and medulla
Lamina terminalis	Closed rostral end of the neural tube
Stria terminalis	Connects amygdala → hypothalamus
Stria medullaris	Connects the septal area, hypothalamus, olfactory area, and anterior thalamus → habenulum
Fornix	Connects hippocampus to: Precommissural — septal nuclei, hypothalamus, mamillary bodies, and anterior thalamus Postcommissural — cingulate gyrus
Ansa lenticularis	GP interna → thalamus (goes *around* the internal capsule)
Lenticular fasciculus FFH2	GP interna → thalamus (goes *through* the internal capsule)
Thalamic fasciculus FFH1	Combination of ansa lenticularis, lenticular fasciculus, and cerebellothalamic tract → VA and VL thalamus.
Mammillothalamic tract	Connects mamillary body → anterior thalamic nucleus
Fasciculus retroflexus	Connects habenulum → midbrain and interpeduncular nuclei
Diagonal band of Broca	Connects septal nuclei → amygdala
Corpus callosum	Connects most of the two hemispheres Covered with indusium griseum, which contains medial and lateral longitudinal striate that connects medial olfactory area with hippocampus
Tapetum	Fibers in the corpus callosum that connect the temporal and occipital lobes
Uncinate fasciculus	Connects anterior temporal lobe → orbitofrontal gyrus
Arcuate fasciculus	Connects the frontal, parietal, and temporal lobe (Wernicke's area to Broca's area)
Anterior commissure	Anterior portion — connects the two olfactory bulbs Posterior portion — connects the two inferior and middle frontal gyri, putamen, GP, external capsules, and claustrum

Inferior collicular commissure	Connects the inferior colliculi
Posterior commissure	Crossing fibers from the pretectal nucleus for the light reflex
Brachium conjunctivum	Superior cerebellar peduncle
Brachium pontis	Middle cerebellar peduncle
Restiform and juxtarestiform bodies	Inferior cerebellar peduncle
Trapezoid body	Connects ventral cochlear nuclei → contralateral superior olive

Abbreviations: FFH1, Forel's field H1 (thalamic fasciculus); FFH2, Forel's field H2 (lenticular fasciculus); GP, globus pallidus; VA, ventroanterior; VL, ventrolateral; VPM, ventroposteromedial

B. Nuclei and ganglia

Nuclei and Ganglia	Functions
Medial geniculate body	Auditory relay nucleus
Lateral geniculate body	Visual relay nucleus
Superior colliculus	Coordination of head/eye movements with visual system
Inferior colliculus	Auditory relay and processing
Superior olive	Auditory relay and processing
Inferior olivary complex	Cerebellar input
Ciliary ganglion	Parasympathetic from oculomotor nerve
Gasserian ganglion (semilunar ganglion)	Trigeminal nerve
Geniculate ganglion	Sensation and taste → facial nerve
Sphenopalatine ganglion (pterygopalatine ganglion)	Lacrimal and nasal glands from the facial nerve
Submandibular ganglion	Submandibular and sublingual glands from facial nerve
Spiral ganglion	Hearing to the cochlear nerve
Scarpa's ganglion Superior and inferior vestibular ganglia	Vestibular function → vestibular nerve Utricle → superior ganglion Saccule → inferior ganglion
Otic ganglion	Parotid secretion from glossopharyngeal nerve
Inferior ganglion of cranial nerve (CN) IX (petrosal)	Taste, carotid sinus/body → glossopharyngeal nerve
Superior ganglion of CN IX	Ear sensation → glossopharyngeal nerve
Inferior ganglion of CN X (nodose)	Taste and visceral sensation → vagus nerve
Superior ganglion of CN X (jugular)	Ear sensation → vagus nerve

C. Sympathetic and parasympathetic nerves

Nerve	Function
Short ciliary nerves	Parasympathetic fibers from the ciliary ganglion → eye Contains some sympathetic fibers Fibers enter the orbit with cranial nerve (CN) III (inferior division).
Long ciliary nerves	Sympathetic fibers from nasociliary branch of CN V_1 → eye
Splanchnic nerves	Preganglionic fibers passing through the sympathetic chain → adrenal medulla
Nervi erigentes	Parasympathetic nerves (S2–4) → genitals, bowel, and bladder
Pelvic plexus	Sympathetic nerves (T10–12) → genitals, bowel, and bladder
Hypogastric nerves	Sympathetic nerves (T10–12) → genitals, bowel, and bladder
Pudendal nerve	Somatic nerve → genitals, external anal and bladder sphincters, and perineum

D. Miscellaneous sensory nerves

    1. T12 — subcostal

    2. L1— iliohypogastric and ilioinguinal

    3. L1, L2 — genitofemoral

2 Physiology

Associate Editor, **Demitre Serletis**

I. Cellular Molecular Transport

A. Cell membrane — a semipermeable lipid bilayer containing channel and carrier proteins that regulate the flow of ions and other molecules across the membrane. It also functions as a capacitor to store charge.

B. Simple diffusion — characterized by kinetic movement of ions or molecules across the cell membrane without the necessity for binding to carrier proteins in the membrane. It may occur either directly through the lipid bilayer of the membrane or through protein channels that are highly selective for specific ions/molecules based on their shape, size, and charge. Simple diffusion is limited to small ions/molecules (e.g., H_2O) and lipid-soluble molecules (e.g., O_2, N_2, CO_2, and alcohols). Other molecules exhibit limited diffusion owing to their larger size (e.g., glucose) or electrostatic charge.

C. Selective permeability — the highly selective property of protein channels to transport specific ions/molecules across the membrane based on shape, size, and charge. For example, Na^+ channels are small in diameter and contain a negatively charged inner surface to attract positively charged Na^+ ions. Once a Na^+ ion is inside the channel, it may then diffuse out in either direction. In contrast, K^+ channels are not negatively charged and are even smaller than Na^+ channels. These properties confer selective permeability to the channels for the transport of their specific ionic species.

D. Gating — mechanism responsible for controlling the permeability of a protein channel to the passage of ionic or molecular species. Gates are structural components of the protein molecule that may open or close over the opening of a channel in response to conformational changes in the protein molecule. The opening or closing of these gates is dictated by either voltage changes or the binding of ligands.

   1. Voltage-gated channels — The ion passage of voltage-gated channels (e.g., Na^+, K^+, Ca^{2+}) is regulated via conformational changes of the gate arising in response to the electrical potential across the membrane (V_m). Not all channels that pass Na^+, K^+, or Ca^{2+} are voltage-gated but for the subtypes that are, they tend to remain closed if there is a sufficiently negative charge inside the cell, and open when V_m becomes less negative (i.e., depolarized).

   2. Ligand-gated channels — Ligand-gated channels open following the binding of a specific molecule (i.e., ligand) to the receptor protein. For example, acetylcholine (ACh) binds the ACh receptor, causing the gate of this channel to open; in fact, this is an important mechanism underlying the transmission of action potentials (AP) within the synapse and neuromuscular junction (NMJ).

E. Facilitated diffusion — used to transport glucose and most amino acids. It involves carrier-mediated transport such that a molecule binds to a receptor protein, inducing a conformational change that carries the molecule into the cell where it is released. Upon release, the receptor protein then reverts to its original shape. The rate of diffusion is dependent upon the rate of conformational change and the number of receptors and is maximal when all carrier proteins are filled.

F. Net rate of diffusion — influenced by the selective permeability of the membrane and the electrochemical gradient (which is itself dependent upon the electrical potential difference, concentration gradient, and pressure gradient across the membrane). The steady-state is achieved when the electrical and concentration forces across the membrane are balanced.

G. Active transport — transport of ions/molecules (e.g., Na^+, K^+, Ca^{2+}, H^+, Cl^-, I^-, uric acid, sugars, and many amino acids) across the cell membrane, against an electrical, chemical, or pressure gradient. This process is energy-dependent (e.g., adenosine triphosphate [ATP]).

  1. Primary active transport — uses ATP-derived energy for the transport of Na^+, K^+, Ca^{2+}, H^+, and Cl^-. The Na^+/K^+ pump is a carrier protein comprising two protein subunits; the larger subunit contains three receptor sites on the intracellular side for Na^+, and the smaller one contains two receptor sites on the extracellular side for K^+. The intracellular portion exhibits ATPase activity, such that one ATP molecule is cleaved to drive three Na^+ ions out and two K^+ ions into the cell.

  2. Secondary active transport — uses the gradient of one compound (created by previous ATP cleavage) to drive the transport of another compound either down its electrochemical gradient (i.e., cotransport) or against it (i.e., countertransport). This process is mediated by a carrier protein.
     a. For example:
       (1) Cotransport — Na^+ cotransport of glucose or amino acids
       (2) Countertransport — Na^+ countertransport of Ca^{2+} or H^+

II. Membrane Potentials and Action Potentials

A. Membrane potential (V_m) — established by selective permeability to Na^+ and K^+ ions

B. Nernst equation — used to determine the electric potential of a cell membrane with respect to one type of ion. Nernst potential = $\pm 61 \log C_i/C_o$, whereby C_i is the intracellular ionic concentration and C_o is the extracellular ionic concentration. Note that the sign of the potential is positive when the ion is negative (e.g., Cl^-), and negative when the ion is positive (e.g., Na^+, K^+, Ca^{2+}). The following table illustrates ionic concentrations and equilibrium potentials.

Ion	Extracellular (mEq/L)	Intracellular (mEq/L)	Equilibrium Potential (mV)
Na^+	142	14	+61
K^+	4	140	−94
Cl^-	103	4	−86
Ca^{2+}	2.4	0.0001	+267

C. Equilibrium potential — V_m at which no net diffusion of the ion occurs because of balanced electrical and chemical gradients, such that the net current of the ion across the membrane is 0.

D. Goldman equation — used to determine the potential across a cell's membrane taking into account all of the ions that are permeable through that membrane: $V_m = -61 \log ([Na^+]_i \times P_{Na+} + [K^+]_i \times P_{K+} + [Cl^-]_o \times P_{Cl-})/([Na^+]_o \times P_{Na+} + [K^+]_o \times P_{K+} + [Cl^-]_i \times P_{Cl-})$. V_m is dependent on electrical charge, concentration, and permeability (P).

E. Resting membrane potential (RMP) — is equal to −90 mV in large myelinated peripheral nerves and in skeletal muscle. The RMP is determined largely by the equilibrium potential of K^+ (−94 mV) because K^+ is 100 times more permeable than Na$^+$ (which has an equilibrium potential of +61 mV). Ca^{2+} ions are not very permeable and have little effect on RMP. RMP is approximately –65 mV in the soma of the neuron and –55 mV in small nerve fibers and smooth muscle.

F. Action potential — All-or-none, propagated phenomenon characterized by rapid changes in V$_m$, which alter permeability of Na$^+$ and K$^+$ voltage-gated channels.

1. Resting state — The RMP is –90 mV, primarily maintained by leaky K$^+$ channels.
    a. Na$^+$ and K$^+$ permeability is dependent on changes in V$_m$ during the AP, although Cl$^-$ permeability does not change much. At rest, K$^+$ conductance is higher than Na$^+$ conductance because the membrane leaks K$^+$ ions to a greater extent than it does Na$^+$ ions.

2. Depolarization state — When a stimulus increases V$_m$ sufficiently (i.e., by 15 to 30 mV, attaining a threshold level of approximately –65 mV), the membrane suddenly becomes permeable to Na$^+$, resulting in further depolarization to +35 mV in large fibers and 0 mV in smaller fibers. This initiates the AP, which subsequently propagates along the neuronal axon.
    a. Approximately 40 to 80 excitatory postsynaptic potentials (EPSPs) are required to induce an AP. Inhibitory postsynaptic potentials (IPSPs) open K$^+$ or Cl$^-$ channels, whereas EPSPs open Na$^+$ channels.
    b. Only a small number of ions present in the cell need to cross the membrane (1/100,000,000) to depolarize it from –90 to +35 mV.
    c. Different neurons exhibit varying thresholds for excitation, baseline RMP, and different frequency of discharges.
    d. Membrane accommodation to a stimulus occurs by a slow rise in the membrane potential that allows some Na$^+$ gates to deactivate while others open. Thus, either a larger amplitude or a faster rise of depolarization is required to trigger an AP.
    e. The AP starts at the neuronal axon hillock, which contains sevenfold more voltage-gated Na$^+$ channels; hence, it is more easily depolarized than the neuronal soma (+30 mV increase is required at the soma, compared with +20 mV at the hillock, to depolarize the membrane potential to –45 mV).
    f. The AP propagates as adjacent neuronal segments undergo local changes in membrane potential. Ion channels open and the impulse moves ahead in both directions. The velocity of the AP increases with increased transmembrane resistance, decreased internal resistance, and decreased membrane capacitance. Myelin further increases transmembrane resistance, decreases membrane capacitance, and is responsible for saltatory conduction of the AP.
    g. During the AP, many negatively charged molecules remain intracellular (i.e., proteins, phosphates, and sulfates).

3. Repolarization state — Following depolarization, the membrane repolarizes in 1/10,000th of a second as Na$^+$ channels close and K$^+$ channels open.
    a. "Positive after-potential" represents the overshoot hyperpolarization to –100 mV, secondary to K$^+$ channels remaining transiently open following repolarization.

G. Voltage-gated Na$^+$ channels — contain an outer activation gate and an inner inactivation gate. At RMP, the inactivation gate is open and the activation gate is closed. The activation gate opens when V$_m$ attains –70 to –50 mV, allowing a Na$^+$ influx. Both gates remain open for a few 10,000ths of a second (allowing for transient depolarization to +35 mV), after which the inactivation gate closes. The inactivation gate does not open again until the RMP is restored and the activation gate is closed.

H. Voltage-gated K$^+$ channels — open slowly as the membrane depolarizes such that K$^+$ efflux occurs as the Na$^+$ inactivation gate closes, thereby leading to repolarization.

I. Tetrodotoxin — voltage-gated Na^+ channel blocker

J. Tetraethylammonium (TEA) — voltage-gated K^+ channel blocker

K. Cl^- ions — passively leak into the cell (i.e., they are not actively pumped). Little change in Cl^- conductance occurs during the AP. The intracellular concentration of Cl^- is low because the −90 mV RMP repels them (i.e., negative charge). The Nernst potential for Cl^- is −86 mV.

L. Ca^{2+} pump and voltage-gated Ca^{2+} channels — a Ca^{2+} pump actively transports Ca^{2+} out of the cell or into the endoplasmic reticulum, creating a Ca^{2+} gradient. Voltage-gated Ca^{2+} channels, also permeable to Na^+, are also referred to as Ca^{2+}–Na^+ channels. These are slow channels, unlike the fast voltage-gated Na^+ channels. When less Ca^{2+} is in the interstitial fluid, Na^+ channels open sooner (as low as −80 mV); thus, the membrane is more excitable and may reach tetany. Alternatively, increased levels of Ca^{2+} result in Ca^{2+} binding to Na^+ channel proteins, which require larger depolarizing voltages to open.

M. Patch clamp technique — used to record ion current flow (through either single or multiple channels) or potentials across membranes. Involves the approximation of a micropipette (with diameter as low as 1–2 mm) onto a cell surface, forming a membrane patch either on or off the cell. One can "clamp" the system to set a constant voltage or current.

N. Heart muscle — Action potentials have a longer depolarization and plateau phase owing to the activity of fast voltage-gated Na^+ channels, slow voltage-gated Ca^{2+} channels, and K^+ channels that do not open until the end of the plateau.

O. Rhythmicity — repetitive, self-induced discharges of cardiac muscle, smooth muscle, and some neurons. It is characterized by a depolarized resting state (RMP of −60 to −70 mV) and a decreased threshold for AP initiation secondary to membrane permeability to Na^+ or Ca^{2+}.

  1. Normally, the delay in subsequent depolarization is due to an overshoot of K^+ efflux causing hyperpolarization. As K^+ conductance decreases, the membrane depolarizes, and then K^+ conductance increases. The AP occurs when K^+ conductance is at its lowest.

P. Sphingomyelin (i.e., myelin) — insulating layer of phospholipid that surrounds the axons of many neurons and contributes to faster neuronal conduction. Peripheral nerves have twice as many unmyelinated fibers than myelinated fibers. Nodes of Ranvier are 3 µm-long unmyelinated segments occurring every 1–3 mm along the axon. Saltatory conduction occurs between these nodes in myelinated fibers, making them faster and more energy efficient. Moreover, myelinated fibers exhibit faster repolarization than unmyelinated fibers; this repolarization is so fast that K^+ channels minimally contribute to it — rather it occurs mainly via the closing of Na^+ channels.

Q. Conduction velocity — In small, unmyelinated nerve fibers, it is ~0.5 m/s; in large, myelinated nerve fibers, velocity is as high as 120 m/s.

R. Excitation of a cell — Occurs following either mechanical stimulation (e.g., secondary to pressure or stretch of the skin), a chemical interaction (e.g., in interneurons and certain sensory receptors), or an electrical stimulation (e.g., in excitable cells such as neuronal, cardiac, or smooth muscle cells).

S. Refractory period — occurs following depolarization, when Na^+ channels (and certain Ca^{2+} channels) remain inactivated such that no amount of stimulus will trigger an AP to fire.

  1. Absolute refractory period — During this period, the neuron will not fire. It lasts 1/2500th of a second in large, myelinated fibers.

2. Relative refractory period — During this period, the neuron requires a supranormal stimulus to fire. It lasts ¼ to ½ as long as the absolute refractory period.

T. Membrane stabilizers — agents that decrease excitability. They include increased serum Ca^{2+}, decreased serum K^+ (as in familial periodic paralysis), certain local anesthetics (e.g., procaine), acidosis (pH < 7.0), and hypoxia.

U. Membrane destabilizers — agents that increase excitability. They include decreased serum Ca^{2+}, increased serum K^+, alkalosis (pH > 7.8, thus explaining why seizures are induced by hyperventilation), caffeine, and strychnine.

III. Synapses and Neurotransmitters

A. Synapse — junction between neurons, or between a neuron and muscle fiber, where impulse conduction occurs. A synapse functions to either transmit an impulse, block it, change it from a single event to repetitive impulses, or integrate it with other impulses.

   1. Chemical synapse — most common type of synapse in the central nervous system (CNS), exhibiting unidirectional flow. Approximately 50 chemical neurotransmitters have been found to date.

   2. Electrical synapse — tubular protein channel (i.e., gap junction) between cells allowing the direct spread of ionic current from one cell to another. Typically found in cardiac and smooth muscle (but rarely in the mammalian CNS), they exhibit bidirectional flow.

   3. 80–95% of axons synapse onto dendrites; 5–20% synapse onto the neuronal soma.

B. Synaptic cleft — 20–30 nm space separating the presynaptic and postsynaptic terminals

C. Presynaptic terminal — contains synaptic vesicles and mitochondria to generate ATP for neurotransmitter synthesis. The presynaptic membrane also contains many voltage-gated Ca^{2+} channels that open with depolarization, allowing an influx of Ca^{2+} ions that induce neurotransmitter release by binding to release sites inside the terminal membrane. This stimulates neurotransmitter-containing vesicles to bind and fuse with the presynaptic membrane, leading to the exocytosis of a few vesicles per AP.

   1. Synaptic vesicle — Each vesicle contains 10,000 molecules of ACh, or 1 quantum. The release of 1 quantum produces a miniature end-plate potential (MEPP).

   2. Following the AP, Ca^{2+} ions are removed from the presynaptic terminal via active transport, bound to cytosol proteins and transported to storage vesicles. Upon fusing with the membrane, these vesicles reform intracellularly.

   3. Presynaptic inhibition — inhibitory effect following the discharge of inhibitory synapses (mediated by the neurotransmitter gamma-aminobutyric acid [GABA]) present on presynaptic terminal nerve fibrils just proximal to their termination on postsynaptic neurons. Anion channels, namely Cl^-, open and allow Cl^- into the terminal fibrils to inhibit subsequent excitation. This mechanism is typically seen in sensory pathways of the CNS.

D. Postsynaptic terminal — contains receptors with a binding component (for the neurotransmitter) and an ionophore component. The latter comprises either a chemically activated ion channel (Na^+, K^+, or Cl^-) or a second-messenger system that activates an internal reaction within the postsynaptic neuron.

1. Second messenger system — may activate adenylate cyclase to produce cyclic adenosine monophosphate (cAMP), protein kinases, or increased gene expression; may increase or decrease receptor numbers; or may alter synaptic reactivity. Neurotransmitters that rely on this mechanism are modulators used for various functions, including memory.

E. Synaptic activity — dependent on the overall effect of excitatory and inhibitory input from presynaptic neurons onto the postsynaptic neuron

1. Excitation — follows opening of Na^+ channels, closing of K^+ or Cl^- channels, increasing excitatory or decreasing inhibitory receptor numbers, or modifying intracellular metabolic activity

2. Inhibition — follows opening of K^+ or Cl^- channels or modifying excitatory or inhibitory receptor numbers

3. Summation — the additive effect of EPSPs and IPSPs, whose net effect is either to increase or decrease ion permeability in the membrane. This phenomenon may last for 1–2 ms and typically resolves within 15 ms. Each axon terminal releases substances that induce a 0.5–1 mV change in V_m; 20 mV is needed to attain the depolarization threshold required to trigger an AP. Summation may occur either in the spatial or the temporal domain.
   a. Spatial summation arises when presynaptic terminals residing in different parts of the neuron are stimulated simultaneously.
   b. Temporal summation is the additive effect of postsynaptic potentials over time. A neuron is considered "facilitated" if an EPSP puts it closer to threshold.

4. Decremented conduction — Many dendrites are unable to generate APs because they have too few voltage-gated channels, yet electrotonic current may spread to the axon by means of the cytosol. Decremented conduction occurs because changes in V_m more distal on the dendrite have less effect on the soma due to current leaking out along the way.

5. Fatigue — when repetitive stimulation leads to a decreased frequency of discharge. This is a protective mechanism against excessive neuronal activity. It arises following exhaustion of neurotransmitter stores in presynaptic terminals (because neurons only store sufficient transmitter for ~10,000 synaptic transmissions), progressive inactivation of postsynaptic receptors and by accumulation of postsynaptic Ca^{2+}, which opens Ca^{2+}-activated K^+ channels that hyperpolarize the membrane.

6. Posttetanic facilitation — occurs in the context of repetitive impulses inducing an excitatory response, followed by a transient period of rest during which the synapse remains more responsive to subsequent stimulation than is normally the case. This occurs because repetitive stimuli lead to Ca^{2+} build-up in the presynaptic terminals, ultimately causing increased neurotransmitter release.

7. Synaptic delay — the time for synaptic transmission (of an AP) to occur from presynaptic to postsynaptic terminal; typically 0.5 ms duration

8. Approximately 50 synaptic transmitters have been identified; these are classified as (1) small-molecule, rapidly acting neurotransmitters, and (2) neuropeptides.

F. Small-molecule neurotransmitters — rapidly acting substances that account for most of the acute reactions in the CNS. They are produced in the cytosol of presynaptic terminals and are actively transported into vesicles, a few of which are released per AP. These agents usually act upon ion channels, a process that occurs within milliseconds. They may also activate receptor-linked enzymes and are ultimately recycled via active transport into presynaptic terminals (i.e., reuptake) for subsequent use. Only a single type of small-molecule neurotransmitter is released per neuron, yet the same neuron may also release more than one neuropeptide.

1. Four classes of small-molecule neurotransmitters — ACh constitutes class 1; amines (i.e., norepinephrine [NE], epinephrine [EPI], dopamine [DA], serotonin [5-hydroxytryptamine; 5-HT] and histamine) are class 2; amino acids [i.e., GABA, glycine, glutamate, and aspartate] constitute class 3; and nitric oxide (NO) is class 4.

    a. Acetylcholine — usually excitatory. ACh is produced in the presynaptic terminal from acetyl-coenzyme A (CoA) and choline, and is stored in vesicles. Upon release, it is split in the synaptic cleft by acetylcholinesterase. ACh is found in the motor cortex, skeletal muscle, preganglionic autonomic nerves, postganglionic parasympathetic nerves, and postganglionic sympathetic nerves supplying sweat glands.

    b. Norepinephrine — usually excitatory; found in the pontine locus ceruleus and postganglionic sympathetic nerve fibers

    c. Dopamine — inhibitory; found in the neurons of the substantia nigra (SN) that project to the putamen and caudate. Synthesis occurs following conversion of tyrosine to 3,4-dihydroxy-L-phenylalanine (DOPA) by the enzyme tyrosine hydroxylase (i.e., the rate-limiting step), followed by conversion to DA. This is subsequently converted to NE, and finally to EPI.

    d. Glycine — inhibitory; found in the spinal cord (Renshaw cells)

    e. GABA — inhibitory; found in the cortex, basal ganglia, cerebellum (Purkinje cells), and spinal cord

    f. Glutamate — excitatory; found in the cortex, dentate gyrus of the hippocampus, striatum, and cerebellar granule cells

    g. Serotonin — inhibitory; found in brainstem nuclei (median raphe nuclei) that project to the hypothalamus and spinal cord (dorsal horns). It acts to inhibit pain pathways, induces sleep, and affects mood. It is used by the pineal gland to synthesize melatonin, which is released in a diurnal fashion.

2. Small-molecule neurotransmitter receptors

    a. ACh receptors

       (1) Nicotinic receptors — Stimulated by nicotine, they are located in the NMJ and preganglionic endings of both sympathetic and parasympathetic fibers. Autonomic nicotinic receptors are composed of five subunits (i.e., 2 alpha, [α_2], one beta [β], one gamma [γ], and one delta [δ]). The α-subunit is composed of four hydrophobic transmembrane proteins and serves as the binding site for ACh; hence, each receptor binds two ACh molecules. Stimulation of the receptor generates a fast EPSP. The receptor is blocked by hexamethonium in a depolarizing fashion that cannot be reversed by anticholinesterase. The nicotinic receptor at the NMJ consists of only two α-subunits, and stimulation of the receptor elicits a slow EPSP (by opening both Na$^+$ and Ca^{2+} channels) and a slow IPSP (by opening K$^+$ channels).

       (2) Muscarinic receptors — Stimulated by muscarine, they are located in postganglionic parasympathetic endings and postganglionic sympathetic endings innervating sweat glands. The receptors' effects are mediated by a G protein via a second messenger system, and activation of one G protein inhibits all other G proteins in the cell. These receptors are blocked by pertussis toxin.

    b. Adrenergic receptors — NE stimulates α-receptors to a greater extent than β-receptors. EPI stimulates α- and β-receptors to the same extent. See Chapter 6 (Critical Care) for more details.

    c. DA receptor — DA1 receptor functions via cAMP (i.e., second messenger).

    d. Glycine receptor — inhibitory; involves Cl$^-$ channels and is bound by strychnine (i.e., competitive antagonist). Mutations cause increased muscle rigidity (as in stiff person syndrome).

e. GABA receptors — GABA-A increases Cl⁻ channel permeability; GABA-B increases K⁺ conductance. GABA-A receptors are composed of five subunits with a central Cl⁻ channel (i.e., α_2, β_2, and either γ or δ). The type A receptor (i.e., GABA-A) is more common than the type B receptor (i.e., GABA-B), which uses a G protein as a second messenger. The GABA-A receptor's α and β subunits bind barbiturates, whereas the γ subunit binds benzodiazepines. The β subunit binds GABA as well. Therefore, barbiturates and benzodiazepines are both GABA-A agonists, whereas baclofen is a GABA-B agonist. Barbiturates prolong the duration of Cl⁻ channel opening, and benzodiazepines increase the frequency of Cl⁻ channel opening. GABA receptors are blocked by picrotoxin, resulting in seizure-like activity.

f. Glutamate receptors — Linked to cell death (via Ca^{2+} influx) and synaptic plasticity, these receptors are either ligand-gated (e.g., metabotropic) or a combination of ligand- and voltage-gated [e.g., N-methyl-D-aspartic acid (NMDA), α-amino-3-hydroxy-5-methylisoxazole-4-propionic acid (AMPA)/quisqualate, and kainate]. Some are blocked by Mg^{2+}. The NMDA receptor is one type of glutamate receptor. It is voltage-regulated because at RMP, Mg^{2+} blocks the channel, whereas with depolarization, Mg^{2+} is driven out and the channel opens. It is also ligand-gated by glutamate and permeable to Ca^{2+}, Na^+, and K^+. It requires glycine as a coagonist for activation. Non-NMDA glutamate receptors do not require glycine for activation. The AMPA/quisqualate and kainate receptors are permeable to monovalent cations (e.g., Na^+ and K^+).

G. Neuropeptide neurotransmitters — higher molecular weight and slow-acting. These transmitters are produced in the soma and packaged by the endoplasmic reticulum and Golgi apparatus after being cleaved from larger peptides. Vesicles of these transmitters are then transported to presynaptic membranes via axonal streaming, at a rate of a few cm/day. The vesicles are not recycled, and although fewer are released in comparison to small-molecule transmitters, they are longer-acting and significantly more potent. Neuropeptides close Ca^{2+} channels and alter metabolic machinery and receptors. They can diffuse into tissues and are typically destroyed within minutes to hours. Examples include hypothalamic-releasing hormones, pituitary peptides, cholecystokinin (CCK), and bradykinin.

H. Intracellular second messengers

1. cAMP — increased with DA1 receptor stimulation

2. Cyclic guanosine monophosphate (cGMP) — involved with photoreception; increased by NO

3. Inositol triphosphate (IP_3) — hydrolyzed by phospholipase C; opens Ca^{2+} release channels in the endoplasmic/sarcoplasmic reticulum, thereby increasing Ca^{2+} in the cytosol

4. Diacylglycerol (DAG) — synergistically activates protein kinase C with Ca^{2+}

5. Ca^{2+} — binds calmodulin

6. G proteins — see Section VII

I. Axonal transport — may be slow (several mm/day) or fast (200–400 mm/day, via microtubular mechanisms) and either anterograde or retrograde. The proteins kinesin and dynein mediate anterograde and retrograde axonal transport, respectively.

IV. Sensory Receptors

A. Sensory receptors (**Fig. 2.1**)

1. Mechanoreceptors — sense mechanical deformation

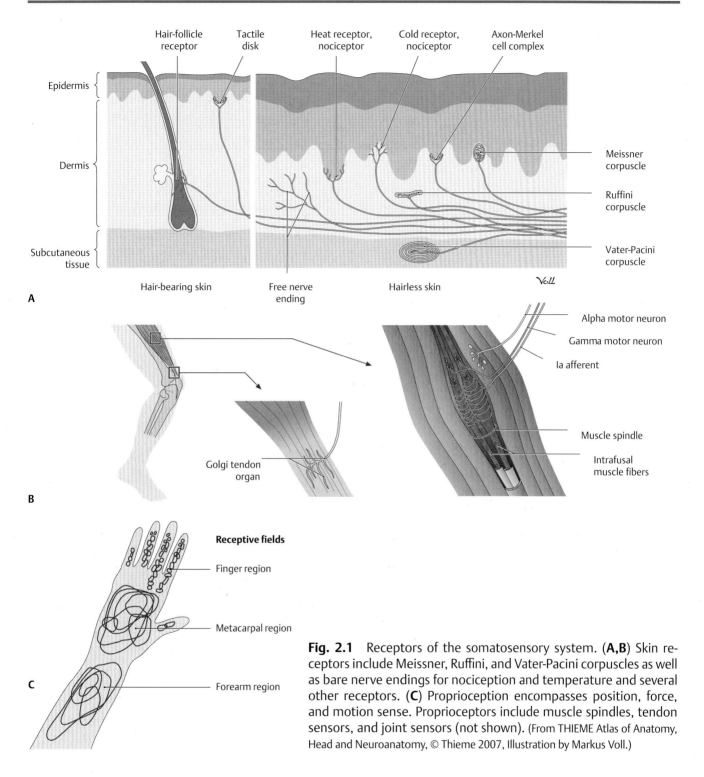

Fig. 2.1 Receptors of the somatosensory system. (**A,B**) Skin receptors include Meissner, Ruffini, and Vater-Pacini corpuscles as well as bare nerve endings for nociception and temperature and several other receptors. (**C**) Proprioception encompasses position, force, and motion sense. Proprioceptors include muscle spindles, tendon sensors, and joint sensors (not shown). (From THIEME Atlas of Anatomy, Head and Neuroanatomy, © Thieme 2007, Illustration by Markus Voll.)

2. Thermoreceptors — sense changes in temperature; may be specific for heat or cold

3. Nociceptors — generate sensation of pain in the context of tissue damage or physical/chemical changes

4. Electromagnetic receptors — detect light in the retina

5. Chemoreceptors — detect various chemicals pertaining to taste, smell, arterial O_2 and CO_2, blood osmolarity, etc.

B. Labeled-line principle — Different sensory modalities are regulated in different parts of the brain; in other words, each type of sensory nerve terminates in specific CNS regions.

C. Receptor potential — When the receptor potential rises above threshold, an AP is generated. A higher receptor potential elicits increased impulse frequency but does not change impulse amplitude. The receptor potential is graded and nonpropagated, in contrast to the AP, which is a propagated, all-or-none response.

D. Receptor potential changes via different mechanisms

   1. Mechanoreceptors — react as deformation stretches the membrane and opens ion channels
      a. For example:
         (1) The Pacinian corpuscle consists of a central nerve fiber surrounded by concentric capsular layers. Mechanical compression (i.e., elongation, bending, denting, etc.) induces changes in the central fiber. As the fiber's unmyelinated tip deforms, Na^+ conductance increases, a receptor potential is generated, and an AP ensues if the receptor potential is sufficiently large to reach threshold. The frequency of the AP is initially proportional to the amplitude of the receptor potential but plateaus at high levels.

   2. Chemical receptors — stimulated by certain chemical agents, thereby triggering specific ion channels to open

   3. Temperature receptors — react to temperature changes by directly opening ion channels or indirectly altering membrane ion permeability

   4. Electromagnetic energy — directly opens ion channels or indirectly alters membrane ion permeability

E. Adaptation — occurs when a sensory receptor decreases its firing rate in the context of continuous sensory stimulation

   1. For example, a Pacinian corpuscle adapts as follows:
      a. Following the initial pressure wave, fluid within the corpuscle is evenly distributed such that firing ceases even though the corpuscle is still compressed; another signal develops when the compression is removed. Such adaptation occurs in 1/100 second.
      b. Accommodation via the gradual inactivation of Na^+ channels — This adaptation is much slower. Both the receptor and the terminal nerve fibers can adapt via this mechanism.

   2. Mechanoreceptors may adapt completely; pain receptors tend to adapt to a lesser extent and chemoreceptors vary in their ability to adapt.

   3. Rapidly adapting (phasic) versus slowly adapting (tonic) receptors
      a. Pacinian corpuscles and hair receptors are phasic receptors; they react only to changes in stimulus strength and are incapable of transmitting continuous signals. Moreover, they increase their firing rate in response to increased rates of change in stimulation and can rapidly adapt.
      b. Joint capsules, muscle spindles, vestibular maculae, pain receptors, baroreceptors, chemoreceptors, Ruffini end organs, and Merkel disks are tonic receptors. They adapt slowly, transmit impulses for many hours, and rarely adapt to extinction.

V. Nerve Transmission

A. Neuronal axon fibers are 0.2–20 mm in diameter. The velocity of transmission ranges from 0.5–120 m/s and is fastest in large fibers. Of interest, large fibers conduct impulses over a distance equivalent to the length of a football field per second, while small fibers require up to 2 seconds to transmit impulses from the big toe to the spinal cord.

B. Types of sensory nerve fibers

1. Ia (α-type A) — annulospiral endings of muscle spindles; largest (i.e., 17 μm diameter) and fastest (120 m/s)

2. Ib (α-type A) — Golgi tendon organs; 16 μm in diameter

3. II (β- and γ-type A) — flower-spray endings of muscle spindles and cutaneous tactile receptors; 8 μm in diameter

4. III (δ-type A) — temperature, crude touch, and pricking pain; 3 μm in diameter

5. IV (type C) — unmyelinated fibers relaying pain, itch, temperature, and crude touch sensations; 0.5–2 μm in diameter

C. Types of motor nerve fibers

1. Skeletal muscle — α-type A (myelinated; fastest fibers)

2. Muscle spindle — γ-type A (myelinated)

3. Sympathetic — type C (unmyelinated; slowest fibers)

D. Neuronal circuits and information processing

1. Receptive field of a nerve fiber — the surface area it innervates. Each nerve fiber has multiple endings and most are in the center of the receptive field.

2. Spatial summation of a stimulus — The more intense a given stimulus, the greater the number of sensory nerve fibers activated. Thus, increased signal strength is relayed via progressively larger numbers of activated fibers.

3. Temporal summation — occurs when increased stimulus intensity increases the rate of neuronal firing

4. Neuronal pool — refers to a specifically organized, collective group of input and output neuronal fibers that processes signals in its own distinct way. Input fibers may have sufficiently extensive branches to relay suprathreshold stimuli into the center of the stimulatory field supplied by the neuronal pool, yet relay only subthreshold (i.e., facilitated) stimuli to the periphery. The center of the stimulatory field is the "liminal" or "stimulated zone" and the peripheral area is the "subthreshold" or "subliminal zone."

5. Divergence — occurs when an input fiber activates greater numbers of nerve fibers leaving the neuronal pool. In other words, one neuron synapses onto multiple cells, either amplifying a signal in one tract (e.g., one motor neuron stimulating 10,000 muscle fibers) or multiple tracts (e.g., dorsal column input into the cortex and cerebellum).

6. Convergence — occurs when multiple different neuronal fibers, either from similar or different sources, synapse onto one neuron. Rarely, a single presynaptic neuron is able to sufficiently stimulate a postsynaptic neuron to elicit an AP (e.g., Purkinje cells synapsing onto deep nuclei in the cerebellum).

7. Reciprocal inhibitory circuit — an axonal branch that stimulates an interneuron in the pathway, which subsequently inhibits an antagonist muscle group while simultaneously stimulating an agonist muscle group

8. After discharge — arises in the context of long-acting neurotransmitters, when lingering stimulatory input continues to elicit APs despite removal of the initial signal

9. Oscillatory (reverberatory) circuit — a circuit whose neuronal output feeds back to reactivate the circuit. A longer period between initial activation and the feedback cycle develops if more interneurons are integrated into the circuit. Synaptic fatigue ultimately stops the reverberatory cycle.

10. Signal output occurs either continuously or rhythmically.
    a. Continuous signal output arises with increased neuronal excitability caused by low RMPs (e.g., cerebellar neurons and spinal cord interneurons) and in reverberating circuits where input either increases or decreases the frequency of AP firing (e.g., autonomic nervous system).
    b. Rhythmic signal output occurs in reverberating circuits (e.g., respiratory center of the pons and medulla).

11. Neuronal circuit stability — Neuronal activity is organized and controlled by a combination of excitatory and inhibitory circuits; otherwise, signal transmission would be disrupted and hyperexcitability (i.e., seizures) could develop. Inhibitory mechanisms include
    a. Inhibitory (i.e., negative feedback) circuits that inhibit input neurons or interneurons
    b. Synaptic fatigue arising from ionic changes (in the short term) and upgrading/downgrading of receptor proteins (in the long term)

VI. Somatic Sensations

A. Tactile senses — touch, pressure, vibration, and tickle senses. Touch, pressure, and vibration use the same receptor pathways.

B. Position senses — static position and rate of movement senses

C. Somatic sensory receptors

   1. Free nerve endings — respond to pain, touch, and pressure

   2. Meissner corpuscles — respond to touch. These are rapidly-adapting receptors located superficially in dermal papillae of non-hairy skin (e.g., fingertips, lips). They have small receptor fields and transmit signals via large, myelinated β-type A fibers.

   3. Merkel disks (i.e., expanded tip tactile receptors) — respond to touch and pressure. These are slowly-adapting receptors with small receptive fields, located superficially in the dermal papillae of hairy and non-hairy skin. Merkel disks typically group together to fill a single receptor organ underneath the epithelium, the Iggo dome receptor, which is innervated by a single, myelinated, β-type A fiber.

   4. Pacinian corpuscles — respond to vibration (i.e., high-frequency stimulation). These are rapidly-adapting receptors and are located in superficial and deep tissues.

   5. Ruffini end organs — respond to heavy touch and pressure. These are slowly-adapting receptors located in deep layers (i.e., subcutaneous tissue and joint capsules) and exhibit large receptive fields.

   6. Hair end organs — respond to touch. These are rapidly-adapting receptors located at the base of hair follicles.

D. Somatic nerve fibers

   1. Touch — mostly relayed by β-type A fibers at speeds of 30–70 m/s. Free nerve endings also transmit touch sensations via myelinated δ-type A fibers at speeds of 5–30 m/s and tickle sensations via unmyelinated C fibers at speeds of 62 m/s. Crude pressure, poorly localized touch, and tickle sensations are relayed via smaller, slower fibers occupying less space in the nerve bundle.

   2. Vibration — relayed by β-type A fibers. All tactile receptors contribute, each at different frequencies (e.g., Pacinian corpuscles at 30–800 cycles/s, Meissner corpuscles at 80 cycles/s).

3. Tickle and itch — sensed by free nerve endings located superficially in the skin and relayed via C fibers. Itch impulses diminish either if the stimulant is removed or with scratching, which activates pain receptors thereby resulting in inhibition.

4. Pain — sensed by free nerve endings and is transmitted via C fibers. See the following sections for more detail.

5. Peripheral sensory or mixed nerves — contain fourfold more unmyelinated fibers than myelinated fibers. The unmyelinated fibers are C fibers; the myelinated fibers are δ-type A fibers. Proprioceptive fibers travel with motor nerves. Each axon connects to several receptors of one type.

E. Anterolateral ascending sensory system — contains smaller myelinated fibers that conduct at speeds of 2–40 m/s. It relays warm, cold, pain, crude touch, tickle, itch, and sexual sensations. These sensations do not require discrete localization, and thus they have poor spatial localization and intensity grading and slow signal repetition. Crude touch originates from laminae 1, 4, 5, and 6 in the dorsal horns. Fibers ascend in the anterior (i.e., ipsilateral) and lateral (i.e., contralateral, due to crossing of fibers in the anterior commissure, within three levels) spinothalamic tracts to the ventroposterolateral (VPL; body), ventroposteromedial (VPM; face), and posterior thalamic nuclei for touch and temperature sensations. Fibers also relay impulses in the spinoreticular tract to the intralaminar thalamic nucleus for pain.

F. Dorsal column system — contains large myelinated fibers that conduct at speeds of 30–110 m/s. It relays fine touch, vibration, position, and pressure sensations. Moreover, its fibers exhibit a greater extent of spatial orientation (i.e., somatotopic organization).

1. Axons enter the spinal cord and divide into a medial branch that travels up the dorsal column (25% of fibers) and a lateral branch (75% of fibers) with multiple synapses in the dorsal horn for reflexes. Second-order neurons are located in the medulla, within the medially situated nuclei gracilis (responsible for the lower limbs) and laterally situated nuclei cuneatus (responsible for the upper limbs). Arcuate fibers cross to form the medial lemniscus (ML), joining fibers from the main sensory nucleus of the trigeminal nerve (V) and the upper spinal nucleus of V to terminate in the thalamic VPL (body) and VPM (face).

2. The ventrobasal complex (VPL, VPM, and the posterior thalamic nucleus) sends fibers to the cortical somatosensory areas S1 and S2. A somatotopic organization exists with the lower limbs represented medially in the spinal cord, laterally in the thalamus, and medially again in the cortex (**Fig. 2.2**).

3. Position sense — static and kinesthetic proprioception to detect joint angles in all directions and the positional rate of change, respectively

4. Proprioceptive impulses — begin at the muscle spindles, Pacinian corpuscles, Ruffini end organs, and Golgi tendon organs of the extremities. Lower limb proprioception is conveyed within the lateral column from Clarke column neurons through the dorsal spinocerebellar tract to the cerebellum (i.e., not in the posterior columns). Upper extremity proprioception is conveyed through the posterior columns in the fasciculus cuneatus prior to synapsing onto the accessory cuneate nucleus in the caudal medulla, before being relayed to the cerebellum via the cuneocerebellar tract.

G. Sensory cortex — Neuronal cells are arranged in vertical columns of 10,000 neurons, each column of diameter 0.3–0.5 mm and able to detect one sensory modality. Different modality columns are interspersed with one another.

1. Six layers of neurons in the cerebral cortex
   a. Layers 1 (most superficial) and 2 receive diffuse, nonspecific input from the lower brain and may control the excitability of a region.

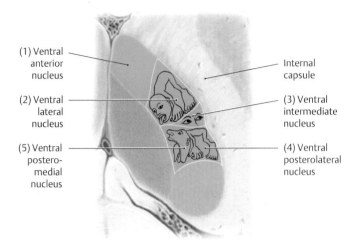

(1) Ventral anterior nucleus

(2) Ventral lateral nucleus

(5) Ventral postero-medial nucleus

Internal capsule

(3) Ventral intermediate nucleus

(4) Ventral posterolateral nucleus

Fig. 2.2   Somatotopic organization of specific thalamic nuclei. Transverse section. Ventrolateral thalamic nuclei receive afferents from the crossed superior cerebellar peduncle and relay to the cortex. The lateral part of the ventrolateral nucleus relays impulses from the extremities and the medial part relays impulses from the head. The ventral intermediate nucleus receives vestibular input. The posterior column input is via the medial lemniscus to the ventral posterolateral nucleus, and trigeminal fibers from the head enter the ventral posteromedial nucleus. (From THIEME Atlas of Anatomy, Head and Neuroanatomy, © Thieme 2007, Illustration by Markus Voll.)

   b. Layers 2 (association fibers) and 3 (association and commissural fibers) relay axons to other cortical areas.

   c. Layer 4 of each column does not interact with the other columns, whereas other layers do. Afferent fibers arrive in layer 4 and either spread up or down a column.

   d. Layers 5 and 6 (projection fibers) disperse axons to distant parts of the nervous system. Layer 5 is larger and connects to the brainstem and spinal cord, whereas layer 6 is smaller and connects to the thalamus.

2. Different somatic cortical regions regulate different areas of the body; the size of these cortical regions is dependent upon sensory receptor numbers in these various body sites. Furthermore, all sensory pathways contribute to lateral inhibition of adjacent neurons, either via interneurons or presynaptic inhibition, to increase the degree of contrast between activated and inhibited neuronal pools in that region.

3. Intensity discrimination — decreases as stimulus intensity is increased. However, percent change is more important than total stimulus intensity; thus, in the context of an increased intensity of stimulation, a greater percent change in stimulus is required for that stimulus to be detected.

4. Primary somatosensory area (S1, Brodmann areas 1, 2, 3) — localizes sensations and detects pressure, weight, shapes, and textures. No pain or temperature loss arises if S1 is removed; however, localization is diminished. The facial region above the nose is represented bilaterally; also, the lips have the largest area of representation. Brodmann area 1 receives input from rapidly-adapting skin receptors; area 2 from deep pressure and joint position receptors; area 3a (located anterior and deep in the central sulcus with connections to the motor cortex) from muscle, tendon, and joint stretch receptors; and area 3b from both slowly- and rapidly-adapting skin receptors. Activation of these receptors elicits contralateral sensory perception.

5. Secondary somatosensory area (S2) — located posterolateral to S1 on the superior bank of the sylvian fissure. It has poor primary sensory representation but is required for shape discrimination, at least in animals. The lower limbs are represented medially. Stimulation elicits bilateral sensory perception in this region.

6. Somatic association areas (Brodmann areas 5, 7) — located behind S1 and above S2. Receives input from S1, ventrobasal thalamus (VPL, VPM, posterior thalamic nucleus), visual cortex, and auditory cortex. Stimulation elicits complex body sensations. A lesion in this region results in amorphosynthesis

(i.e., the inability to recognize or detect objects sensed contralaterally) and astereognosia. This region contributes to two-point discrimination (1 mm in the finger, 30–70 mm in the back).

7. Thalamus — discriminates pain and temperature (and to a lesser extent, touch). Inhibitory corticofugal fibers synapse onto peripheral relay nuclei in the thalamus, medulla, and spinal cord to regulate sensitivity to input, to decrease lateral spread (and thus increase signal contrast), and to maintain the sensory system in an appropriate operating range of sensitivity.

H. Pain and temperature sensation

1. Pain serves a protective function and, unlike sensations other than vision (otherwise one would be blind in continuous light), is nonadapting. It may be classified as follows:
    a. Fast pain — occurs in 0.1 second, travels 6–30 m/s, and is sharp and electric in quality. It is relayed via δ–type A fibers and is detected by mechanical and thermal receptors in the skin.
    b. Slow pain — occurs after 1 second but increases over seconds to minutes, travels 0.5–2 m/s, and is burning, aching, and/or throbbing. It is transmitted by C fibers, detected by all receptors in the skin and deep tissues, and generally associated with tissue destruction.

2. Pain receptors — free nerve endings located in the skin, periosteum, arterial walls, joint surfaces, and dura. They respond to mechanical, thermal, and chemical stimuli to varying degrees and exhibit very little adaptation to these stimuli. In fact, pain receptors may even become more sensitive (i.e., hyperalgesic) to persistent stimuli. Furthermore, increased pain intensity reflects increased tissue damage.

3. Pain pathway mediators — bradykinin, 5-hydroxytryptamine (5-HT; serotonin), histamine, K^+, acids, acetylcholine (ACh), and proteolytic enzymes all activate pain receptors. Prostaglandins enhance pain receptor sensitivity but do not themselves excite these receptors.

4. Potential causes of pain
    a. Thermal pain — activated at $\geq 45°C$, at which point tissue damage begins
    b. Tissue ischemia — Pain results from altered tissue metabolism, likely attributed to the production of lactate (i.e., acidosis).
    c. Spasm of a muscle, artery, or hollow viscus — induces pain by stimulating mechanoreceptors or indirectly compressing blood vessels, resulting in ischemia. Spasmodic activity increases metabolism in muscle tissue, contributing to ischemia and releasing chemical mediators of pain.
    d. Neurogenic inflammation — elicited by antidromic APs from spinal ganglia stimulating the release of substance P from C fiber terminals in the skin. Erythema and edematous changes ensue following histamine release.

5. Relevant anatomy
    a. Afferent pain fibers — enter the spinal cord to ascend/descend 1–3 segments in Lissauer tract (i.e., posterior to the dorsal horn), prior to terminating in the dorsal horn itself
    b. Neospinothalamic tract — relays fast pain with better localization than for slow pain (but only to ~10 cm, unless tactile sensation is also activated). It is composed of δ-type A fibers receiving sensory input from mechanical and thermal receptors and relays impulses (via glutamate, a fast-acting transmitter) to second-order neurons in lamina 1 (i.e., lamina marginalis). These cross in the anterior commissure of the spinal cord, ascend in the anterolateral tracts to synapse onto third-order neurons in the ventrobasal thalamus, and then continue on to fourth-order neurons in the somatosensory cortex.
    c. Paleospinothalamic tract — transmits slow pain with poor localization, due to its diffuse connectivity. It consists of C fibers synapsing onto second-order neurons in laminas 2 and 3 (i.e., substantia gelatinosa) via glutamate and substance P (i.e., a slow-acting transmitter), ultimately

relaying signals to laminas 5–8. From here, impulses cross in the anterior commissure (although some remain ipsilateral) and ascend to third-order neurons in the reticular formation, tectum, and periaqueductal gray matter; only 10–25% continue to terminate in the thalamus. The reticular formation then relays fibers to the thalamic intralaminar nuclei, hypothalamus, and basal brain, accounting for the strong arousal (and suffering) associated with pain. Note that conscious pain may be perceived without cortical processing of painful stimuli, but the cortex likely helps to qualify such sensations.

6. Analgesia system

    a. Periaqueductal gray matter and periventricular hypothalamus — contain neurons whose axons release enkephalins onto the nucleus raphe magnus (lower pons and upper medulla) and the nucleus reticularis paragigantocellularis (lateral medulla). Secondary neurons release 5-HT to a pain inhibition complex in the dorsolateral spinal cord. Ultimately, the analgesia system blocks pain before it is relayed to the brain.

        (1) Enkephalins cause presynaptic inhibition of C and δ-type A fibers in the dorsal horns by blocking Ca^{2+} channels. These enkephalins mediate presynaptic pain inhibition, particularly in laminas 1, 2, and 5. Neurons in laminas 1 and 5 possess presynaptic and postsynaptic opiate receptors. NE from the pons also decreases pain, thus accounting for stress-induced analgesia.

        (2) Endogenous opiates — β-endorphin (i.e., hypothalamus and pituitary), met-enkephalin and leu-enkephalin (i.e., spinal cord system), and dynorphin (200 times more potent than morphine)

    b. "Gate control" theory — introduced by Melzack and Wall in 1965. Large myelinated fibers have negative dorsal root potentials, and smaller C fibers have positive potentials. Stimulation of the larger fibers prevents transmission of pain impulses in the smaller fibers by maintaining a negative potential in the dorsal horns. One problem with this theory is that the loss of large myelinated fibers does not result in increased pain. However, electrical stimulation of large fibers by transcutaneous electrical nerve stimulation (TENS) units, spinal cord stimulators, or deep brain stimulators does appear to cause lateral inhibition of pain. Acupuncture may also work via this mechanism, as well as by endogenous opiates and psychogenic input.

    c. Medical treatment for pain — Amitriptyline decreases pain by stimulating 5-HT release from the descending pathway and increasing NE release. Nonsteroidal antiinflammatory drugs (NSAIDs) decrease the production of pain-stimulating prostaglandins.

    d. Deep brain stimulation of the periventricular and periaqueductal gray matter has been used to treat chronic pain. Side effects of periaqueductal gray matter stimulation are diplopia, oscillopsia, fear, and anxiety. Stimulation of periventricular gray matter is much better tolerated.

7. Referred pain — Visceral pain fibers synapse onto the same secondary neurons in the spinal cord (lamina 5) as do fibers from the skin, such that they conduct via the same central pathway. The only visceral receptors that reach consciousness are for pain.

    a. Visceral pain — different from surface pain. Focal injuries are not very painful, but diffuse injuries (e.g., ischemic gut) certainly are, mediated by pain-relaying C fibers that travel with sympathetic (occasionally parasympathetic) nerves.

    b. Visceral pain is triggered by ischemia, chemical damage, spasm, distention, and ligamentous stretching. Spasm and distention cause both mechanical pain and ischemia. The liver parenchyma and lung alveoli are insensitive to pain, but the bronchi, parietal pleura, liver capsule, and bile ducts are all sensitive.

c. Parietal pleura, peritoneum, and pericardium — Referred pain from parietal surfaces is sharp and relayed by spinal nerves innervating the parietal surface overlying a particular viscus.

d. From an embryological standpoint, the heart originates in the neck/upper thorax of the embryo; thus, visceral pain is referred to C3–T5 (i.e., neck, shoulder, and arm). Pain is also more frequently left-sided than right-sided because left-sided vessels (e.g., aorta) are more often occluded by coronary artery disease.

e. Visceral pain is localized by two transmission pathways.

   (1) "True" visceral pain — referred pain to body surface areas, dependent on sensory C fiber transmission to autonomic nerves

   (2) Parietal sensations — Irritated parietal surfaces relay pain directly into spinal nerves. For example, appendicitis typically begins with periumbilical pain from C fibers, progressing to right-sided, lower-quadrant pain from δ-type A fibers. These help to localize the pain once the inflamed appendix irritates the overlying peritoneum.

8. Pain syndromes

  a. Hyperalgesia — increased sensitivity (i.e., decreased threshold) to pain

    (1) Primary hyperalgesia — increased sensitivity of receptors (e.g., sunburn, due to histamine release from damaged tissue)

    (2) Secondary hyperalgesia — due to facilitation resulting from lesions in the spinal cord or thalamus

  b. Hyperpathia — increased reaction to pain, but with increased threshold

  c. Allodynia — pain triggered by typically nonpainful stimuli (e.g., light touch)

  d. Reflex sympathetic dystrophy — may develop following neuronal damage, with the sprouting of axons that are sensitive to EPI or NE

  e. Phantom pain — may arise in the absence of normal input, when pain-related neurons in lamina 5 (and later the thalamus) fire spontaneously

  f. Thalamic pain (Dejerine–Roussy) syndrome — usually due to a posteroventral thalamic stroke causing ataxia and contralateral hemianesthesia, which in subsequent weeks to months is characterized by a return of crude sensation, but also increased pain and affective, unpleasant feelings. It may be caused by facilitation of the medial thalamic nucleus with increased transmission of reticular formation pain.

  g. Shingles (herpes zoster) — Pain is triggered by irritation of the dorsal root ganglion cells, following localized infection with the herpesvirus.

9. Headache — caused by referred pain from sinuses, temporomandibular joint, ocular structures, dura, blood vessels, or other deep structures. The brain itself is insensitive to pain, but the sinuses, tentorium, dura, and vessels are all sensitive.

  a. Innervation

    (1) Supratentorially — by the trigeminal nerve; manifests as frontal headache

    (2) Infratentorially — by C2, cranial nerve (CN) IX, and CN X; manifests as occipital and retroauricular headache

  b. Postlumbar puncture headache — caused by a decreased cerebrospinal fluid (CSF) volume that allows the weight of the brain to stretch blood vessels bridging from the surface of the brain to the skull

  c. Migraine headaches — likely a vascular phenomenon; caused by reflex spasm of intracranial arteries leading to ischemia, followed by dilatation for 24–48 hours, with increased blood flow and arterial wall stretching that produces a throbbing type of headache

  d. Postethanol or "hangover" pain — due to chemical irritation of the meninges

e. Constipation pain — occurs even with a transected spinal cord, possibly via absorbed toxins or circulatory system changes

f. Muscle spasms — produce referred pain over the scalp

g. Nasal structures — may become inflamed, causing headache

h. Eye activity — Ciliary muscle contraction (i.e., attempting to obtain focused vision) and reflex vasospasm may cause a retroorbital headache.

10. Thermal sensation — detected by three receptors:

a. Cold receptors — more numerous; consist of myelinated δ-type A fibers terminating in the basal epidermal cells, and some free C fiber endings

b. Warm receptors — free nerve endings from C fibers; stimulated if the temperature is >30 °C

c. Pain receptors for extreme temperatures (i.e. <10 °C or >45 °C) — These receptors are in the subcutaneous tissue and separate from each other. The receptive field is 1 mm in diameter and detects a change in temperature with slow adaptation, activating receptors by changing the metabolic rate of neurons. Fibers enter the spinal cord, travel in the Lissauer tract; synapse in laminas 1, 2, and 3 (i.e., same as pain); cross to the contralateral side; and ascend to the reticular formation, ventrobasal thalamus, and S1 cortex.

VII. Vision

A. Physics of vision

1. Speed of light — 300,000 km/s in a vacuum; slightly less in air and much less in a liquid or solid

2. Refraction — bending of light rays at an interface between substances of different density. Refraction depends on the angle between the interface and the wave front (e.g., no refraction occurs if these are perpendicular), and the ratio of the two refractive indices. Refractive index = Velocity in air/velocity in a substance. The refractive index of air is 1.

3. Convex lens — Rays converge at a focal point beyond the lens.

4. Concave lens — Rays diverge, with the focal point before the lens.

5. Focal length (f) — determined via the equation: $1/f = 1/a + 1/b$, where a = distance from a point source to the lens and b = distance of focus

6. Refractive power — increases as the lens bends rays to a greater extent. It is measured in diopters (D) = $1/f$ (in meters). +1 D means the focal point is 1 m beyond a convex lens, +2 is 0.5 m, and +10 is 0.1 m. With a concave lens, the diopter number is negative.

7. The eye functions as a camera with four refractive indices: air/cornea, cornea/aqueous humor, aqueous humor/lens, and lens/vitreous humor. Most refraction occurs at the air/cornea interface because the other components are similar in density. The lens is less refractive as it is surrounded by fluid, but it is necessary for accommodation. The image on the retina is inverted and reversed. The eye unit has a maximum refraction of 59 D. Refractive power in children ranges from 20 to 34 D, with an accommodation of 14 D.

8. Depth perception is achieved by:

a. Subconsciously comparing a visualized object's size against the expected size

b. Moving parallax — Nearby objects move more in the visual field when the head is turned.

c. Stereopsis — binocular vision, whereby an image strikes both eyes at different retinal sites

9. Intraocular pressure — normally 12–20 mm Hg. A tonometer works by resting a plunger on the eye and measuring the displacement that ensues with the application of a defined pressure.

B. Anatomy of the eye

1. Lens — a strong, elastic capsule filled with proteinaceous transparent fibers. When it is relaxed, it is spherical in shape. Seventy ligaments (zonules) are radially attached to the lens and the ciliary body at the anterior border of the choroid, to provide constant tension to maintain the lens in a flat shape.

2. Ciliary body — has ciliary muscles with two sets of fibers: meridional fibers that attach to the corneo-scleral junction, and circular fibers that are sphincter-like around the eye.

3. Ciliary muscle contraction — causes the eyeball to become narrower and thus decreases tension on the lens, allowing it to become more spherical. When the ciliary muscle relaxes, the lens is pulled flat. The ciliary muscle is innervated by parasympathetic nerves and serves to increase the eye's refractive power for accommodation to focus on closer objects.

4. Pupil — When the pupil is small, the eye's focus is better because most of the light enters at a fairly straight trajectory and less refraction is needed.

5. Eye fluid — maintains distention of the eye
    a. Vitreous humor — a gelatinous mass held by a fibrillary network of proteoglycans. It does not flow, but some diffusion occurs.
    b. Aqueous humor — free-flowing fluid. A balance of production and reabsorption regulates intra-ocular pressure. The ciliary body's ciliary processes secrete aqueous humor by active Na^+ secretion that draws in Cl^-, HCO_3^-, and H_2O. Aqueous humor flows out of the pupil through small trabeculae at the iris–corneal junction and through the Schlemm's canal into the venous system.

6. Layers of the eye — sclera, choroid (vascular layer), and retina

7. Retina — composed of outer-pigmented layer, rods and cones, outer limiting membrane, outer nuclear layer (containing cell bodies of the rods and cones), outer plexiform layer, inner nuclear layer, inner plexiform layer, ganglionic layer, optic nerve fiber layer, and inner limiting membrane. The outer pigment layer contains black melanin to prevent light reflection and stores large quantities of vitamin A for exchange with the rods and cones. It is absent in albinism, causing those affected to have poor visual acuity.

8. Retinal blood supply — The inner layers are supplied by the central retinal artery that enters through the optic nerve; the outer layers are adherent to the choroid and are supplied by diffusion from the choroid to the outer segments of the rods and cones.

9. Macula — the region of the retina with the highest visual acuity, measuring 61 mm²

10. Fovea — the center of the macula that contains only cones, with the inner layers set aside to provide improved vision

11. Blind spot — 15 degrees lateral to central vision, due to the medial location of the optic disk in the retina

12. Rods and cones — Rods have outer segments containing light-sensitive rhodopsin with transmembrane proteins and multiple membrane folds shaped into disks. Cones contain other types of photochemicals. Cones are 300 times less sensitive than rods, so color vision is poor in dim lighting. The rod pathway connects to bipolar cells, then to amacrine cells, and finally to ganglion cells. The cone

pathway, however, is phylogenetically newer, faster, and uses larger cells and fibers; the cone pathway connects to bipolar cells and then to ganglion cells. The neurotransmitter of rods and cones is glutamate. Amacrine cells have at least eight types of neurotransmitters; all of them are inhibitory.

13. Innervation of the eye
    a. Parasympathetic innervation — begins at the Edinger–Westphal nucleus, transmitting via the third nerve → ciliary ganglion behind the eye → short ciliary nerves → ciliary muscle (for accommodation) and iris sphincter (for miosis)
    b. Sympathetic innervations — from the T1 level → sympathetic chain → superior cervical ganglion, up along the carotid artery to the small vessels, and then as the long and short ciliary nerves to the eye's radial iris fibers (for mydriasis), to the Müller muscle of the eyelid and weakly to the ciliary muscle
    c. Accommodation — from Brodmann areas 18/19 to the pretectal/Edinger–Westphal area, and on to the ciliary muscle. The accommodation reflex elicits slight pupillary constriction. If there is no response to light, yet the accommodation reflex is intact, this is called an Argyll–Robertson pupil (as seen with syphilis).
    d. The pupil is innervated at the iris sphincter by parasympathetic nerves, and at the radial iris muscles by sympathetic nerves. The light reflex is activated by impulses from the retina → optic tract → pretectal nucleus → Edinger–Westphal nucleus → third nerve → iris sphincter. It is decreased in syphilis, ethanol intoxication, etc.

C. Visual conditions

1. Presbyopia — caused by lack of accommodation as the lens becomes larger, thicker, and less elastic with advancing age, causing the eye to remain permanently focused at a certain distance. Bifocals are required for near and far clarity. At 45 years of age, only 2 D of change is present; at 70 years, usually no change is present.

2. Hyperopia (farsightedness) — caused by either a short eyeball or a weak lens that does not curve sufficiently when the ciliary body is relaxed (i.e., the ciliary muscle is contracted). Near vision is difficult. This condition is treated with a convex lens.

3. Myopia (nearsightedness) — caused by an eyeball that is too long or a lens that is too strong. Light focuses in front of the retina because the lens is unable to straighten sufficiently despite a relaxed ciliary muscle. Far vision is difficult. This condition is treated with divergence of rays by a concave, spherical lens.

4. Astigmatism — caused by refractive error of the lens system from an oblong cornea (rarely from the lens). Rays focus at one distance in one plane, and another in another plane. It is treated with spherical and cylindrical lenses of a certain axis.

5. Cataracts — opacities of the lens due to build-up of coagulated, denatured protein. They are treated by removal of the lens.

6. Glaucoma — increased intraocular pressure; levels of 60–70 mm Hg commonly cause blindness, although even levels slightly > 20 mm Hg may compromise vision. The elevated pressure on the optic disk causes atrophy. It is caused by decreased trabecular aqueous humor outflow, as occurs in acute inflammation or chronic fibrosis. It is treated with drops to decrease aqueous humor formation or to increase its absorption. It may also be treated surgically to open the outflow pathway.

7. Retinal detachment — retinal separation from the pigment epithelium; occurs with trauma (i.e., when blood or fluid accumulates behind the retina) or by uneven contractures of fine collagen fibrils in the vitreous humor, causing the retina to pull away. The retina maintains its own blood supply for a few days, affording a window for surgical repair; if this is delayed, it degenerates and never regains function.

8. Scotoma — an area of decreased vision surrounded by preserved vision in the visual field. Causative etiologies include lead, tobacco, retinal disease, glaucoma, macular degeneration, retinal ischemia, and trauma.

9. Strabismus (cross-eyed) — when eye fusion mechanisms are not coordinated. It may be horizontal, vertical, or torsional (rotational). One eye may eventually become suppressed, leading to decreased acuity during development.

10. Horner syndrome — caused by impaired sympathetic input resulting in miosis, ptosis (i.e., sympathetic nerves innervate the smooth muscle of the eyelid), anhidrosis, enophthalmos, and dilated facial vessels

D. Photochemistry

1. Important molecules
   a. Rhodopsin — light-sensitive pigment; combination of scotopsin + 11-cis-retinal. When light energy is absorbed, rhodopsin decomposes via photoactivation of an electron in the retinal component, converting it to the trans form, which pulls away from scotopsin (i.e., rhodopsin + light → bathorhodopsin → lumirhodopsin → metarhodopsin-1 → metarhodopsin-2 → scotopsin and all-trans-retinal). Rhodopsin is reformed by all-trans-retinal → 2-cis-retinal + scotopsin → rhodopsin; it is also reformed by all-trans-retinal → all-trans-retinol (vitamin A) → 2-cis-retinol → 2-cis-retinal → rhodopsin.
   b. G protein — Each G protein is regulated by many receptors and itself regulates many effectors. The α-subunit binds guanosine triphosphate (GTP); the β- and γ-subunits hold the α-subunit to the plasma membrane and modulate GTP/ guanosine diphosphate (GDP) exchange. The conversion from GTP to GDP inactivates the G protein. β and γ subunits stabilize GDP binding and inhibit the binding of GTP to inactivate the G protein. When it is activated, the α-subunit has decreased affinity for the β- and γ-subunits. Activation of the G protein inhibits others in the membrane.
   c. Vitamin A (all-trans-retinol) — contained in the cytoplasm of rods and the pigment layer of the retina. Retinal (a light-sensitive pigment) can be converted to retinol (i.e., vitamin A) for storage.

2. Phototransduction — occurs as activated rhodopsin (i.e., metarhodopsin-2) initiates a G protein-mediated pathway, wherein cGMP phosphodiesterase converts cGMP to 5′GMP (thus decreasing the concentration of cGMP). This decreases current through cGMP-activated Na^+ channels, leading to hyperpolarization. The resting membrane potential is –40 mV because the outer portion is leaky to Na^+, whereas the inner segment actively pumps it out. The activated membrane potential is –80 mV, at maximal light intensity. Light only has to activate the receptor for 0.0001 milliseconds, but the receptor potential persists for longer than 1 second. The receptor potential is proportional to light intensity. There is an amplifying cascade effect, such that one photon of light causes the movement of millions of Na^+ ions. Rhodopsin kinase inactivates rhodopsin within a fraction of a second.

3. Night blindness — due to a severe vitamin A deficiency, leading to inadequate amounts of photosensitive pigment to detect light in dim/dark settings. This may be cured within an hour with intravenous vitamin A.

4. Sensitivity of rods and cones — proportional to opsin concentration. If one remains in bright light for a prolonged length of time, most of the photochemicals are reduced to retinal and opsins; retinal is converted to vitamin A to decrease the sensitivity for light adaptation. If one moves into the dark for a time, the number of active photopigments is increased (i.e., dark adaptation). Cones adapt first (within 10 minutes), up to 100-fold; rods (which take 40 minutes to adapt) become 25,000 times more sensitive. Light adaptation also depends on pupillary size (up to 30-fold change in sensitivity) and neural adaptation (through decreased firing).

5. Color vision — relies on photopsins that are sensitive to red, green, and blue, with peak absorptions at specific wavelengths. Color is interpreted by the percent stimulation of each color cone (e.g., orange color results from stimulation of 99% of red cones, 42% of green cones, and 0% of blue cones). White light is produced by the equivalent stimulation of red, green, and blue cones. Color constancy relates to the brain's ability to detect an object's natural color even after it undergoes color illumination by another colored light source. Color blindness is due to the absence of a single or multiple groups of cones. Red or green color blindness is X-linked; rarely is blue missing. Color blindness is tested using Ishihara (color spot) charts.

6. Cell types
   a. Retinal cells — conduct signals by electrical conduction, not APs (except for ganglion cells). This allows for graded conduction of signal strength with increased light intensity, leading to greater hyperpolarization. Retinal cells consist of 100 million rods, 3 million cones, and 1.6 million ganglion cells. Each optic nerve fiber receives input from ~60 rods and 2 cones. Near the fovea, rods and cones are more slender and there are fewer of them per ganglion cell (increasing the visual acuity). No rods are in the fovea. The peripheral retina is more sensitive to weak light than the fovea because the rods are 300 times more sensitive than the cones, and 200 rods provide input to each ganglion cell.
   b. Photoreceptor cells — connect to bipolar and horizontal cells
   c. Horizontal cells — transmit signals horizontally within the outer plexiform layers. Their afferent fibers arrive from rods/cones, and their efferent fibers relay to bipolar cells (contributing to lateral inhibition to increase contrast).
   d. Bipolar cells — Afferent fibers arrive from rods, cones, and horizontal cells; efferent fibers relay to the inner layer amacrine and ganglion cells. Impulses either depolarize or hyperpolarize to affect lateral inhibition.
   e. Amacrine cells — Afferent fibers arrive from bipolar cells; efferent fibers relay to ganglion cells and horizontal cells in the inner plexus layer.
   f. Ganglion cells — relay their axons through the optic nerve. W cells make up 40% of the fibers, are small, slow (8 m/s), synapse with rods, supply large fields, and are used for directional and dark vision; X cells make up 55%, are medium-sized, travel at 14 m/s, supply small fields, synapse with cones, and serve accurate color vision; Y cells make up 5%, are the largest and fastest (50 m/s), have wide fields, and detect changes in fields and black and white vision. There are continuous impulses in the background (5–40/s). Ganglion cells respond to borders of vision by excitatory/inhibitory bipolar cells. If light hits all the cells, stimulation and inhibition cancel each other out, and no firing occurs. Each ganglion cell is stimulated or inhibited by specific colors.
   g. Interplexiform cells — run from the inner plexiform layer to the outer plexiform layer, and laterally inhibit to increase contrast

E. Visual pathway's optic tract projections (**Fig. 2.3**)

   1. Suprachiasmatic nuclei of the hypothalamus — for circadian rhythms

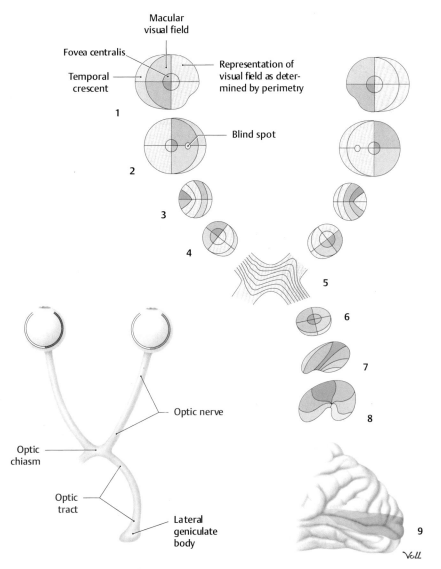

Fig. 2.3 Topographic organization of the visual pathways. The fovea centralis has the maximal visual acuity and highest receptor density. Accordingly there are more axons from this part and greater representation in the visual cortex. The diagram shows the left half of the complete visual field subdivided into four quadrants (clockwise from top left in (1): upper temporal, upper nasal, lower nasal, and lower temporal. This representation is carried through to the visual cortex. (1) The three zones that make up a particular visual hemifield (in this case the left) are indicated by color shading of decreasing intensity. The smallest, darkest is the fovea centralis, the next is the macular zone, and the outermost is the temporal crescent. The lower nasal quadrant of each visual field is indented by the nose. (2) The visual fields are reversed after passing through the lens of the eye. (3, 4) In the initial part of the optic nerve, the fibers that represent the macular visual field first occupy a lateral position (3) and then move toward the center of the nerve (4). (5) In traversing the optic chiasm, the nasal fibers of the optic nerve cross the midline to the opposite side. (6) At the start of the optic tract, the fibers from the corresponding halves of the retinae unite. The fibers from the right visual field terminate in the left striate cortex. (7) At the end of the optic tract, just before the lateral geniculate body, the fibers collect to form a wedge. (8) In the lateral geniculate body, the wedge shape is preserved, the macular fibers occupying almost half the wedge. The fibers relay to a fourth neuron and project to the visual cortex. (From THIEME Atlas of Anatomy, Head and Neuroanatomy, © Thieme 2007, Illustration by Markus Voll.)

2. Pretectal nuclei — for eye and pupillary reflexes

3. Superior colliculi — for conjugate eye movements in response to head movements

4. Ventral lateral geniculate bodies (LGBs) — to basal brain for behavioral functions

5. Dorsal LGBs — to relay organized visual fibers to the cortex and gate input (all inhibitory) by corticofugal and midbrain reticular fibers. The LGB layers 1 and 2 contain magnocellular large neurons with input from Y cells and detect black and white vision only. Layers 3 to 6 are parvicellular (smaller cells) and receive input mostly from the X cells; they transmit color vision. The LGB input is from the contralateral eye to layers 1, 4, and 6 and from the ipsilateral eye to layers 2, 3, and 5.

F. Visual cortex

1. Primary visual (striate) cortex — Brodmann area 17, located above and below the calcarine fissure in the medial occipital lobe. The macular field is represented at the pole, with peripheral fields located more anteriorly. The upper field is represented inferiorly, and the right field is represented on the left-hand side.

2. Ocular dominance columns — several million columns, each 40 μm wide, containing 1000 neurons each. The signals from each eye alternate as they enter these columns. No ocular dominance columns exist for the monocular temporal crescent or the blind spot (because these are only detected by one eye).

3. The cortex has six layers. Afferent input from the geniculocalcarine tract is to layer 4, just as in all sensory systems. This layer has thin stripes from alternating eyes, called the lines of Gennari, and they eventually blend together. The secondary visual area/visual association area (Brodmann areas 18 and 19) are anterior to the primary visual area, used to analyze visual information.

4. Cortical processing — There are concentric receptive fields with either on-center or off-center projections from the retinal ganglion cells or lateral geniculate cells.
   a. Simple cells of the primary visual cortex — have a rectangular field
   b. Complex cells — no clear border, and orientation is more important than position
   c. Color blobs — interspersed among the primary visual columns for color depiction. Three-dimensional position, form, and motion are detected in black and white by the Y cells, and relayed to the middle posterotemporal and occipitoparietal cortex. Detail and color are relayed to the inferior ventromedial occipitotemporal cortex.
   d. Cortex and ganglion cells — exhibit maximal excitation at the borders of a pattern. Serial analysis occurs from simple to complex to hypercomplex cells, with increasing detail. There is parallel analysis of different information at different sites.

G. Eye fixation

1. Voluntary fixation — used to locate objects; initiated by the premotor cortex in the middle frontal gyrus

2. Involuntary fixation — used to keep an object in the foveal field; controlled by the tertiary visual area (Brodmann area 19). The eyes exhibit continuous tremor, slow drift, and flicker. The reflex is from area 19 to the superior colliculus, to the reticular formation, and finally to the extraocular muscle nuclei.

3. Saccades — shifting of the eyes from one point to the next in a moving field

4. Pursuit movements — keep the eyes fixed on a moving object. Even if the visual cortex is destroyed, the superior colliculus (with visuotopic representation) turns the head toward a visual disturbance by medial longitudinal fasciculus (MLF) input.

5. Superior colliculus — orients the eyes to visual, auditory, and somatic input, thus allowing the eyes to track head movements

VIII. Hearing

A. Inner anatomy of the ear

1. Tympanic membrane — attached to the malleus, incus, and then the stapes that lies against the oval window of the cochlea. The handle of the malleus is constantly pulled inward. The tympanic membrane is kept tense by the tensor tympani muscle (innervated by a branch of V3).

2. Ossicles — malleus, incus, and stapes. Do not change the amplitude of the sound wave, but they increase the force by a factor of 1.3. Because the surface area of the tympanic membrane is 55 mm^2 and that at the base of the stapes is 3.2 mm^2, the 17-fold amplification imposes a 22-fold (i.e., 17 × 1.3) pressure increase on the cochlea compared with the tympanic membrane.

3. Cochlea (**Fig. 2.4** and **Fig. 2.5**) — consists of three side-by-side coiled tubes that rotate 2.5 times, with the scala media in the center. Sound vibrations enter the scala vestibuli and the scala media (owing to

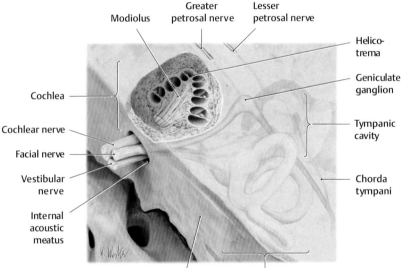

A

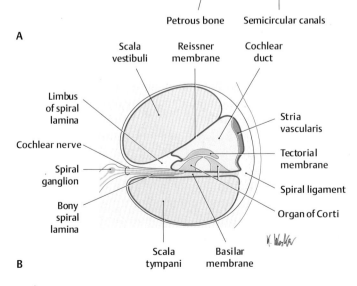

B

Fig. 2.4   The location and structure of the cochlea. (**A**) Cross-section through the cochlea. (**B**) The three compartments of the cochlear canal. The bony canal of the cochlea is 30–35 mm long and makes 2.5 turns around its bony-axis, the modiolus, which contains the spiral ganglion (**A**). A cross-section through the cochlear canal displays the three membranous compartments arranged in three levels (**B**). The upper and lower compartments, the scala vestibuli and scala tympani, each contain perilymph; the middle level, the cochlear duct (scala media) contains endolymph. The perilymphatic spaces are interconnected at the apex by the helicotrema, whereas the endolymphatic space ends blindly at the apex. The vestibular Reissner membrane separates the cochlear duct from the scala vestibuli, and the basilar membrane separates the cochlear duct from the scala tympani. (*Continued on page 136*)

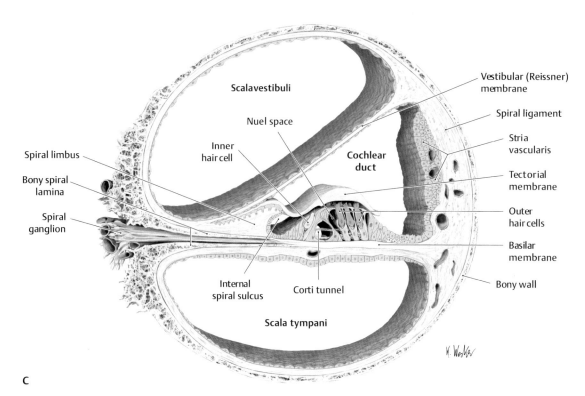

C

Fig. 2.4   The location and structure of the cochlea. (*Continued from page 135*) (**C**) Cochlear turn with sensory apparatus. A magnified cross section of a cochlear turn shows the stria vascularis, a layer of vascularized epithelium in which the endolymph is formed. This endolymph fills the membranous labyrinth (appearing here as the cochlear duct). The organ of Corti is located on the basilar membrane. It transforms energy of the acoustic traveling wave into electrical impulses, which are carried by the cochlear nerve. (From THIEME Atlas of Anatomy, Head and Neuroanatomy, © Thieme 2007, Illustration by Karl Wesker.)

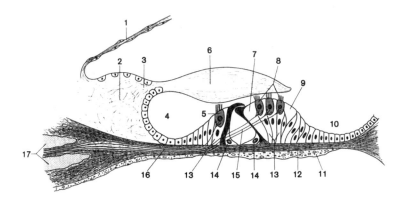

Fig. 2.5   The cochlea. 1. Vestibular (Reissner) membrane. 2. Limbus of osseous spiral lamina. 3. Vestibular lip. 4. Internal spiral sulcus. 5. Inner hair (sensory) cell. 6. Tectorial membrane. 7. Nuel's space. 8. Outer hair (sensory) cells. 9. Outer tunnel. 10. External spiral sulcus. 11. Lining tissue of scala tympani. 12. Basilar membrane. 13. Outer phalangeal (Deiter) cells. 14. Pillar cells. 15. Nerve fibers in inner tunnel. 16. Dendrites of cell bodies located in spiral ganglion. 17. Osseous spiral lamina. (From Frick H, Leonhardt H, Starck D. Human Anatomy 2. New York, NY: Thieme, 1991. Reprinted by permission.)

the flexibility of the Reissner's membrane). The basilar membrane is a fibrous membrane separating the scala media and scala tympani, made of 25,000 fibers extending from the bony center of the cochlea (i.e., modiolus) to the outer wall. These fibers are reed-like and fixed at the modiolus, yet free at their outer ends to enable them to vibrate. The basilar fibers also get longer and narrower and thus less stiff as they approach the apex of the cochlea. Near the oval window, they are stiff and short and detect higher frequencies. Vibrations at the apex have lower frequencies. The cochlea is bounded on all sides by bony walls; if the stapes and the oval window move inward, the round window pushes outward and the basilar reeds move inward. Sound waves proceed forward until they meet reeds with the same frequency, which then vibrate with ease until the sound dies out. High-frequency waves only travel short distances in the cochlea.

4. Organ of Corti — hearing receptor that senses vibration, located on the surface of the basilar membrane. It has internal and external hair cells. The bases and sides of the hair cells synapse with cochlear nerve endings that have cell bodies in the spiral ganglion within the modiolus at the center of the cochlea. Axons from the spiral ganglion constitute the cochlear nerve.
   a. One hundred stereocilia project from each of the hair cells into the gel of the tectorial membrane in the scala media. Depending on how they bend, they induce either hyperpolarization or depolarization. The tectorial membrane remains still while the basilar membrane shifts in response to vibrations.
   b. Depolarization — occurs by increased K^+ conductance into the stereocilia; the scala media contains endolymph, whereas the scala vestibuli and the scala tympani contain perilymph that communicates with the CSF and the perilymph of the vestibular organs.
   c. Endolymph — secreted by the stria vascularis; contains high K^+ and low Na^+ (i.e., more like intracellular fluid, unlike perilymph). The scala media's endolymph potential is +80 mV compared with that of the perilymph, due to the inwardly-directed active pumping of K^+. This establishes the endocochlear potential.
   d. The body of each hair cell resides in the perilymph and has a potential of –70 mV with respect to the perilymph; the cilia of each hair cell, however, lies in the endolymph and has a potential of –150 mV; this high (i.e., negative) potential makes the cilia extremely sensitive.

5. Acoustic reflex — Loud sounds are attenuated by a reflex from the superior olivary nucleus. The tensor tympani (V3) tightens the tympanic membrane and pulls the malleus inward, whereas the stapedius (VII) pulls the stapes outward to make a rigid system that effectively protects the cochlea. This masks low-frequency sounds in a loud environment and decreases the hearing of one's own speech (activated with speech production).

B. Sound interpretation — relies on the "place" principle, in which stimulation of different cochlear areas causes different nerves to fire, thereby determining the overall frequency (i.e., pitch). The cochlear nucleus may still distinguish different frequencies if part of the cochlea is removed. Loudness is detected by increased amplitude, causing an increased frequency of hair cell firing and spatial summation as more cilia are being moved. Humans are able to distinguish 1 dB change in sound intensity. One can hear high-frequency sounds at low intensities, but low-frequency sounds require higher intensities. The frequency range in humans lies between 20–20,000 cycles/s (i.e., Hz); below 60 dB, only 500–5000 cycles/s are detectable.

   1. The elderly lose high-frequency discriminatory abilities. Chronic exposure to loud noises results in high-frequency hearing loss; in contrast, ototoxic medications induce hearing loss at all frequencies.

C. Auditory pathway (see Chapter 1) — relays from the spiral ganglion (first-order neurons) → dorsal and ventral cochlear nuclei (second-order neurons) in the medulla → contralateral (some ipsilateral) superior olivary nucleus (third-order neurons) → lateral lemniscus and the nucleus of the lateral lemniscus (fourth-order neurons) → inferior colliculus (fifth-order neurons) → medial geniculate body (sixth-order neurons) → auditory cortex (seventh-order neurons)

1. The fibers from the dorsal cochlear nuclei bypass the superior olivary nucleus and the nucleus of the lateral lemniscus to synapse onto the neurons in the inferior colliculus (third-order neurons). Fibers cross to the contralateral side from the ventral cochlear nuclei by way of the trapezoid body (to the superior olivary nucleus), in the nucleus of the lateral lemniscus by way of the commissure of Probst, and in the inferior colliculus by way of the inferior collicular commissure.

2. There is bilateral representation with slightly greater hearing on the contralateral side. Crossover pathways render unilateral hearing loss uncommon with lesions in the brainstem or more proximally. There are collateral fibers to the reticular formation, the vermis, and the spinal cord. Tonotopic orientation is maintained in the tracts. The superior olivary nucleus inhibits the hair cells to isolate specific sounds.

D. Primary auditory cortex (Brodmann area 41) — receives afferent fibers from the medial geniculate body. The auditory association area (Brodmann area 42) receives afferent fibers from the primary auditory cortex and the thalamic association areas. There is tonotopic organization based on sound frequency and location. Lateral inhibition sharpens sound detection but decreases the frequency range detected by the cochlea.

1. Cortex — necessary for tonal and sequential sound pattern discrimination. If the primary auditory cortex is destroyed, there is decreased spatial localization because both sides compare the intensity of low-frequency input and the time difference of arrival with high-frequency input. If the secondary auditory cortex is destroyed, there is decreased sensitivity. If the association areas are destroyed, sound agnosia ensues.

2. Localization — achieved by the medial superior olivary nucleus (which detects the time lag between the ears) and the lateral superior olivary nucleus (which detects the intensity change between the ears)

IX. Taste

A. Taste — conveyed by the combination of activated taste buds, smell, and texture. From an evolutionary perspective, it functions to help one choose safe and nutritious foods. The taste sensation is dependent on activation of receptors for Na^+, K^+, H^+, Cl^-, adenosine, inosine, glutamate, and sweet or bitter chemicals. The sensation is intense at first, but adaptation is rapid; the chemical is eventually washed away with saliva. Most sensory systems adapt at the receptors, but taste has 50% adaptation at the receptors and 50% in the CNS.

B. Four major taste sensations:

1. Sour — responds to acids, is proportional to H^+ concentration, and is detected on the lateral aspect of the tongue

2. Salt — responds to Na^+ and K^+ and is detected on the tip of the tongue

3. Sweet — responds to sugar, alcohol, and many organic chemicals; detected on the tip of the tongue

4. Bitter — responds to organic molecules, especially long chains with nitrogen and alkaloids (e.g., caffeine, nicotine, quinine, and deadly plant toxins); detected on the posterior aspect of the tongue and palate

C. Anatomy of taste

1. Taste buds — Adults have ~10,000 taste buds, but this number decreases with age. Taste buds are composed of ~50 epithelial cells, consisting of sustentacular cells and taste cells that are constantly regenerating to replace old ones (with newer, dividing cells at the center). Microvilli project from taste cells into the taste pore, sampling the contents in the mouth.

2. Taste nerve fibers — stimulated by taste receptor cells capable of detecting more than one stimulus. Taste cells bind to chemicals, increasing Na^+ conductance and resulting in depolarization and impulse generation.

3. The anterior of the tongue is innervated for sensation by CN VIII (i.e., lingual nerve) and taste by CN VII (i.e., chorda tympani). The posterior of the tongue is innervated for sensation and taste by CN IX. The base of the tongue and pharynx are innervated by CN X for both sensation and taste. Ultimately, fibers from CNs VII, IX, and X relay in the nucleus solitarius (with fibers from CN VII positioned most rostrally) and then to the thalamic VPM nucleus and cortex.

4. Taste impulses are relayed within the brainstem from the tractus solitarius to the superior/inferior salivatory nuclei, and on to the submandibular, sublingual, and parotid glands to control salivary release.

X. Smell

A. Seven known olfactory stimulants — camphoraceous, musky, pungent, putrid, floral, peppermint, and ethereal. There may be many more, however. Many people cannot detect certain odors because they are missing a receptor. Moreover, an affective component of smell may alter sex drive and appetite.

B. Only a small range of intensity is detected. It is more important that the smell is present than how much is present.

C. Anatomy of smell

1. Olfactory membrane — Located in the superior nasal cavity; the olfactory cells are bipolar cells from the CNS (~100 million) that are embedded in the olfactory epithelium and supported by sustentacular cells. The mucosal surface of the cell has 6–12 olfactory cilia projecting into the mucus secreted by Bowman glands. These cilia project odor-binding proteins through their membranes that may sense smell by changing ion flow or by cAMP formation. Detected substances must be volatile and may be water- (i.e., mucous) or lipid- (i.e., membrane) soluble.

2. Olfactory pathway — The olfactory bulb lies over the cribriform plate. Axons from the olfactory cells (first-order neurons) relay to the glomeruli in the olfactory bulb (second-order neurons). There are 25,000 axons per glomerulus, which is composed of 25 mitral cells and 60 tufted cells. The glomeruli relay axons to the CNS via the olfactory tract (i.e., CN I), and are tonically active with specific glomeruli detecting specific smells. The olfactory tract divides into medial and lateral olfactory striae that travel to medial and lateral olfactory areas.
   a. Medial olfactory area — contains the septal nuclei anterior and superior to the hypothalamus. It is phylogenetically old and is used for primary reflexes such as salivation, licking, and emotion.
   b. Lateral olfactory area — lies in the prepyriform and pyriform cortex, as well as in the cortex over the amygdala nucleus. It has efferents to the limbic system, particularly to the hippocampus, creating a strong association between smell and memory. This correlates with learning and previous aversion to foods (e.g., nausea, vomiting). These structures correlate with the older paleocortex;

newer structures include the dorsomedial (DM) thalamus, which connects to the posterolateral, orbitofrontal cortex for conscious analysis of odor.

3. The RMP is –55 mV and there is continuous firing. Stimulation increases the AP rate in proportion to the stimulus strength. Adaptation of 50% occurs within 1 second and then gradually continues to baseline. Adaptation is at the level of the granule cells (i.e., inhibitory) in the olfactory bulb.

4. The cortex sends impulses to the granule cells to inhibit mitral and tufted cells, sharpening the distinction of smells.

5. Smell is the only sensation not directly connected to the thalamus.

XI. Motor Systems

A. Organization within the spinal cord

1. Topographical representation — in the vermis and intermediate zone of the cerebellum, sensory and motor cortices, basal ganglia, red nucleus, and reticular formation

2. The spinal cord has many preset activities that the brain modulates. However, the walking reflex is contained within the spinal cord; thus, animals can still walk after the cervical cord is severed. In a decerebrate animal, the lower midbrain is severed to remove inhibition of the reticular formation and the vestibular nuclei inputs.

3. Anterior motor neurons are divided into two types:
   a. Alpha motor neurons — larger. They innervate skeletal muscle by sending α-type A fibers to large skeletal muscle fibers within the motor unit.
   b. Gamma motor neurons — smaller. They are 50% less numerous and relay γ-type A fibers to the intrafusal fibers of the muscle spindle.

4. Interneurons — smaller, very excitable, and have many connections; almost all of the corticospinal tract fibers synapse first onto interneurons. Very few sensory axons synapse directly onto anterior motor neurons.

5. Renshaw cells — located in the anterior horn. An α motor neuron's axon sends a branch to a Renshaw cell, which uses the neurotransmitter glycine to inhibit nearby α motor neuron synergists and inhibit antagonizing inhibitors. This creates a negative feedback loop that sharpens signals (i.e., similar to lateral inhibition).

6. Propriospinal fibers — connect various spinal cord segments and constitute more than 50% of the spinal cord fibers

B. Feedback during movement — from muscle spindles and Golgi tendon organs

1. Muscle spindles — located within the muscle belly; detect length and velocity of change in length of the muscle. Each spindle is activated by movement of the midportion of the spindle, such that stretching increases firing and contraction decreases it.
   a. Muscle spindles lie in parallel with muscle fibers and are each composed of 3–12 intrafusal muscle fibers attached to larger extrafusal fibers. The central part of each spindle lacks actin and myosin and thus does not contract; rather, it functions as a sensory receptor. The terminal ends of each spindle receive motor neuron input and are stimulated to contract.
   b. Two sensory ending types in the receptor area of each muscle spindle:

          (1) Primary ending (annulospiral ending) — type Ia fiber encircling each intrafusal fiber; relays impulses at 70–120 m/s, and is the fastest sensory fiber in the body

          (2) Secondary ending (flower-spray ending) — type II fiber located on the receptor site on one side of the primary ending, and conducts more slowly

    c. Two types of intrafusal fibers:

          (1) Nuclear bag fibers — 1–3/spindle; innervated by primary sensory endings

          (2) Nuclear chain fibers — 3–9/spindle; these are smaller and innervated by both primary and secondary sensory endings

    d. Gamma motor neurons — innervated by the bulboreticular facilitory region, cerebellum, basal ganglia, and cortex. Gamma motor neurons exhibit decreased activity with cerebellar lesions, resulting in decreased tone; 31% of motor nerve fibers are from γ motor neurons. Coactivation occurs as the γ motor neuron is stimulated at the same time as the α motor neuron; this maintains the fibers at an equivalent loading force and prevents opposition to initial contraction.

    e. Impulses are proportional to the degree of stretching. The "static" response is transmitted by nuclear chain fibers that fire tonically when a muscle remains stretched. The "dynamic" response is initiated by nuclear bag fibers, which sense an increase or decrease in the rate of change of tonic firing with either increasing or decreasing stretch in muscle.

    f. Muscle spindle-related reflexes

          (1) Myotactic (muscle stretch) reflex — When a muscle is stretched, impulses travel from the spindle's type Ia fibers to the α motor neuron; this induces contraction via a monosynaptic reflex. A damping mechanism smooths contractions from multiple sources to produce fluid (i.e., not jerky) movement.

          (2) Servo-assist mechanism — During contraction against a load, intrafusal fibers become shorter than extrafusal fibers; this reflexively increases muscle activity to render the contraction less load-sensitive.

          (3) Stretch reflex — upon stimulation, identifies the degree of tone (i.e., input) the brain relays to the spinal cord. The cortex inhibits the reflex, whereas the brainstem increases it. Damage to the cortex causes hyperreflexia; damage to the brainstem causes hyporeflexia.

          (4) Clonus — oscillation of the muscle jerk response arising from intermittent stretch on the spindle. It is increased if the reflex is sensitized by facilitory impulses in the brain (e.g., decerebrate state).

2. Golgi tendon organs — encapsulated receptors with bundles of tendon fibers passing through them, located at the muscle–tendon junction. They are oriented in series with muscle fibers. Each tendon organ detects the tension within 10–15 contained muscle fibers. The latter increase their firing rate with active contraction and passive stretch. The afferent signal is mediated from type Ib fibers to interneurons that decrease α motor neuron output. The reflex is not monosynaptic. It prevents muscle tearing and serves to equalize forces in the muscle, such that tense fibers are allowed to relax.

3. Dorsal spinocerebellar tracts — transmit signals from muscle spindles and Golgi tendon organs to the reticular formation and cortex, at ~120 m/s.

C. Many reflexes are programmed within the spinal cord; these are characterized by the entry of sensory fiber branches into the spinal gray matter and include:

1. Flexor (withdrawal) reflex — seen in spine-injured or decerebrate animals. This occurs when stimulus applied to a limb elicits withdrawal. It is evoked more by pain than touch and relies on divergence of interneurons (with reciprocal inhibition of antagonists) and circuits to prolong the discharge after the stimulus has gone. Longer durations are associated with increased signal intensity, lasting 1–3 seconds.

2. Crossed extensor reflex — when the opposite limb extends 0.2–0.5 seconds after the flexor reflex to push the body from the stimulus; mediated by interneurons

3. Positive supportive reaction — when pressure on the footpad of a spine-injured or decerebrate animal causes limb extension and standing

4. Cord righting reflex — enables a spine-injured animal to stand up, reflexively

5. Rhythmic stepping reflex — refers to flexion then extension of a limb, controlled by oscillating circuits with reciprocal inhibition of agonists and antagonists. It does not require sensory input, but sensation may increase or decrease the rate.

6. Rhythmic walking reflex — enables both sides of the spinal cord to coordinate both limbs

7. Rhythmic galloping reflex — in animal models, allows front and hind legs to move together

8. Scratch reflex — triggered by itch and tickle

D. Autonomic reflexes — alter vascular tone to control body temperature, sweating, and blood pressure (BP). Peritoneointestinal reflexes decrease gut motility with peritoneal irritation. Evacuation reflexes exist for the bladder and colon. The mass reflex in the spine-injured animal occurs when strong pain or increased filling of the bladder or gut induce flexor-type body spasms, evacuation of the bladder and colon, increased BP and sweating.

E. Control of motor function at higher levels

1. Primary motor cortex — Brodmann area 4; the homunculus was mapped by Penfield and Rasmussen and >50% is dedicated to hand and face function. Betz cells are large pyramidal neurons found only in the primary motor cortex; they relay impulses at 70 m/s (i.e., the fastest fibers from the brain to the spinal cord) and constitute 3% (i.e., 34,000 of 1 million fibers) of the corticospinal tract.
   a. Efferent fibers from the motor cortex — collateral fibers to the cortex (for lateral inhibition), caudate and putamen, red nucleus (rubrospinal fibers), reticular formation (reticulospinal, cerebellar fibers), vestibular system (vestibulospinal, cerebellar fibers), and inferior olive (olivocerebellar fibers)
   b. Afferent fibers to the motor cortex — input from somatosensory systems (e.g., muscle spindles), visual cortex, auditory cortex, frontal cortex, contralateral motor cortex (via the corpus callosum), ventrobasal thalamus, ventrolateral (VL) and ventroanterior (VA) thalamus (with input from the cerebellum and basal ganglia), and intralaminar nuclei of the thalamus (which regulate the level of excitability).
   c. Neurons of the motor cortex are arranged in vertical columns, each functioning as a unit. There are six layers, including layers 2–4 (which receive input), layer 5 (which contains Betz pyramidal cells mediating corticospinal output), and layer 6 (responsible for corticothalamic communication). Note that 50–100 Betz cells are required to contract one muscle. "Dynamic" neurons develop force, whereas "static" neurons maintain it.

2. Premotor area — Brodmann area 6; located anterior to area 4. It has the same layered organization as area 4 and contains patterns for specific tasks. A circuit exists whereby the premotor cortex relays to the basal ganglia, thalamus, and area 4.
   a. Broca's area (Brodmann area 44) — posteroinferior frontal gyrus; functions in selecting correct words and coordinating breathing with speaking
   b. Frontal eye field (Brodmann area 8) — just above Broca's area, in the middle frontal gyrus; controls eyelid movements (i.e., blinking) and horizontal saccadic eye movements to the opposite side. If it is damaged, one may still lock onto targets via occipital cortical function.

    c. Head rotation area — just above the eye field; functions to turn the head with eye movements

    d. Hand skill area — just above the head rotation area, anterior to the primary motor hand area; a lesion here results in motor apraxia

3. Supplemental motor area (Brodmann area 6) — located anterior and superior to the premotor cortex. It is mainly along the medial side of the hemisphere (adjacent to the longitudinal fissure), extending slightly over the superior surface of the hemisphere. The lower limb area lies posteriorly; the facial area lies anteriorly. This cortical region requires a stronger stimulus to elicit contraction than other areas and stimulation elicits bilateral contractions. It serves to set complex actions that serve as a background for finer actions. Injury causes decreased voluntary movement and speech output and usually resolves within 6 weeks.

4. Corticospinal (pyramidal) tract — most important output pathway from the motor cortex; contains 1 million fibers (30% from area 4, 30% from premotor and supplementary motor cortices (area 6), and 40% from sensory fibers). It travels in the posterior limb of the internal capsule and down through the brainstem, forming the medullary pyramid; most fibers then cross and descend in the lateral cortico-spinal tract. They terminate on interneurons (in cord gray matter), sensory relay neurons (in the dorsal horn), and anterior motor neurons. Some fibers, however, remain ipsilateral; these descend in the ventral corticospinal tract, ultimately crossing at lower levels within the spinal cord. These fibers are used for bilateral postural control, relaying impulses from the supplementary motor area.

5. Red nucleus — participates in an accessory route of corticospinal transmission between the motor cortex and spinal cord. It receives afferent input from corticospinal and corticorubral fibers, relaying to the magnocellular area that contains large Betz-like neurons. Efferent fibers are conducted in the rubrospinal tract, which crosses just anterior to the corticospinal tract. There is also afferent input from the dentate and nucleus interpositus and efferent fibers to the nucleus interpositus. Further, it is also connected to the reticular formation.

6. Lateral motor system of the spinal cord — includes the corticospinal tract and the rubrospinal tract. These have direct connections with α motor neurons in the cervical cord to regulate fine motor control of the hand.

    a. The spinal cord helps to grade power with the servo-assist mechanism; it has reciprocal antagonistic reflexes such that the brain only requires a simple command to accomplish a complex task.

    b. If the primary motor cortex is removed, there are no voluntary fine movements of the hand and tone is decreased (because the corticospinal tract normally provides tonic excitatory input to the spinal cord).

    c. Damage to the basal ganglia, deep structures, and adjacent cortex results in increased tone because tonic inhibition to the vestibular system and reticular formation is removed.

    d. The Babinski response is present only if there is damage to the corticospinal tract or the primary motor cortex. The corticospinal tract delivers fine control and evolved more recently than other primitive systems (e.g., rubrospinal tract), which it overrides. The noncorticospinal tracts are older systems, used for pain avoidance by withdrawal mechanisms. When the corticospinal system is damaged, however, the older systems take over.

7. Medial motor system of the spinal cord — includes the vestibulospinal and reticulospinal tracts to the axial and limb-girdle muscles

    a. Pontine reticular nucleus — laterally situated, extends up to the midbrain and excites antigravity muscles via the lateral reticulospinal tract (by synapsing onto medial anterior horn cells). It is stimulated by the vestibular nucleus and the cerebellum.

b. Medullary reticular nucleus — ventromedial; inhibits antigravity muscles by means of the medial reticulospinal tract (lateral fibers). It is stimulated by the corticospinal and rubrospinal tracts, along with other motor groups.

c. Vestibular nucleus — stimulates antigravity muscles to maintain equilibrium, with the aid of the pontine reticular formation. The lateral vestibular nucleus sends fibers to the lateral and medial vestibulospinal tracts.

F. Clinical considerations

1. Muscle spasm — response to pain; decreased with analgesics or antispasmodics. A cramp is a reflex contraction triggered in response to pain, cold, or decreased blood flow; it is treated via reciprocal inhibition by contracting antagonist muscles.

2. Spinal shock — refers to the loss of spinal cord function and reflexes following injury; associated with an immediate decrease in mean BP to 70–80 mm Hg due to the loss of sympathetic tone and skeletal muscle reflexes, with unopposed vagal tone. The spinal cord is normally under tonic stimulation from the corticospinal, reticulospinal, and vestibulospinal tracts. After transection, within hours to weeks, spinal neurons may regain partial excitability. The first reflexes to return are stretch reflexes (e.g., bulbocavernosus reflex). The bulbocavernosus reflex may return within hours of injury; however, more complex reflexes may take up to weeks. Increased extracellular K^+ in the spinal cord is believed to be an important mechanism of spinal shock.

3. Decerebrate rigidity — ensues following injury to the brainstem region between the pons and the midbrain. There is increased antigravity muscle action of the neck, trunk, and lower limb muscles. This type of lesion blocks normal stimulatory input to the medullary reticular formation from the cortex, red nucleus, and basal ganglia. This allows the pontine reticular nucleus and lateral vestibular nucleus to take over, with increased and unopposed antigravity tone.

a. The increased spasticity (i.e., resistance to change in muscle length) occurs following increased γ motor neuron stimulation compared with α motor neuron stimulation from the pontine reticular and vestibular nuclei.

b. If the anterior lobe of the cerebellum is destroyed, this impairs Purkinje cell–mediated inhibition of the lateral vestibular nucleus, resulting in increased extensor tone.

4. Spasticity and rigidity (Chapter 4 section XXIII)

a. Spasticity — characterized by unidirectional resistance to change, velocity dependency, and increased reflexes

b. Rigidity — characterized by bidirectional resistance to change, is not velocity dependent, and is not associated with hyperreflexia

XII. Vestibular System

A. Anatomy of the vestibular system (**Fig. 2.6**)

1. The bony labyrinth surrounds the membranous labyrinth.

2. Macula — sensory organ of the utricle and saccule; contains hair cells with cilia embedded in a gelatinous layer containing calcium carbonate otoliths. The hair cells synapse with the vestibular nerve. Each hair cell has 50–70 stereocilia and one large kinocilium. All cilia are connected via filaments at the tip in the gel layer and gradually become longer until they reach the kinocilium. When they bend toward the kinocilium, there is increased Na^+ conductance, causing depolarization. When they bend away, there is decreased Na^+ conductance, causing hyperpolarization. There is a baseline firing rate of 100

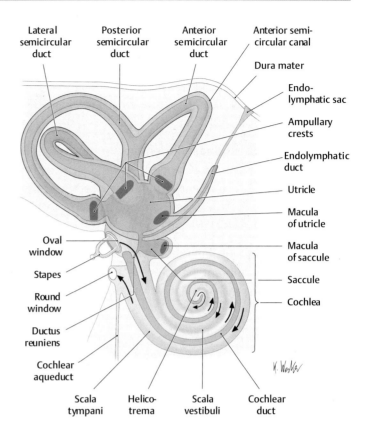

Lateral semicircular duct

Posterior semicircular duct

Anterior semicircular duct

Anterior semi-circular canal

Dura mater

Endo-lymphatic sac

Ampullary crests

Endolymphatic duct

Utricle

Macula of utricle

Macula of saccule

Saccule

Cochlea

Oval window

Stapes

Round window

Ductus reuniens

Cochlear aqueduct

Scala tympani

Helico-trema

Scala vestibuli

Cochlear duct

Fig. 2.6 Schematic diagram of the inner ear. The inner ear is embedded in the petrous part of the temporal bone. It comprises the membranous labyrinth inside the similarly shaped bony labyrinth. The auditory part is the cochlear labyrinth with the membranous cochlear duct. The membranous duct and its bony shell make up the cochlea, which contains the organ of Corti. The vestibular apparatus includes the vestibular labyrinth with three semicircular canals, a saccule, and a utricle, each housing a sensory epithelium. The bony labyrinth contains perilymph (beige), and the membranous labyrinth, containing endolymph (blue-green), floats in this. The endolymphatic spaces of the auditory and vestibular apparatus communicate via the ductus reuniens and are connected by the endolymphatic duct to the endolymphatic sac. (From THIEME Atlas of Anatomy, Head and Neuroanatomy, © Thieme 2007, Illustration by Karl Wesker.)

impulses/s that either increases to several hundred impulses/s or decreases to virtually zero. These hair cells face various directions, such that some depolarize with forward-bending, whereas others depolarize with backward- or lateral-bending.

3. Utricle — contains its macula in the horizontal plane. It senses the direction of gravitational force when one is upright.

4. Saccule — contains its macula in the vertical plane. It functions when one is lying horizontal.

5. Three semicircular canals (anterior, posterior, and lateral) — at right angles to each other, enabling them to detect motion in any of three planes. If the head is bent forward from the horizontal by 30 degrees, the lateral canal is horizontal with respect to the earth's surface, the anterior canal is forward and 45 degrees lateral, and the posterior canal is backward and 45 degrees lateral.

6. Ampulla — a dilatation at the end of each semicircular canal, filled with endolymph. It contains the crista ampullaris, the sensory organ of the semicircular canals, which has ciliated hair cells that project into a gelatinous body, the cupula. Na^+ conductance is dependent upon the direction of bending. The rate of AP generation is proportional to the direction of rotation. With head rotation, the endolymph remains stationary while the semicircular canals move, bending the hair cells' cilia in the cupula. Rotation to the left causes the cilia to bend to the right.

7. Vestibular nerve — relays impulses to the vestibular nucleus and cerebellum, which connects to the reticular formation and spinal cord. The flocculonodular lobe functions with the semicircular canals to detect rapid changes in direction; the cerebellar uvula maintains static equilibrium. The cerebellum and vestibular system provide input to the MLF to control eye movement and to the primary equilibrium cortex in the parietal lobe (deep in the sylvian fissure, opposite the auditory cortex of the superior temporal gyrus).

8. Superior and medial vestibular nuclei — involved with eye reflexes. They receive afferent input from the semicircular canals and transmit efferent fibers to the MLF (for the control of eye movement) and to the medial vestibulospinal tract (for the control of head and neck motion). The medial vestibular nucleus is the largest vestibular nucleus and relays crossed fibers to all extraocular nerve nuclei and to the cerebellum. The superior vestibular nucleus sends uncrossed fibers by way of the MLF to the nuclei of CNs III and IV.

9. Lateral vestibular nucleus (Deiter nucleus) — involved with posture. It receives afferent fibers from the utricle (from the superior vestibular ganglion) and the saccule (from the inferior vestibular ganglion), and relays efferent fibers to the lateral vestibulospinal tract which function in lower limb extension and upper limb flexion (i.e., for postural control). It stimulates both α and γ motor neurons and is tonically inhibited by Purkinje cells; thus, removal of the anterior lobe of the cerebellum results in spasticity.

10. Inferior vestibular nucleus — integrates input from the vestibular system and the cerebellum. It receives afferent input from the semicircular canals and the utricle and relays efferent fibers to the cerebellum and reticular formation.

B. Detection of motion

1. Macula — detects static and linear acceleration (but not velocity). When the head moves forward, the otoliths move backward in relative fashion because they have more inertia than the surrounding fluid.

2. Semicircular canals — detect angular acceleration because endolymph in the ducts remains relatively stationary (due to inertia) during head movement. The semicircular canals predict a fall by detecting head rotation, allowing for an early adjustment to be made; the utricle, in comparison, only acts after falling has begun. If the flocculonodular lobe is removed, impaired function of the semicircular canals ensues (interestingly, the macula is spared).

C. Other vestibular mechanisms

1. Postural reflex — rapid changes in spatial orientation elicit a postural reflex. This functions to achieve and preserve balance as appropriate postural adjustments are made.

2. Stabilizing the eyes — The semicircular ducts cause the eyes to move in a direction equal and opposite to the head by means of the MLF.

3. The vestibular apparatus only detects head movements, whereas the orientation of the head against the neck and the body is detected by proprioceptive inputs to the vestibular system, the reticular formation, and the cerebellum.

4. It is interesting to note that visual mechanisms are effective in preserving equilibrium in the absence of a functioning vestibular apparatus.

D. Stereotyped body movements — stored in various parts of the CNS

1. Forward flexion, extension, and rotation — midbrain and lower thalamus

2. Rotational eye movement and head movement — interstitial nucleus of the midbrain, near the MLF

3. Raising of the head and body — prestitial nucleus, at the junction of the midbrain and thalamus

4. Flexion of the head and body — nucleus precommissuralis, at the level of the posterior commissure

5. Turning of the body — pontine and midbrain reticular formation

XIII. Cerebellum

A. Anatomy of the cerebellum

    1. Cerebellum — controls the timing of motor movements and the rapid progression of agonist/antagonist interplay. It sequences and corrects activities, compares intention with action by means of sensory input and aids the cortex in planning the next movement. It is theorized to have memory for learning by mistakes. Stimulation elicits no motor or sensory activity.

    2. Vermis — coordinates the axial body (i.e., neck, shoulders, and hips). It receives afferent inputs from the motor cortex, brainstem, and spinal cord. Efferent fibers relay to the motor cortex, red nucleus, and reticular formation.

    3. Intermediate zone — controls the distal limbs. It has similar afferent and efferent connections as the vermis.

    4. Lateral zone — involved with planning of sequential motor movements. There is no known topographic representation. It is connected to the association areas of the cortex (i.e., premotor, somatic, and somatic association).

    5. Afferent tracts
        a. Inferior cerebellar peduncle
            (1) Juxtarestiform body
                (a) Vestibulocerebellar pathway — vestibular nucleus to the fastigial nucleus of the flocculonodular lobe
            (2) Restiform body
                (a) Olivocerebellar pathway — motor cortex, basal ganglia, reticular formation, and spinal cord to the inferior olive and on to the cerebellum
                (b) Reticulocerebellar pathway — reticular nucleus to the vermis
                (c) Dorsal spinocerebellar pathway — from the muscle spindles, Golgi tendon organs, tactile and joint receptors → Clarke column → dorsal spinocerebellar tract → inferior cerebellar peduncle → ipsilateral vermis and intermediate zone. The spinocerebellar tracts conduct impulses at 120 m/s and are the fastest fibers in the CNS.
        b. Middle cerebellar peduncle
            (1) Corticopontocerebellar pathway — from the motor, premotor, and sensory cortices to the pontine nucleus and on to the contralateral cerebellar hemisphere
        c. Superior cerebellar peduncle
            (1) Ventral spinocerebellar pathway — from anterior motor neurons through the superior peduncle to the cerebellum (bilaterally); relays to the cerebellum those motor signals received in the spinal cord from the corticospinal and rubrospinal tracts
        d. Deep nuclear input — from both the cortex and the sensory afferent tracts
        e. In general, incoming fibers to the cerebellum divide, with one fiber relaying to the deep nuclei and one to the cortex.

    6. Efferent tracts
        a. Inferior cerebellar peduncle
            (1) By way of the juxtarestiform body
                (a) Flocculonodular lobe to the lateral vestibular nucleus — A lesion along this pathway produces nystagmus.

   (b) Vermis to the fastigial nucleus, to the pons and medulla — pathway for equilibrium and posture. A lesion here causes truncal ataxia and scanning speech.

  b. Superior cerebellar peduncle

   (1) Intermediate zone to the interposed nuclei → VL and VPL thalamus → cortex, thalamus, basal ganglia, red nucleus (mainly), and midbrain reticular formation; participates in distal limb agonist/antagonist control. A lesion along this pathway causes appendicular ataxia.

   (2) Lateral zone → dentate nucleus → VL and VPL thalamus → cortex (area 4) — coordinates sequential action. A lesion here produces an intention tremor.

  c. In general, injury to the vermis or intermediate zone produces decreased tone.

7. Cerebellar neuronal circuits — The cerebellum has 30 million functional units, each centered around a Purkinje cell. The cortex has a molecular layer (with basket and stellate cells), a Purkinje layer, and a granular layer (with granule and Golgi type 2 cells). These are all inhibitory except for the granule cells. The output of this functional unit is conveyed to cells of the deep nuclei, which are excitatory by nature; these are inhibited by Purkinje cells and excited by peripheral afferents (i.e., climbing and mossy fibers).

  a. Climbing fibers — excitatory; transmit from the inferior olivary complex to the Purkinje cells and deep nuclear cells. One fiber predominantly stimulates 10 Purkinje cells via 300 synapses in the molecular layer but also multiple deep nuclear cells.

  b. Mossy fibers — excitatory; conduct from all other afferent sources (i.e., cortex, brainstem, spinal cord, etc.) to the deep nuclear cells and granular layer

  c. Granule cells — excitatory; mediated by glutamate (i.e., neurotransmitter). They project to the molecular layer, where the axon bifurcates and forms parallel nerve fibers that travel parallel to the axis of the folia. They form 80,000–200,000 synapses with each Purkinje cell. Each fiber contacts 250–500 Purkinje cells. There are 500–1000 granule cells per Purkinje cell. The Purkinje cells and the deep nuclear cells fire continuously at 50–100/s.

  d. Basket and stellate cells — inhibitory; these cells lie along the parallel fibers and are stimulated by them to inhibit nearby Purkinje cells

  e. Golgi type II cells — inhibitory; located in the granular layer and inhibit the granule cells, thereby decreasing the duration of an excitatory response

8. Flocculonodular lobe — important for mediating rapid changes in body position, as detected by the vestibular apparatus. It computes the velocity and direction of movement and ascertains how the body should move to preserve equilibrium.

9. Intermediate zone — compares the intentions of the cortex and red nucleus (by way of impulses from α motor neurons through the ventral spinocerebellar tract) with actual performance (as detected by the peripheral nervous system). It transmits corrective impulses to the thalamic relay path to the cortex and on to the red nucleus. It also has a damping function that prevents overshoot by anticipating momentum; hence, damage to the intermediate zone causes intention tremor by allowing overshoot in each direction. It also controls ballistic movements, short actions, and fast actions (i.e., no time for feedback). These are preplanned motions (e.g., eye saccades, finger typing). In this context, damage to the intermediate zone results in slow movements in the absence of cerebellar agonistic activity, causing decreased force and slowing of the ability to stop a particular action.

10. Lateral zone — receives no input from peripheral receptors or the primary motor cortex but only from the premotor and association areas. It is involved with the planning and time sequencing of movements. Damage here results in dyscoordination of speech and limbs. Planning is accomplished via a two-way connection between the premotor cortex, basal ganglia, and sensory cortex. The dentate nucleus contains information about a subsequent action to follow, not what is going on at the time.

Damage will alter the control of timing, making one unable to determine when a movement will end, and preventing a smooth transition to the next movement. An extramotor function predicts information from auditory and visual stimuli (e.g., how fast something is approaching).

B. Cerebellar learning — mediated by climbing fibers as they adjust the sensitivity of the Purkinje cells. They fire strong excitatory impulses at a rate of 1 per second; a rate change, however, alters the long-term sensitivity of the Purkinje cells to the mossy fibers. Once a task is mastered, climbing fibers no longer relay error impulses. The inferior olive compares input from the corticospinal tract and motor centers of intent. If they correlate well, the inferior olive does not alter its firing rate; however, if the act requires modification, the rate of firing is either increased or decreased accordingly.

C. Clinical manifestations of cerebellar disease — In general, a lesion must involve at least one deep nucleus and the cortex to be symptomatic.

1. Dysmetria and ataxia — also seen with spinal cord tract lesions

2. Dysdiadochokinesis — difficulty with rapid alternating movements

3. Dysarthria — decreased coordination of speech

4. Intention tremor — due to overshoot and lack of damping

5. Nystagmus — failure of damping tremors of the eyes, particularly seen in flocculonodular damage

6. Rebound — unable to stop an initiated motion, resulting from the absence of the cerebellar aspect of the stretch reflex. This leads to the inability to stop movement in an unwanted direction.

7. Hypotonia — due to loss of the ipsilateral dentate and interpositus nuclei's tonic discharge to the motor cortex and brainstem.

XIV. Basal Ganglia (Fig. 2.7)

A. Basal ganglia — control the intensity of movement (i.e., scaling) and how fast it is performed (i.e., timing). These features are accomplished by the caudate circuit, with input from the association areas (i.e., the posterior parietal cortex, which provides the spatial relationship of the body to the surroundings). The basal ganglia store learned movements that must be relearned by the cortex in the event of injury.

B. Anatomy of the basal ganglia

1. Putamen circuit — executes motor activity patterns. Premotor cortex, supplementary motor cortex, and S1 relay → putamen, globus pallidus interna (GPi), VA and VL thalamus, and primary motor, premotor, and supplementary motor cortices. There are also three smaller circuits:
   a. Putamen → globus pallidus externa (GPe) → subthalamus (ST) → thalamus → motor cortex
   b. Putamen → GPi → SN → thalamus → motor cortex
   c. GPe → ST → GPe

2. Caudate circuit — involved with the cognitive control of motor patterns. It integrates sensory information with memory to determine motor activity and selects which muscle patterns should be used for each goal. The caudate nucleus extends through all cortices (frontal, parietal, temporal, and occipital) and receives much input from the association areas. The prefrontal, premotor, and supplemental motor cortices and the parietal, temporal, and occipital association areas relay fibers to the caudate and putamen and then to the GPi, to the VA and VL thalamus, and on to the prefrontal, premotor, and supplemental motor cortices (but not primary motor cortex).

C. Neurotransmitters — SN relays dopaminergic fibers to the caudate and putamen; the caudate and putamen relay GABAergic fibers to the globus pallidus (GP) and SN; the caudate relays cholinergic fibers (ACh) to the putamen; the cortex relays cholinergic fibers to the caudate and putamen; the brainstem relays NE, 5-HT, and enkephalins to the basal ganglia. GABA and DA are inhibitory, whereas ACh is excitatory. All basal ganglia circuits to the cortex are inhibitory.

D. Clinical considerations

1. Damage to the GP causes athetosis. Damage to the ST causes hemiballismus. Damage to the caudate and putamen causes chorea. Damage to the SN causes rigidity and tremor.

2. Parkinson's disease (**Fig. 2.7**) — caused by degeneration of the pars compacta of the SN, resulting in decreased release of DA to the caudate and putamen. It is characterized by rigidity, tremor (3–6 cycles/s), akinesia, and postural instability.

   a. Because there is less DA to inhibit the caudate and putamen, there is more GABA to inhibit the GP and decrease the basal ganglia output. This allows for unopposed corticospinal stimulation with increased rigidity and tremor from oscillating circuits.

   b. Akinesia is due to impaired excitation-inhibition of the basal ganglia by decreased levels of DA. Increased ACh leads to increased GABA release from the GP, thereby worsening symptoms.

   c. This disease is treated by raising DA levels (i.e., via 3,4-dihydroxy-l-phenylalanine [l-DOPA]) or by decreasing function of the VL and VA thalamus to inhibit the feedback loops. This last treatment is best for controlling tremors. Other targets include the GPi and the ST. See Chapter 4 for more information.

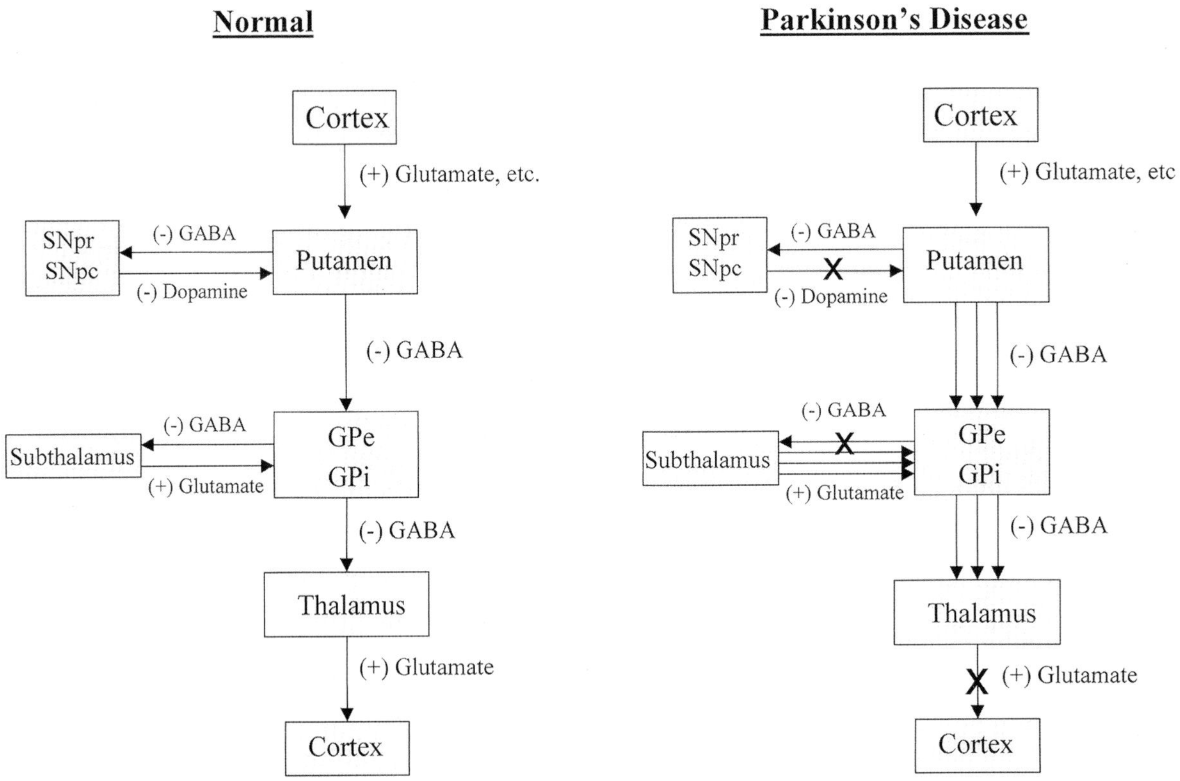

Fig. 2.7 Neurotransmitters in Parkinson's disease. GABA, gamma-aminobutyric acid; GPe, globus pallidus externa; GPi, globus pallidus interna; SNpr, substantia nigra pars reticulata; SNpc, substantia nigra pars compacta

3. Huntington's chorea — caused by the loss of GABAergic neurons in the caudate and putamen, resulting in diminished inhibition of the GP and SN. The associated dementia may be due to ACh changes in the cortex. See Chapter 3 for more information.

XV. Neurotransmitter Changes in Disease

A. Parkinson's disease — DA is decreased.

B. Huntington's disease and dementia — ACh is decreased.

C. Depression — decreased NE, 5-HT, or both in the raphe nucleus and locus ceruleus that transmit to the limbic system and cortex to stimulate the pleasure and well-being centers

   1. Treatment is via monoamine oxidase (MAO) inhibitors to decrease the destruction of NE and 5-HT, tricyclic antidepressants to block the reuptake of NE and 5-HT, or shock therapy to increase NE transmission (which occurs after seizures).

   2. In contrast, manic depression is treated with lithium to decrease the formation and action of NE and 5-HT.

D. Schizophrenia — increased DA; characterized by auditory hallucinations, delusions of grandeur, paranoia, fear, etc. There is overactivity of the ventral tegmentum of the midbrain, medial and superior to the SN (i.e., mesolimbic dopaminergic system) that stimulates mainly the medial and anterior limbic areas.

E. Alzheimer's disease — decreased ACh. There is a 75% loss of neurons in the nucleus basalis of Meynert (beneath the GP in the substantia innominata), which receives input from the limbic system and relays output to the neocortex. ACh activates the neuronal mechanism for storage and recall of memories. Also seen is a decrease in somatostatin and substance P.

XVI. Motor Control

A. Spinal cord — contains local patterns of muscle movement that are stimulated or inhibited by higher centers. Stored movements include reflexes, walking, etc.

B. Brainstem — maintains axial tone for standing and equilibrium, which is then modified by vestibular input

C. Corticospinal tract — issues commands and changes the intensity or timing of movements. It may bypass the spinal cord patterns by inhibition, and can "learn" (unlike the spinal cord).

D. Cerebellum — modifies stretch reflexes to facilitate their load-resisting effects and smoothes out equilibrium movements. It also provides accessory motor commands to enable accurate execution of motor function, and programs subsequent movements in advance (particularly fast movements).

E. Basal ganglia — help the cortex to execute learned movements and are involved with the planning of parallel and sequential patterns of movement, modifying timing/rate and intensity/size, and planning appropriate actions. They require parietal lobe input because loss of either lobe results in contralateral neglect.

XVII. Cortical Functions (Fig. 2.8)

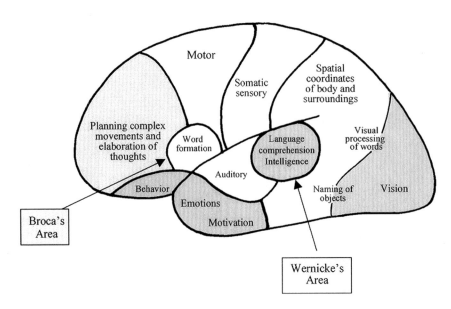

Fig. 2.8   Functional cortical areas.

A. Structure of the cerebral cortex

1. Cortex — 2–5 mm thick; contains 100 billion neurons

2. Three cell types
   a. Granular (stellate) cells have short axons, are intracortical, and are more numerous in sensory and association areas, where processing occurs. They are either excitatory (i.e., release glutamate) or inhibitory (i.e., release GABA).
   b. Fusiform cells yield output fibers.
   c. Pyramidal cells also yield output fibers, are larger and more numerous, and relay large axons to the spinal cord and subcortical association fibers.

3. Incoming sensory signals arrive in layer 4. Output typically leaves from layers 5 (to the brainstem and spinal cord) and 6 (to the thalamus). Layers 1–3 provide intracortical association fibers to adjacent cortical areas.

4. The thalamus and cortex have reciprocal connections and function as a unit.

B. Association areas — distinct from the primary and secondary motor and sensory areas. They receive and analyze impulses from several different cortical and subcortical regions.

1. Parieto-occipito-temporal association cortex — located between the somatosensory, visual, and auditory cortices. It determines the spatial coordinates of the body and its surroundings. Damage leads to neglect of the opposite side of the body/surroundings.
   a. Wernicke's area (Brodmann area 22, 39, 40) — Region of language comprehension; located behind the primary auditory cortex in the posterosuperior temporal lobe and inferior parietal lobe. It is the most important area for higher intellectual function because this is language-based. It is found in the left hemisphere in virtually all right-handed individuals. Stimulation elicits complex thoughts, memory, visual scenes, and auditory hallucinations.
   b. Angular gyrus (Brodmann area 39) — It lies in the posteroinferior parietal lobe and is responsible for the visual processing of words. Damage to the angular gyrus produces dyslexia (inability to

read) without a deficit in understanding spoken language. Damage to the auditory association area results in word deafness. The ability to name a word is dictated by the lateral temporo-ocipital junction.

   c. Nondominant parieto-temporo-occipital cortex — used for music, nonverbal visual expression, spatial relationships, body language, and voice intonations

2. Prefrontal association area — coordinates with the motor cortex to plan complex patterns and sequences. It receives input from the parietal, temporal, and occipital association areas. Output is via the caudate loop for sequential and parallel movement complexes. It is also involved with thought elaboration.

   a. Prefrontal cortex — required to keep track of multiple, simultaneous inputs of information and to recall them as needed. It is used to prognosticate, plan, and delay action until all sensory input is considered, evaluates the consequences of actions, and solves complicated problems.

     (1) After a prefrontal lobotomy, there is impaired complex problem solving, decreased ambition, decreased ability to perform sequential/parallel tasks, aggression (limbic system), decreased social responsiveness (especially with regard to sex and excretion), mood changes, decreased purpose, and decreased attention span. This is due to the fact that this cortex receives input from all areas and normally decides the appropriate motor response.

   b. Broca's area (Brodmann area 44) — controls word formation and execution and coordinates the simultaneous stimulation of respiratory, pharyngeal, and laryngeal muscles. Part of it resides in the prefrontal cortex and part in the premotor cortex.

3. Limbic association area — located in the anterobasal temporal lobe, basal frontal lobe, and cingulate gyrus. It is involved in behavior, motivation, and emotion.

4. Prosoprognosia — inability to recognize faces; caused by bilateral damage to the medial basal occipito-temporal cortex between the limbic cortex in the temporal lobe and the visual cortex in the occipital lobe.

C. Language function

1. Relies on different brain regions, including the Wernicke's area for thought formation and word choosing, the Broca's area for vocalizing, and the motor cortex, cerebellum, basal ganglia, and sensory system to control pharyngeal and laryngeal movements.

2. There is hemispheric dominance for the Wernicke's area, the angular gyrus, speech function, and motor function. The left side is dominant in 95%, there is dual dominance in 5%, and rarely does one find right-sided dominance. Dominance may switch sides if the cortex is injured at a young age (usually before 2 years of age). The left hemisphere is larger at birth 50% of the time. Dominance may develop because one hemisphere becomes larger and attracts more input. The brain focuses on one area at a time, such that the other area becomes silent. Both sides are connected by the corpus callosum; thus, there is no conflicting activity.

3. A major portion of our sensory experience is stored as language equivalents; therefore, the language center develops closer to the temporal lobe than the occipital lobe because children first learn language by hearing before reading.

D. Corpus callosum — connects the respective cortical areas in the two hemispheres except for the anterior temporal lobe and amygdala, which are connected by the anterior commissure. It connects Wernicke's language information with control of the left hand and with left visual and somatic input. The temporal lobe connections of the anterior commissure allow similar bilateral emotional output.

XVIII. Thought and Memory

A. Thought — characterized as a stimulation pattern of many different parts of the cortex in a definite sequence

B. Consciousness — stream of awareness of our thoughts and surroundings

C. The limbic system, thalamus, and reticular formation determine the quality of pleasure and pain and provide crude localization.

D. The cortex determines specific localization, shape, etc.

E. Pain is elicited by midbrain and hypothalamic stimulation but very little by cortical stimulation.

F. Memory results from the altered ability for synaptic transmission from one neuron to the next as a result of previous activity. It induces new pathways to form, referred to as memory traces. Once established, it can be activated by the mind to reproduce memories. Some memories may be stored in the spinal cord and brainstem (e.g., blink reflex). The brain ignores some information, or else its memory capacity would be filled up within minutes. The inhibition of the memory of useless sensory information is called habituation. Pain and pleasure are stored by facilitation of the synaptic pathways (i.e., memory sensitization). The determination of whether to save a memory is made by the basal limbic areas. Each area of the thalamus reverberates with specific cortical areas and may help store memories. There are three types of memory:

   1. Immediate memory (recall) — Lasts up to several minutes, and only while one is thinking of the facts (e.g., a 10-digit numeric sequence). It is maintained by continued activity in a temporary memory trace by means of reverberating neurons. Presynaptic facilitation or inhibition may be involved. Synaptic potentiation occurs because frequent impulses cause an accumulation of Ca^{2+}, which stimulates neurotransmitter release.

   2. Short-term memory — lasts several weeks; caused by chemical or physical changes. The snail *Aplysia* studied by Kandel was used as a model. For up to 3 weeks, a noxious stimulus was capable of stimulating the sensory terminal and inducing the facilitator terminal to store the information. Stimulation of the facilitator terminal at the same time as the sensory terminal was found to stimulate 5-HT release onto the presynaptic terminal by the facilitator nerve ending. This increased cAMP and activated some protein kinases inside the presynaptic sensory terminal, leading to K^+ channel blockade for minutes to weeks. A longer AP was found to increase Ca^{2+} influx and neurotransmitter release, and facilitated transmission.

   3. Long-term memory — lasts longer than 3 weeks; caused by structural changes at the synapses that either increase or decrease conduction. The area of overall vesicle release is increased, leading to increased release of neurotransmitter. There may be an increase in the number of neurotransmitter vesicles in the presynaptic terminals or an increased number of terminals.

G. Synaptic numbers increase with age as a child grows, but decrease in the blind, deaf, etc. Neuronal numbers are highest soon after birth and then gradually diminish if certain neurons are not used; however, they proliferate with rapid learning.

H. The conversion of a memory from immediate to short- or long-term requires "consolidation." This refers to a chemical, physical, or structural change that occurs anywhere between 5 minutes to 1 hour. The brain is better able to store memories with frequent rehearsals, especially with less information and more repetition. Also, memories are better stored/recalled if categorized based on similarities or differences.

I. The hippocampus stores new memories and is an important output area for the reward/punishment region of the limbic system. Motivation from a happy or sad experience excites the brain to store the experience as a memory. The decision as to what is to be remembered is made by the hippocampus and DM thalamus. Removal of both hippocampi decreases long-term memory storage (i.e., anterograde amnesia) for verbal and symbolic memories.

J. Damage to the amygdala impairs new memory formation.

K. The temporal lobe and Wernicke's area are required for normal consolidation/analysis.

L. Retrograde amnesia — affects more recent memories to a greater extent because older memories are rehearsed so much that they become stored in many different parts of the brain. A hippocampal lesion may cause both anterograde and retrograde amnesia. A thalamic lesion only causes retrograde amnesia because it is used to help search the storehouses of memory.

M. Reflexive learning — a type of learning that does not rely on verbal or symbolic intelligence (i.e., declarative learning), but more on physical skills (e.g., hand skills). It is not affected by damage to the temporal lobe. Reflexive learning occurs by repetitive physical activity, not by symbolic rehearsal in the mind.

XIX. Reticular Activating System and Neurotransmitters (Fig. 2.9)

A. Reticular activating system

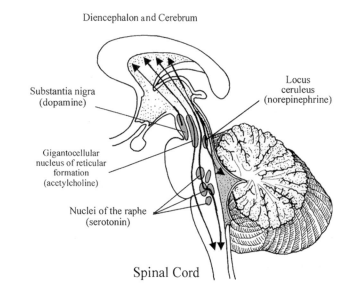

1. Input from the reticular activating system keeps the brain "on." If it is damaged or the brainstem is transected above the fifth cranial nerve, the patient lapses into a coma.

2. The reticular activating system is located in the middle/lateral pons and midbrain, and relays signals upward, but also downward to the spinal cord (to maintain tone in antigravity muscles and to activate spinal reflexes).

3. The system's output is conveyed to all of the subcortical structures, but particularly to the thalamus. Large cells relay rapid, transient signals via ACh to the thalamus. Small cells relay slow fibers to the intralaminar nuclei

Fig. 2.9   Brainstem neurotransmitters.

of the thalamus and reticular nuclei over the thalamic surface; these convey longer impulses that regulate background excitability.

4. There is increased output with increased sensation, particularly with pain. Positive feedback is relayed by the cortex to the reticular system when it is active.

B. Inhibitory reticular formation — located in the lower brainstem, in the medial ventral medulla. Mediated by 5-HT, it reduces the tonic signals sent from the pons to the spinal cord to stimulate antigravity muscles. It requires cortical input to function.

C. Brain activity is also controlled by excitatory and inhibitory neurotransmitters that are directly released into the brain or at synapses with longer duration (minutes to hours).

  1. NE — excitatory, released diffusely and distributed by neurons arising from the locus ceruleus

  2. 5-HT — inhibitory, released in the midline and derived from the raphe nucleus

  3. DA — either excitatory or inhibitory and mainly contained in neurons of the basal ganglia and SN

  4. ACh — excitatory and released from the basal nucleus of Meynert and gigantocellular nucleus of the reticular formation

D. Locus ceruleus — located bilaterally at the posterior pontine–midbrain junction. It relays diffuse projections that are predominantly excitatory (via NE), although a few areas are inhibitory by other receptors.

E. Substantia nigra — projects inhibitory fibers that release DA to the caudate and putamen. However, note that DA is excitatory in the hypothalamus and limbic system.

F. Raphe nucleus in the lower pons/medulla — inhibits via 5-HT; mostly influences the thalamus (for sleep and restful functions), but also the cortex (for sleep) and spinal cord (to decrease pain).

G. Gigantocellular layer of the reticular activating system in the pons/midbrain — stimulates via ACh; neurons relay one branch to the cortex and one branch to the reticulospinal tract.

H. Other neurotransmitters — GABA, enkephalin, angiotensin-2, endorphins, EPI, adrenocorticotropic hormone (ACTH), glutamate, and others

XX. Limbic System, Hypothalamus, and Hippocampus

A. Limbic (border) system — hypothalamus, septal area, paraolfactory area, epithalamus, anterior thalamic nucleus, hippocampus, and amygdala

B. Orbitofrontal cortex — relays fibers → subcallosal gyrus → cingulate gyrus → parahippocampus and the uncus

C. Medial forebrain bundle — bidirectional tract connecting the septal nuclei and orbitofrontal gyrus through the middle of the hypothalamus to the reticular formation. It also connects the reticular formation to the thalamus, hypothalamus, and cortex.

D. Hypothalamus — connected to the reticular formation of the midbrain, pons, and medulla, as well as the diencephalon and cortex (especially the anterior thalamic nucleus and limbic cortex); it also connects to the pituitary via the infundibulum. The hypothalamus regulates the cardiovascular, gastrointestinal (GI), and endocrine systems and controls body temperature, body water, and uterine contractility. It also coordinates with associated limbic system structures to regulate behavioral function.

  1. Lateral hypothalamus — regulates thirst, hunger, emotion, and sympathetic output

  2. Medial hypothalamus — controls satiety

  3. Anterior hypothalamic stimulation — decreases temperature, heart rate, and BP while increasing parasympathetic output

  4. Posterior hypothalamic stimulation — increases body temperature, heart rate, BP, and sympathetic tone

  5. Temperature — mainly regulated by the anterior hypothalamus, particularly the preoptic area

6. Body water concentration — a balance between thirst impulses (from the lateral hypothalamus) and renal excretion of water (regulated by antidiuretic hormone [ADH], released from the supraoptic nucleus)

7. Uterine contractility and milk ejection — regulated by the release of oxytocin from the paraventricular nucleus, whose production increases at the end of pregnancy; this stimulates the uterus to contract. Also, the sucking reflex activates oxytocin release, which causes milk to be expelled through the nipples.

8. Feeding habits
    a. Lateral hypothalamus — initiates searching behavior
    b. Ventromedial hypothalamus — controls satiety
    c. Mamillary bodies — control feeding reflexes (e.g., licking of lips, swallowing)

9. Endocrine function — controlled via portal blood, which delivers hypothalamic releasing factors from the hypothalamic arcuate nucleus and median eminence of the infundibulum to the pituitary gland

10. Behavior
    a. Lateral hypothalamus — controls hunger, rage, and level of activity
    b. Ventromedial hypothalamus — controls satiety and peacefulness
    c. Periventricular region, central gray matter of the midbrain — controls fear and punishment
    d. Anterior/posterior hypothalamic nuclei — controls sex drive
    e. Types of behavior
        (1) Rage — caused by stimulation of the lateral hypothalamic nuclei and the periventricular punishment areas; elicits defensive behavior, claw extension, tail lifting, hissing, spitting, growling, pupillary dilatation, eye opening, piloerection, and attacking
        (2) Fear and anxiety — elicited by stimulation of the midline preoptic nucleus. In animals, this produces a flight response. These impulses are counterbalanced by the ventromedial nucleus, amygdala, anterior cingulate gyrus, and anterior subcallosal gyrus.
        (3) Placidity and tameness — elicited by stimulation of the reward centers

E. Limbic system — determines whether a sensation is pleasant or unpleasant and thus controls our drives and motivations. Reward centers are predominantly located in the lateral and ventromedial hypothalamic nuclei, along with the medial forebrain bundle. Strong lateral nucleus stimulation causes rage and punishment (i.e., unpleasant feelings). Reward centers are also located in the septum, amygdala, thalamus, basal ganglia, and midbrain. Punishment is located in the central gray and periventricular hypothalamus, as well as the amygdala and hippocampus. Punishment and fear can override pleasure and reward.

1. Tranquilizers (e.g., chlorpromazine) — inhibit both the reward and punishment centers and decrease motivation

F. Limbic cortex — association area for the control of behavior and functions as the transitional zone from the cortex to the limbic system. The anterior temporal cortex is mostly used in olfactory and gustatory association. The parahippocampal gyri are used in auditory association and complex thought (along with the Wernicke's area). The middle and posterior cingulate gyri are used in sensorimotor association.

1. Ablation of the temporal tip — produces the Klüver–Bucy syndrome

2. Ablation of the posterior orbitofrontal cortex — causes insomnia and restlessness

3. Ablation of the anterior cingulate and subcallosal gyri — causes rage by the release of the septal nuclei and hypothalamus

G. Amygdala — has bidirectional connections with the hypothalamus via stria terminalis. In lower animals, it receives input from the olfactory tract, which relays to the corticomedial nuclei of the amygdala (under the pyriform cortex). The basolateral nuclei are more important in humans and are not olfactory-related. Input is received from the limbic, parietal, temporal, and occipital cortices (particularly the visual and auditory association areas), which serve as the limbic system's window to the outside world. Output is relayed to these same cortical areas, along with the hippocampus, septal areas, thalamus, and hypothalamus.

1. Stimulation of the amygdala — causes all of the hypothalamic effects (i.e. changes in BP, heart rate, GI motility and secretion, defecation, micturition, pupillary changes, and anterior pituitary secretions), tonic movements (i.e., raising the head, bending the body), clonic movements, eating movements (licking, chewing, swallowing), rage, pleasure, sexual feelings, ejaculation, ovulation, uterine contractions, and copulatory movements

2. Bilateral ablation of the amygdala — produces the Klüver–Bucy syndrome, characterized by a tendency to examine objects orally, decreased aggressiveness (i.e., tameness), dietary changes (i.e., patients become carnivorous), psychologic blindness (i.e., loss of ability to determine what an object is used for by sight), increased sex drive (frequently inappropriate), curiosity, fearlessness, and forgetfulness

H. Hippocampus — connects to the cortex and limbic system (i.e., amygdala, hypothalamus, septum, and mamillary bodies). Incoming sensory information is relayed to the hippocampus and then to the anterior thalamus. Stimulation of various areas elicits reactions similar to stimulation of the amygdala.

1. The hippocampus has a low seizure threshold with long output signals. Seizures are psychomotor with associated olfactory, visual, auditory, and tactile hallucinations. The hippocampus may be more excitable because it is a three-layered paleocortex, as opposed to the six-layered cortex.

2. Early on in life, the hippocampus functions as the critical decision maker. It controls hunger, sexual impulses, and detection of danger by smell (with input from the olfactory areas). Later on in life, it contributes to the function of memory. It senses reward/punishment and rehearses immediate memories until they are stored. Without the hippocampus, one is unable to consolidate short-term memories.

3. Bilateral removal impairs the ability to learn new verbal symbolism (i.e., anterograde amnesia), but one may still recall with immediate memory. Also, retrograde amnesia may ensue from bilateral hippocampal resection.

4. Learning — requires either reward or punishment stimulation to be remembered. Otherwise, the stimulus causes habituation and is ignored. If it elicits a reward feeling or punishment, stimulus repetition reinforces memory.

XXI. Brain Activity States

A. Sleep — when one is unconscious but arousable by stimuli

1. Slow-wave sleep alternates with rapid eye movement (REM) sleep throughout the night.
   a. Slow-wave sleep — constitutes 75% of sleep. It is deep and restful, occurs for the first hour, and is characterized by decreased BP, respiratory rate, and basal metabolic rate (BMR). Dreams occur, but are not remembered.
   b. REM sleep — constitutes 25% of sleep; occurs every 90 minutes, lasts 5–30 minutes (shorter if one is more tired, or longer toward the end of the night), is associated with increased dreaming, is harder to awaken with sensory stimuli, and is characterized by decreased muscle tone, irregu-

lar respiratory rate and heart rate, and increased BMR (~ 20%). Electroencephalographic (EEG) activity resembles the awake state (i.e., paradoxical sleep).

2. Stimulus for sleep — The old theory is passive, stating that sleep occurred when the ascending reticular activating system (ARAS) fatigued. The new theory involves active inhibition of the ARAS and is based on the fact that sleep never occurs if the midportion of the pons is severed and removed from cortical control.

3. Muramyl peptides and other sleep factors accumulate when one is awake, and they increase in the CSF and urine in sleep-deprived people.

4. Sleep cycle — may occur by gradual fatigue of the ARAS and an accumulation of sleep factors. Awakening results from a decrease in these sleep factors and a reinvigoration of the ARAS.

5. Raphe nucleus in the midline lower pons and upper medulla — connected to the reticular formation, thalamus, cortex, hypothalamus, limbic system, and dorsal horns of the spinal cord (for pain modulation). The raphe nucleus uses serotonin as its neurotransmitter; stimulation elicits sleep.

6. Stimulation of the solitary tract nucleus (which receives visceral sensory input via CNs VII, IX, and X) increases sleep, but not if the raphe nucleus is destroyed.

7. Other structures involved with sleep — rostral hypothalamus (suprachiasmatic portion) and intralaminar thalamic nuclei

8. Lesion of the locus ceruleus — decreases REM sleep because it activates certain cortical areas during REM sleep without causing wakefulness

9. Sleep deprivation — causes psychosis, decreased thought, increased sympathetic output, decreased parasympathetic output but no physical harm to the body

B. Brain waves/EEG (**Fig. 2.10**)

1. Brain waves — amplitude of 0–200 mV, and frequency range of 0.3–750 waves/s; usually without a pattern. Brain waves only form when many neurons fire synchronously and are mainly derived from cortical layers 1 and 2. Increased activity causes increased wave frequency but decreased voltage because they are more asynchronous.

2. Alpha waves — 8–13 waves/s and an amplitude of 50 mV. They occur when one is awake and quiet, mostly in the occipital lobes. They are suppressed with eye opening or thought and disappear during

Brain Waves during Wakefulness and Sleep

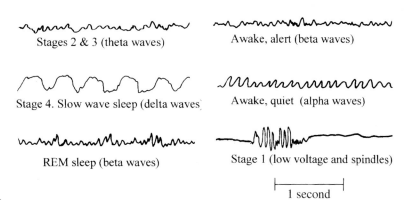

Stages 2 & 3 (theta waves)

Awake, alert (beta waves)

Stage 4. Slow wave sleep (delta waves)

Awake, quiet (alpha waves)

REM sleep (beta waves)

Stage 1 (low voltage and spindles)

1 second

Fig. 2.10   Sleep waves.

sleep. They are changed to asynchronous beta waves when attention moves elsewhere (i.e., increased frequency and decreased voltage). They will not form without a corticothalamic connection because they are elicited by the spontaneous firing of nonspecific thalamic nuclei.

3. Beta waves — 14–80 waves/s, but with decreased amplitude. They occur in the frontal and parietal areas when one is active.

4. Theta waves — 4–7 waves/s, with increased amplitude; occur in the parietal and temporal areas in children. They may occur with stress in adults and are increased in various brain disorders.

5. Delta waves — less than 3.5 waves/s, with increased amplitude. They occur in deep sleep (which functionally separates the cortex from underlying control), infancy, brain disease, and subcortical transection separating the cortex from the thalamus.

6. Four stages of slow-wave sleep
   a. Stage 1 — very light sleep with elimination of alpha waves
   b. Stage 2 — characterized by sleep spindles (short alpha bursts) and K complexes; moreover, stages 2 and 3 may exhibit theta waves
   c. Stages 3 and 4 — characterized by slow-wave, high-amplitude delta waves

7. REM sleep — beta waves that are desynchronized, as in the awake state

C. Epilepsy

1. Seizure — sudden, excessive and/or synchronous alteration of brain electrical activity, resulting from increased excitability of part or all of the CNS
   a. Types of seizures
      (1) Generalized tonic/clonic (grand-mal) seizure — involves the entire brain; begins with tonic activity that transitions into tonic/clonic activity, with high-frequency, high-voltage, synchronized discharges. They may occur by activation of the reticular formation or the thalamus. Overall prevalence of epilepsy is 1–2% of the population. Seizure frequency is increased with emotion, alkalosis, drugs, fever, loud noise, flashing light, and trauma. They are caused by reverberating circuits and terminate via fatigue or active inhibition.
      (2) Absence (petit mal) seizure — 3–30 seconds of unresponsiveness, followed by blinking and head twitching; activated by the basal forebrain and more common in late childhood to 30 years of age. There is a typical 3 per second spike and dome waveform on EEG. They rarely initiate a generalized tonic/clonic seizure.
      (3) Focal seizure — caused either by congenital circuit derangements, a variety of brain injuries that cause gliosis and neuronal damage, tumors, infection, trauma with contusion, or stroke. Occurs due to local reverberating circuits and may spread from the upper limbs to the mouth and lower limbs (i.e., Jacksonian march). May lead to midbrain excitement, which elicits a grand mal seizure. Psychomotor seizures are characterized by amnesia, rage, anxiety, and incoherent speech.

XXII. Autonomic Nervous System

A. Sympathetic nervous system — Each sympathetic pathway is composed of two neurons: a pre- and a postganglionic neuron.

1. Preganglionic fibers — Each preganglionic fiber originates in the spinal cord from a cell body in the intermediolateral cell column (extending from T1–L2) and passes through the anterior root of the cord to

a spinal nerve. From there, preganglionic fibers conduct through the white ramus to the paravertebral sympathetic chain of the ganglia, where they synapse within the ganglia (including the prevertebral ganglia, such as the celiac or hypogastric plexuses) onto postganglionic fibers; however, they may also relay upward/downward within the paravertebral chain.

2. Postganglionic fibers — originate in either sympathetic chain ganglia or prevertebral ganglia and relay to tissues/organs. Some postganglionic fibers relay back to spinal nerves via the gray ramus.

3. Sympathetic fibers — small, type C fibers that distribute to the body in skeletal nerves; in fact, 8% of fibers in the skeletal nerves are sympathetic fibers. They mediate control of BP, sweating, and piloerection.

4. Splanchnic nerves — preganglionic fibers that pass through the sympathetic chain directly to the adrenal medullae without synapsing; there they act upon postganglionic cells that release mainly EPI and NE

5. The sympathetic system does not have as many segments as the spinal nerves. Its distribution is determined by the initial embryonic location of an organ (e.g., the heart in the neck or the abdominal contents in the lower thorax). There is sympathetic innervation to the entire body via the peripheral nerves; sympathetic nerves only travel with blood vessels in the head and neck. Fibers from T1 pass up the sympathetic chain to the head; T2 supplies the neck; T3–T6 supply the thorax; T7–T11 pass into the abdomen; and T12–L2 supply the lower limbs.

B. Parasympathetic nervous system — relies on preganglionic and postganglionic nerve fibers; however, aside from certain cranial parasympathetic nerves, these preganglionic fibers typically synapse onto postganglionic fibers in the walls/substance of end organs

1. Parasympathetic fibers are found in CNs III, VII, IX, and X (~75%) and in the sacral nerves, S1–S4.

2. Unlike the sympathetic system, the parasympathetic system only innervates part of the body. Parasympathetic nerves supply the head, neck, and viscera (but not the limbs).

3. The oculomotor nerve (CN III) supplies the pupillary sphincter and ciliary muscle. The facial nerve (CN VII) innervates the lacrimal, nasal, submandibular, and sublingual glands. The glossopharyngeal nerve (CN IX) innervates the parotid gland. The vagus nerve (CN X) provides parasympathetic innervation to the body, down to the mid-colon level.

4. Sacral roots relay to the nervi erigentes (i.e., pelvic nerves), which exit the sacral plexus to supply the descending colon, bladder, lower uterus, and external genitalia.

5. Parasympathetic stimulation — elicits copious secretions from the mouth and stomach, whereas the intestines are mainly controlled by local factors.

C. Neurotransmitters of the autonomic nervous system

1. All preganglionic fibers are cholinergic.

2. Postganglionic parasympathetic fibers are cholinergic.

3. Most postganglionic sympathetic fibers are adrenergic (NE), except for certain cholinergic fibers regulating sweat, piloerectors, and blood vessels (via muscarinic receptors).

4. Acetylcholine
   a. Produced in nerve terminal endings from acetyl-CoA + choline, by choline acetyltransferase
   b. It is broken down by acetylcholinesterase to choline + acetate.

c. Receptors

(1) Nicotinic receptors — located in the NMJ and preganglionic terminals of sympathetic and parasympathetic fibers; consisting of five subunits, α_2, β, γ, δ. The α-subunit is the ACh binding site; each receptor may therefore bind two ACh molecules, and is composed of four hydrophobic transmembrane proteins. Blocked by hexamethonium (depolarizing, not reversible with anticholinesterase) and stimulated by nicotine.

(2) Muscarinic receptors — located in all postganglionic parasympathetic fiber terminals and postganglionic sympathetic terminals (sweat glands, piloerectors, and blood vessels). Blocked by pertussis toxin; stimulated by muscarine.

5. Norepinephrine

a. Synthesis begins in the axoplasm of terminal endings (from tyrosine to DOPA and then to DA) and is completed in the vesicles (DA to NE and then to EPI).

b. Its removal occurs via presynaptic reuptake (50–80%), diffusion into blood (20–50%), and destruction by MAO. It is rapidly cleared and lasts 10–30 seconds in the blood before catechol O-methyltransferase destroys it in the liver.

c. Adrenergic receptors — NE stimulates $\alpha > \beta$; EPI stimulates α and β equally.

6. Receptor proteins for each transmitter undergo conformational changes upon binding, resulting in increased ion permeability or enzyme activation (e.g., EPI causes an increase in cAMP that either increases/decreases different reactions). The reaction in each organ depends on the receptor protein activated.

7. Examples

a. Sweat — mainly controlled by the sympathetic system (with ACh as the postganglionic neurotransmitter, in this rare instance), except for parasympathetic innervation to the palms of the hands. Thick apocrine secretions occur purely by sympathetic impulses.

b. Adrenal medulla — accounts for 80% EPI and 20% NE. Its effects last 5–10 times longer than other sympathetic stimulation because its products are cleared slowly; this produces more systemic effects, including increased BMR. Both the hormonal and direct stimulation of the sympathetic system work together.

D. The autonomic nervous system works with a low stimulation rate of 10–20 impulses/s, as opposed to the 50–500 impulses/s required for muscle stimulation. It is always active with a basal rate of sympathetic and parasympathetic tone, allowing one system to increase or decrease activity for control. There is also a basal secretion rate of EPI and NE from the adrenal gland. After sympathetic and parasympathetic input is severed from an organ, it gradually compensates with intrinsic tone to a level near baseline. The organ also develops denervation supersensitivity with increased responses to NE, EPI, and ACh.

E. Autonomic reflexes

1. Baroreceptor reflex — specific organs sense stretch in the aorta, carotid, etc., reflecting increased BP. Stretch elicits decreased sympathetic tone, lowering BP.

2. GI reflexes — The smell of food, or its presence in the mouth, stimulates the vagal, glossopharyngeal, and salivatory nuclei to increase oral and gastric secretions. Feces in the rectum causing distention elicit an impulse to the spinal cord to activate parasympathetic system activity, thereby inducing peristalsis to empty the bowel. Accumulation of urine in the bladder elicits a similar response.

3. Mass response (sympathetic) — Stress can cause increased BP, increased blood flow to the muscle, decreased blood flow to the GI tract and kidney, increased BMR, increased serum glucose and glycolysis, increased muscle strength and mental activity, and increased blood coagulation.

4. Focal response (sympathetic) — Change in body temperature alters sweating and blood flow to skin. Some reflexes do not involve the spinal cord but may only relay to the ganglia.

5. Parasympathetic responses — typically more specific

F. Drugs that affect the autonomic system

1. Sympathomimetics — act on the adrenergic receptors. Phenylephrine stimulates α receptors. Isoproterenol activates β_1 and β_2. Albuterol stimulates β_2. NE release is increased by ephedrine, tyramine, and amphetamine.

2. Reserpine — blocks NE synthesis and storage; causes release from the vesicles. It prevents DA uptake into vesicles.

3. Guanethidine — decreases NE release

4. α blockers — phenoxybenzamine and phentolamine

5. β_1 and β_2 blockers — propranolol

6. β_1 blockers only — metoprolol

7. Sympathetic and parasympathetic ganglionic blockers — hexamethonium, tetraethylammonium (TEA), and pentolinium. These are more effective on the sympathetic system, resulting in an overall decrease in BP.

8. Muscarinic receptor agonists (parasympathetic) — pilocarpine and methacholine. These also cause sweating from sympathetic organs, and vasodilation.

9. Muscarinic ACh receptor blockers — atropine, pertussis toxin, and scopolamine

10. Anticholinesterases (reversible) — neostigmine, pyridostigmine, and physostigmine

11. Anticholinesterase (irreversible) — organophosphates

12. Nicotinic ACh receptor agonists — ACh, nicotine, and methacholine

13. Nicotinic ACh ganglionic receptor blockers — hexamethonium; depolarizing and not reversible by anticholinesterase

14. Depolarizing nicotinic ACh receptor blockers — succinylcholine and decamethonium; nonreversible with anticholinesterase. Their action is amplified with decreased muscle temperature.

15. Nondepolarizing nicotinic ACh receptor blocker — α-bungarotoxin (curare); competitive inhibition

16. Botulism toxin — decreased ACh release from the presynaptic terminal, also seen with aminoglycosides and Eaton–Lambert syndrome

17. Cholera toxin — decreased GTP hydrolysis

18. Tetanus toxin — blocks exocytosis by preventing fusion of the vesicle with the cell membrane, e.g., blocks glycine release from Renshaw cells

19. Diphtheria toxin — inactivates tRNA transferase

20. Strychnine — glycine antagonist; increases muscle rigidity

21. Cocaine — α_1-uptake inhibitor; blocks DA and NE uptake

22. TEA — blocks voltage-gated K^+ channels

23. Tetrodotoxin — blocks voltage-gated Na^+ channels

24. Cyanide — blocks the Na^+/K^+ pump, disrupting active transport

XXIII. Cerebral Blood Flow (CBF)

A. Cessation of blood flow to the brain for 5–10 seconds causes unconsciousness; neurons need O_2.

B. CBF — normally 50–55 mL per 100 g/min

  1. Neuronal function is impaired if CBF is <23 mL per 100 g/min.

  2. Irreversible damage occurs when CBF <8 mL per 100 g/min, due to ionic pump failure.

  3. Autoregulated at mean arterial pressures of 60–140 mm Hg, assuming normal intracranial pressure (ICP)

  4. Increased by elevated P_aCO_2 or serum H^+ and lowered by decreased P_aO_2
      a. $CO_2 + H_2O \rightarrow H_2CO_3$ (carbonic acid) $\rightarrow H^+ + HCO_3^-$. Increased H^+ leads to vasodilation, thus increasing CBF.

  5. Normally accounts for 15% of cardiac output (CO). Moreover, the brain consumes 20% of O_2 in the body (oxygen consumption = 3.5 mL O_2 per 100 g/min).

  6. CBF and cerebral metabolic rate of O_2 ($CMRO_2$) — highest in the gray matter (fourfold greater than that in white matter)

  7. Posterior pituitary gland receives the highest blood flow.

C. Ischemic penumbra — the zone of neurons receiving 8–23 mL per 100 g/min of blood flow and exhibiting isoelectric silence. Neurons are still salvageable with the return of blood flow. This also depends on duration of ischemia, temperature, glucose concentration, location, and other factors.

D. Sympathetic fibers — innervate the brain's blood vessels, but usually exert little effect as local autoregulation maintains the CBF in a normal range. However, increased BP with exercise or other causes activates the sympathetic system, which decreases CBF in the face of higher systemic pressures.

E. The brain's mass accounts for 2% of body mass, yet the organ accounts for 15% of its total metabolism. Anaerobic glycolysis does not occur in neurons, and only low stores of glycogen and O_2 are present. Thus, neurons require a constant supply of O_2 and glucose. All cells, except neurons, require insulin for glucose uptake; glucose crosses the blood–brain barrier (BBB) via facilitated transport.

F. Blood–brain barrier

  1. Permeable to H_2O, CO_2, O_2, and lipid-soluble compounds; impermeable to plasma proteins and organic compounds; some permeability to ions, however

  2. Capillary endothelial cells are joined via tight junctions; podocytes of astrocytic cells form a continuous covering along the external wall of the capillary.

XXIV. Skeletal Muscle (Fig. 2.11)

A. Structural components of skeletal muscle

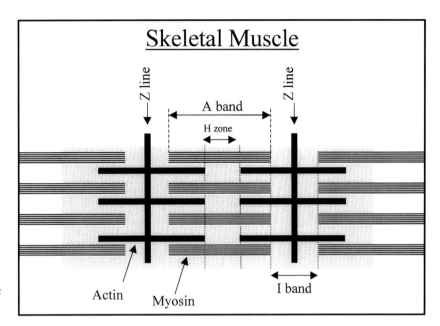

Fig. 2.11 Skeletal muscle structure of contractile apparatus.

1. Each muscle fiber is innervated by one nerve ending that synapses near the longitudinal midpoint of the fiber.

2. One myofibril contains 1500 myosin and 3000 actin filaments.

3. Light and dark bands — Light bands contain only actin; dark bands contain both myosin and actin. I bands only contain actin and are isotropic to polarized light. A bands contain actin and myosin and are anisotropic to polarized light. H bands only contain myosin.

4. Sarcomere — muscle unit that lies between two Z disks

5. Myofibrils of actin and myosin reside in the sarcoplasm of the muscle fiber.

6. Sarcoplasmic reticulum (SR) — extensive endoplasmic reticulum in muscle (skeletal, cardiac or smooth muscle)

7. Myosin molecule — has two heads, each of which expresses ATPase activity; there are 200 myosin molecules per myosin filament

8. Actin filament — composed of actin, tropomyosin, and troponin C (which binds four Ca^{2+} ions)

B. Sliding filament mechanism — accepted model for muscle contraction

1. ACh receptors open Na^+ channels, producing an AP. This depolarizes the cell, along with adjacent SR (at the muscle triads).

2. The SR releases Ca^{2+}, which binds troponin, and shifts tropomyosin off actin's binding site for myosin.

3. Myosin heads bind to actin and pull it along in a ratchet-like fashion. ATP cleavage on the myosin head causes it to become cocked before binding to actin. Upon binding to actin, a power stroke pulls the tilted myosin head, releasing ADP and a phosphate and causing actin and myosin to slide along each other.

4. ATP then binds the myosin head and is cleaved, causing the myosin head to release actin and to reset. Both the attachment and detachment of myosin to actin require ATP.

5. After contraction, there is active pumping of Ca^{2+} back into the SR, where it is stored with calsequestrin such that very little is left in the cytosol. The Ca^{2+} pulse and contraction last 1/20th of a second.

C. Muscle contraction

1. Muscle contraction occurs when the fiber's membrane becomes depolarized and current spreads along the membrane and opens Ca^{2+} release channels on the SR, which releases Ca^{2+}. The RMP is –80 to –90 mV (the same as large myelinated nerve fibers). The duration of the AP is 1–5 milliseconds (5 times as long as in myelinated fibers). Impulse velocity is 3–5 m/s (1/18th that of nerve speed). Current spreads inside the muscle cell to all the fibrils by means of transverse (T) tubules, which are extensions of the cell membrane filled with extracellular fluid and abutting the SR.

2. Maximum contraction — occurs with maximal actin/myosin overlap of 2.0–2.2 mm. Normal resting muscle length, which is around the midpoint of the muscle length spectrum, has the highest force of contraction. The velocity of contraction decreases with increasing load.

3. Muscle requires energy, which is used by the myosin ATPase head, the Ca^{2+} SR pump, and the cell membrane Na^+/K^+ pump. Phosphocreatine and ATP stores last 8 seconds. Glycogenolysis is depleted at 60 seconds. Oxidative metabolism supplies energy over longer periods by use of carbohydrates and proteins (in the short term) and fats (over the long term).
   a. 25% of energy released is used for work; 75% is dissipated as heat.

4. Isometric versus isotonic contractions
   a. Isometric — no change in muscle length
   b. Isotonic — no change in muscle tension

5. Motor unit — consists of 1 α motor neuron and numerous muscle fibers (ranging from 1600 in the quadriceps to 6 in the extraocular muscles, where fine control is required). Current spreads among other motor units to coordinate their actions.

6. Multiple fiber summation — occurs because the smaller and weaker motor units are more excitable and are thus stimulated first. This provides a gradation of force development. Units contract asynchronously, and movement is smooth.

7. Frequency summation may occur, and overlap may cause tetany.

8. Muscle fibers hypertrophy by increasing the number of intracellular fibrils, not the number of cells (i.e., true hyperplasia does not occur).

9. Denervation — results in atrophy and replacement of muscle by fat or fibrous tissue. Fibrous replacement may shorten muscle fibers, resulting in contractures (e.g., a "frozen" shoulder that occurs following brachial plexus injury). Thus, one must be sure to apply stretch to the muscle during the healing process.

10. Reinnervation — no longer occurs after 1–2 years due to loss of muscle fibers. Exemplified in poliomyelitis, where axons sprout to cover other muscle units and form macromotor units with decreased fine control.

D. More skeletal muscle physiology — innervated by large myelinated nerves. The motor end plate is insulated from the extracellular fluid by Schwann cells. The synaptic cleft is 20–30 nm wide. There are 300,000 ACh-containing vesicles at the axon terminal per motor end plate. Each AP releases 300 vesicles into the synaptic cleft. Each vesicle contains 1 quantum = 10,000 ACh molecules. The AP in the axon terminal causes increased

Ca^{2+} conductance by opening voltage-gated Ca^{2+} channels. This causes ACh-containing vesicles to fuse to the membrane for exocytosis.

1. Vesicles — formed in the neuronal cell body by the Golgi apparatus and transported to the axon terminal via axonal transport. ACh is synthesized in the cytosol and actively transported into vesicles. Occasionally, a vesicle fuses spontaneously with the membrane surface, producing an MEPP. A full end-plate potential surpasses the threshold for depolarization, producing an AP in the muscle fiber.

2. After the axon depolarizes and releases ACh to the NMJ, ACh is broken down by acetylcholinesterase or cleared by diffusion. Choline is reabsorbed by the axon terminal for reuse. The entire sequence occurs in 5–10 milliseconds. The vesicle membrane is retrieved from the cell membrane by endocytosis, resulting from the contraction of clathrin protein-coated pits.

3. The muscle membrane at the NMJ contains subneural clefts to increase its surface area. ACh receptors are located near these clefts and form channels through the cell membrane, which are opened by ACh. Na^+, K^+, and Ca^{2+} can move through the channel, but not Cl^- (because a negative charge is present in the channel opening). Only Na^+ moves in, however, generating an MEPP. If depolarization is sufficient, an AP develops.

4. Important pharmacologic agents — Curare blocks the ACh receptor. Botulism toxin decreases ACh release. Both cause paralysis. Neostigmine blocks acetylcholinesterase for several hours. Fluorophosphate irreversibly blocks acetylcholinesterase for weeks and is treated with 2-pyridine aldoxime methochloride (PAM).

5. Myasthenia gravis (MG) — caused by antibodies to the ACh receptor. Treatment is an acetylcholinesterase inhibitor (e.g., neostigmine).

XXV. Smooth Muscle

A. Structural components of smooth muscle

1. Types of smooth muscle
   a. Multi-unit smooth muscle — Multiple, independent fibers innervated by a single nerve ending. Individual smooth muscle cells are connected via gap junctions (i.e., electrical synapses), which permit synchronous contraction of cells. No APs or spontaneous contractions are present. Examples include the ciliary muscle, iris, and piloerectors.
   b. Single-unit smooth muscle — syncytial, with a mass of fibers that contract together. Cell membranes are adherent, and gap junctions permit ion flow between cells. These units may depolarize with or without an AP and thus may develop spontaneous contractions. Examples include the walls of the gut, uterus, and blood vessels.

2. Smooth muscle cells — smaller than skeletal muscle fibers. Smooth muscle cells do not contain troponin. They contain 15 times more actin than myosin. A dense body attached to the cell membrane acts like a Z disk to anchor the actin. Smooth muscle cells exhibit slower and longer contractions, slower cycling of cross-bridges (due to decreased ATPase activity), increased time of cross-bridge attachment (i.e., increased force), lower energy requirements, slower onset of contraction and relaxation, and greater shortening than skeletal muscle with generation of full force. Skeletal muscle only contracts usefully over ⅓ of its length. Smooth muscle contracts over ⅔ of its length because it contains interspersed units (unlike skeletal muscle) and longer actin filaments.

3. Smooth muscle NMJ — formed by autonomic nerves that branch to yield diffuse junctions that secrete neurotransmitters into the interstitial fluid a few nanometers away. These transmitters diffuse to the outer cell and inside the inner cell or produce an AP. No branching end-feet are present as in skeletal muscle nerves, but instead varicosities are evident. Some lie on the fiber membrane to form contact junctions that enable faster transmission.

B. Muscle contraction — does not involve troponin; regulated by increased intracellular Ca^{2+} caused by nerve stimulation, hormonal activation, mechanical stretching, or chemical changes. Ca^{2+} binds calmodulin (each calmodulin molecule binds four Ca^{2+} ions), and this complex binds to and activates myosin light chain kinase; phosphorylation of the myosin heads ensues, generating a contraction cycle. As the Ca^{2+} ion concentration decreases, this process is reversed, and myosin phosphatase cleaves the phosphorus and enables muscular relaxation. Relaxation time is proportional to the concentration of myosin phosphatase.

C. More smooth muscle physiology

1. ACh and NE — either stimulatory or inhibitory via different membrane receptors controlling ion channel permeability

2. RMP is –50 to –60 mV. APs only occur in the single-unit type (i.e., visceral smooth muscle). APs primarily occur due to increased Ca^{2+} conductance because there are few voltage-gated Na^+ channels. They open more slowly than Na^+ channels; thus, the APs are slower.

3. Slow-wave potentials resulting from decreased outward pumping of Na^+ ions may produce spontaneous APs at –35 mV, allowing the cell to function as a pacemaker.

4. Excitation occurs with stretching, which depolarizes the cell via stretch-activated ion channels.

5. Multiunit smooth muscle depolarizes without an AP in response to a nerve stimulus because its fibers are too small to generate a sustaining AP.

6. Most smooth muscle contraction does not occur in response to APs or neural input but due to local tissue factors. These include decreased O_2, increased CO_2, increased H^+, adenosine, lactate or K^+, and decreased Ca^{2+} or temperature. All these factors produce vasodilation. Furthermore, hormones such as NE, EPI, ACh, 5-HT, histamine, angiotensin, and ADH affect smooth muscle if the appropriate chemically-gated receptor is present.

7. Ca^{2+} for skeletal muscle contraction is derived mostly by release from the SR. In smooth muscle, it is derived both by influx from the extracellular space and release from the SR. Smooth muscle has a rudimentary SR. Serum Ca^{2+} concentration has no effect on skeletal muscle, but if it is low, it decreases smooth muscle contraction. Furthermore, slow Ca^{2+}-clearing pumps allow for longer contractions in smooth muscle.

XXVI. Cardiac Muscle

A. Structure of cardiac muscle

1. Striated muscle with cells separated by intercalated disks exhibiting minimal resistance to electricity passing through gap junctions via ionic flow. A syncytium permits easy flow of current.

2. Atrial syncytium — separated from ventricular syncytium by a fibrous bundle around the valves, such that the only pathway for current flow is by way of the atrioventricular (AV) node and associated conducting system.

3. Sinoatrial (SA) node — Located in the superior lateral wall of the right atrium, it contains no contractile elements. It has the fastest automatic rhythm and controls the heart rate. RMP is –55 mV because of a natural leak to Na^+; at –40 mV, Ca^{2+} channels open. Repolarization occurs via opening of K^+ channels. Fast Na^+ channels are blocked at > –60 mV, where only slow Ca^{2+} and Na^+ channels open. The SA node exhibits slow AP activity and slow recovery.

4. Atrioventricular (AV) node — prevents reentry; it is located in the posterior septal wall of the right atrium. A fibrous barrier prevents ventriculoatrial spread of impulses. The AV node self-fires at 40–60 impulses/min; in contrast, Purkinje cells self-fire at 15–40 impulses/min, and the sinus node self-fires at 70–80 impulses/min. The ventricular escape rhythm is 15–40 impulses/min and is due to septal Purkinje fibers taking over rhythm generation.

5. Current spreads from the sinus node more quickly through anterior, middle, and posterior internodal pathways to the AV node, and more slowly along atrial fibers to the AV node. The AV node further delays impulse transmission by 0.13 seconds. This delay is caused by slow transmission due to small fiber size, fewer gap junctions, and low RMPs.

6. Impulses then travel along Purkinje fibers in the right and left bundle branches, which are large fibers with rapid transmission and increased numbers of gap junctions.

B. Muscular contraction

1. Excitation-contraction coupling occurs via T tubules that spread APs to myofibrils and via longitudinal SR tubules that release Ca^{2+}. Unlike skeletal muscle, cardiac muscle exhibits an important inward Ca^{2+} influx; also, there are fewer SR Ca^{2+} stores but more T-tubules in cardiac muscle. Note that T-tubules contain mucopolysaccharides with negative charges to attract Ca^{2+} ions.

2. The AP, with its plateau, lasts longer than in skeletal muscle because of increased conductance through slow Ca^{2+}, slow Na^+, and fast Na^+ channels, and due to an initially diminished K^+ conductance. Thus, it exhibits a slower velocity than in skeletal muscle.

C. More cardiac muscle physiology

1. RMP in cardiac cells is –85 to –95 mV, compared with –90 to –100 mV in Purkinje cells.

2. The atria have shorter refractory time than the ventricles and hence can beat faster. The duration of the AP and contraction is 0.2 seconds in the atria and 0.3 seconds in the ventricle.

3. Parasympathetic system — innervates the SA and AV nodes and blocks both by increasing K^+ conductance, producing hyperpolarization of the cell membrane

4. Sympathetic system — innervates the entire heart, whereby NE increases Na^+ and Ca^{2+} conductance. It increases the rate of contraction threefold and contractility twofold.

5. Adams–Stokes syndrome — intermittent sudden AV block, with a 5- to 30-second delay before the Purkinje system initiates its own beat; patients either faint or die.

XXVII. Circulation

A. Circulatory system — exhibits intrinsic control via local factors and extrinsic control via the nervous system. Parasympathetic input is only important for cardiac function. The sympathetic system, however, innervates the entire circulatory system.

1. The sympathetic chain relays sympathetic fibers to the viscera and spinal nerves to the periphery. The sympathetic system innervates all vessels except capillaries, precapillary sphincters, and arterioles. Small arteries respond by changing the rate of blood flow; large veins affect blood volume.

2. Normal sympathetic (vasoconstrictor) tone contributes 50% of total vessel tone; thus, a sympathetic block may lower BP by 50%.

B. Vasomotor center — located in the reticular formation of the medulla and caudal pons. It is affected by the reticular formation of the diencephalon, mesencephalon, and pons (superolateral aspect is excitatory; the inferomedial aspect is inhibitory). The hypothalamus and limbic system either excite or inhibit this region.

1. Vasoconstrictor area (C-1) — located in the anterolateral upper medulla; relays NE to the spinal cord

2. Vasodilator area (A-1) — located in the anterolateral lower medulla; projects up to the vasoconstrictor area for inhibition

3. Sensory area (A-2) — located in the tractus solitarius, in the posterolateral pons and medulla; receives input from CN IX and X. Each area originates bilaterally.

C. Lateral and medial vasomotor centers

1. Lateral vasomotor center — relays sympathetic input to the heart

2. Medial vasomotor center — relays parasympathetic input to the heart

D. Sympathetic outflow — constricts almost all arterioles and increases peripheral vascular resistance, constricts veins, increases heart rate and contractility, and is the fastest way to increase BP

E. Baroreceptor reflex — uses spray-type nerve endings in the walls of arteries, especially in the carotid sinus (above the common carotid artery bifurcation and in the aortic arch). Stretching of the carotid sinus stimulates Hering's nerve (CN IX), which synapses in the solitary tract. There is progressively increased firing as the mean BP increases from 60 to 180 mm Hg. Aortic receptors stimulate the vagus nerve (relaying to the solitary tract), to inhibit the vasoconstrictor center and stimulate the vasodilatory center if the mean BP is between 90 and 210 mm Hg (normal is 100 mm Hg). The firing rate increases with higher pressures and faster rates of change. Each system is activated with postural changes and resets in 1–2 days to whatever pressure the body is currently at.

F. Chemoreceptors — detect a decrease in O_2, and an increase in CO_2 and H^+. They consist of several small organs (1–2 mm in size), located in the two carotid bodies (at the bifurcations) and aorta. Afferent input from the carotid bodies is via Hering's nerve (CN IX); that from the aortic bodies occurs via the vagus nerve.

G. CNS ischemic response — elicited by an increase in P_aCO_2, as detected by the vasomotor center. It is a very powerful sympathetic response and only reacts if the mean arterial pressure is < 60 mm Hg (mainly at 20 mm Hg, for emergencies only).

H. Regulation of body water

1. Body water is controlled by the anterior hypothalamus, whose supraoptic nucleus secretes ADH to decrease renal H_2O excretion; the lateral hypothalamus, which increases H_2O intake via thirst mechanisms; and the anteroventral third ventricular (AV-3V) region, which detects serum osmolarity.

2. Osmolarity receptors — detect increased serum osmolarity and serum Na^+. This stimulates ADH secretion, resulting in loss of Na^+ and other osmolar substrates into the urine, while H_2O absorption is enhanced in the distal tubules. ⅚ of ADH derives from the supraoptic nuclei; ⅙ from the paraventricular nuclei.

3. Serum osmolarity — regulated by the AV-3V region; the superior aspect comprises the subforniceal organ, and the inferior part constitutes the organ vasculosum of the lamina terminalis. Between these two regions lies the median preoptic nucleus, with connections to both the supraoptic nucleus and BP control centers. There is no BBB in this location, and cells themselves act as receptors (e.g., they shrink in the presence of increased serum Na+ or decreased K$^+$). Moreover, they respond to increasing thirst and ADH secretion.

4. Thirst — inhibited by drinking and stomach distention. If there is no change in serum Na$^+$, the thirst sensation returns every 15–30 minutes; upon fluid consumption, it takes 1 hour to absorb the fluid for osmolarity to equalize. If thirst is not satiated before equalization, overshoot compensation may lead to hyponatremia. The threshold for drinking is attained when Na$^+$ rises at least 2 mEq/L above normal, or the osmolarity rises 4 mEq/L above normal. Arterial baroreceptors and atrial volume receptors also increase the thirst sensation and ADH release.

XXVIII. Respiration

A. Important features of the respiratory center — bilateral center in the medulla and pons

1. Dorsal respiratory group — located in the dorsal medulla; controls inspiration. It is the main respiratory center. Input arrives from neurons in the nucleus of the solitary tract, as well as from chemoreceptors and baroreceptors. There are repetitive inspiratory APs in which one set of neurons fires and inhibits the next. There is also a "ramp" signal to the inspiratory muscles, with a gradual increase in force followed by complete cessation for 3 seconds, and then another cycle begins. This allows for steady inhalation without gasps.

2. Ventral respiratory group — located in the ventrolateral medulla, in the nucleus ambiguus and retroambiguus; controls both inspiration and exhalation. It is not active in normal breathing, where the dorsal nuclear group stimulates the diaphragm in inspiration, and exhalation occurs via recoil of the lung and chest. It contributes to larger respiratory efforts, from abdominal muscle exhalation and strong inhalation.

3. Pneumotaxic center — located in the dorsal superior pons, in the nucleus parabrachialis; controls the rate and pattern of breathing. It supplies continuous impulses to the inspiratory area to switch it off to shorten a breath and start exhalation. Increased input causes rapid breathing; decreased input produces long, drawn-out breathing.

B. Control of respiration

1. Chemical control of respiration — used to correct O_2, CO_2, and H$^+$

2. Direct control of respiration — mediated by CO_2 and H$^+$. The chemosensitive area of the ventral medulla is located just below the brainstem surface. It excites the respiratory center if H$^+$ is increased, and to a lesser extent, if CO_2 is increased. pH has less effect on respiration because H$^+$ has more affinity for the receptor but does not cross the BBB. CO_2 is a weaker stimulant but crosses the BBB; together with H_2O, it forms HCO_3^- and H$^+$. P_aCO_2 is important in the CSF because it is minimally buffered. Changes in P_aCO_2 are therefore associated with rapid changes in CSF H$^+$. The response to changes in CO_2 decreases within hours to days, to ⅕ of its initial effect; this occurs partly by renal clearance of H$^+$, by increasing HCO_3^- binding to H$^+$ in the CSF. P_aCO_2 causes potent acute respiratory changes but not chronic ones.

3. Indirect control of respiration — occurs via O_2, which does not directly stimulate the respiratory center. The peripheral chemoreceptor system detects O_2, CO_2, and H$^+$. There are multiple receptors relaying to the dorsal respiratory area: the carotid bodies, which relay impulses via the Hering's nerve (CN IX); and

the aortic bodies, which relay through CN X. The carotid and aortic bodies receive arterial blood and relay increased impulses when P_aO_2 is decreased (i.e., 30–60 mm Hg). Increased signals are also relayed with elevated P_aCO_2 or H^+, but receptors to these stimuli are sevenfold weaker than central receptors (although they are faster). This particular system minimally affects CO_2 and H^+ control of respiration.

4. During exercise — O_2 consumption and CO_2 formation increase 20-fold. Ventilation increases to match supply with demand. As muscle is stimulated by the brain, collateral fibers relay to the respiratory and BP control centers to perform the correct responses (these may be learned). Also joint receptors stimulate respiration. Hence, both chemical and neuronal factors regulate respiration, especially with exercise.

5. Hering–Breuer inflation reflex — stimulated by stretch receptors in the bronchi and bronchioles. Afferent fibers travel in the vagus nerve to inhibit the dorsal respiratory nucleus to stop respiratory inspiration if the lungs are overly distended. It does not fire until the tidal volume is 71.5 L and it serves a protective function.

XXIX. Gastrointestinal Tract

A. Important features of the GI tract

1. The GI tract has its own nervous system in the gut wall extending from the esophagus to the anus. This contains 100 million neurons (the same number as the spinal cord) and controls GI tract movements and secretions.

2. Two plexuses
   a. Auerbach myenteric plexus — located between the longitudinal and circular layers of muscle; controls GI movements
   b. Meissner submucosal plexus — located in the submucosa; controls secretions and blood flow

3. Sensory nerve endings from the epithelium relay to both plexuses, the sympathetic ganglia, spinal cord, and parasympathetic fibers in the spinal cord and brainstem.
   a. Parasympathetic system — innervates the gut from the esophagus down to the first half of the colon, by means of the vagus nerve. It also innervates from the sigmoid colon to the anus via S2–S4 fibers. Postganglionic neurons are retained within the myenteric and submucosal plexuses.
   b. Sympathetic system — input from T5–L2, relaying to the celiac and mesenteric ganglia, to the postganglionic fibers that travel as separate nerves, to the intestine's enteric plexus. It acts to decrease movement and smooth muscle contraction (except for the muscular mucosal layer).

B. Reflexes — either purely enteric or relaying from the intestine to the autonomic system and back to the intestine (e.g., gastrocolic defecation reflex or enterogastric and coloileal reflexes to slow transit); or relaying from the intestine to the spinal cord or brain and back to the intestine (e.g., for pain or defecation).

C. Two types of movement in the GI tract:

1. Propulsive movement — peristalsis; a contractile ring propels forward as a result of stimulation by local reflexes of distention/irritation, in response to parasympathetic input. It requires the myenteric plexus to contract and moves forward because the plexus is polarized.

2. Mixing — occurs in the mouth (i.e., chewing), stomach, and intestine

D. GI-related functions

1. Intake — stimulated by hunger. One craves food when the stomach contracts. The lateral hypothalamus generates the stimulus to eat and increases the emotional drive for food. The ventromedial hypothalamus causes satiety and inhibits the feeding center. The amygdala also contributes input in conjunction with the olfactory system and prefrontal cortex. The mechanism for intake resides in the brainstem; the amount of intake is regulated by the hypothalamus. It is stimulated by glucose, amino acid, and lipid levels; thus, nutrient stores dictate overall appetite. Appetite decreases with GI distention, CCK (stimulated by the fat in food), glucagon, insulin, and the oral meter of intake (with chewing and salivation for short-term control).
   a. Obesity — Nutrient stores do not shut off the hunger center; may be psychogenic, hypothalamic (i.e., different set point of nutrient stores), or genetic.

2. Salivation — controlled by the salivatory nuclei at the medulla/pons junction. The superior nucleus relays to the facial nerve, to the submandibular ganglion, and on to the submandibular and sublingual glands. The inferior nucleus relays to CN IX, to the otic ganglion, and on to the parotid gland. It is increased by certain tastes (especially sour) and tactile stimulation (i.e., increased with "smooth," and decreased with "rough" textures). Salivation is controlled by higher areas (i.e., increased with disliked food) and gastric stimulation (i.e., increased with irritation).

3. Chewing — stimulated by the reticular formation, hypothalamus, amygdala, and cortex, with final input into the trigeminal motor nucleus. A reflex is initiated by a bolus of food causing the jaw to stretch; this stimulates the muscles of mastication to contract.

4. Swallowing (deglutition) — voluntary stage (i.e., tongue movement) and involuntary stage (i.e., passage from the pharynx into the esophagus). The soft palate pulls up to block the nasal passage, the trachea closes, the esophagus opens, and a fast wave propels the food bolus to the esophagus. The tonsillar pillars contain afferent fibers from CN V and IX that relay to the solitary tract; reticular formation swallowing center; CNs V, IX, X, XII; and the cervical roots. The esophageal (i.e., involuntary) stage has both afferent and efferent fibers from CN X.

5. Gastric secretions — increased with ACh (which effectively increases all secretions, namely gastrin, pepsinogen, mucus, and HCl), gastrin, and histamine (mainly acid). Acid secretion occurs via local reflexes (50%) and by the dorsal CN X nucleus relaying to CN X, to the enteric system, and on to the gastric glands (50%). The main neurotransmitter is ACh except for gastrin-releasing peptides. Input arrives from the limbic system and stomach.
   a. Stimulated by stomach distention, tactile sensation in the stomach, and various chemicals (i.e., amino acids, peptides, and other acids). Increased gastrin secretion is stimulated by the vagus nerve acting on parietal cells that produce HCl. Also, gastrin secretion is increased by histamine release from the gastric mucosa.
   b. Three phases of gastric secretions:
      (1) Cephalic phase — from the cortex or appetite center in the amygdala or hypothalamus to the dorsal motor nucleus of CN X
      (2) Gastric phase — from vago-vagal input, local reflexes, and gastrin release
      (3) Intestinal phase — mediated by gastrin

6. Intestinal secretions — mainly controlled by local reflexes. These include mucus (to lubricate feces, allowing them to slide) and electrolyte solutions (for absorption and transport).

7. Defecation — initiated by a stimulus in the rectum; controlled by the internal (voluntary, smooth muscle) and external anal sphincters (voluntary, striated muscle innervated by the pudendal nerve). The reflex returns impulses to the myenteric plexus to increase peristalsis and relax the sphincters. The urge

sensation is increased by the parasympathetic defecation reflex from the pelvic nerves. If one voluntarily counteracts the reflex, it will not occur again until more stool accumulates in the rectum. Sensory fibers distinguish between gas, liquid, and solid.

XXX. Genitourinary Tract

A. Micturition — involves the bladder detrusor (i.e., smooth) muscle and internal sphincter (which are involuntary) and the external sphincter (which is voluntary). The parasympathetic system supplies sensation and motor function to the bladder via pelvic nerves from S2–S3. Stretch is detected by sensory parasympathetic fibers, which relay to the spinal cord and on to the detrusor for contraction. The pudendal nerve functions to provide voluntary control to the external sphincter. There is sympathetic innervation from L2 via hypogastric nerves to regulate pain and blood vessels; however, this does not contribute to bladder contraction or internal sphincter relaxation.

B. Micturition reflex — self-regenerating; an initial contraction causes increased sensory input from stretch fibers, leading to increased urge and tonic contraction that transiently subsides but ultimately increases in frequency until the bladder is emptied. The reflex lies within the spinal cord, but there is upper control by the pons and cortex. The reflex is initiated by a Valsalva maneuver to increase the stretch reflex. Residual bladder volumes should be less than 10 mL.

C. Atonic bladder — caused by decreased sensory input to the spinal cord, resulting in overflow incontinence. This is seen with syphilis or lower motor neuron injuries.

D. Spastic bladder — characterized by a lack of neuronal input above the sacral level. Following spinal cord injury, patients develop spinal shock and lose reflexes, necessitating insertion of a catheter. If reflexes return, bladder function may be normal or hyperactive. It may require skin stimulation or suprapubic pressure (Credé maneuver) for initiation of micturition.

XXXI. Temperature

A. Temperature — autoregulated in dry air (60–130°F) to preserve body temperature at 97–100°F, via a homeostatic, hypothalamic-neuronal mechanism

B. Detection — occurs in the anterior hypothalamus and preoptic areas, which exhibit increased firing mostly with heat (but also with cold), thereby inducing sweating and vasodilatation; and by cold and warm receptors in the skin and deep tissues. Cold stimulation produces increased shivering to generate heat, along with decreased sweating and vasoconstriction to conserve heat.

C. Both the anterior hypothalamus and skin receptors relay signals to the posterior hypothalamus to activate heat-generating mechanisms.

D. Lowering of body temperature — occurs by vasodilatation, decreasing sympathetic tone, sweating, and decreasing heat production (i.e., decreased shivering and chemical thermogenesis)

E. Raising body temperature — occurs by vasoconstriction (i.e., increased sympathetic tone), piloerection (to increase insulation), shivering (to increase heat production), and increased BMR (via thyroxine). The primary motor center for shivering is in the posterior dorsomedial hypothalamus, which is under tonic inhibition by the heat center in the anterior hypothalamus. Stimulation by cold signals from the periphery results in increased body tone and increased heat production. Sympathetic input increases cell metabolism for chemical thermogenesis and uncouples oxidative phosphorylation. Body temperature is increased further with brown fat, which contains special mitochondria for heat production (only found in animals and neonates). Body temperature also increases with acclimation to cold. Moreover, thyroxine aids in thermogenesis by producing a delayed increase in cell metabolism; for example, there are increased levels in chronically cold animals (e.g., goiters are more common in a colder climate).

F. Set-point — 37°C; fever ensues when there is a change in the set-point by proteins, chemicals, or toxins (i.e., pyrogens). Gram-negative bacterial endotoxin is taken up by white blood cells (WBCs); this produces increased interleukin-1, which causes increased prostaglandins, leading to the onset of fever (as regulated by the hypothalamus) within 8 hours. Treatment of fever is by blocking prostaglandin formation with acetylsalicylic acid. Fever may also be generated in the context of tumors or surgery near the hypothalamus.

XXXII. Endocrine

A. Relevant anatomy

1. Pituitary gland — secretes eight hormones; six from the anterior pituitary and two from the posterior pituitary gland

2. Hypothalamus — gathers information (pain, smells, electrolytes, etc.) and relays it to the pituitary gland

3. Primary capillary plexus — The primary capillary plexus of the median eminence of the hypothalamus and the tuber cinereum drains into the hypothalamic–hypophyseal portal system, with sinuses to the anterior pituitary gland.

4. The hypothalamic cell bodies are diffusely spread out, but axons relay to the median eminence. The hypothalamus secretes releasing and inhibiting hormones: thyrotropin, corticotrophin, growth hormone and gonadotropin-releasing hormones, somatostatin, and DA. Somatostatin inhibits growth hormone and thyrotropin-releasing hormones.

5. Posterior pituitary gland — secretes oxytocin and ADH, which are synthesized in the cell bodies of the supraoptic and paraventricular nuclei of the hypothalamus; they are coupled to neurophysins (carrier proteins), placed in vesicles, and transported along the axons to the posterior pituitary gland, where they are identified as Herring bodies.

B. Hormones of the pituitary gland

1. All anterior pituitary hormones (aside from growth hormone [GH]) act on target organs.

2. GH — promotes infant-to-child and child-to-adult growth by increasing bone and tissue growth. Bones stop growing when epiphyseal cells are used up. GH also mediates metabolic functions (e.g., increasing protein formation and fat consumption and decreasing carbohydrate use). Somatomedin C is synthesized in the liver in response to GH, acts on end organs, and provides negative feedback by increasing somatostatin levels and decreasing GH levels. A GH deficiency early in life produces dwarfism. However, an excess early in life causes gigantism; later on in life, it causes acromegaly.

3. Thyroid-stimulating hormone (TSH) — increases the rate of body metabolism and heat production. Hypothyroidism early in life causes cretinism.

4. ACTH — stimulates the production of cortisol in response to stress. It also stimulates aldosterone production (which is also controlled by Na⁺, K⁺, and angiotensin). ACTH decreases protein formation and increases metabolism, using amino acids elsewhere to repair damage or as energy to make carbohydrates. Furthermore, it increases fat and glucose consumption.

5. Prolactin (PR) — increased levels in pregnancy, causing an increase in breast size and milk secretion. Prior to birth, it is inhibited by estrogen and progesterone. However, it is activated by the sucking (spinal cord) reflex, and tonically inhibited by DA. Stress may decrease the secretion of PR and cause a mother to stop secreting milk.

6. Luteinizing hormone (LH) — contributes to ovulation; also stimulates the secretion of female sex hormones by the ovaries and activates Leydig cells to proliferate and produce testosterone. However, testosterone inhibits hypothalamic gonadotrophin-releasing hormone, thereby decreasing LH secretion in the testes.

7. Follicle-stimulating hormone (FSH) — induces growth of follicles in the ovaries, prior to ovulation; also promotes the formation of sperm in the testes. Spermatogenesis in the testes causes Sertoli cells to secrete inhibin, decreasing FSH release by the anterior pituitary and inhibiting Sertoli cells; this prevents the overproduction of sperm.

8. ADH — Secreted when an increase in the osmolarity or Na^+ is detected by receptors in the supraoptic nucleus. It causes increased distal tubule H_2O reabsorption and NaCl loss. Most is secreted from the supraoptic nucleus; the rest is from the paraventricular nucleus. Its release is stimulated by warm skin, vomiting, decreased blood volume, pain, narcotics, and angiotensin-2. Its release is decreased by ethanol and cold. Corticotropin-releasing hormone inhibits ADH.

9. Oxytocin — mostly secreted by the paraventricular nucleus; causes uterine contractions at the end of pregnancy. Secretion is increased with cervical stimulation, which provides positive feedback. Sucking causes oxytocin secretion, resulting in contraction and excretion of milk from myoepithelial cells in the breast glands.

C. Female sexual response — Gonadotropin-releasing hormone is secreted mainly by the arcuate nucleus in the medial basal hypothalamus. Low estrogen levels and high progesterone levels decrease FSH/LH secretion, mainly at the anterior pituitary gland (but also at the hypothalamus). Inhibin secreted by the corpus luteum decreases FSH and some LH secretion. There are increased LH levels 48 hours before ovulation, accompanied by a slight increase in FSH.

1. In the first half of the cycle, estrogen imposes positive feedback and increases FSH/LH. Also, progesterone from the corpus luteum increases the LH surge for ovulation.

2. After ovulation, the corpus luteum increases the level of progesterone, estrogen, and inhibin to decrease FSH/LH. Three days before menstruation, the corpus luteum involutes and decreases estrogen/ progesterone secretion, causing an increase in FSH/LH, and promoting menstruation.

3. The peak estrogen level is 13 days after the start of menstruation. Twelve days after the onset of menstruation, the FSH and LH that were slowly decreased by estrogen's negative feedback increase significantly via positive feedback, increasing the LH and FSH surge for ovulation and corpus luteum formation.

4. Menarche — occurs at 13 years. Menopause occurs at 40–50 years and is associated with decreased estrogen production by the ovaries. In this context, there is no inhibition or surge of FSH and LH.

5. The female sexual response requires psychological and local stimulation. There is increased desire at ovulation, with peak levels of estrogen.
    a. Input — from the pudendal nerve to the spinal cord and brain
    b. Output — by means of the sacral plexus to the nervi erigentes of the parasympathetic system to the erectile tissue of the clitoris. It also tightens the vagina around the penis to increase pleasure for both.

  c. There is increased Bartholin gland secretion of mucus under the labia minora. Fluid is also secreted by the vaginal wall and by the male.

  d. The sympathetic system is involved in orgasm, which helps promote fertilization by increasing uterine and fallopian tube motility and increasing cervical dilatation. It also causes perineal contraction, and increased oxytocin production activates uterine contraction. This facilitates sperm transport to the uterus.

D. Male sexual response — involves afferent fibers from the pudendal nerves to the sacral plexus and on to the spinal cord and brain. Irritation or full sensation of the sexual organs causes increased sexual desire (i.e., aphrodisiac).

 1. The sexual act is completely coded in spinal reflexes (i.e., input above the lumbar level is not necessary), although psychological factors can influence it.

 2. Parasympathetic input — generates an erection (simply remember the "p" in "point"); the spinal cord supplies the penis via the nervi erigentes, causing an increase in blood flow.

 3. Increased mucus is secreted by the urethra and bulbourethral glands for lubrication.

 4. Sympathetic input — causes ejaculation (simply remember the "s" in "shoot"); arrives from the L1–L2 levels to the hypogastric and pelvic plexuses. Emission occurs from the vas deferens and ampulla, which contract to secrete sperm into the urethra. The prostate and seminal vesicle, under muscular contraction, secrete fluid to form semen, which mixes with urethral mucus.

 5. Ejaculation — Pudendal nerves relay to the spinal cord, causing rhythmic contraction of the genital organs, and the ischiocavernosus and bulbocavernosus muscles. This also stimulates pelvic thrusts.

3 Pathology and Radiology

Associate Editor, **Charles Matouk**

I. General Neuropathology

A. Neural stains — hematoxylin and eosin stain (H&E) for general pathologic examination, the Nissl stain for neuron cell bodies (binds nucleic acid), and the silver stain for cell processes. Lipofuscin accumulates in central nervous system (CNS) neurons with aging. Neuromelanin accumulates in neurons (especially the substantia nigra [SN] and locus ceruleus) and is a catecholamine waste product (it is not made by tyrosinase). True melanin is made by tyrosinase and is located in the leptomeningeal melanocytes of the ventral medulla and cervical cord. These cells form the primary CNS melanomas.

B. Edema (increased brain water)

    1. Vasogenic edema — due to increased blood–brain barrier (BBB) permeability to proteins and macromolecules. It is caused by vessel damage, inflammation, and neovascularity. It is the most common type of edema, is extracellular, and affects the white matter more than the gray matter. Corticosteroids decrease the edema.

    2. Cytotoxic edema — caused by an impaired Na^+/K^+ pump caused by decreased adenosine triphosphate (ATP) delivery during hypoxia and ischemia. Water and electrolytes accumulate in the cell, but not plasma proteins. It is intracellular, affects both the gray and white matter, and is not associated with computed tomographic (CT) or magnetic resonance imaging (MRI) enhancement because of the intact BBB. Steroids do not decrease the edema.

    3. Interstitial edema — the transependymal shift of fluid caused by cerebrospinal fluid (CSF) accumulation (hydrocephalus) and is extracellular

C. Lethal neuronal injury — characterized by ischemic necrosis. The cytoplasm that was slightly basophilic becomes eosinophilic (red is dead) and the nucleus becomes shrunken and dark. Changes can be seen within 6 hours. Ferrugination occurs when dead neurons become encrusted with Fe^{2+} and Ca^{2+} salts.

D. Progressive or reversible neuronal injury is characterized by

    1. Central chromatolysis — occurs after an injury to an axon near the cell body. The Nissl substance disappears, the nucleus becomes eccentric, and the cell body enlarges. It is seen in the anterior horn cells with anterior nerve root compression and Guillain–Barré syndrome. The cells may progress to death or recover.

    2. Neurofibrillary tangles — Argyrophilic linear densities accumulate in the cell bodies and processes. They can be detected on silver stain. The neurofibrils are made up of hyperphosphorylated tau proteins, neurofilaments, and microfilaments (actin). They are much more numerous with Alzheimer disease, postencephalitic Parkinson disease, progressive supranuclear palsy, and aluminum toxicity.

    3. Neuronal storage of lipids or carbohydrates — The cell body enlarges, the nucleus becomes eccentric, and the cytoplasm becomes foamy.

4. Inclusion bodies
    a. Viral
        (1) Intranuclear — herpes simplex virus 1 (HSV-1; Cowdry type A, eosinophilic, in neurons, astrocytes, and oligodendrocytes; seen early in the disease), cytomegalovirus (CMV), and measles (subacute sclerosing panencephalitis [SSPE])
        (2) Intracytoplasmic — rabies (Negri bodies), SSPE, and CMV
    b. Degenerative/metabolic (all intracytoplasmic) — Pick bodies (in Pick disease, round stain with silver), Lewy bodies (in Parkinson disease, have a halo), Lafora bodies (in Lafora disease, periodic acid Schiff [PAS] positive, basophilic, have a dense core), Hirano bodies (eosinophilic, most in hippocampus, made of actin, seen in the elderly and increased number with Alzheimer disease), and Bunina bodies (eosinophilic, increased with amyotrophic lateral sclerosis [ALS])

5. Marinesco bodies are seen in normal brain. They are eosinophilic and contain chiefly ubiquitin. They are located mainly in the nucleus of melanin cells of the brainstem.

E. Neuronal atrophy — occurs with degenerative diseases and has been postulated to be due to either excitatory amino acids, subcellular injuries by free radicals, or gene-directed apoptosis. Neuronal atrophy is associated with proliferation of astrocytes and microglia.

F. Hamartoma — disorganized cells in the proper location for that cell type

G. Choristoma — correctly organized cells in the wrong location

H. Brain herniation changes — Kernohan notch (the contralateral cerebral peduncle is compressed against the incisura with ipsilateral weakness producing a false localizing sign), posterior cerebral artery (PCA) stroke, Duret hemorrhages of the midbrain and pons (by arteriole stretching), CN III palsy, and hydrocephalus (by compression of the cerebral aqueduct).

II. Glial Cell Response to Injury

A. Astrocytes — either protoplasmic (mainly in the gray matter) or fibrillary (mainly in the white matter). Glial fibrillary acidic protein (GFAP) is the main component of astrocytic intermediate filaments.

B. Astrocytic reaction to injury

1. Secondary (reactive) astrocytosis — occurs after stroke, degenerative diseases, etc. There rarely are mitotic figures unless there is neoplastic disease. Gemistocytic astrocytes are large reactive astrocytes with eccentric nuclei. Fibrillary astrocytes appear later, have smaller cell bodies, and more fibers. Rosenthal fibers are eosinophilic masses in the astrocytic processes and are increased with Alexander disease, pilocytic astrocytomas, and reactive astrocytosis.

2. Primary astrocytosis — the proliferation of astrocytes after astrocytic disease such as hepatic encephalopathy with Alzheimer II astrocytes (large nuclei, gray, glycogen inclusions) (**Fig. 3.1**)

C. Microglia — macrophages from outside the CNS. With mild injury, there may be rod cells with cigar-shaped nuclei.

D. Oligodendrocytes — proliferate around multiple sclerosis plaques and are increased in size with bizarre shapes around the periphery in progressive multifocal leukoencephalopathy (PML)

E. Ependymal cells — do not proliferate with injury but when damaged are replaced by subependymal astrocytes

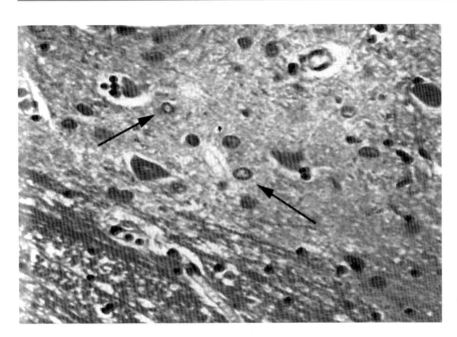

Fig. 3.1 Alzheimer type II astrocytes (hematoxylin and eosin [H&E] stain) with large vesicular nuclei and cyto-plasm (*arrows*).

III. General Neuroradiology

A. Conventional x-rays — usage largely supplanted by the widespread availability and rapidity of CT scans. In the pediatric population skull x-rays continue to have a defined role in the evaluation of minor head trauma and suspected child abuse, metallic foreign objects implanted in the skull, abnormal head shape, and integrity of ventricular shunt tubing as part of a "shunt series." Spinal x-rays continue to be performed in the preliminary evaluation of spinal trauma and to assess spinal stability.

B. Multislice CT scans — x-ray-based method remains investigation of choice for preliminary radiographic evaluation of the CNS. Particularly well suited for identifying bony lesions and acute hemorrhage, for example, in the evaluation of trauma and stroke. The ability of modern scanners to perform 3D-reconstruction is particularly advantageous in the evaluation of traumatic spinal injuries.

   1. CT angiography (CTA) — involves administration of iodinated contrast agent; well-suited for evaluation of carotid and vertebral atheromatous disease and dissection, cerebral aneurysms, and acute thrombi within intracranial vessels

   2. CT perfusion (CTP) — involves administration of iodinated contrast agent and can be rapidly performed on any standard helical CT scanner. Its main usage is distinguishing between "at risk" and infarcted brain in stroke patients. The following perfusion parameters are typically measured: cerebral blood volume, cerebral blood flow (CBF), mean transit time, and time to peak enhancement.

C. MRI — the modality of choice for resolution of anatomic detail and subtle disease processes. Unlike CT scans, it does not use ionizing radiation. MRI is based on electromagnetic fields generated by hydrogen nuclei. Prior to the application of an external magnetic field, the magnetic axes of hydrogen nuclei are randomly aligned. Upon exposure to an external magnetic field, these axes are forced into alignment with the external source to produce a net magnetization vector. When a radiofrequency (RF) pulse is then applied, the net magnetization vector tilts to produce a vector with two constituent components — a longitudinal vector and a transverse vector. The transverse vector contributes to the return RF pulse, or "echo," to generate the MR signal. When the RF pulse is turned off, the net magnetization vector realigns with the external source. This occurs through two simultaneous processes: T1 recovery and T2 decay. T1 recovery is the time constant for the "recovery" of magnetization along the longitudinal axis. T2 decay reflects the concomitant decrease in magnetization along the transverse axis. Different tissues have different T1 and T2 values, which serve as the basis for tissue contrast in all MR imaging. Moreover, tissue contrast may be preferentially dependent on either T1 recovery or T2 decay, and images can be generated that are relatively T1- or T2-weighted to maximize these contrasts.

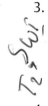

1. Conventional spin-echo sequences — typically used to generate T1- and T2-weighted MRIs. T1-weighted MRIs provide the best depiction of anatomy; T2-weighted MRIs provide the best depiction of disease processes characterized by high water content (which appears bright on T2-weighted MRIs).

2. Fluid-attenuated inversion-recovery (FLAIR) — special spin-echo sequence that eliminates signal from CSF. FLAIR MRI is most useful in the delineation of cystic lesions and tumors abutting sulci or the ventricles.

3. Gradient echo (GRE) sequences — extremely fast sequence that is particularly sensitive to magnetic field inhomogeneity that results in a local loss of signal. This sequence is well suited for the detection of hemorrhage, e.g., cerebral contusions, cavernous malformations, where the iron in hemoglobin causes its own magnetic field. GRE sequences form the basis of MR perfusion studies (which require the administration of a gadolinium-based contrast agent) and functional MRI (fMRI, discussed below).

4. Diffusion-weighted imaging (DWI) — distinguishes rapid (unrestricted diffusion) and slow diffusion of protons (restricted diffusion). When coupled with apparent diffusion coefficient (ADC) maps, this technique allows determination of stroke age. Acute stroke will appear bright on DWI and dark on ADC maps. The reverse is true for chronic stroke.

5. MR angiography (MRA) — useful for visualization of the cerebral vasculature
   a. Time-of-flight (TOF) — a rapid sequence that does not require intravenous (IV) administration of a contrast agent. The technique involves suppression of MR signal from stationary tissues so that flowing blood appears relatively hyperintense.
   b. Contrast-enhanced MRA — requires IV administration of a gadolinium-based contrast agent. The paramagnetic contrast agent serves to shorten the T1 of blood, which results in high signal intensity on T1-weighted MRIs.

6. MR spectroscopy (MRS) — a water suppression technique that permits the detection of brain metabolites. MRS can be performed at the same time as conventional MRI with appropriate software. Clinically, it is most useful in the differentiation of tumor from nonneoplastic processes such as abscess, tumefactive demyelination, and subacute infarcts. Brain tumors typically demonstrate reduced N-acetylaspartate (NAA) and creatine levels and increased choline levels compared with normal brain.

7. fMRI — used for functional mapping of the brain, in particular, preoperative mapping of eloquent cortex (e.g., primary motor, sensory, and language cortex). The underlying premise of fMRI is the observation that increased neuronal activity is associated with increased CBF and oxygen delivery out-of-proportion to the tissue's capacity to consume the increased oxygen. The result is a local increase in the concentration of intravascular oxyhemoglobin (nonparamagnetic substance) and a concordant decrease in the concentration of deoxyhemoglobin (paramagnetic substance). The locally decreased concentration of a paramagnetic substance allows for less severe local magnetic field distortions and an increased MRI signal. fMRI does not require IV administration of a contrast agent.

D. Digital subtraction angiography (DSA) — prior to CT scans and MRI, DSA (an x-ray-based technique that involves the administration of iodinated contrast agent) was the test-of-choice in the evaluation of suspected intracranial tumors whose mass effect caused the displacement of cerebral vascular structures. Today DSA remains the gold standard in the evaluation of cranial and spinal vascular disease. Therapeutic neurointerventional radiology involves the deployment of coils, embolic materials, and stents for the treatment of aneurysms, vascular malformations (arteriovenous malformations [AVMs], dural arteriovenous fistulas), and carotid atheromatous disease. Preoperative tumor embolization is sometimes a useful surgical adjunct in the treatment of meningiomas.

E. Positron emission tomography (PET) — useful in the study of brain function, in particular, metabolism and CBF. The technique involves the administration (usually IV) of a metabolically active, radioactive tracer that spontaneously decays to release positrons (similar to electrons, but positively charged). These positrons travel short distances (a few millimeters) into adjacent tissue where they are annihilated by reacting with electrons. This annihilation reaction results in the release of paired, high-energy photons that travel in opposite directions from each other and are detected simultaneously by the PET scanner (a "coincidence event"). This information serves as the basis for localization of positron annihilation events and the computer-assisted generation of a PET scan. Currently, PET imaging is largely investigational with the greatest clinical potential in neurooncology, ischemic cerebrovascular disease, and epilepsy.

1. Brain tumors — increased tumor metabolic rate, as measured by the uptake of a glucose analog, ^{18}F-2-deoxy-D-glucose, may help differentiate low- versus high-grade gliomas, tumor recurrence versus radiation necrosis and primary CNS lymphoma versus toxoplasmosis in acquired immunodeficiency syndrome (AIDS) patients. It may also be useful in monitoring subclinical response to radiation and chemotherapy and assessing for malignant transformation of low-grade lesions. Other radioactive tracers, e.g., radiolabeled amino acids, have shown early promise in the evaluation of brain tumors.

2. Epilepsy — clinical utility generally restricted to patients with focal epilepsy being evaluated for surgical therapy. Interictal PET demonstrates lesional reduced glucose metabolism and CBF. An opposite pattern is seen during an ictal event. Interictal PET may also be useful in localization of eloquent cortex.

3. Emerging areas — early diagnosis of Alzheimer disease and other dementia syndromes, diagnosis and differentiation of Parkinsonian syndromes, evaluation of "at-risk brain" in patients with cerebral ischemia

IV. Nervous System Development

A. 3% of newborns have major structural abnormalities, and most involve the CNS.

B. The brain and spinal cord are formed from neuroectoderm at 3 to 8 weeks. Primary neurulation occurs at 3 to 4 weeks with formation of the neural plate, neural groove, and neural folds. The primitive streak forms at postovulatory day 13. The notochord forms at day 17 and induces the primitive streak to form the neural plate that later develops the neural groove and neural folds. The neural folds fuse at 22 days to form the neural tube, with the proximal two thirds forming the brain and the distal one third forming the spinal cord. It closes like a zipper starting at the hindbrain with the anterior neuropore closing first at 24 days (forming the lamina terminalis) and the posterior end closing second (to L1/2) at 26 days. A problem at this stage causes neural tube defects and Chiari malformations.

C. Dysjunction — the separation of ectoderm from neuroectoderm after the neural tube forms. The mesenchyme in between the two layers forms dura, neural arches, and paraspinal muscles. If dysjunction occurs too early, the mesenchyme can enter the neural tube and form lipomas and lipomyelomeningoceles. Focal failure of dysjunction causes an epithelial-lined dermal sinus tract. More widespread failure of dysjunction may cause a myelocele or a myelomeningocele.

D. Secondary neurulation — occurs at 4–5 weeks as the mesoderm forms the dura, skull, vertebrae, and distal spine. Defects of secondary neurulation cause spinal dysraphism below L1/2.

E. Ventral induction — occurs at 5–10 weeks as the primary vesicles form from the neural tube (see following). Abnormalities at this stage cause holoprosencephaly, septooptic dysplasia, and Dandy–Walker malformation. Induction is the growing brain's influence on the overlying mesoderm causing it to grow.

F. Neuronal proliferation and differentiation — occur at 2–4 months. A problem at this stage causes vascular malformations and neurocutaneous syndromes.

G. Cellular migration — occurs at 2–5 months with migration of cells from the deeper layers to more superficial layers, except for the outer cortical layer. A problem at this stage causes callosal agenesis, schizencephaly, and heterotopias.

H. Neuronal organization and myelination — occur from 5 months to the postnatal period as the synapses form. Myelination begins in the fifth fetal month and proceeds caudad to cephalad, dorsal to ventral, central to peripheral, and sensory before motor. Most is completed by 2 years. At birth, the cortex/white matter signals on MRI are reversed because of the paucity of myelination and increased water content of the cortex compared with the white matter.

I. At 4–5 weeks, the prosencephalon, mesencephalon, and rhombencephalon form. The prosencephalon then divides into (1) the telencephalon that forms the hemispheres, caudate, putamen, fornices, anterior commissure, corpus callosum, and hippocampus; and (2) the diencephalon that forms the thalamus, globus pallidus (GP), posterior hypophysis, infundibulum, optic nerve, retina, posterior commissure, and habenular commissure. The mesencephalon forms the midbrain. The rhombencephalon divides into (1) the metencephalon that forms the pons, fourth ventricle, and cerebellum; and (2) the myelencephalon that forms the medulla.

J. The germinal matrix — forms at 7 weeks and produces neurons and glia. At 30 weeks, the germinal matrix involutes (although some clusters exist until 39 weeks).

K. The commissures — form at 8–17 weeks. The corpus callosum forms from front to back except for the rostrum that forms last, so partial agenesis always includes the rostrum and splenium.

L. Cells proliferate in the walls of the neural tube and form a pseudostratified columnar layer with ventricular and subventricular zones (precursors of neurons and glia). Processes of these cells go from the lumen to the external basement membrane forming the marginal zone with an underlying intermediate zone. Most cells proliferate in the ventricular zone and migrate outward by ameboid movement guided by glial processes that extend from the ventricular zone to the pial surface of the marginal zone. The migration is dictated by intercellular adhesion molecules and integrins (cell surface receptors). The cells mature, selectively die, group together, and form connections.

M. Brainstem — forms between 2–6 months. The basal plate has (medial to lateral) somatic efferent, special visceral efferent, and general visceral efferent nuclei. The alar plate has (medial to lateral in the plate and lateral to medial in the final position) general visceral afferent, special visceral afferent, and somatic afferent nuclei. Both efferent and afferent somatic nuclei are the most medial of their groups in the full-term human.

N. Spinal cord — has a sulcus limitans that forms between the dorsal (alar) and ventral (basal) plates. The connections form at 2–4 months.

O. Caudal spinal cord — forms separately by retrograde differentiation at 4–8 weeks as the caudal cell mass forms and cavitates.

P. Neural crest — the group of cells at the neural tube/somatic ectoderm junction. It forms the leptomeninges, Schwann cells, sensory ganglia of the cranial nerves, dorsal root ganglia (DRG), autonomic nervous system ganglia, the adrenal medulla, melanocytes, and amine precursor uptake and decarboxylation (APUD) cells.

Q. Ectodermal placodes (overlying the neural tube) — form the olfactory epithelium and cranial nerve (CN) V and CN VII to CN X ganglia.

R. Notochord remnants — form the nucleus pulposus of the intervertebral disks. They are also believed to be the cells of origin of chordomas.

S. Dura — formed from mesodermal elements, and the pia/arachnoid is formed from neuroectoderm

T. Full-term brain — weighs 400 g and is 90% water (the adult brain is 70% water). It has larger nuclei with less arborization. The anterior and lateral corticospinal tracts are incompletely myelinated. The corpus callosum and the fornix are completely unmyelinated. There may be myelination glia where immature oligodendrocytes in the site of myelination may appear like reactive astrocytes. There frequently is a cavum septum pellucidum. The immature cells around the lateral ventricles and the external granular layer of the cerebellum are gone after 12–15 months.

U. Suture closure — Metopic suture closes around the first year of life.

V. The anterior fontanelle closes by 2.5 years of life. The posterior and sphenoid fontanelles close by 2–3 months of life. The mastoid fontanelle closes by 1 year of life.

V. Developmental Pathology

A. Malformation — occurs when an organ is not formed properly. Dysplasia occurs when a tissue is not formed properly. Developmental injury may be caused by genetic abnormalities, chromosomal aberrations, or environmental factors (infections, drugs, chemicals, malnutrition, and maternal illness).

B. Neural tube defects (dysraphism) — caused by failure of fusion of the neural tube.

   1. During neurulation (occurs at 17–30 days) — failure of fusion produces open defects by failure of dysjunction of the neural and cutaneous ectoderm. The risk is increased with a neural tube defect in a sibling or maternal folate deficiency. Maternal serum α–fetoprotein (AFP) usually is increased. This group includes spina bifida aperta, meningomyelocele, myelocele, anencephaly, and cranioschisis.

   2. Postneurulation (occurs at 26–60 days or even near birth) — Failure of fusion produces closed, skin-covered deficits such as spina bifida occulta, holoprosencephaly, encephaloceles, hydrocephalus, diastematomyelia, lipoma, meningocele, and Chiari malformations (**Fig. 3.2**).

   3. Anencephaly — the most common congenital malformation. It occurs in 0.03–0.7% of births in the United States and most commonly affects Caucasian females. 95% of cases occur without a family history of neural tube defects. After one affected child, the risk increases to 2–5%. It is caused by chromosomal abnormalities or mechanical problems from adhesions to the placenta. The risk is increased with twins, polyhydramnios, hyperthermia, and decreased maternal folate, zinc, or copper. The neonates tend to be stillborn or to die within 2 months. They may have brainstem activity. Anencephaly is associated with the absence of scalp and skull. The brain consists of an exposed mass of tissue with a cerebrovascular area containing vessels, neural tissue, choroid, optic nerves, eyes, some cranial nerves, and brainstem. Craniorachischisis totalis occurs when the entire neuraxis is involved. 15–40% have other organ malformations. Amniotic fluid has increased AFP and acetylcholinesterase.

   4. Exencephaly — occurs when the cerebral hemispheres are present but disorganized. There is also absent calvaria and abnormalities of the skull base.

   5. Myelomeningocele occurs in 0.07% of births in the United States and is more common in females. It is related to genetic and environmental factors. Risk factors include parental consanguinity, affected

siblings, decreased vitamin A or folate, and use of valproic acid or carbamazepine. It is usually in the lumbar spine, with absent arachnoid and adjacent hydromyelia. It is associated with Chiari II malformation (100%), hydrocephalus (80%), lipoma (75%), syringomyelia (50%), diastematomyelia (40%), scoliosis (20%), kyphosis (10%), orthopedic deformities, and callosal dysgenesis (**Fig. 3.3**).

6. Meningocele — 10% as common as myelomeningocele and has no gender predilection. It is rarely associated with other anomalies and is covered with skin.

7. Cephaloceles — include meningocele and meningoencephalocele. In the United States, they are occipital (80%), parietal (10%), frontal (10%), and rarely basal.

    a. Occipital cephalocele — the most frequent among Caucasians and in Europe and North America. There is a female predilection. The cephalocele protrudes between the foramen magnum and the lambdoid suture. It is associated with myelomeningocele (7%), diastematomyelia (3%), Chiari II and III malformations, Dandy–Walker malformation, and Klippel–Feil syndrome (**Fig. 3.4**).

    b. Parietal cephalocele — accounts for 10% of cases in the United States. There is a male predilection. The cephalocele protrudes between the lambda and bregma. It is associated with midline

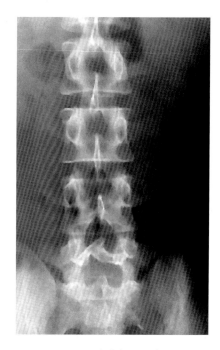

Fig. 3.2 Spina bifida occulta. Anteroposterior lumbar spine x-ray film demonstrates an L5 bifid spinous process.

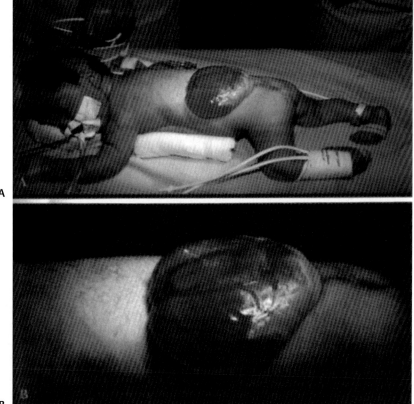

Fig. 3.3 Myelomeningocele. (**A**) Neural placode noted on center of dorsal aspect in this neonate prepared for surgery. Note foot deformities and preparation being made for ventriculoperitoneal shunt. (**B**) Close-up image of the myelomeningocele.

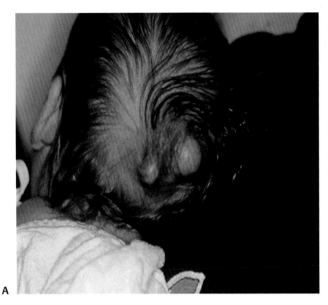
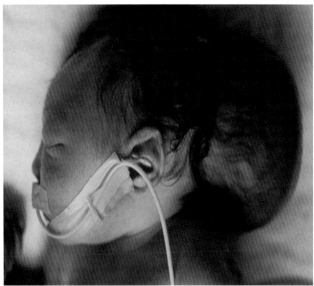

A   B

Fig. 3.4   Encephaloceles. (**A**) Two small occipital encephaloceles, and (**B**) large occipital encephalocele.

anomalies, agenesis of the corpus callosum, lobar holoprosencephaly, Dandy–Walker malformation, and Chiari II malformations.

c. Transsphenoidal cephalocele — rare, associated with sellar abnormalities, endocrine dysfunction,
   and agenesis of the corpus callosum
d. Sincipital (frontoethmoidal) cephalocele — the most frequent type in Southeast Asia and Austra-
   lian aborigines. There is a male predilection. The cephalocele protrudes between the nasal and
   ethmoid bones and is not associated with neural tube defects.
e. Sphenoethmoidal (nasal) cephalocele — the crista galli is absent or eroded and the foramen cecum
   is enlarged. The dural diverticulum normally regresses, but if it does not, it may form a dermal
   sinus tract. They are associated with dermoids, epidermoids, and nasal gliomas (dysplastic or heterotopic glial tissue). If the crista galli is split, there is likely to be a dermoid present (**Fig. 3.5**).
f. Meckel–Gruber syndrome — cystic dysplastic kidneys, cardiac anomalies, orofacial clefting, and
   cephaloceles. It is associated with maternal hyperthermia on days 20–26 of gestation.

8. Dermal sinus tracts — epithelium-lined tracts caused by faulty segmental disjunction. 60% extend from
   the skin to the spinal canal, although they may end in the subcutaneous tissue, dura, spinal cord, or
   nerve roots. 50% end in epidermoids or dermoids. More than 50% are lumbar and the next most frequent site is occipital. There is no gender predilection. Symptoms are mainly a result of infection. They
   are associated with skin dimples, hyperpigmentation, hairy nevi, and capillary malformations.

C. Cleavage disorders ("the face predicts the brain") — Cleavage of the telencephalon and development of midline facial structures are dictated by the prechordal mesoderm.

   1. Holoprosencephaly (**Fig. 3.6**)
      a. Alobar — completely undivided forebrain, severe craniofacial abnormalities (i.e., cyclopia), ab-
         sence of olfactory nerves, abnormal optic nerves, monoventricle, fused basal ganglia and thala-
         mus, absence of corpus callosum, septum pellucidum, falx, and fornix. It is associated with tri-
         somy 13, 14, 15, and 18, polydactyly, renal dysplasia, and maternal diabetes.
      b. Semilobar — monoventricle with forebrain divided by partial falx and interhemispheric fissure,
         partially separated thalamus and basal ganglia, and variable craniofacial abnormalities (i.e., hy-
         potelorism and cleft lip)

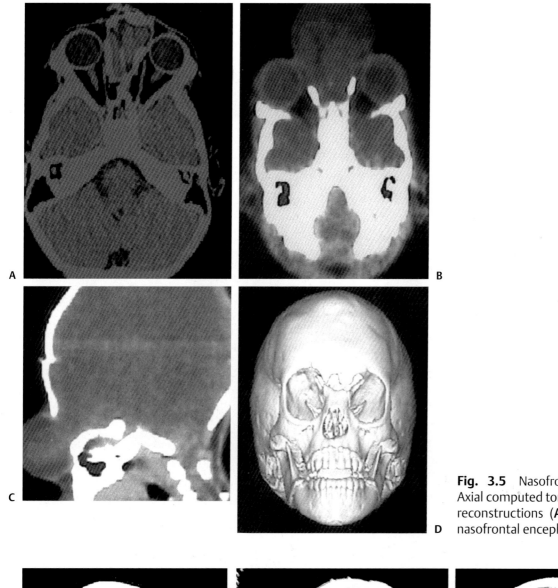

Fig. 3.5 Nasofrontal encephalocele. Axial computed tomographic scans and reconstructions (**A–D**) demonstrate a nasofrontal encephalocele.

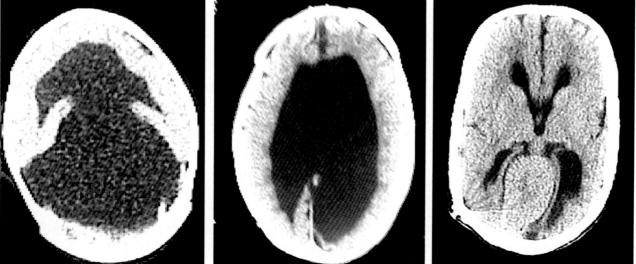

Fig. 3.6 Holoprosencephaly. Axial computed tomographic scans demonstrate (**A**) alobar, (**B**) semilobar, and (**C**) lobar holoprosencephaly with progressively more cleavage.

c. Lobar — squared frontal horns, absence of the septum pellucidum but falx and interhemispheric fissure are present; hemispheres are separated by thalamus and basal ganglia. There is gray matter that extends across the midline. The corpus callosum is still missing and there are no craniofacial abnormalities.

2. Arrhinencephaly — the absence of the olfactory bulbs and tracts with normal cortex and gray matter in place of the corpus callosum. It is associated with holoprosencephaly and Kallmann syndrome (anosmia, hypogonadism, and mental retardation).

3. Septooptic dysplasia (de Morsier syndrome) — occurs with mild lobar holoprosencephaly, absence of the septum pellucidum, schizencephaly, and hypoplastic optic nerves. It is associated with seizures, visual symptoms, hypothalamic–pituitary dysfunction (precocious puberty), enlarged ventricles, and hypotelorism (**Fig. 3.7**).

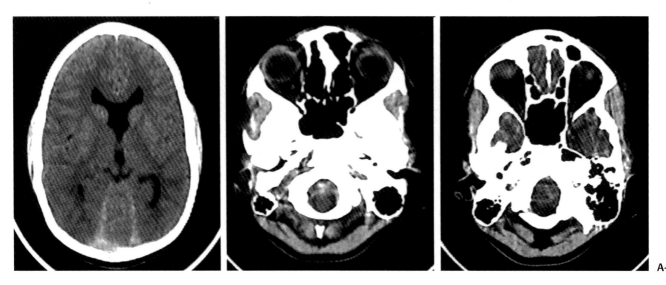

A–C

Fig. 3.7 Septooptic dysplasia. Axial computed tomographic scans demonstrate (**A**) absence of the septum pellucidum and (**B, C**) thin optic nerves.

4. Cleidocranial dysostosis — occurs with retention of mandibular teeth, delayed closure of fontanelles, wormian bones, and midline defects

D. Migrational disorders

1. Normal neuronal migration occurs between the second to fifth gestational months.

2. Heterotopias — normal neurons in abnormal CNS locations (i.e., in the centrum semiovale, along the lateral ventricles or in the cerebellar white matter). They may be laminar or nodular and usually do not enhance (**Fig. 3.8**).

3. Ectopias — neurons in locations brain tissue should not be in (i.e., the subarachnoid space). They are associated with dysraphism and hydranencephaly.

4. Lissencephaly — smooth brain. In the complete form, the cerebral hemispheres have no sulci. In the incomplete form, there are several shallow sulci. It is associated with in utero infections.

5. Pachygyria — overall decreased number of gyri and those that are present are enlarged

6. Polymicrogyria — wrinkled-appearing brain with many small gyri. It forms occasionally after neuronal migration from neural injury. Usually, there are only four layers of cortex in the abnormal gyri. It may be focal or widespread.

7. Schizencephaly — a gray matter–lined cleft extending from the pia to the ventricle. The cleft may be filled with CSF (opened lip) or collapsed (closed lip) (**Fig. 3.9**).

8. Porencephaly — a cleft not lined with gray matter but by gliotic white matter that forms after an insult to an otherwise normal brain

9. Unilateral megalencephaly — hamartomatous overgrowth of one hemisphere with ipsilaterally enlarged ventricle and cortex. It is associated with seizures.

10. Agenesis of the corpus callosum — the corpus callosum forms from anterior to posterior, but the rostrum forms last so the splenium and rostrum are almost always involved with agenesis. Agenesis may be complete or partial. It is characterized by a high-riding third ventricle, radial spoke-like gyri, Probst bundles (longitudinal white matter tracts indenting the medial ventricles), and colpocephaly. Occasionally, the cingulate gyrus, anterior commissure, or fornix may be absent. 50% have associ-

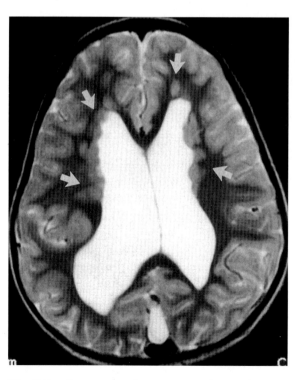

Fig. 3.8 Gray matter heterotopias (*arrows*). (From Albright AL, Pollack IF, Adelson PD, eds. Principles and Practice of Pediatric Neurosurgery. New York, NY: Thieme; 1999. Reprinted by permission.)

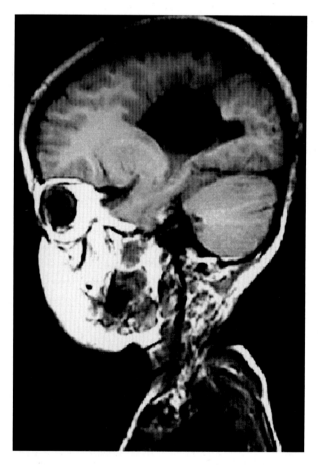

Fig. 3.9 Schizencephaly. Sagittal T1-weighted magnetic resonance image demonstrates gray matter-lined cleft extending from the subarachnoid space to the lateral ventricle.

ated abnormalities such as Chiari II malformation, Dandy–Walker malformation, migrational disorders, cephalocele, holoprosencephaly, lipomas, and an azygous anterior cerebral artery (ACA). Aicardi syndrome has a female predominance and consists of callosal agenesis, ocular abnormalities, and infantile spasms (**Fig. 3.10**).

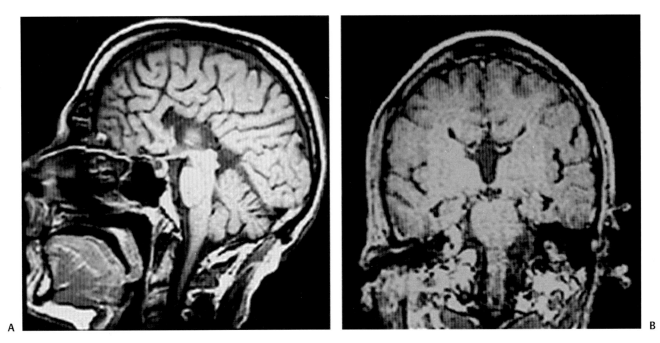

Fig. 3.10   Agenesis of the corpus callosum. (**A**) T1-weighted sagittal and (**B**) coronal magnetic resonance images demonstrating absence of the corpus callosum with characteristic "Viking helmet" ventricles on coronal view.

E. Other developmental syndromes

    1. Congenital hydrocephalus — commonly due to aqueductal stenosis, Chiari II malformation, Dandy–Walker malformation, infection, and intraventricular hemorrhage (IVH)

    2. Chiari I malformation (**Fig. 3.11**) — peg-like tonsils extending below the foramen magnum (6 mm below the foramen magnum at age < 10 years, 5 mm <30 years, 4 mm <80 years, and 3 mm <90 years). If the tonsils extend >12 mm below the foramen magnum, all are symptomatic and from 5–10 mm, 70% are symptomatic. Chiari I malformation is occasionally acquired after frequent lumbar punctures or placement of a lumboperitoneal shunt. Chiari I malformation is not associated with other brain abnormalities, but is associated with skeletal abnormalities in 25% of cases: basilar invagination (25–50%), Klippel–Feil syndrome with fused cervical vertebrae (5–10%), atlantooccipital fusion (5%), and cervical spina bifida occulta (5%). It presents in early adulthood with pain, occipital headache, Lhermitte sign, long tract signs, syringomyelia (20–40%; with 60–90% of symptomatic cases), and hydrocephalus (25%). Chiari malformations of all types present differently at different age groups.

        a. Infants — hydrocephalus and brainstem compression with apnea, decreased gag reflex, nystagmus, and spasticity

        b. Children — nystagmus, spastic paralysis, and bulbar dysfunction

        c. Adolescents — progressive spasticity and cape-like pain and temperature loss in the upper limbs

        d. Adults — occipital headache, neck and arm pain, and nystagmus (**Fig. 3.11**)

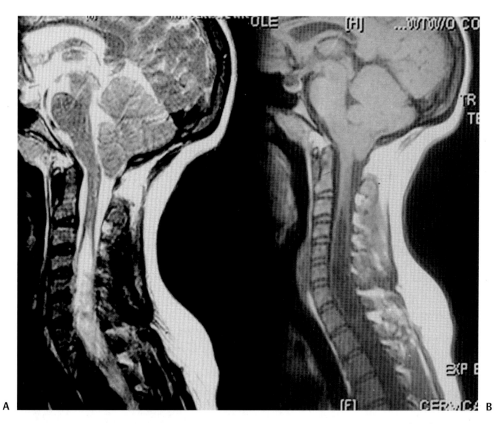

Fig. 3.11 Chiari I malformation. (**A**) Sagittal T2- and (**B**) T1-weighted magnetic resonance image demonstrates peg-like tonsils extending below foramen magnum with associated syringomyelia.

3. Chiari II malformation — thought to develop when the neural folds do not completely meet and there is abnormal ventricular CSF flow into the amnion with collapse of the ventricles. A small posterior fossa develops and as the cerebellum grows, it herniates upward forming a large tentorial incisura and downward pushing the vermis and brainstem through the foramen magnum. It presents in neonates and is associated with many abnormalities (**Fig. 3.12**).

   a. Skull and dura — lacunar skull ("lückenschädel," with scooped out appearance), small posterior fossa, low-lying torcula and transverse sinus, large foramen magnum, concave petrous temporal bones, short concave clivus, and a thin falx cerebri with occasional interdigitating gyri through fenestrations in the falx cerebri (**Fig. 3.13**)

   b. Hindbrain — herniation of the vermis, nodulus, uvula, and pyramis through the foramen magnum, medullary kinking (70%), enhancing ectopic choroid, upward cerebellar herniation, and tectal beaking

   c. CSF spaces — tubular fourth ventricle, large third ventricle with enlarged massa intermedia, colpocephaly (large atria and occipital horns), aqueductal stenosis, small cisterna magna, and hydrocephalus (90%)

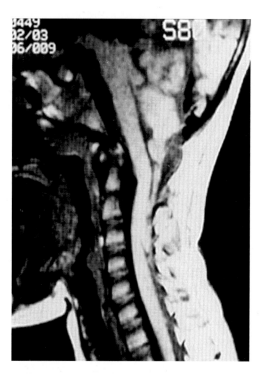

Fig. 3.12 Chiari II malformation. Sagittal T1-weighted magnetic resonance image with tectal beaking, low-lying torcula, and vermian descent.

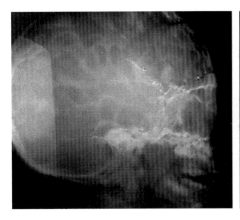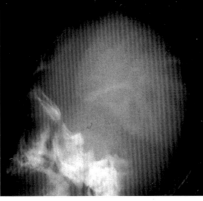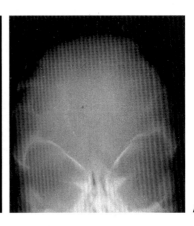

A–C

Fig. 3.13   Lückenschädel skull. (**A, B**) Lateral and (**C**) anteroposterior skull x-ray films demonstrate the scooped out appearance with myelomeningocele.

    d. Cerebral hemispheres — heterotopias, polymicrogyria, and callosal dysgenesis

    e. Spine—myelomeningocele (100%), syringomyelia (50–90%), diastematomyelia, and incomplete C1 arch (70%). It is not associated with lipomyelomeningocele.

4. Chiari III malformation — hindbrain herniation into an encephalocele, usually occipital or high cervical (**Fig. 3.14**)

5. Chiari IV malformation — cerebellar hypoplasia, an entity distinct from the other Chiari malformations

6. Dandy–Walker malformation — posterior fossa cyst continuous with the fourth ventricle with partial or complete vermian absence. It may be due to failure of development of the superior medullary velum (roof of the fourth ventricle) combined with fourth ventricle outlet atresia. It is associated with a large posterior fossa, high tentorium and transverse sinus, lambdoid-torcula inversion, hydrocephalus (80%), callosal agenesis (25%), heterotopias, schizencephaly, cephaloceles, dolichocephaly, cardiac abnormalities, and polydactyly (**Fig. 3.15**).

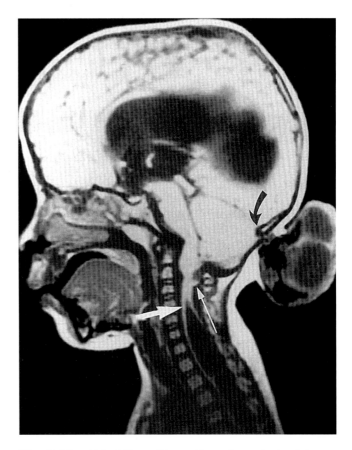

Fig. 3.14   Chiari III malformation characterized by an occipital encephalocele (*curved black arrow*) and syringomyelia (*thick white arrow*). (From Ramsey RG. Teaching Atlas of Spine Imaging. New York, NY: Thieme; 1999. Reprinted by permission.)

7. Dandy–Walker variant — mild inferior vermian hypoplasia with open communication between the fourth ventricle and the cisterna magna through an enlarged vallecula. The fourth ventricle is enlarged, but the posterior fossa is normal size. There may be associated hydrocephalus.

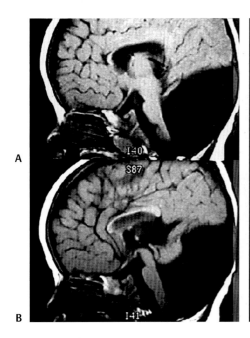

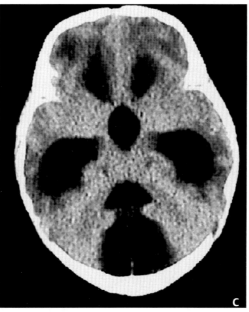

Fig. 3.15 Dandy–Walker malformation. (**A, B**) Sagittal T1-weighted magnetic resonance images and (**C**) axial computed tomographic scan demonstrate vermian agenesis and connection of the fourth ventricle to a posterior fossa cyst.

8. Mega cisterna magna — posterior fossa CSF accumulation in an enlarged cisterna magna. There is a normal fourth ventricle and no hydrocephalus. It fills with intrathecal contrast.

9. Posterior fossa arachnoid cyst — posterior fossa CSF accumulation with a normal cerebellum and fourth ventricle. There may or may not be hydrocephalus. The cyst does not fill with intrathecal contrast.

10. Lhermitte–Duclos disease — hypertrophied cerebellar granular cell layer and increased myelin in the molecular layer of the cerebellum with thick folia. There is mass effect on the fourth ventricle. The lesion is considered a hamartoma. There may be calcifications, hydrocephalus, and folia with increased signal intensity on T2-weighted MRI. It is associated with Cowden syndrome where patients have facial trichilemmomas, fibromas of the oral mucosa, hamartomatous polyps of the gastrointestinal (GI) tract and breast, and thyroid tumors. Cowden syndrome is due to mutations of the phosphatase and tensin (PTEN) gene on chromosome 10q.

11. Hydromyelia — a distended central canal of the spinal cord lined by ependymal cells. It is associated with Chiari II malformations and myelomeningoceles.

12. Syringomyelia — a fluid-filled cavity in the spinal cord lined by astrocytes

13. Syringobulbia — a fluid-filled cavity in the brainstem

14. Fetal alcohol syndrome — characterized by growth retardation, craniofacial dysmorphism, CNS and visceral malformations, mental retardation, and microcephaly. It is associated with migrational defects, hydrocephalus, schizencephaly, callosal agenesis, and neural tube defects. The incidence is increased if the mother uses drugs, has poor nutrition, or smokes tobacco.

15. Colpocephaly — dilated occipital horns associated with agenesis of the corpus callosum and periventricular leukomalacia, mental retardation, and seizures.

16. Craniosynostosis — premature fusion of the sutures causing abnormal skull growth and shape. Surgical treatment to open the sutures and reshape as needed usually is done between 3–6 months and is generally performed for cosmetic purposes.

a. Sagittal synostosis — most common (50%), male predominance, causes scaphocephaly or dolichocephaly (**Fig. 3.16**)
b. Unilateral coronal synostosis — 25%, causes anterior plagiocephaly, female predominance (**Fig. 3.17**)
c. Bilateral coronal synostosis — usually genetic, causes brachycephaly, associated with Apert and Crouzon syndromes (**Fig. 3.18**)

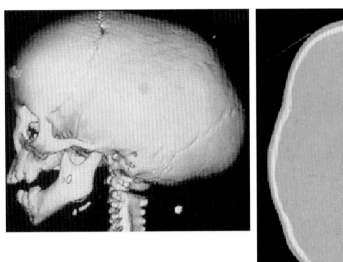

A

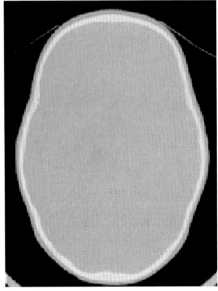

B

Fig. 3.16 Sagittal synostosis (scaphocephaly, dolichocephaly). (**A**) Computed tomographic (CT) reconstruction and (**B**) axial CT.

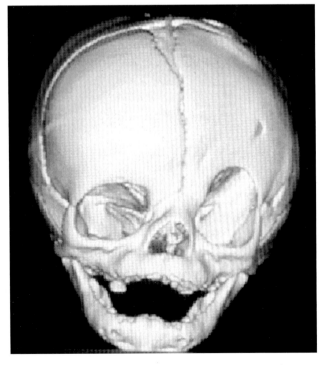

Fig. 3.17 Unilateral left coronal synostosis. Computed tomographic reconstruction with "harlequin eye" on the left.

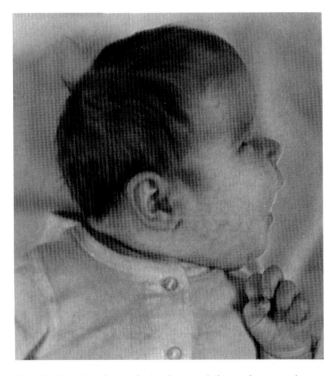

Fig. 3.18 Brachycephaly due to bilateral coronal synostosis.

d. Unilateral lambdoid synostosis — 1.3%, male predominance, causes posterior plagiocephaly and must be distinguished from the much more common positional plagiocephaly resulting from a baby lying on one side too often. Differentiating the two conditions can often be accomplished by history and physical examination (true synostosis is present at birth, positional is not). In positional plagiocephaly, a parallelogram-type deformity is appreciated when the head is viewed from above and associated with the following: unilateral flattening of the occiput, ipsilateral frontal/parietal bossing, ipsilateral cheekbone prominence, ipsilateral anterior displacement of the ear, and contralateral occipital bossing. This is treated initially by changing the infant's sleeping position, not by surgery. Unilateral lambdoid synostosis is also characterized by unilateral flattening of the occiput, ipsilateral frontal/parietal bossing (typically less severe), and contralateral occipital bossing. In contradistinction, the ipsilateral ear is typically posteriorly and inferiorly displaced and the posterior skull base is tilted with an unusually prominent ipsilateral mastoid process (**Fig. 3.19**).

e. Metopic synostosis — 5%, causes trigonocephaly (**Fig. 3.20**)

f. Turricephaly — 5–10%, synostosis of both coronal sutures and the sphenofrontal sutures, causes a tall broad head

g. Oxycephaly — 5–10%, synostosis of multiple sutures, causes a cone-shaped head

h. Pansynostosis — causes Lückenschädel head

i. Crouzon syndrome — most frequent craniofacial syndrome, autosomal dominant or sporadic inheritance, shallow orbits, exophthalmos, midface hypoplasia, malformed ears, agenesis of the corpus callosum, less severe mental retardation than with Apert syndrome, and increased incidence of hydrocephalus. More than one suture is involved, and they may have oxycephaly, turricephaly, or dolichocephaly. The sphenofrontal synostosis produces exophthalmos; associated with mutations of the fibroblast growth factor receptor 2.

j. Apert syndrome — second most common craniofacial syndrome, autosomal dominant or sporadic inheritance, turricephalic head, maxillary hypoplasia, orbital hypertelorism, syndactyly, mental retardation, deafness, flat nose, and vertebral and skeletal abnormalities. Only the coronal suture is involved. There are GI, GU, and cardiac abnormalities, and increased incidence of frontal encephaloceles; also associated with mutations of the fibroblast growth factor receptor.

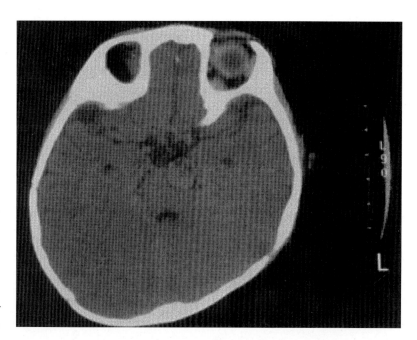

Fig. 3.19 Lambdoid synostosis as demonstrated on axial computed tomographic scan.

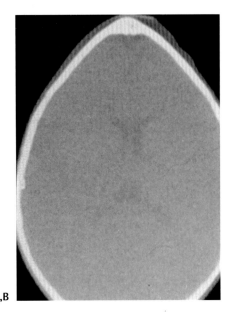
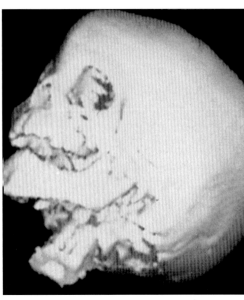

A,B

Fig. 3.20 Metopic synostosis (trigonocephaly); (**A**) axial computed tomographic (CT) scan and (**B**) CT reconstruction.

17. Klippel–Feil syndrome — congenital fusion of the upper cervical vertebrae; associated with Sprengel deformity (elevation of the scapula) and Chiari I malformation (**Fig. 3.21**)

F. Chromosomal disorders

1. Trisomy 13 (Patau syndrome) — female predominance, hypotelorism, holoprosencephaly, microcephaly, microphthalmia, cleft palate and lip, polydactyly, dextrocardia, and ocular abnormalities. Death ensues before 9 months.

2. Trisomy 18 (Edward syndrome) — female predominance, gyral dysplasia, callosal agenesis, Chiari II malformation, dolichocephaly, cerebellar hypoplasia, hypertelorism, microphthalmia, syndactyly, rocker bottom feet, and ventricular septal defects. Less than 10% live 1 year.

3. Trisomy 21 (Down syndrome) — most frequent of the chromosomal abnormalities and occurs in 0.1% of births. Varieties include (1) sporadic trisomy (95%) (increased risk with maternal age >35 years), (2) Robertson translocation 21q and 14 or 21q and 22q in 4% (not associated with age), and (3) mosaic (1%). It is characterized by brachycephaly, hypotelorism, hypoplastic maxilla and nose, simian crease, epicanthal folds, skull base abnormalities, cervical stenosis, atlantoaxial instability, underdeveloped inferior temporal gyrus, narrow superior temporal gyrus, flattened occipital pole, mental retardation, lens opacities, congenital heart disease (increased risk of brain abscess), and Alzheimer disease (by 40 years). Recall: Amyloid precursor protein is found on chromosome 21.

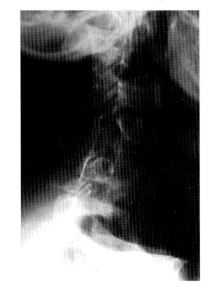

4. 5p deletion (cri-du-chat syndrome) — mental retardation, microcephaly, hypertelorism, and congenital heart disease

5. 15q deletion (Prader–Willi syndrome) — mental retardation, truncal obesity, short stature, and hypogonadism

6. Fragile X syndrome — the most frequent hereditary cause of mental retardation. It is more common (and severe) in males (1 in 4,000)

Fig. 3.21 X-ray showing Klippel-Feil syndrome.

than females (1 in 8,000). There is a dysmorphic appearance with long face, large testicles, and vermian hypoplasia. The syndrome is caused by mutation of a single gene, the *FMR1* (Fragile X Mental Retardation 1) gene. This mutation is characterized by massive expansion of a trinucleotide repeat that leads to transcriptional shutdown of the gene.

7. Ataxia-telangiectasia — cerebellar atrophy, lentiform nucleus calcifications, pachygyria, impaired immune system, increased lymphoreticular carcinoma, and defective deoxyribonucleic acid (DNA) repair

VI. Perinatal Brain Injuries

A. Perinatal brain injury — may be caused by birth or other trauma, infection, metabolic disorders, or maternal intoxications

B. Caput succedaneum — cutaneous hemorrhagic edema in the skin over the calvarium caused by pressure during birth with vascular stasis. It crosses sutures and resolves in 48 hours.

C. Subaponeurotic hemorrhage — Blood accumulates under the aponeurosis.

D. Cephalohematoma — subperiosteal blood that does not cross suture lines. It is usually parietal and may calcify.

E. Epidural hematoma (EDH) — rare, associated with fractures

F. Subdural hematoma (SDH) — rare, caused by mechanical trauma from a small birth canal, rapid or prolonged labor, abnormal presentation, premature birth with increased skull compliance, large head, and forceps deliveries. It forms from tearing of the bridging veins over the convexity, tentorium, or skull base (**Fig. 3.22**). Occipital osteodiastasis is the traumatic separation of the squamous and lateral occipital bone with tearing of the occipital sinus and bleeding in the posterior fossa. Laceration of the falx or inferior sagittal sinus causes bleeding over the corpus callosum. There is a subgroup of falcine or tentorial SDH associated with asphyxia or mechanical trauma that are usually small and rarely have clinical significance.

G. Subarachnoid hemorrhage (SAH) — caused by hypoxia or trauma and usually has a good outcome

H. Intraparenchymal hemorrhage — caused by coagulation defects, vitamin K deficiency, trauma, vascular malformation, tumor, or stroke

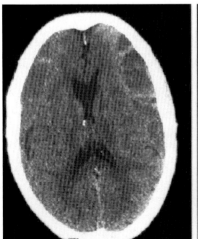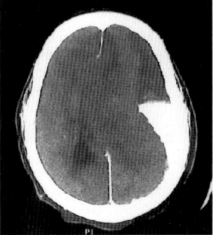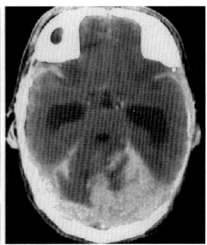

A–C

Fig. 3.22 Subdural hematoma (SDH). Nonenhanced computed tomographic scans demonstrate (**A**) bilateral subacute SDH, (**B**) chronic left SDH with acute hemorrhage (fluid-fluid level), and (**C**) posterior fossa SDH.

I. Periventricular/IVH — occurs in 40% of births <35 weeks and 3–7% of full-term births. There is increased incidence with prematurity and acute respiratory distress syndrome. It develops an average of 72 hours postpartum in the subependymal germinal matrix near the foramen of Monro or the body of the caudate. In full-term births, the hemorrhage develops in the choroid plexus of the lateral ventricle. Mortality is 20–60% and morbidity is 15–40% (mainly motor deficits and mental retardation). Hydrocephalus may be by obstruction at the aqueduct, fourth ventricular outlet, or arachnoid granulations.

J. Delivery trauma — usually causes SDH (interhemispheric or tentorial) and less frequently posterior fossa SAH that results from the sudden frontooccipital shortening that may tear a sinus or vein. The risk increases with cephalopelvic disproportion or abnormal presentation.

K. Hypoxic/ischemic perinatal brain injury

1. Acute injury
    a. Periventricular leukomalacia — increased incidence with prematurity, congenital heart disease, shock, sepsis, and respiratory distress syndrome. It occurs within 72 hours and causes lower extremity weakness and visual problems.
    b. Gray matter necrosis — seen in full-term births with perinatal asphyxia and mainly affects the subthalamus, lateral geniculate body, inferior colliculus, cranial nerves, dentate nuclei, Purkinje cells, and the cortical internal granular layer

2. Chronic injury
    a. Ulegyria — parietooccipital mushroom-like atrophic gyri with atrophy in sulcus valleys
    b. Status marmoratus — the thalamus, neostriatum, and cortex develop irregular intersecting bands of myelin and astrocytic fibers that grossly resemble marble caused by cell loss followed by remyelination

3. Kernicterus — caused by increased unbound unconjugated bilirubin staining the gray matter and causing neuronal necrosis. It affects predominantly the GP, thalamus, subthalamus, and CNs III and VIII nuclei, causing symmetric cell loss with extrapyramidal motor signs. Treat the elevated bilirubin with phototherapy using ultraviolet light, but if the bilirubin is >20 with associated sepsis, prematurity, acidosis or low albumin, treat with an exchange transfusion.

4. Cavitary encephalopathies — caused by infections, genetic defects, or toxic gases
    a. Porencephaly — a cavity that extends from the leptomeninges to the ventricles or superficial white matter lined by white matter (as opposed to schizencephaly, which is a cleft lined by gray matter).
    b. Hydranencephaly — most of the cortex is replaced by CSF, may result from cerebral ischemia (internal carotid artery [ICA] occlusions) or infection (e.g., CMV or toxoplasmosis) (**Fig. 3.23**).
    c. Multicystic encephalopathy — ACA and middle cerebral artery (MCA) distribution, multiple cavities

VII. Infectious Diseases

A. Meningitis

1. Etiologies — the most frequent pathogen overall is *Haemophilus influenzae*, and the most frequent cause in adults is *Streptococcus pneumoniae*. The subarachnoid space near the blood vessels fills first with neutrophils and fibrin, then macrophages, and then it eventually fibroses. Meningitis is associated with arteritis, phlebitis, superior sagittal sinus thrombosis, and hydrocephalus. The three most common causes of meningitis (*H. influenzae, S. pneumoniae,* and *Neisseria meningitidis*) all normally colonize

the nasopharynx. The fourth most common pathogen is *Listeria*, which causes opportunistic infections. *Staphylococcus aureus* is associated with postoperative infections, and *S. epidermidis* is the most common cause of shunt infections. The mortality from various types of meningitis is 10% (*H. influenzae* and *N. meningitidis*), 25% (*S. pneumoniae*), and 50% (neonatal, with 50% of survivors having permanent sequelae).

2. Neonate (0–4 weeks) — the most frequent organisms are (1) group B streptococcus with acute onset <5 days postpartum with sepsis and pneumonia. It is associated with intrapartum infection and has a 15–30% mortality; (2) *Escherichia coli* is the most frequent cause in Latin America, especially with the K1 capsular antigen; and (3) *Listeria*. Sequelae include hydrocephalus, encephalomalacia at the border zones, and in the white matter, seizures, deafness, mental retardation, and focal deficits. The overall morbidity and mortality is 30–50%. Risk increases with prematurity, prolonged membrane rupture, traumatic delivery, congenital malformations (myelomeningocele or dermal sinus), and acquired respiratory, GI, and umbilical infections.

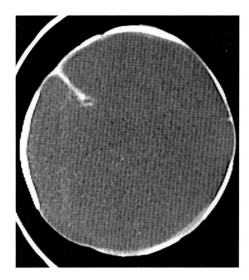

Fig. 3.23 Hydranencephaly; axial computed tomographic scan demonstrates a very thin rim of brain.

3. 4 to 12 weeks — The most common pathogen is *S. pneumoniae.*

4. 3 months to 3 years: The most common pathogen is *H. influenzae*, although it rarely occurs after 5 years; 85% are type b. It develops from nasopharyngeal colonization that leads to sepsis followed by meningitis. Blood cultures are positive in 70%. The bacteria need X and V growth factors to grow. It is associated with bilateral subdural effusions (usually culture negative because they are due to increased permeability of blood vessels, also seen with *S. pneumoniae* infections) and frequently causes seizures. Treatment is with third-generation cephalosporins. Concomitant use of steroids has been shown to decrease the incidence of deafness in children.

5. Children and young adults — the most frequent pathogen is *N. meningitidis*, and the meningitis occurs in epidemics. It develops from nasopharyngeal colonization that leads to hematologic dissemination and meningitis. The risk increases with decreased complement and in patients with systemic lupus erythematosus (SLE). It is associated with cutaneous eruptions (60%), arteritis, and cardiac deaths. The Waterhouse–Friderichsen syndrome is meningococcemia with vasomotor collapse, shock, diffuse intravascular coagulation, and diffuse hemorrhages, especially in the adrenal glands. *N. meningitidis* is a gram-negative intracellular diplococcus. Treatment is with penicillin or chloramphenicol.

6. Elderly — the most common pathogen is *S. pneumoniae*. It is more common in the elderly (because of age-dependent immune decline) and alcoholics (ethanol induces a chemotaxis defect and impairs phagocytosis). Risk is increased with trauma (it is the normal flora of the mastoid, ear, sinus, and nose), infection and sickle cell disease (caused by impaired splenic filtering, the risk is not increased in adults). Detection uses the Quellung reaction. Treatment is with penicillin.

B. Brain abscess (**Fig. 3.24** and **Fig. 3.25**)

1. Etiologies — the most common pathogen is *Streptococcus* and the most common cause is adjacent ear or sinus infection (40%), with spreading along the valveless venous channels (frontal sinus to frontal lobe, sphenoid sinus to temporal lobe, and ear to cerebellum or temporal lobe). 33% are from hematogenous

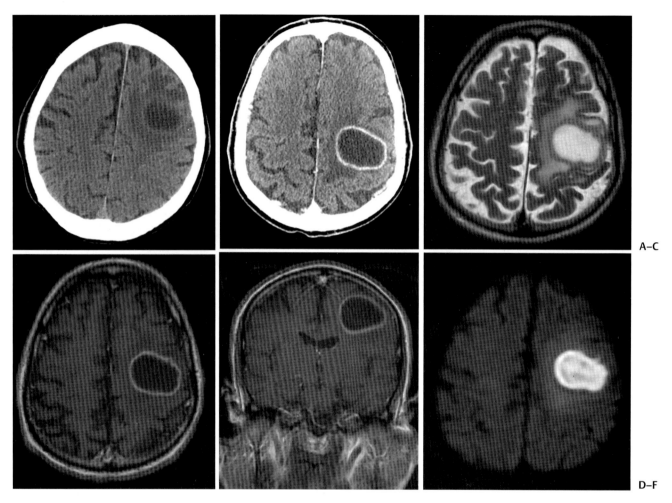

A–C

D–F

Fig. 3.24 Brain abscess. (**A**) Nonenhanced and (**B**) enhanced axial computed tomographic scans demonstrate a smooth ring-enhancing lesion. (**C**) T2-weighted magnetic resonance image demonstrates the characteristic hypointense capsule and surrounding hyperintensity, which is the associated edema. (**D,E**) There is a thin enhancing rim on T1-weighted MRI with gadolinium and (**F**) restricted diffusion on the diffusion-weighted image.

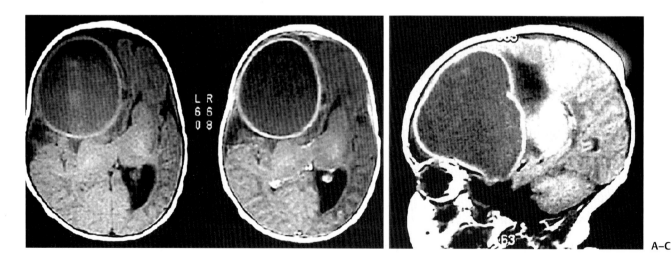

A–C

Fig. 3.25 Neonatal brain abscess. (**A**) Axial T1-weighted nonenhanced and (**B**) enhanced magnetic resonance images (MRIs) and (**C**) enhanced sagittal T1-weighted MRI demonstrate a massive cystic abscess cavity.

spread from another infected site (usually lung, dental disease, or trauma, more likely multiple; and usually in the distal MCA territory at the gray/white matter junction); 20% have no identifiable cause.

2. Risk — increases with cyanotic heart disease (5% incidence of brain abscesses, accounts for 60% of abscesses in children and is due to decreased pulmonary blood filtration and lower oxygen tension in the brain) and pulmonary AVMs (5% incidence of abscesses, associated with Rendu–Osler–Weber [hereditary hemorrhagic telangiectasia] disease).

3. Neonates — The most common causes are *Citrobacter, Bacteroides, Proteus*, and gram-negative bacilli. (**Fig. 3.25**).

4. Trauma — The most frequent cause is *Staphylococcus*, and with otitis, enteric bacilli are common.

5. Subacute bacterial endocarditis (SBE) — with streptococcal deposits on the valves usually causes ischemic stroke, but not abscesses. 10% of SBE cases develop infectious aneurysms. Acute endocarditis caused by *Staphylococcus* or hemolytic *Streptococcus* may be associated with multiple abscesses. There are mixed species in 30%.

6. Brain abscesses occur most commonly at the gray–white matter junction and are multiple in 35%. The abscess has a tendency to rupture into the ventricle because the capsule is thinner medially where there is decreased collagen formation. This has been postulated to be due to increased oxygen content near the cortex that stimulates the fibroblasts to develop. The mortality is 5% and is mainly from brain herniation or abscess rupture into the ventricles.

7. Pathologic stages — (a) early cerebritis (up to 5 days), (b) late cerebritis (5 days–2 weeks); (c) early capsule formation (2–3 weeks); and (d) late capsule formation (>3 weeks, there is a firm capsule around the abscess).

C. Encephalitis — commonly by *Legionella* (CSF culture is usually negative), *Mycoplasma, Listeria* (in neonates and immunosuppressed, CSF culture is usually positive), and *Brucella*

D. Subdural empyema — mainly caused by *Streptococcus* and *Bacteroides* from an adjacent infection. Treat with antibiotics and drainage with multiple burr holes or osteoplastic flap and consider antibiotic therapy alone if asymptomatic (**Fig. 3.26**).

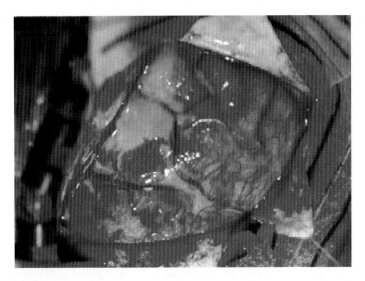

Fig. 3.26 Subdural empyema; thick pus collection over the convexity.

E. Epidural abscess — most commonly caused by *S. aureus, Streptococcus*, gram-negative bacilli, and tuberculosis (TB). It is usually secondary to an associated osteomyelitis or sinusitis and most frequently occurs in the thoracic, lumbar, or sacral spine (**Fig. 3.27**).

F. Osteomyelitis — most commonly caused by the same bacterial species as epidural abscesses and occurs with sinusitis (**Fig. 3.28**), after craniotomy or by hematologic spread. It is characterized by moth-eaten cortical bone with poor margins and soft tissue swelling. X-ray films may appear similar to metastatic lesions. Gradenigo syndrome is petrous apex osteomyelitis with CN VI palsy and retroorbital pain and may occur in children from extension of severe otitis.

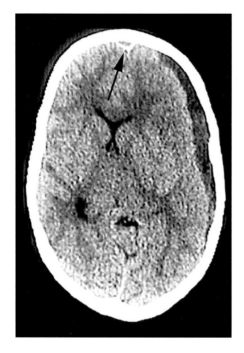

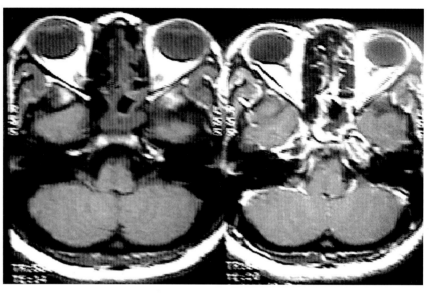

Fig. 3.28 Sphenoid sinusitis. (**A**) Axial nonenhanced and (**B**) enhanced T1-weighted magnetic resonance images demonstrating thickened enhancing mucosa.

Fig. 3.27 Epidural abscess and subdural empyema. Enhanced computed tomographic scan demonstrates a large convexity, low-density subdural collection and a small anterior rim-enhancing epidural lesion (*arrow*).

VIII. Infectious Pathogens

A. Mycobacterial infections

    1. TB — caused by *Mycobacterium tuberculosis*

        a. CSF — increased lymphocytes, decreased glucose (but not as low as with pyogenic infections) and increased protein up to 200 mq/dL. Acid-fast bacilli are seen in the CSF in <25% of cases and require up to 4 weeks to grow in culture. It is diagnosed by positive purified protein derivative (PPD) skin test and TB lesions found elsewhere in the body.

        b. TB meningitis — characterized by a thick basilar exudate, small miliary granulomas on the convexities, and frequent vascular occlusions. Morbidity is 80% and mortality is 30%. It usually results from hematogenous spread. Pathologic examination (**Fig. 3.29**) demonstrates granulomas with caseating necrosis, lymphocytes, and Langerhans giant cells.

        c. Tuberculomas — In the brain, parenchyma are rare in the United States, but are common intracranial masses in India and Mexico. They may be solid or cystic, 30% are multiple; in children, two thirds are infratentorial.

        d. Miliary TB — has innumerable small lesions, is rare, and is more frequently seen in children

        e. Two-thirds of cases have active TB infections elsewhere in the body. Treatment is with 24 months of triple antibiotics.

    2. Leprosy — caused by *Mycobacterium leprae*. It most frequently occurs in tropical climates, California, Texas, New York, and Louisiana. In the United States, it is primarily brought in by travelers. There are two types:

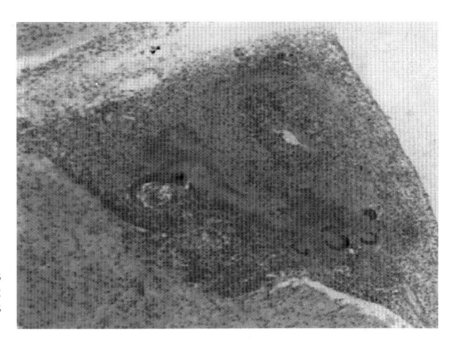

Fig. 3.29 Tuberculous meningitis (hematoxylin and eosin [H&E] stain); caseating granuloma with Langerhans giant cells.

    a. Lepromatous form seen with low host resistance and has lepra cells that are plump histiocytes filled with organisms. Lesions are located in the skin on cooler parts of the body (i.e., hands, feet, head, peripheral nerves, anterior eyes, upper airways, and testes). The lepromin skin test is negative.

    b. Tuberculoid form is seen with maximal host resistance, and there are areas of hypesthetic skin, inflamed swollen nerves, caseating granulomas, and occasional gram-negative bacilli seen on histologic examination. The lepromin skin test is positive.

B. Other granulomatous disease

    1. Sarcoid is a systemic granulomatous disease of unknown cause that involves lymph nodes (especially hilar), lungs, skin, eyes, salivary glands, and liver. The nervous system is involved in 5% of cases with cranial nerve palsies (especially CN VII), aseptic meningitis, pituitary dysfunction, hydrocephalus, and noncaseating granulomas at the base of the brain (especially the hypothalamus). It may also cause myelopathy, neuropathy, and myopathy. Sarcoid is most common in African Americans. The serum angiotensin converting enzyme (ACE) level usually is elevated. Treatment is with steroids (**Fig. 3.30**).

    2. Whipple disease — a chronic multisystem disease caused by *Tropheryma whippelii*. It is characterized by weight loss, abdominal pain, diarrhea, lymphadenopathy, arthralgia, and Alzheimer disease–like neurologic symptoms (10%). Pathologic examination demonstrates foamy macrophages with PAS-positive granules. These are degenerating bacilli. Treatment is with tetracycline.

C. Spirochetes

    1. Neurosyphilis — a sexually transmitted disease caused by *Treponema pallidum*. A genital lesion (chancre) forms 3 weeks after infection and secondary lesions develop several weeks later. 25% of cases involve the CNS, but usually after 3 years. Treatment is with penicillin and CSF testing at 6 months and 1 year for evaluation of treatment success. There are four types of neurosyphilis:

        a. Meningovascular syphilis (lues) — occurs after 7 years and is characterized by subacute or chronic meningitis with perivascular lymphocytes, Huebner arteritis with intimal proliferation and vessel obliteration, and multiple ischemic strokes in the basal ganglia and MCA territory.

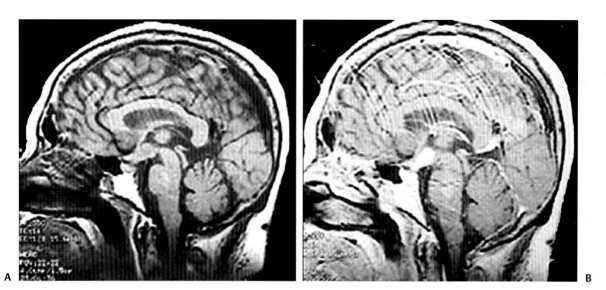

Fig. 3.30 Neurosarcoid. (**A**) Nonenhanced and (**B**) enhanced sagittal T1-weighted magnetic resonance imaging scans demonstrate the sellar and suprasellar enhancement.

    b. General paresis of the insane — occurs after 15 years and is characterized by invasion into the parenchyma with chronic encephalitis, atrophy, and gummas with nonsuppurative necrotic debris, progressive physical and mental deterioration, and Argyll Robertson pupils.

    c. Tabes dorsalis — occurs after 15–20 years and is characterized by myelopathy from meningeal fibrosis. There is mainly dorsal root and posterior column involvement, W-shaped demyelination in the thoracic and lumbar spinal cord from the posterior horns inward, lightning-like pains, sensory ataxia, urinary incontinence, decreased lower limb deep tendon reflexes, decreased proprioception and vibratory sense, positive Romberg test, Argyll Robertson pupils (90%), ptosis, optic atrophy, and Charcot joints of the hip, knee, and ankle.

    d. Congenital syphilis — includes Hutchinson triad of notched teeth, deafness, and interstitial keratitis. This is also associated with meningovascular syphilis.

  2. Lyme disease — caused by *Borrelia burgdorferi*, a tick-borne spirochete that causes erythema migrans (70%). 15% have neurologic symptoms such as aseptic meningitis, cranial neuritis (especially CN VII), encephalitis, myelopathy, radiculopathy, and peripheral neuropathy. It is most frequently seen from May through July in New England, along the Pacific coast, and in Wisconsin and Minnesota. Symptoms are caused by immune complexes and vasculitis with a postviral-type demyelination and perivascular infiltration. Diagnosis is by enzyme-linked immunosorbent assay (ELISA) and treatment is with tetracycline.

D. Other bacterial infections

  1. Actinomyces — a branched filamentous bacterium that looks like a fungus. It is rare in the CNS, contains sulfur granules, and is acid fast bacillus (AFB) negative.

  2. Nocardia — an opportunist infection that usually infects the lungs, although the CNS is involved in 30% of cases. It forms multiple abscesses and is AFB positive.

E. Fungal infections

  1. Mycotic infections — usually occur in immunosuppressed patients and result from hematologic spread from the lungs. They cause basilar meningitis (with cranial neuropathies, hydrocephalus, and arteritis causing strokes) or abscesses with granulomas. CSF reveals increased lymphocytes and decreased glu-

cose. All fungi stain with methenamine silver. The true pathogens are *Histoplasma, Blastomyces*, and *Coccidiomycoses*; all others only infect the immunosuppressed.

2. Candidiasis — caused by *Candida albicans*. It is the most frequent CNS fungal infection. *C. albicans* is normal flora of the GI tract, skin, and genitals. Risk of infection increased with antibiotics, steroids, IV lines, diabetes mellitus, burns, immunosuppression, and IV drug abuse. It forms multiple microabscesses with granulomas and rarely causes meningitis. It also infects the urine, blood, skin, heart, and lungs. Treatment is with amphotericin B.

3. Histoplasmosis — caused by *H. capsulatum* from the soil of the Ohio, Mississippi, and St. Lawrence River valleys. It frequently causes pulmonary infections and only rarely CNS infections with basilar meningitis and occasional parenchymal granulomas.

4. Blastomycosis — caused by *B. dermatidis* from the soil of the eastern United States. The CNS is involved in less than 5% of cases. Abscess is more frequent than meningitis. Culture demonstrates a single, budding yeast.

5. Cryptococcosis — caused by *C. neoformans* from soil contaminated with bird feces. It is the most frequent fungal meningitis and the second most frequent CNS fungal infection. There are rarely cryptococcomas in the parenchyma. CSF cultures are positive (75%), Cryptococcus antigen is positive (90%), and India ink stain is positive (**Fig. 3.31**) (50%), with a single budding yeast with a thick capsule. The capsule disappears during the tissue preparation to form the characteristic halo. Treatment is with amphotericin B and fluconazole.

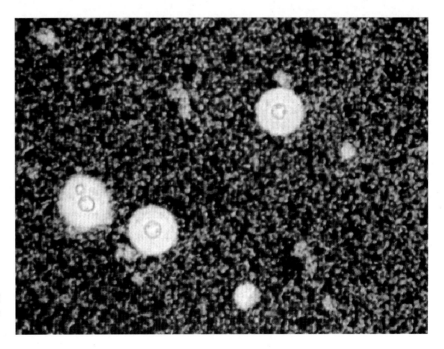

Fig. 3.31 Cryptococcus (India ink stain); yeast organism surrounded by clear halos.

6. Coccidioidomycosis — caused by *C. immitis* from the soil of the Southwest United States, especially in California (the San Joaquin Valley) and Arizona. The CNS is involved in 63% of cases with meningitis or cerebritis with granulomas. There are large sporangia filled with endospores. Treatment is with intrathecal amphotericin B and mortality is 50%.

7. Aspergillosis — caused by *Aspergillus fumigatus* or *A. flavus* from the soil. It is the third most frequent fungal CNS infection. It is named from its sporangia that resemble a container of holy water and only

forms when growing with contact to air. It is rarely diagnosed before death. It is angioinvasive causing hemorrhagic cerebritis and rarely meningitis. It has branching septate hyphae. Treatment is with amphotericin B and 5-fluorocytosine (**Fig. 3.32** and **Fig. 3.33**).

8. Mucormycosis — the fungus is from the soil. Rhinocerebral involvement is most common in diabetic patients with acidosis or dehydrated children with diarrhea and immunosuppression who develop acidosis. It causes periorbital swelling, proptosis, and nasal discharge. It spreads by direct extension from the sinuses through the veins to the orbit, cavernous sinus, and the brain. There is also spread from the lungs. It is angioinvasive causing deep hemorrhagic necrosis and ischemic strokes. It has nonseptate right-angle branching hyphae. Treatment is with amphotericin B.

F. Parasites

1. Nematodes (roundworms)

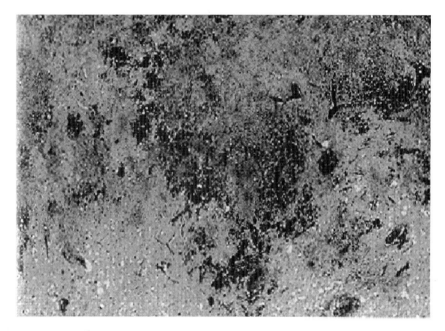

Fig. 3.32 Aspergillus encephalitis (hematoxylin and eosin [H&E] stain); hemorrhagic cerebritis with branching septate hyphae.

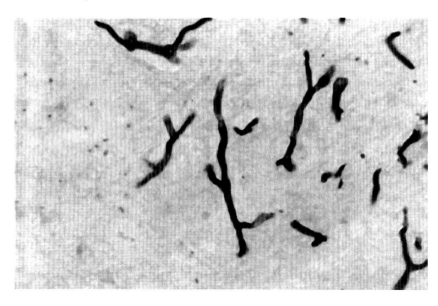

Fig. 3.33 *Aspergillus* (silver stain); branching septate hyphae.

    a. Trichinosis — caused by *Trichinella spiralis*. There are only about a dozen cases reported per year in the United States. It is obtained by ingestion of undercooked pork that contains infectious cysts. Lesions occur mainly in the skeletal muscle but occasionally in the CNS causing meningitis. Treatment is with thiabendazole and steroids.

    b. *Angiostrongylus cantonensis* — a rat lung worm that involves the CNS causing eosinophilic meningitis

    c. Strongyloidiasis — caused by the roundworm, *Strongyloides stercoralis*. This worm can carry bacteria with it to the CNS and cause mixed meningitis

2. Platyhelminth (flatworms)

    a. Cestodes (tapeworms)

      (1) Cysticercosis — caused by *Taenia solium*, the pork tapeworm. It is the most frequent CNS parasitic disease in the world. The human is the definitive host of the adult worm. Cysticercosis occurs when a human serves as the intermediate host and the cysticerci accumulate in the subcutaneous tissue, skeletal muscles, eyes, and CNS. It may cause meningitis, seizures, parenchymal or intraventricular abscesses. Taeniasis (tapeworm infection) is contracted by ingestion of undercooked pork, whereas cysticercosis is contracted by ingestion of food with fecal contamination. Treatment is with praziquantel or albendazole (**Fig. 3.34–Fig. 3.36**).

      (2) Echinococcus (hydatid disease) — caused by *E. granulosa*, a dog tapeworm. The intermediate host is sheep. Each cyst contains multiple larvae (hydatid sand), and rupture can lead to further cyst formation. Cysts form in the liver (65%), lung (20%), and brain (2%). Treatment is with mebendazole.

    b. Trematodes (flukes)

      (1) Schistosomiasis — caused by *S. haematobium* and *S. mansoni*, which can infect the spinal cord and by *S. japonicum*, which can infect the brain. They live in blood vessels and the snail is the intermediate host. Treatment is with praziquantel.

      (2) Paragonimiasis — caused by a fluke that resides in the lung and rarely enters the brain (1%) by way of the basal foramina. It can be acquired by ingestion of raw fish.

G. Protozoa

1. Toxoplasmosis — caused by *T. gondii*, an obligate intracellular organism. The definitive host is the cat. Human infection is caused by ingestion of cat feces or raw meat. Serum antibodies are seen in 30% of the normal population. The cyst may lie dormant until the host becomes immunocompromised. It is

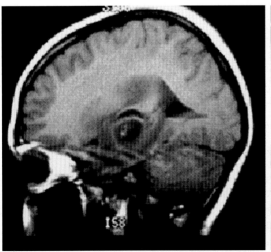
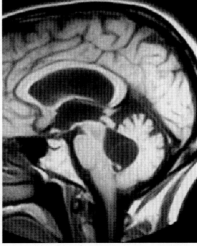

A,B

Fig. 3.34 Cysticercosis. Nonenhanced sagittal T1-weighted magnetic resonance images demonstrate cystic lesions with a scolex (**A**) in the left temporal lobe and (**B**) in the fourth ventricle.

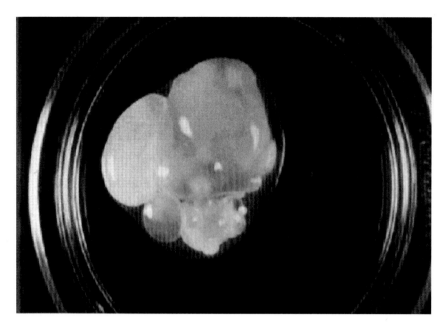

Fig. 3.35 Cysticercosis (gross); cyst with larva.

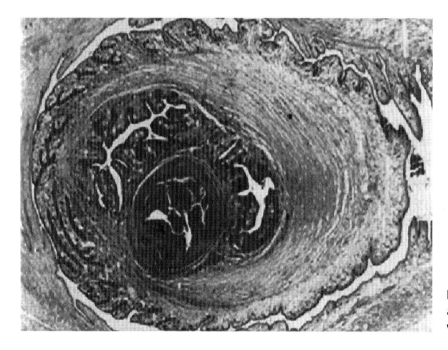

Fig. 3.36 Cysticercosis (hematoxylin and eosin [H&E] stain); encysted larva with scolex.

the most frequent mass lesion in the brain in patients with AIDS. It is hypoactive on thallium-201 single photon emission CT. The cyst is full of and is surrounded by free tachyzoites that can be seen on H & E. Infection of the mother during pregnancy causes congenital lesions such as brain necrosis, periventricular calcification, hydrocephalus, hydranencephaly, chorioretinitis, and hepatosplenomegaly. Acquired infection may cause meningoencephalitis or abscesses. Treatment is with 4 weeks of sulfadiazine and pyrimethamine with leucovorin (to rescue the cells from the antifolate effects) or for the remainder of life in AIDS patients (**Fig. 3.37**).

2. Amoebic meningoencephalitis — caused by (1) *Naegleria fowler* from freshwater ponds or lakes that enters the skull through the cribriform plate and causes basilar hemorrhagic meningitis that may be rapidly fatal, (2) *Acanthamoeba* from contact lenses that gets in the corneal stroma (treatment may require a corneal transplant), and (3) *Entamoeba histolytica* that also may cause meningoencephalitis.

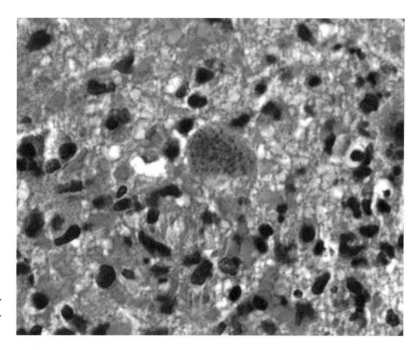

Fig. 3.37 Toxoplasma. Pseudocyst and multiple free tachyzoites in the brain (hematoxylin and eosin [H&E] stain).

3. Malaria — caused mainly by *Plasmodium falciparum*, but also by *Plasmodium vivax*, *Plasmodium malariae*, and *Plasmodium ovale*. One to 10% of cases involve the CNS and manifest as acute encephalopathy, fever, decreased mental status, seizures, and focal deficits. Symptoms may be due to cerebral hypoxia from capillary obstruction by infected erythrocytes.

4. Trypanosomiasis — caused by (1) *Trypanosoma brucei* that causes African sleeping sickness, a meningo-encephalitis transmitted by the tsetse fly; (2) *T. rhodesiense* that causes a more severe meningoencephalitis; (3) *T. gambiense* that is more chronic; and (4) *T. cruzi* that causes Chagas disease in South America, which is transmitted by the reduviid bug and causes cardiomyopathy, megacolon, and congenital CNS lesions in children.

H. Viruses

1. Viruses — obligate intracellular parasites that depend on the host cell for protein synthesis and energy. They may contain either DNA or ribonucleic acid (RNA). They have no organelles or nucleus and are not cells. They are surrounded by a capsid with protein subunits (capsomeres).

2. Neurotropic RNA viruses — picornavirus (poliomyelitis), togavirus (Eastern and Western equine encephalopathy and rubella), flavivirus (St. Louis encephalopathy), paramyxovirus (measles, SSPE), rhabdovirus (rabies), arena (lymphocytic choriomeningitis), bunyavirus (California group encephalitis), and retrovirus (human immunodeficiency viruses [HIV])

3. Neurotropic DNA viruses — papovavirus (PML) and the herpes group with HSV-1 and 2, varicella-zoster, and CMV

4. Infection transmission
   a. Respiratory route — measles, mumps, and varicella-zoster
   b. GI route — poliovirus
   c. Subcutaneous inoculation — rabies and arbovirus

5. Virus access to the CNS
   a. Blood — poliovirus
   b. Peripheral nerves — rabies

6. DNA viruses
   a. Circular without envelope — papovavirus JC and SV40
   b. Circular with envelope — poxvirus
   c. Linear without envelope — adenovirus
   d. Linear with envelope — herpesvirus

7. RNA viruses
   a. Single strand, with sense, without envelope — picornavirus (poliovirus, echovirus, and Coxsackie virus)
   b. Single strand, with sense, with envelope — togavirus (rubella and eastern, western, and Venezuelan equine encephalopathies), retrovirus (HIV), and flavivirus (St. Louis and Japanese encephalopathies)
   c. Single-strand, without sense, with envelope — paramyxovirus (measles, SSPE, mumps), rhabdovirus (rabies), bunyavirus (California encephalopathy), orthomyxovirus (influenza), and arenavirus (lymphocytic choriomeningitis)

8. Virus detection — by in situ hybridization with radioactive complementary DNA or RNA or by polymerase chain reaction (PCR) used to amplify their DNA segments. HSV is persistent so it can always be recovered. Varicella-zoster becomes latent so it is intermittently recovered.

9. Viral (aseptic) meningitis — 70% are caused by enterovirus (picornavirus: polio, echovirus, Coxsackie virus) and mumps. It is self-limited and usually lasts up to 1 week.
   a. Symptoms — fever, headache, and nuchal rigidity. There are no features of encephalitis such as decreased mental status, seizures, or focal deficits.
   b. CSF evaluation — lymphocytic pleocytosis, normal protein, and glucose (except decreased glucose with mumps and lymphocytic choriomeningitis virus in rodent handlers) and no bacteria or fungus on culture.
   c. Epidemiology — it is most common in August and September. Nonviral aseptic meningitis may be caused by an adjacent sinus or mastoid bacterial infection, syphilis, *Cryptococcus*, TB, *Borrelia*, leukemia, lymphoma, and Behçet disease.

10. Viral encephalitis — the most frequent epidemic cause is arbovirus and the most frequent sporadic cause is HSV-1. In immunocompromised patients, the most common viruses are HIV, CMV, and papovavirus (there are also infections from *Toxoplasma, Aspergillus*, and *Listeria*). Symptoms include seizures, decreased mental status, and focal deficits. There is a 5–20% mortality (HSV has 50% mortality) and 20% incidence of permanent sequelae.

11. Arboviruses — "Arthropod borne" by mosquitoes, ticks, etc. Reservoirs are birds, small mammals, and horses. Humans are dead-end hosts. They include togavirus, flavivirus, bunyavirus, and reovirus.
    a. Eastern encephalopathy — the most severe and occurs in late summer on the eastern seaboard of the United States and has a 70% mortality
    b. Western encephalopathy — milder and occurs on the west coast of Canada, the United States, and Central America
    c. Venezuelan equine encephalopathy — mild, occurs in Central and South America and has <1% mortality
    d. LaCrosse encephalitis — the second most frequent encephalitis in the United States after enterovirus, has a low mortality, and occurs in the Midwest and New York
    e. St. Louis encephalitis — transmitted by birds and occurs in the summer in the Midwest and South

   f. Japanese encephalitis — the most frequent epidemic encephalitis in the world and has a 50% mortality rate

   g. Pathologic findings of all these viruses — perivascular mononuclear infiltrates

12. Herpes encephalitis

   a. HSV — enters through the eye, mouth, and genitals and reaches the CNS by the peripheral nerves. In the CNS, it remains relatively shielded from the host's immune system.

      (1) The virus may travel from the skin to the olfactory nerve, trigeminal nerve, or trigeminal ganglion. It rarely spreads hematogenously. It is found in the trigeminal ganglion in 50% of normal adults and reactivates after trauma or immunosuppression.

      (2) Findings — aseptic meningitis, encephalitis, myelitis, keratitis, skin lesions, and hemorrhagic necrosis of the basal frontal and medial temporal lobes (**Fig. 3.38**)

      (3) It is generally held that in children, the virus reaches the CNS by means of the olfactory mucosa and in adults by means of the trigeminal ganglion to the middle fossa. HSV-1 is the most frequent cause of sporadic encephalitis.

      (4) It usually affects those older than neonates, frequently involves limbic structures, and sequentially becomes bilateral. HSV-2 encephalitis affects mainly neonates and is more diffuse.

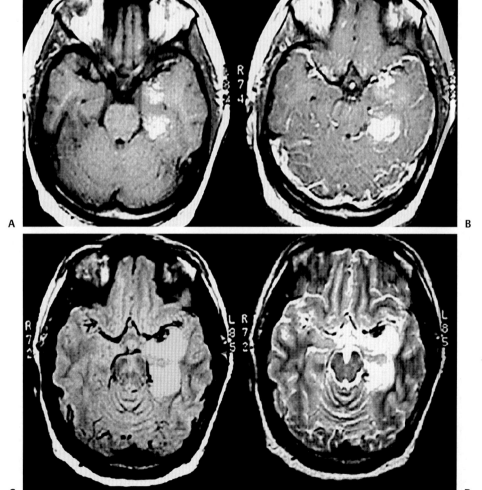

Fig. 3.38 Herpes encephalitis. Axial magnetic resonance images (MRIs) demonstrate hemorrhagic and edematous left medial temporal lobe lesion. (**A**) Nonenhanced T1-weighted MRI, (**B**) enhanced T1-weighted, (**C**) proton density, and (**D**) T2-weighted MRIs.

(5) Diagnosis — by PCR to detect viral nucleic acid in the CSF (must be in first few days) or biopsy and culture of the anterior inferior temporal gyrus.

(6) Pathologic examination (**Fig. 3.39**) — demonstrates Cowdry type A inclusions (intranuclear eosinophilic masses with a surrounding halo found in neurons, oligodendrocytes, and astrocytes). These inclusions are best seen in the first few days of the infection. The CSF culture is usually negative. Mortality is 50–60%. Treatment is with steroids and acyclovir IV for 14 days.

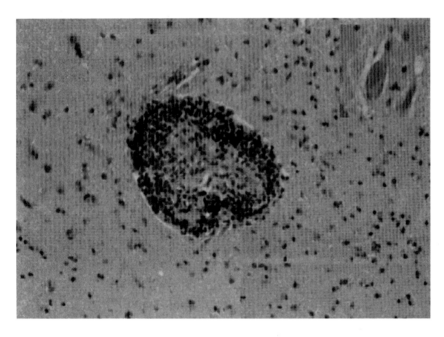

Fig. 3.39 Herpes simplex virus-1 encephalitis (hematoxylin and eosin [H&E] stain); lymphocytic perivascular cuffing. Inset with Cowdry A eosinophilic intranuclear inclusions.

b. CMV —the largest herpesvirus. It is commonly found in all body fluids. It also produces Cowdry type A and intracytoplasmic inclusions. Diagnosis is by culture and in situ hybridization. Intrauterine infections cause congenital malformations such as microcephaly, hydrocephalus, chorioretinitis, and microphthalmia (**Fig. 3.40**).

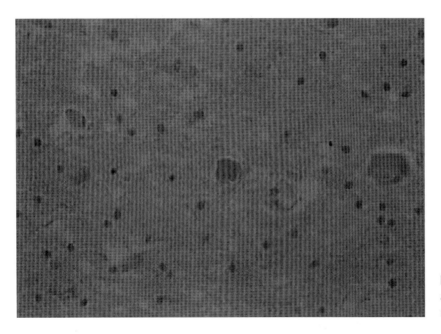

Fig. 3.40 Cytomegalovirus (hematoxylin and eosin [H&E] stain); eosinophilic intranuclear and intracytoplasmic inclusions.

   c. Varicella zoster — the primary infection is varicella after which the virus becomes latent in the DRG. A reactivation is zoster (shingles) that mainly affects the elderly and immunocompromised. Two-thirds of cases are levels T5–T9, and 15% of cases involve CN V1 (trigeminal ophthalmic branch).

     (1) Herpes infection of the geniculate ganglion (Ramsay Hunt syndrome) — may cause dysfunction of CN VII with altered sensation of taste, facial weakness, and vesicular eruptions on the pinna and in the external auditory canal

     (2) Pathologic examination — intranuclear inclusions in the DRG and the posterior horn gray matter, posterior roots, and meninges

     (3) Treatment — skin lotions (calamine), capsaicin, acyclovir (must be given within 48 hours of rash formation to decrease the duration of disease, use 7-day oral course or 10-day IV course for immunocompromised patients or if >3 dermatomes involved) and topical acyclovir for the eye with a V1 infection. Postherpetic pain is treated (although it responds poorly) with amitriptyline, carbamazepine, gabapentin, pregabalin, and time.

13. Rabies — acquired from the bites of skunks, foxes, coyotes, and bats. It may also be transmitted by aerosolized vectors inside caves where bats live. The virus travels through the peripheral nerves to the CNS and has an incubation period of 1 to 3 months.

   a. The prodrome phase is followed by either a paralytic (Guillain–Barré-like) form or encephalitic (more frequent) form that progresses to coma and death 2 to 25 days after the onset of symptoms.

   b. The virus destroys mainly limbic neurons. Negri bodies (intracytoplasmic eosinophilic collections of ribonucleoproteins) are seen in 80% of cases and are especially prominent in the cerebellum (Purkinje cells), brainstem, and hippocampus (**Fig. 3.41**).

   c. Symptoms — anxiety, dysphagia, and spasms of the throat when attempting to swallow (hydrophobia)

   d. Treatment — washing the wound with soap, water, and benzyl ammonium chloride (inactivates virus) and watching the biting animal for 10 days. If it becomes symptomatic, it should be euthanized and the brain examined. If there are signs of rabies, treat with rabies immune globulin to provide 10 to 20 days of passive immunization. If one is at high risk, consider a vaccine.

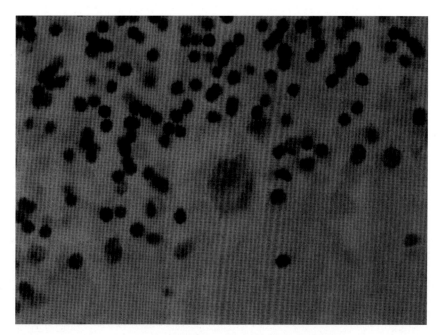

Fig. 3.41 Rabies (hematoxylin and eosin [H&E] stain. Large intracytoplasmic eosinophilic Negri body in Purkinje cell between the granular and molecular layers.

14. Enteroviruses (poliovirus, Coxsackie virus, and echoviruses; the human GI tract is the reservoir); most common cause of viral meningitis
    a. Poliovirus (single-stranded RNA virus)
       (1) There are <10 cases/year in the United States and they are mostly vaccine related. Incubation is 7 to 21 days. 10% of cases develop viremia.
       (2) Most infections are subclinical (nonparalytic form). The CNS is involved in 0.1–1% of cases with aseptic meningitis, encephalitis, and paralysis.
       (3) Anterior horn cells—the most susceptible because they have increased numbers of viral receptors on their surface. The virus may also infect Betz cells and brainstem nuclei (10–35% of patients develop bulbar palsy).
       (4) Pathologic examination reveals perivascular mononuclear infiltrates and neuronophagia. There is no virus detected in the CSF.
       (5) The risk of paralytic disease with the live attenuated oral vaccine is 1 in 2.5 million.
       (6) Mortality is 5–10%. Motor strength usually returns in 4 months.
    b. Coxsackie and echoviruses — cause meningoencephalitis and polymyositis. They may be cultured from the CSF. The incidence is increased in patients with humoral immunity deficiencies.

15. Mumps — 10% of the patients with mumps parotiditis develop meningitis. Before the routine use of the mumps vaccine, it accounted for 25% of viral encephalitis cases. It can be cultured from the CSF.

16. Measles — a postinfectious encephalomyelitis develops after the rash in 1 in 1000 cases. It is immune mediated and not directly caused by the virus.
    a. SSPE — occurs in children and adolescents (ages 5–15 years) after a measles infection that has usually occurred before 2 years of age.
    b. Chronic encephalitis develops with deteriorating school performance and behavioral changes followed by myoclonus, seizures, weakness, and death in 1–3 years.
    c. It affects both the gray and white matter with perivascular lymphocytes, neuronophagia, demyelination, and oligodendrocyte destruction.
    d. There are intranuclear and intracytoplasmic inclusions in the neurons and oligodendrocytes. The CSF has oligoclonal antibodies to the measles virus, no cells, and increased protein (**Fig. 3.42**).
    e. Diagnosis can be made by periodic 2–3 electroencephalographic (EEG) spikes per second, increased CSF immunoglobulin, and increased serum and CSF measles antibody titers.

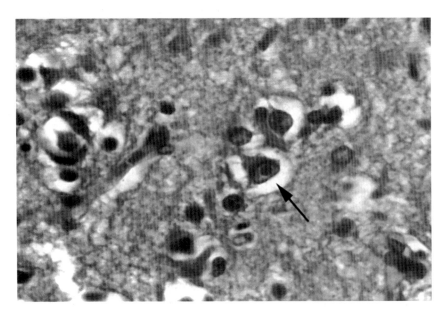

Fig. 3.42 Subacute sclerosing panencephalitis (hematoxylin and eosin [H&E] stain); eosinophilic intranuclear and intracytoplasmic inclusions (*arrow*).

17. PML — from the papovavirus family that includes (1) the papillomavirus (associated with warts and cervical carcinoma), (2) the polyoma BK virus (associated with hemorrhagic cystitis), and (3) the JC and SV40 viruses (associated with PML)

    a. The JC virus normally resides in the kidney. PML occurs in immunocompromised people and is found in 2% of AIDS autopsies.

    b. Typically, CT and MRI demonstrate patchy hypodense white matter changes without enhancement or mass effect (**Fig. 3.43**).

    c. It is bilateral, asymmetric, subcortical, spares the cortex, and usually starts in the posterior centrum semiovale. There is minimal cellular infiltration, central destruction of oligodendrocytes, demyelination, and peripheral swollen irregular oligodendrocytes with ground-glass nuclei and intranuclear inclusions of "stick-and-ball" viral particles. CSF is normal (**Fig. 3.44** and **Fig. 3.45**).

    d. Death occurs within a few months.

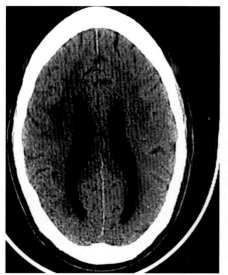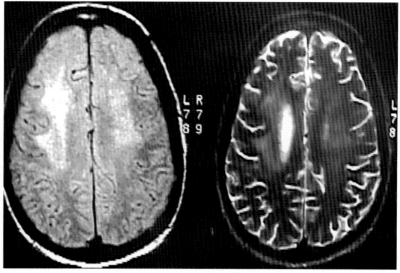

A–C

Fig. 3.43 Progressive multifocal leukoencephalopathy. (**A**) Computed tomographic, (**B**) proton density, and (**C**) T2-weighted magnetic resonance images demonstrating patchy white matter degeneration.

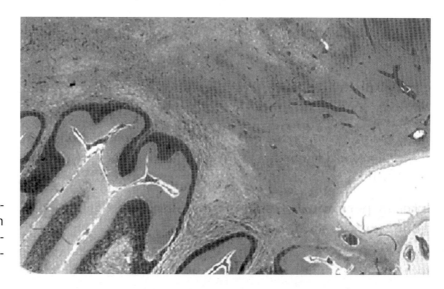

Fig. 3.44 Progressive multifocal leukoencephalopathy (hematoxylin and eosin [H&E] stain); low-power view demonstrates demyelination in cerebellar subcortical white matter.

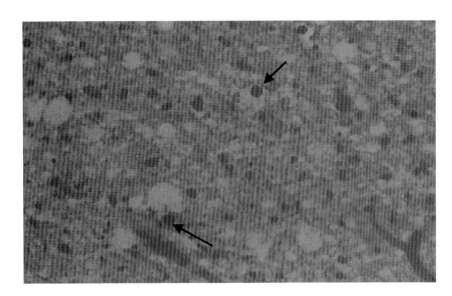

Fig. 3.45 Progressive multifocal leuko-encephalopathy (hematoxylin and eosin [H&E] stain). High-power view demonstrates demyelination with surrounding enlarged bizarre oligodendrocyte nuclei (*arrows*).

18. Transmissible spongiform encephalitis — The incubation is months to years, but once deterioration is started it progresses rapidly to death. These are a heterogeneous collection of probable infections caused by SSPE and HIV, but most commonly prions.

19. Prions — These are not viruses because they are protein without nucleic acid. They are resistant to nucleases, ultraviolet light, and radiation. They can be inactivated with autoclaving for 1 hour at 132°C or immersion in 1N NaOH for 15 minutes or 0.5% sodium hypochlorite for 1 hour.
    a. A protease-resistant protein is coded on chromosome 20 and the production may be released by a DNA configuration change.
    b. Prion diseases — kuru (in cannibals of New Guinea), scrapie (in sheep), chronic wasting disease in elk and mink, fatal familial insomnia, Creutzfeldt–Jakob disease (CJD), and Gerstmann–Sträussler syndrome. CJD occurs in 50- to 65-year-old people and manifests as myoclonus, pyramidal, and extrapyramidal degeneration, dementia, ataxia, and visual deterioration.
    c. There is a characteristic EEG with bilateral sharp waves of 1–2 waves/s that resemble periodic lateralized epileptiform discharges, but are reactive to painful stimuli.
    d. May have positive CSF immunoassay for 14-3-3 protein; fairly sensitive and specific
    e. Pathologic examination — demonstrates spongiform changes with astrocytosis but no inflammation most prominently in the cortex, putamen, and thalamus (**Fig. 3.46**). 5–10% of patients develop amyloid kuru plaques. Death occurs in less than 1 year.
    f. Gerstmann–Sträussler syndrome — ataxia, dysarthria, hyporeflexia, and cognitive decline, without myoclonus. Transmission is both autosomal dominant and sporadic, and Kuru plaques are seen in the cerebellum. These diseases can be transmitted to laboratory animals that develop the same microscopic changes.
    g. Fatal familial insomnia — sleep disturbance, agitation, mild cognitive changes, and dysautonomia; characterized by thalamic atrophy

20. Acquired immune deficiency syndrome
    a. Acquired immune deficiency syndrome (AIDS) — caused by a retrovirus that contains RNA. It requires reverse transcriptase to convert its RNA to DNA and allow replication.
    b. HTLV-1 (human T cell lymphotropic virus) — causes a chronic myelopathy with spastic paresis, but no sensory deficit and involves the anterior and lateral columns. It occurs mainly in the Tropics (tropical spastic paraparesis) and Japan.

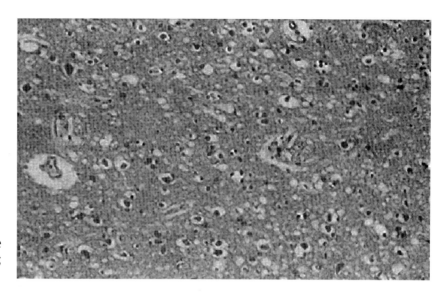

Fig. 3.46 Creutzfeldt–Jakob disease (hematoxylin and eosin [H&E] stain); spongiform changes.

 c. HTLV-2 — associated with chronic T cell leukemia and lymphoma

 d. HIV (HTLV-3) — a lentivirus with a surface molecule that interacts with T4. It is associated with *Pneumocystis* infections and Kaposi sarcoma. Viral latency is 8 years, and once AIDS ensues, 50% die in <1 year and most in <3 years if untreated. 50% of cases develop neurologic symptoms and 80% have CNS abnormalities. CNS complications at various stages include

  (1) Seroconversion — aseptic meningitis, acute encephalitis, and myelopathy

  (2) HIV-positive — asymptomatic or AIDS-related complex with aseptic meningitis

  (3) AIDS — aseptic meningitis, AIDS dementia complex, lymphoma, and vacuolar myelopathy

 e. AIDS dementia complex — the most frequent AIDS disorder seen in 50% of patients. It is believed to be caused by encephalitis or the viral impact on the neurons. It consists of a triad of cognitive dysfunction (subcortical dementia), behavioral changes (psychoses and hallucinations), and motor deficits (by centrum semiovale and brainstem involvement).

 f. Congenital lesions — atrophy, hydrocephalus ex vacuo, microcephaly, facial dysmorphism, and basal ganglia calcifications

 g. HIV encephalitis — pathologic examination demonstrates microglial nodules in the white matter and subcortical gray matter with focal demyelination, neuronal loss, reactive astrocytosis, and calcifications in the parenchymal blood vessels and basal ganglia. There are characteristic multinucleated giant cells that are unique to HIV in the CNS and are of macrophage origin (**Fig. 3.47**).

 h. Vacuolar myelopathy — mainly involves the posterior and lateral columns of the low thoracic levels. Pathologic examination demonstrates vacuolar changes with lipid-laden macrophages. It is detected in 50% of AIDS autopsies, but less often clinically.

 i. Peripheral neuropathy — seen in 5–38% of AIDS cases and is caused by didanosine, demyelination, and arteritis

 j. Myopathy — seen in 20% of AIDS cases, is characterized by inflammation, atrophy, polymyositis, and azathioprine-induced mitochondrial changes

 k. Toxoplasmosis — seen in 10% of autopsy cases. It is the most frequent cause of focal neurologic symptoms in AIDS. Toxoplasmosis may cause focal or diffuse lesions and predominantly causes basal ganglia and gray/white matter junction lesions. The serum IgG level is increased with infection, and pathologic examination demonstrates a mononuclear inflammation with extracellular tachyzoites and encysted bradyzoites (**Fig. 3.37**). Treatment is with pyrimethamine and sulfadiazine for 14 days.

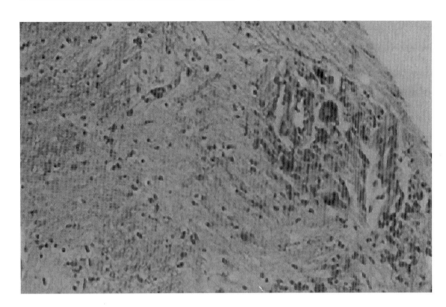

Fig. 3.47 Human immunodeficiency virus encephalitis (luxol fast blue-hematoxylin and eosin [H&E] stain). Microglial nodule with characteristic multinucleated giant cells.

l. CMV — seen in 30% of AIDS autopsies, but only 10% are symptomatic with necrotizing encephalomyelitis. Pathologic examination demonstrates microglial nodules, mainly in the gray matter and rarely in the white matter (unlike HIV). There are Cowdry type A intranuclear and intracytoplasmic inclusions in the neurons and astrocytes.

m. PML — described above.

n. Primary CNS lymphoma — seen in 5% of autopsies. It is invariably of B cell origin with large or mixed large/small cell types. They are usually periventricular with perivascular spread. Epstein–Barr virus (EBV) is frequently detected in the cells and may play a role in the development of the lymphoma.

o. Cryptococcus — in the normal population it causes meningitis, whereas in immunocompromised patients it causes encephalitis and cryptococcomas in the basal ganglia and midbrain

p. AIDS symptomatic infections — HIV encephalitis (60%), toxoplasma (30%), Cryptococcus (5%), PML (4%), and less frequently lymphoma (not an infection), TB, syphilis, varicella-zoster, and CMV

21. Rasmussen chronic encephalitis — occurs in childhood and causes progressive deficits and seizures (classically complex partial status epilepticus) with unilateral atrophy. It may be caused by CMV infection or antibodies to glutamate receptors.

22. Postinfectious encephalitis

a. SSPE — It develops several years after a measles infection. There are increased neutralized measles virus immunoglobulin titers in the serum and CSF. Pathologic examination demonstrates atrophy, perivascular lymphocytosis, demyelination, and increased eosinophilic intranuclear and intracytoplasmic inclusions in the neurons and oligodendrocytes. It affects children and young adults and develops in 1 in 1,000,000 cases of measles. Findings are as described above. Death occurs within 1–3 years.

b. Acute disseminated encephalomyelitis — immune-mediated disease that occurs after a viral infection or a vaccination

(1) It most commonly occurs after varicella-zoster, measles, upper respiratory infection, rabies vaccination, diphtheria, smallpox, tetanus, typhoid, and influenza.

(2) Pathologic examination demonstrates perivascular mononuclear infiltrates with a zone of demyelination along the course of the venules.

(3) All ages are affected, but it usually occurs in children and young adults.

(4) Symptoms occur 1–3 weeks after the infection. It follows a rapid course, although some patients survive.

(5) Treatment is with steroids. Mortality is 20–50%.

23. CSF glucose — low with fungal infections, TB, carcinomatous meningitis, and sarcoid.

24. Interleukin-1 — released in response to endotoxins and stimulates the interleukin cascade to increase T cell proliferation

25. Tumor necrosis factor — stimulates interleukin-1 production and activates neutrophils

IX. Congenital Infections (Torch)

A. Congenital infections are acquired three ways:

1. Hematogenous spread through the placenta (toxoplasma and viruses)

2. Ascending from the cervix (bacteria)

3. During passage through the birth canal (herpes, this mechanism causes neonatal rather than true congenital infection)

4. They may cause developmental changes or tissue destruction. Larger organisms such as bacteria, fungus, and protozoa are unable to enter the embryo before 3 to 4 months, but viruses may pass through the placenta.

5. The usual time frame for congenital infections is first trimester (rubella), 4 months (syphilis), 5 months (toxoplasma), perinatal (bacteria, HIV), during passage through birth canal (HSV-2, HIV).

B. Cytomegalovirus

1. CMV is the most frequent congenital CNS infection.

2. It causes migration disorders during the first or early second trimester. Transmission is transplacental. 75% of women have serum CMV antibodies (which are protective), 1% of newborns have CMV detected in the urine, and 10% of these have CNS infection.

3. It affects the brain, heart, liver, and spleen. The virus has an affinity for the germinal matrix and causes perivascular necrosis and calcifications.

4. Premature infants may have hepatosplenomegaly, jaundice, thrombocytopenia, chorioretinitis, seizures, mental retardation, optic atrophy, impaired hearing, and hydrocephalus.

5. Diagnosis is made by cultures, immunoglobulin levels, and intracellular (intranuclear and intracytoplasmic) inclusions on biopsy specimens.

6. Radiographs may demonstrate microcephaly and periventricular eggshell calcifications.

C. Toxoplasma

1. Toxoplasma is the second most frequent congenital CNS infection.

2. It occurs in 1 in 1000 to 1 in 10,000 pregnancies and is acquired by hematogenous spread through the placenta. There may be giant cell granulomas with atrophy of the basal ganglia, periventricular white matter, and cortex.

3. Unlike CMV, there are no migrational disorders or periventricular calcifications. The infection is significant if acquired before 26 weeks gestation.

4. Findings include seizures, microcephaly, and spontaneous abortions. A classical triad includes hydrocephalus, bilateral chorioretinitis, and cranial calcifications. Deafness is the most common late manifestation.

5. Treat with spiramycin if the mother seroconverts in 2–3 months. If the mother seroconverts after 4 months, use pyrimethamine and sulfadiazine.

D. Rubella

1. Rubella is transmitted transplacentally.

2. The virus inhibits cell multiplication to cause an insufficient number of cells in the brain (less neurons, astrocytes, and oligodendrocytes) and also is teratogenic and destructive.

3. The infection may cause meningoencephalitis, vasculopathy with ischemia and necrosis, microcephaly, decreased myelin, and cortical and basal ganglia calcifications. If the infection occurs before 12 weeks, the effects are very severe and spontaneous abortion is likely. If it occurs after 12 weeks, the infection is less severe.

4. Congenital rubella syndrome occurs with infection in the first trimester and includes chorioretinitis, cataracts, glaucoma, microphthalmia, microcephaly, mental retardation, and deafness.

5. During infection, the CSF has increased mononuclear cells and IgM; prevent with maternal vaccination before pregnancy.

E. Herpes simplex virus

1. HSV is transmitted transvaginally.

2. It occurs in 1 in 200 to 1 in 5000 births. 85% are caused by HSV-2 and rare early lesions cause death, chorioretinitis, and microcephaly. The virus has a predilection for vascular endothelial cells and causes thrombosis and hemorrhagic stroke that develops 2–4 weeks postpartum.

3. Pathologic examination demonstrates microglial nodules and intranuclear inclusions. The infection is diffuse and causes white matter edema without the temporal localization.

4. The most frequent manifestations are skin, eye, and mouth lesions, but if no treatment is given, the infection may disseminate with an 80% mortality (only 50% with treatment).

5. The CNS is involved in 30% and produces fever, seizures, and lethargy. HSV-1 affects older children.

F. Human immunodeficiency virus

1. HIV can be transmitted perinatally. 30% of HIV mothers transmit the virus to the children.

2. Pathologic examination demonstrates brain atrophy and basal ganglia calcifications.

3. Symptoms include weight loss, failure to thrive, diarrhea, and fever. Most die in 1 year.

G. Syphilis

1. Syphilis has transplacental transmission at 4–7 months.

2. Hutchinson triad — dental disorders, bilateral deafness, and interstitial keratitis

3. The other symptoms of syphilis are the same as in adults, but occur much earlier at 9–15 years. Hydrocephalus and stroke may occur.

4. The child should be treated with penicillin until the CSF is acellular and has a normal protein.

H. Listeria — causes increased abortions and premature deliveries

I. Calcifications — caused mainly by CMV (periventricular) and toxoplasma (disseminated)

J. Cardiac malformations — caused by rubella

K. Deafness — caused by rubella, syphilis, and CMV

X. Oncology

A. General Neurooncology

1. Primary brain tumors are less common than metastatic tumors. The most frequent is glioblastoma multiforme (GBM) followed by meningioma. Gliomas are more common in males, and meningiomas are more common in females.

2. Children — Brain malignancies are the second most common cancer after leukemia. 70% are infratentorial. The most frequent types are cerebellar astrocytoma (33%), brainstem glioma (25%), medulloblastoma (25%), and ependymoma (12%). 20% of brain tumors occur before 15 years of age. The most frequent supratentorial tumors in children are low-grade astrocytomas (50%), craniopharyngiomas (12%), and optic gliomas (12%).

3. Neonates and infants (<2 years) — Brain tumors are rare and usually congenital. Two thirds are supratentorial. The most common is teratoma, followed by primitive neuroectodermal tumors (PNETs), high-grade astrocytoma, and choroid plexus papilloma. Findings include macrocephaly, hydrocephalus, split sutures, seizures, and focal deficits. Most of the tumors are highly malignant and have a poor prognosis.

4. Older children — Most brain tumors are infratentorial. The most common types are astrocytoma (50%), PNET (15%), craniopharyngioma (10%), ependymoma (10%), and pineal tumor (3%).

5. Adults — Primary tumors are less common than metastatic tumors in clinical series. 70% are supratentorial. The most frequent tumors are GBM, metastases, anaplastic astrocytoma, meningioma, pituitary tumors, and vestibular schwannomas. The most frequent infratentorial tumors are metastases, schwannoma, meningioma, epidermoid, hemangioblastoma (the most frequent primary intraaxial posterior fossa tumor), and brainstem glioma.

6. In the spinal cord — The most frequent epidural lesions are metastatic. The most frequent intradural/extramedullary lesions are schwannoma and meningioma. The most frequent intramedullary lesions are astrocytoma and ependymoma.

7. Causes of tumors
   a. Radiation — associated with meningiomas, fibrosarcomas, and gliomas
   b. Immunosuppression — associated with lymphomas
   c. Viruses — EBV is associated with Burkitt lymphoma and nasopharyngeal carcinoma, and the human papillomavirus is associated with cervical carcinoma.
   d. Chemotherapy — nitrosoureas
   e. Genetics — as seen in phakomatoses and Turcot syndrome (APC gene mutation on chromosome 5q with familial polyposis, colorectal cancer, and primary brain tumors)

8. Prognosis of gliomas depends on (1) age, (2) histologic findings (especially necrosis), (3) Karnofsky score, (4) neurologic deficit, and (5) extent of resection.

9. Analysis of tumors — light microscopy, electron microscopy, immunohistochemistry, and in situ messenger RNA hybridization

10. Immunohistochemical stains
    a. AFP — embryonal carcinoma, endodermal sinus tumor
    b. CEA – carcinoembryonic antigen
    c. Chromogranin — pituitary adenoma
    d. Common leukocyte antigen — lymphoma, germinoma
    e. Cytokeratin — carcinoma, craniopharyngioma, chordoma
    f. Desmin — rhabdosarcoma, teratoma
    g. Epithelial membrane antigen (EMA) — carcinoma, meningioma, epithelial cysts
    h. GFAP — astrocytomas, other glial tumors
    i. Human melanoma black (HMB) — melanoma
    j. Beta human chorionic gonadotrophin (HCG) — choriocarcinoma and the syncytiotrophoblastic variant of germinomas
    k. Immunoglobulins kappa and lambda chains — lymphomas
    l. Neurofilament and synaptophysin — ganglioglioma, PNET
    m. Pituitary hormones — pituitary adenoma
    n. Prostate specific antigen — prostate carcinoma
    o. S100 — schwannoma, neurofibroma, glioma, PNET, chordoma, melanoma, renal cell carcinoma
    p. Synaptophysin — tumors with neurons (ganglioglioma, central neurocytoma, etc.)
    q. Transthyretin — choroid plexus tumors
    r. Vimentin — meningioma
    s. Many tumors have unexpected overlaps.

11. Assessment of proliferative capacity
    a. G1 phase — preparation for DNA synthesis (susceptible to radiation)
    b. S phase — DNA synthesis (resistant to radiation)
    c. G2 phase — preparation for mitosis
    d. M phase — mitosis (susceptible to radiation)
    e. G0 phase   nondividing quiet phase of cell cycle

12. Only a small portion of the dividing cells is in the M phase, so the mitotic index is misleading. Flow cytometry is more accurate because it stains DNA and counts the number of cells with double DNA. Also available are cytophotometry, DNA synthesis markers, and proliferation antigens that appear during the cell cycle (Ki67 is expressed in all stages except G0).

13. Oncogenes
    a. Oncogene — overexpression of an oncogene can cause the cell to enter an unrestrained replication cycle (malignant change). They may be introduced by a virus. Examples are *c-myc* oncogene (activation causes Burkitt lymphoma) and *n-myc* oncogene 9 (activation causes neuroblastoma).
    b. Proto-oncogene — a gene locus that becomes an oncogene by deletion or translocation
    c. Tumor suppressor gene — a gene in the normal genome that when lost or mutated allows malignant growth to occur. Tumor suppressor gene loss is associated with gliomas (chromosomes 9, 10, and 17), meningiomas (chromosome 22), and retinoblastomas (chromosome 13). The p53 nuclear protein gene is a tumor suppressor gene on chromosome 17p, and alterations are seen in 33% of astrocytomas.

14. Paraneoplastic syndromes (possibly autoimmune or viral)
    a. Limbic encephalitis — subacute encephalitis. Gross examination appears normal. There are peri-vascular mononuclear infiltrates but no viral inclusions. The medial temporal lobes, cingulate gyrus, and insula are predominantly affected. There are usually bilateral hyperintense lesions on T2-weighted MRI. It is most common in men in their mid-60s and manifests as memory impairment and altered mental status. It may be associated with testicular or lung cancer and anti-Ma protein antibodies. Limbic encephalitis should be differentiated from herpes encephalitis.
    b. Anti-Yo antibodies — cause cerebellar degeneration and are associated with ovarian and breast cancer
    c. Anti-Hu antibodies — cause sensory neuropathy, encephalitis, and cerebellar degeneration. They are associated with oat cell pulmonary carcinoma or lymphoma.
    d. Anti-Ri antibodies — cause opsoclonus and are associated with breast cancer
    e. Eaton–Lambert syndrome — antibodies to the presynaptic voltage-gated Ca^{2+} channels; associated with oat cell (small cell) lung carcinoma. See section XXXIII.
    f. Stiff man syndrome — involuntary muscle spasms and rigidity; 60% have antibodies to glutamic acid decarboxylase

15. Radiation
    a. Radiation-sensitive tumors — Lymphoma and germ cell tumors (mainly germinoma but to some extent the others) are very radiosensitive. Meningioma, pineal tumors, craniopharyngioma, pituitary tumors, vestibular schwannoma, and metastatic tumors are less sensitive.
    b. Standard radiation doses
       (1) Metastatic tumors — 30 Gray (Gy) over 2 weeks
       (2) Gliomas — 6000 centigray (cGy) in 200 cGy daily fractions
       (3) Doses higher than these are much more likely to cause radiation necrosis.
    c. Radiation necrosis — white matter coagulation necrosis or demyelination associated with arterioles with hyalin intimal thickening, fibrinoid necrosis, and thrombosis. The neurons are relatively resistant. Symptoms usually start 3 months–3 years (average 15–18 months) after radiation. Radiation myelopathy is reduced if the daily fraction is kept less than 200 cGy, the weekly fraction less than 900 cGy, and the total dose less than 6000 cGy. Symptoms begin with paresthesias/dysesthesias in the hands or feet and Lhermitte sign. There is no local pain, and it may progress irregularly. T2-weighted MRI demonstrates increased signal intensity, and pathologic examination demonstrates necrosis of the gray and white matter. There is no effective treatment: steroids are sometimes tried (**Fig. 3.48** and **Fig. 3.49**).
    d. Radiation may induce tumor formation such as sarcomas, GBMs, and meningiomas.

B. Glial tumors

1. Astrocyte types are
    a. Fibrillary — more numerous, mainly in the white matter, stains with phosphotungstic acid hematoxylin (PTAH), silver, and GFAP
    b. Protoplasmic — mainly in the gray matter and has a larger nucleus, but less cytoplasm
    c. Gemistocytic — swollen active astrocyte with increased fibers and cytoplasm and appears often with injury, stroke, toxin, infection, or tumor

2. Circumscribed astrocytic tumors — low grade, good prognosis, and frequently cystic
    a. Juvenile pilocytic astrocytoma (grade 1 astrocytoma) — the second most common pediatric brain tumor. It accounts for one-third of pediatric gliomas and 5 to 10% of all gliomas. It is most frequently located in the cerebellum, brainstem, optic pathway, and infundibulum. In adults, it

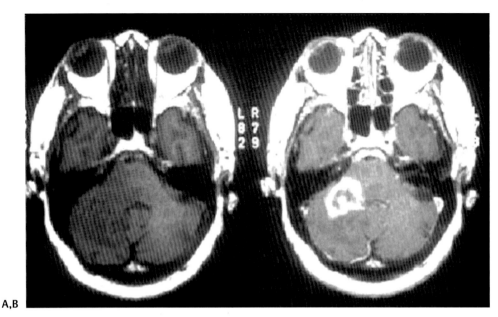

A,B

Fig. 3.48 Radiation necrosis. (**A**) Nonenhanced and (**B**) enhanced axial T1-weighted magnetic resonance images demonstrate the irregularly enhancing low-density lesion.

is more common near the third ventricle. The peak age is 10 years. 60% are cystic and they usually have a mural red-tan nodule. There is a biphasic pattern of loose cells and microcysts and also dense elongated hair-like astrocytes with Rosenthal fibers and eosinophilic granular bodies. They tend to be noncystic in the medulla and optic pathway. Leptomeningeal invasion, nuclear atypia, multinucleated cells, and vascular proliferation are frequently noted but are not adverse prognostic indicators. Approximately 10% contain calcium. The nodule may enhance. There is usually no necrosis. Survival rate is 86–100% at 5 years, 83% at 10 years, and 70% at 20 years (**Figs. 3.50–3.54**).

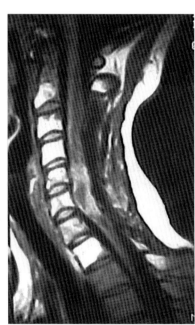

Fig. 3.49 Vertebral body radiation changes. Sagittal T1-weighted magnetic resonance image demonstrates the high-signal intensity changes in the vertebral bodies because of increased fat content.

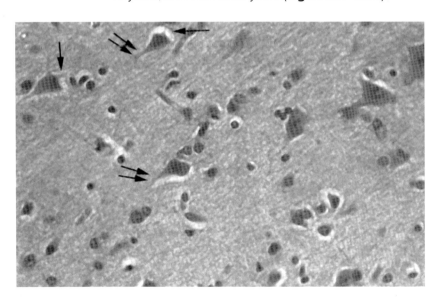

Fig. 3.50 Normal gray matter (hematoxylin and eosin [H&E] stain). Neurons oriented with large apical dendrites (double arrows) toward the pia and axons (*arrows*) toward the ventricles.

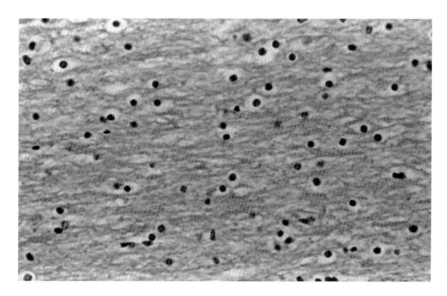

Fig. 3.51 Normal white matter (hematoxylin and eosin [H&E] stain). Normal oligodendrocytes interspersed in a fibrillary background.

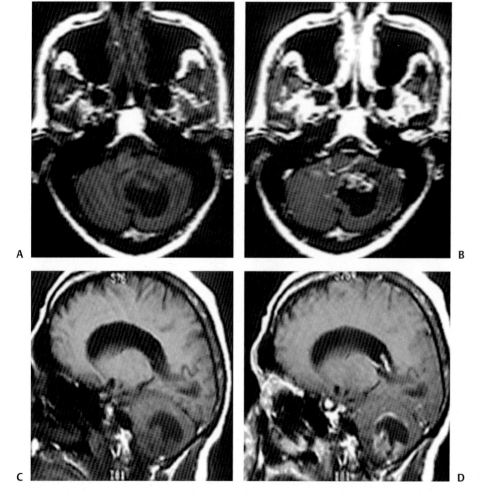

A   B

C   D

Fig. 3.52 Juvenile pilocytic astrocytoma. Axial T1-weighted magnetic resonance image (MRI). (**A**) nonenhanced and (**B**) enhanced, and sagittal T1-weighted (**C**) nonenhanced and (**D**) enhanced MRI scans with an enhancing nodule in a cerebellar cystic lesion.

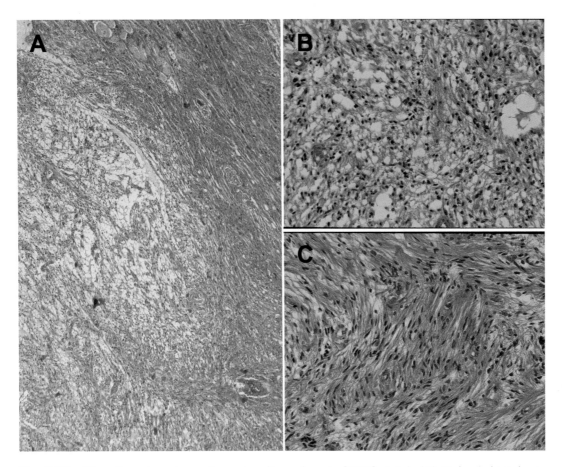

Fig. 3.53 Pilocytic astrocytoma (hematoxylin and eosin [H&E] stain). (**A**) Biphasic histologic pattern of a loose microcystic component and a dense component with higher-power views of the (**B**) loose and (**C**) dense areas.

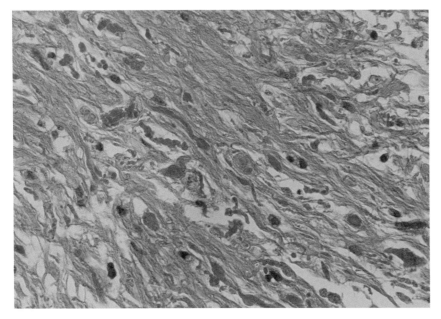

Fig. 3.54 Pilocytic astrocytoma (hematoxylin and eosin [H&E] stain); eosinophilic Rosenthal fibers.

b. Pleomorphic xanthoastrocytoma — the peak age is 7–25 years. Seizures are frequent. There is a temporal lobe predominance. They are usually superficial and involve the cortex and leptomeninges but not the dura. They tend to be cystic with a mural nodule. Pathologic examination demonstrates bizarre pleomorphic astrocytes with xanthomatous fat cells, spindle cells, and multinucleated cells. There are frequent mitoses, calcifications, a rich reticulin network, and no necrosis. They have a good prognosis, and most patients are alive at 17 years. There have been occasional reported transformations to GBM.

c. Subependymal giant cell astrocytoma — the peak age is <20 years. Symptoms are by hydrocephalus and seizures. They are located near the foramen of Monro. They enhance, have frequent calcifications, may be cystic and lobulated, and tend to be well demarcated. Pathologic examination reveals large multinucleated cells and rare mitoses. These tumors are seen in 15% of patients with tuberous sclerosis, and if found in a patient without tuberous sclerosis, it is considered a forme-fruste (**Fig. 3.55** and **Fig. 3.56**).

3. Diffuse astrocytic tumors — infiltrative and carry a worse prognosis. They may be fibrillary (most frequent), protoplasmic, gemistocytic (probably a worse prognosis if > 20% of cells are gemistocytic) or

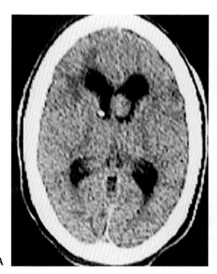
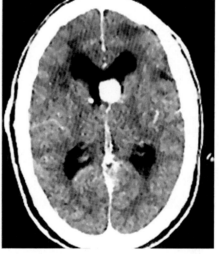

A   **B**

Fig. 3.55 Subependymal giant cell astrocytoma. (**A**) Axial nonenhanced and (**B**) enhanced computed tomographic scans demonstrating a large enhancing mass in the lateral ventricle. Also noted is a calcified tuber on the right lateral ventricular wall.

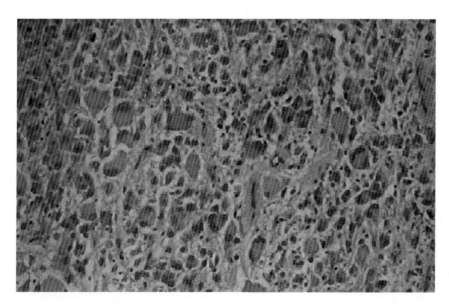

Fig. 3.56 Subependymal giant cell astrocytoma (hematoxylin and eosin [H&E] stain). Enlarged cells with abundant eosinophilic cytoplasm and large nuclei with prominent central nucleoli.

mixed. The grade is determined by the degree of anaplasia with increased cellularity, nuclear pleomorphism, mitoses, endothelial proliferation, necrosis, and to a lesser extent, pseudopalisading features.

    a. Grade II (low-grade astrocytoma) — well differentiated, represent 15% of astrocytomas, peak age is 30 years, male predominance, most frequently in the frontal white matter and most commonly fibrillary. They tend to be hypodense, minimally enhancing, and occasionally cystic. Pathologic examination reveals a gray-colored homogeneous tumor with indistinct borders that expands the white matter. There are no mitoses and only rarely hemorrhage or edema. 15% calcify. It is differentiated from reactive gliosis because it is patternless, violates the gray/white matter junction, has microcysts, microcalcifications, and increased nuclear atypia and pleomorphism. The 5-year survival rate with total resection and radiation is 70% and with subtotal resection and radiation is 38%. Median survival rate is 8.2 years and 50% increase in grade over time (**Fig. 3.57** and **Fig. 3.58**).

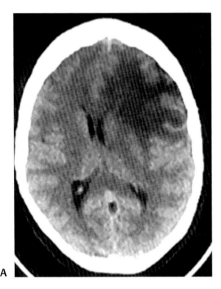 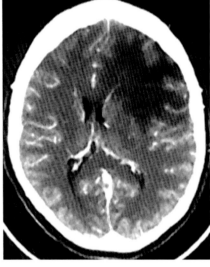

Fig. 3.57 Low-grade astrocytoma. Axial computed tomography scans (**A**) nonenhanced and (**B**) enhanced with nonenhancing left frontal hypodense mass.

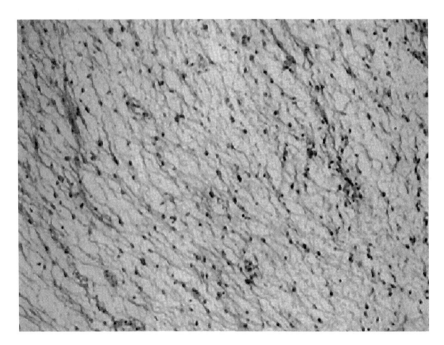

Fig. 3.58 Fibrillary (grade 2) astrocytoma (hematoxylin and eosin [H&E] stain). Patternless but uniform infiltrating cells.

b. Grade III (anaplastic astrocytoma) — represent 30% of astrocytomas; peak age is 40–60 years, with male predominance. CT reveals a mixed density lesion with irregular rim enhancement and edema. Pathologic examination demonstrates increased cellularity, nuclear atypia, mitotic figures, with or without endothelial hyperplasia, and no necrosis. There may be hemorrhages or cysts and rarely calcification. There are frequent gemistocytes (>20 per high power field denotes worse prognosis). They spread through white matter tracts, and there is frequent ependymal and CSF dissemination. Secondary structures of Scherer are located around neurons in the gray matter, the subpial region, and the subependymal zone. The median survival rate is 2–3 years (**Fig. 3.59**).

c. Grade IV (GBM) — represent 50% of astrocytomas, the most frequent primary brain tumor (20%), peak age is 45 to 60 years, with male predominance. GBM and anaplastic astrocytoma are among the four most common CNS tumors.

    (1) The location is most commonly deep frontotemporal. CT reveals a heterogeneous lesion that is cystic in 85% of cases with rare calcifications. Angiogram demonstrates a vascular mass with arteriovenous shunting and early draining veins (**Fig. 3.60**).

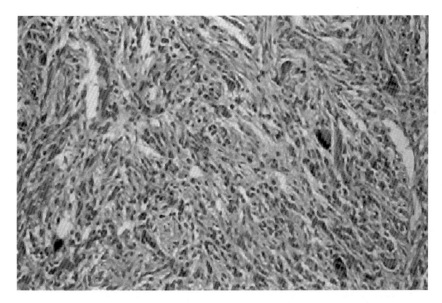

Fig. 3.59 Anaplastic (grade 3) astrocytoma (hematoxylin and eosin [H&E] stain). Increased cellularity with hyperchromatic, pleomorphic nuclei.

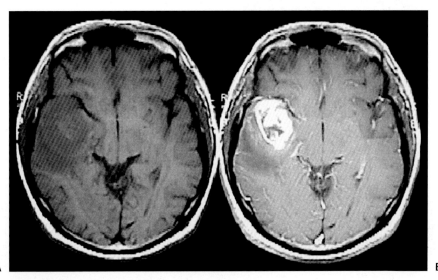

Fig. 3.60 High-grade astrocytoma. (**A**) Axial nonenhanced and (**B**) enhanced T1-weighted magnetic resonance images demonstrating a temporal lesion with irregular cystic enhancement characteristic of a glioblastoma multiforme.

A

B

(2) Pathologic examination is heterogeneous with cysts, degeneration, necrosis, hemorrhages, edema, marked hypercellularity, nuclear atypia, frequent mitoses, pseudopalisading, and endothelial hyperplasia with glomeruloid structures (**Fig. 3.61** and **Fig. 3.62**).

(3) The tumor cells follow white matter tracts (especially the corpus callosum) and may invade dura, disseminate in the CSF, and occasionally produce distant metastases. They are occasionally multicentric (3–6%). GBMs are associated with increased epithelial growth factor receptor (on chromosome 7). The median survival rate is 9–12 months.

(4) Giant cell GBM — has multinucleated giant cells, increased reticulin, and a slightly better prognosis probably because the giant cells can no longer divide. Small cell GBM has a worse prognosis.

(5) Gliomatosis cerebri — one or two diffusely enlarged hemispheres filled with tumor or diffuse enlargement of the cerebellum or brainstem. It is most common at 20–30 years, and there are no focal masses (**Fig. 3.63**).

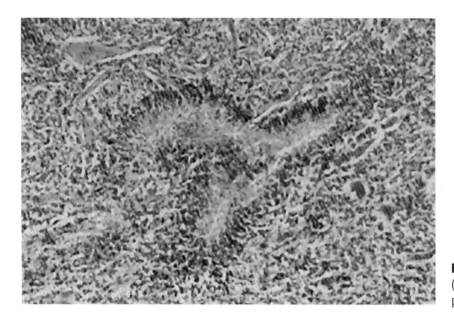

Fig. 3.61 Glioblastoma multiforme (hematoxylin and eosin [H&E] stain); pseudopalisading necrosis.

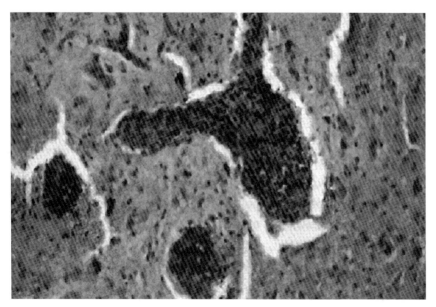

Fig. 3.62 Glioblastoma multiforme (hematoxylin and eosin [H&E] stain); endothelial proliferation.

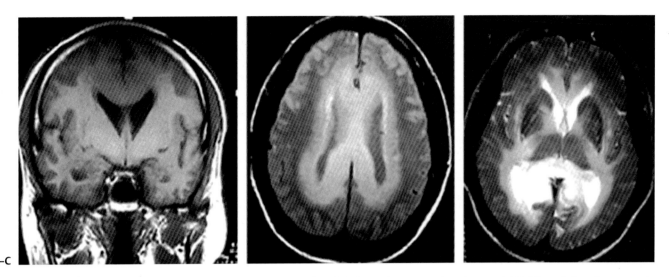

A–C

Fig. 3.63 Gliomatosis cerebri. Coronal (**A**) T1-weighted, (**B**) axial proton density, and (**C**) T2-weighted magnetic resonance images demonstrating diffuse bilateral white matter infiltration by the tumor.

     (6) In addition to maximal surgical resection and external beam radiation, the concomitant use of temozolomide chemotherapy during and after radiation therapy significantly prolongs survival compared with radiotherapy alone in patients with newly diagnosed GBM – representing a new standard of care. Epigenetic silencing (DNA methylation) of the O^6-methylguanine-DNA methyltransferase (MGMT) gene, which encodes a DNA repair protein and represents an important mechanism of chemotherapy resistance, is an independent predictor of improved survival as well as survival benefit from temozolomide.

  d. Protoplasmic astrocytoma — small stellate cells with delicate processes that are predominantly in the gray matter. Prognosis is similar to fibrillary astrocytomas.

  e. Adult pilocytic astrocytoma — unlike the juvenile variety. It is not circumscribed and has a worse prognosis.

  f. Gemistocytic astrocytoma — defined by >20% gemistocytes, contains large cells with eccentric eosinophilic cytoplasm, and has a worse prognosis (**Fig. 3.64**).

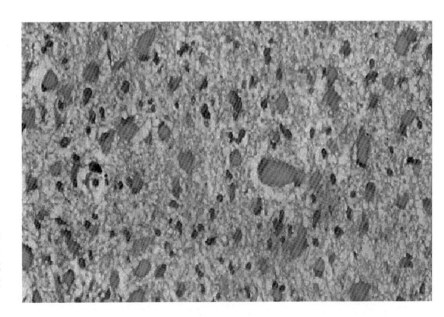

Fig. 3.64 Gemistocytic astrocytoma (hematoxylin and eosin [H&E] stain). Enlarged astrocytes with prominent eosinophilic cytoplasm and eccentric nuclei.

g. Gliosarcoma — represents 2% of GBMs, peak age is 40–60 years. It most commonly involves the temporal lobe superficially with dural invasion. Lesions are firm, circumscribed, lobulated, and contain fascicles of spindle cell sarcoma with interspersed GBM cells. Silver stains the reticulin in the sarcoma component and GFAP stains the GBM component. There are frequent intracranial and extracranial metastases (15–30%). It is postulated that the sarcoma arises from the vascular structures in the GBM or from leptomeningeal fibroblasts. The survival rate is similar to GBM (**Fig. 3.65**).

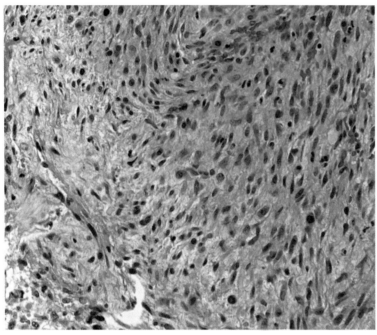

Fig. 3.65 Gliosarcoma (hematoxylin and eosin [H&E] stain). Biphasic pattern of neoplastic glial and mesenchymal cells with reticulin background.

h. Optic glioma — peak age is 3–5 years, female predominance, 20% may act malignantly, associated with neurofibromatosis type I (NF1). Treatment is (1) if distal to the chiasm, remove optic nerve and attached globe; and (2) if the chiasm is involved, resect up to the chiasm preserving vision in the better eye and consider radiation if tumor progression is noted (**Figs. 3.66–3.68**).

i. Brainstem glioma — accounts for 20% of intracranial tumors in children, usually diffusely infiltrates and enlarges the pons, progresses rapidly. The 5-year survival rate is 30%. Symptoms begin with cranial nerve palsies, and hydrocephalus develops late. Treatment is with radiation. The one tumor for which biopsy is usually not necessary because the diffuse pontine lesion (hypointense on T1-weighted MRI and nonenhancing) is very characteristic. The prognosis is better with cystic lesions, dorsal exophytic lesions, and lesions involving the midbrain, medulla, or cervicomedullary junction. These lesions may be amenable to surgical resection (**Fig. 3.69**).

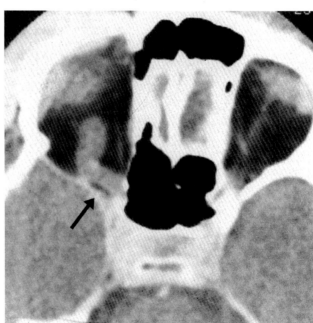

Fig. 3.66 Optic glioma. Nonenhanced axial computed tomographic scan demonstrating thickened right optic nerve (*arrow*). (From Valvassori GE, Mafee MF, Carter BL. Imaging of the Head and Neck. New York, NY: Thieme; 1995. Reprinted by permission.)

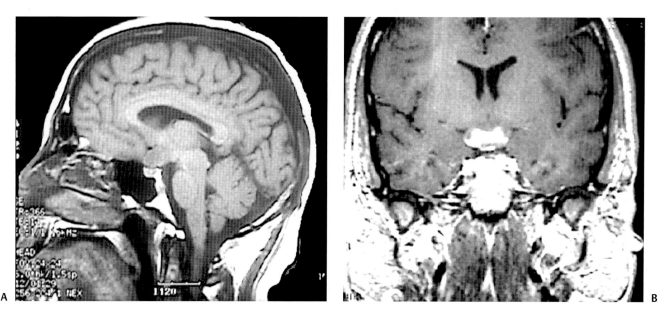

Fig. 3.67 Optic chiasm glioma. (**A**) T1-weighted nonenhanced sagittal and (**B**) enhanced coronal magnetic resonance images demonstrating an expansile enhancing lesion of the optic chiasm.

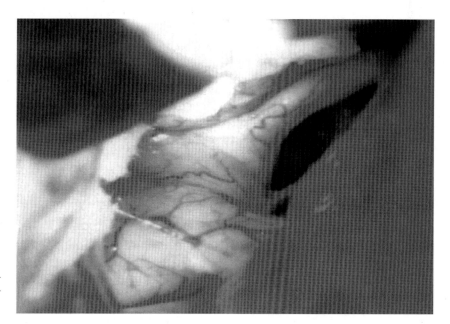

Fig. 3.68 Optic chiasm glioma. Diffuse enlargement with extension under chiasm.

4. Oligodendroglioma
    a. Accounts for 10% of gliomas, peak age incidence is 35–40 years, and there is no sex predominance.
    b. Oligodendrogliomas can be pure or mixed with astrocytic components (i.e., oligoastrocytoma). Histological grade II is pure or mixed and histological grade III is anaplastic.
    c. Symptoms frequently include seizures. They grow from the white matter and infiltrate the cortex. CT demonstrates a hypodense lesion, which is frequently cystic. It has a higher frequency of hemorrhage than other glial tumors (**Fig. 3.70**).
    d. Pathologic examination demonstrates round nuclei with scant cytoplasm, a chicken-wire vascular pattern with thin vessels, occasional serpentine configuration, and an Indian-file lineup of cells

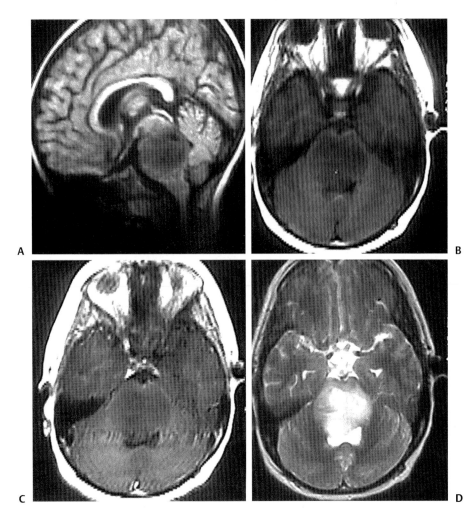

Fig. 3.69 Pontine glioma. (**A**) T1-weighted sagittal, (**B**) nonenhanced and (**C**) enhanced axial, and (**D**) T2-weighted axial magnetic resonance images with low-intensity nonenhancing expansion of the pons.

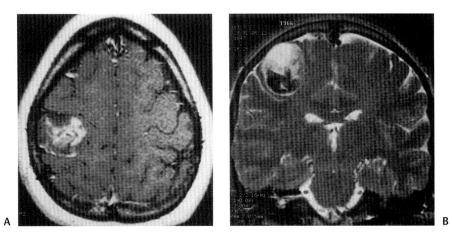

Fig. 3.70 Oligodendroglioma. (**A**) T1-weighted axial enhanced and (**B**) T2-weighted coronal magnetic resonance images demonstrating right posterior frontal hemorrhagic tumor. (From Yasargil MG. Microneurosurgery IV A. New York, NY: Thieme; 1994.)

in the white matter with satellitosis of neurons in the gray matter. The fried egg yolk–appearing cells and nucleus are caused by an artifact from cytoplasmic retraction seen in permanent, but not in frozen sections. 80% have calcifications. Immunohistochemistry is positive for GFAP and S100 (**Fig. 3.71**).

e. Systemic metastases are rare and usually occur after surgery. The 5-year survival rate is better than for astrocytomas. The most important prognostic factor is grade (1–4). The low-grade tumors have a 5-year survival rate of 74% and 10-year survival rate of 46%. The high-grade tumors

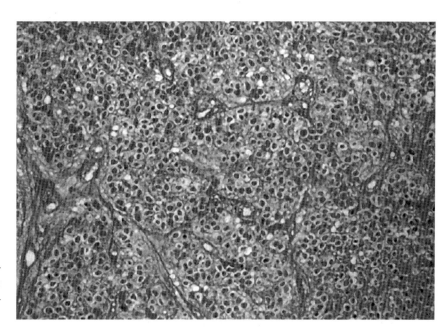

Fig. 3.71 Oligodendroglioma (hematoxylin and eosin [H&E] stain). Uniform "fried-egg" cells with geometric "chicken-wire" arrangement of vessels.

have a 5-year survival rate of 41% and a 10-year survival rate of 20%. Grades 3 and 4 have endovascular proliferation and hypercellularity. PCV (procarbazine, carmustine, and vincristine) or temozolomide chemotherapy is used for oligodendrogliomas.

    f. Combined loss of heterozygosity of chromosomes 1p and 19q (the most common genetic alteration in oligodendrogliomas) is associated with a better response to chemotherapy and improved progression-free and overall survival in patients with anaplastic oligodendrogliomas.

5. Ependymoma
    a. Peak age is 10–15 years, with a large peak at 1–5 years and smaller peak at 35 years. There is no sex predominance.
    b. Location is usually infratentorial. They may grow from the fourth ventricle out through the foramen of Luschka and Magendie. They also account for 60% of intramedullary spinal cord tumors, occurring mostly at the filum.
    c. They are usually pencil-shaped in the spinal cord, often associated with a syrinx, and have a good margin for resection. There may be multiple spinal cord tumors with neurofibromatosis type 2 (NF2). The myxopapillary variety occurs only at the filum (normally it has a good prognosis, but is worse if it invades the conus).
    d. CT and MRI demonstrate a lobulated, circumscribed, cystic, moderately enhancing lesion with calcifications (50%) and only rarely hemorrhage. Grossly it is tan-red in color (**Fig. 3.72**).
    e. Pathologic examination demonstrates various patterns:
        (1) Cellular — a sheetlike growth of polygonal cells with true rosettes (around a central canal), pseudorosettes (around a blood vessel), and blepharoplasts (ciliary basal bodies in the apical cytoplasm) (**Fig. 3.73**).
        (2) Papillary — with typical papillary projections
        (3) Myxopapillary — with intracellular mucin, occurs at the filum and presacral/postsacral area if there is local spread (**Fig. 3.74**)
        (4) Clear cell — with oligodendrocyte-like halos
    f. Immunohistochemistry is positive for GFAP and histochemistry for PTAH. These can be differentiated from (1) medulloblastoma by the smaller nuclei, fewer mitoses, absence of Homer Wright rosettes, positive GFAP, and negative synaptophysin; and (2) choroid plexus papilloma that are PTAH negative and cytokeratin positive.

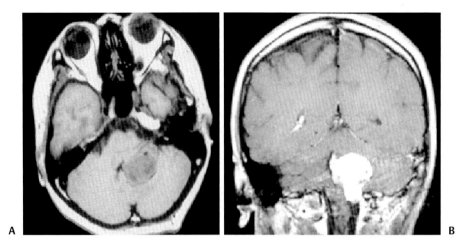

Fig. 3.72 (**A**) Ependymoma. T1-weighted axial nonenhanced and (**B**) coronal enhanced magnetic resonance images demonstrating an enhancing fourth ventricular mass extending through the foramen of Magendie and Luschka.

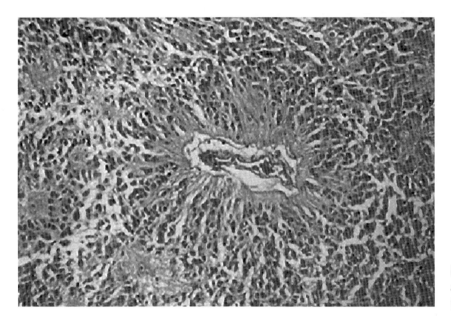

Fig. 3.73 Ependymoma (hematoxylin and eosin [H&E] stain); pseudorosette (around a vessel).

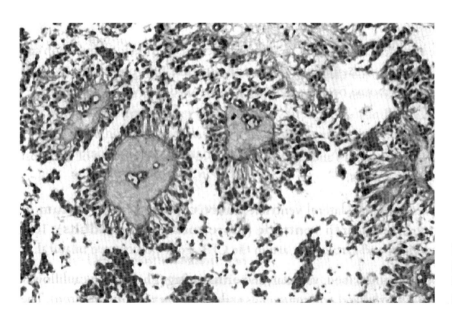

Fig. 3.74 Myxopapillary ependymoma (hematoxylin and eosin [H&E] stain). Cohesive ependymal cells terminating around mucin-rich perivascular spaces.

g. Grades I and II have few mitoses; grade III has frequent mitoses and endovascular hyperplasia; and grade IV has more frequent spinal cord and brain metastases. There is a 45% 5-year survival rate with prognosis influenced by age, location, and grade. Grades I and II are better than III and IV. Radiation helps prolong survival. A cure is usually only possible with the myxopapillary variant (grade I). They frequently seed the CSF, and subtotal resection is associated with local and distant seeding. Rarely, the presacral and postsacral soft tissue tumors may metastasize to the lung.

h. Ependymoblastoma (grade IV) occurs in childhood, is in the PNET group, and is malignant.

i. The normal ependyma consists of a single layer of cuboidal/columnar cells that are ciliated early in life and have microvilli. They have a dual epithelial–glial nature and lie over the subependymal glia.

6. Subependymoma
   a. Peak age is 40–60 years, with male predominance and usually located in the floor of the inferior fourth ventricle or the lateral ventricle.
   b. They arise at the ependymal–subependymal zone and grow slowly. They are benign, avascular, nonenhancing, firm, well circumscribed, hypocellular, and nodular with rests of cells separated by glial fibrils (**Fig. 3.75** and **Fig. 3.76**).

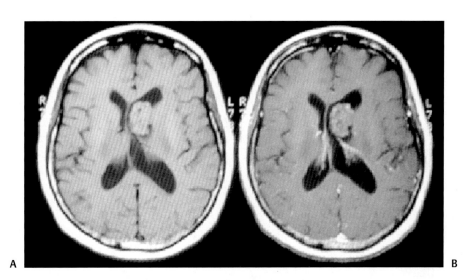

Fig. 3.75 Subependymoma. (**A**) Nonenhanced and (**B**) enhanced T1-weighted axial magnetic resonance images demonstrating a pedunculated nonenhancing lateral ventricular mass (the most common location is the fourth ventricle).

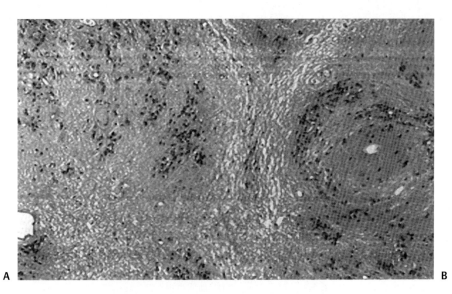

Fig. 3.76 Subependymoma (hematoxylin and eosin [H&E] stain). Hypocellular with small nests of cells separated by broad bands of fibrils

c. They contain both ependymal and astrocytic features with uniform cells, microcysts, calcifications, vascular hyaline, hemosiderin, and mitoses (without prognostic significance). There is no necrosis, rosettes, or seeding.

d. Only 50% become symptomatic, usually by CSF obstruction. A gross total resection can usually be achieved except at the floor of the fourth ventricle. It is postulated that this may be a form of ependymoma because they are often mixed.

7. Choroid plexus papilloma

a. Represents <1% of brain tumors and the peak age is >10 years. It is one of the most frequent tumors before 2 years.

b. 50% are located in the lateral ventricle (more commonly left atrium in children), 40% are in the fourth ventricle (more commonly in adults), 10% is in the third ventricle. Rarely, they occur in the CPA. 4% are bilateral.

c. They tend to be well circumscribed, vascular, and enhancing. They have a cauliflower papillary shape with cuboidal and columnar cells and no cilia (except in children). The cells are piled up on stalks in a single layer unlike the papillary ependymomas that have multiple layers. 25% have calcification. There may be nuclear atypia and rare mitoses, but no mucin. There is rarely bone, cartilage, or melanin formation (**Figs. 3.77–3.79**).

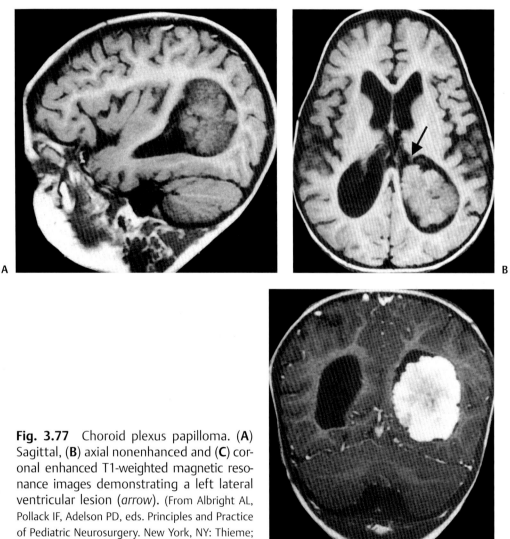

Fig. 3.77 Choroid plexus papilloma. (**A**) Sagittal, (**B**) axial nonenhanced and (**C**) coronal enhanced T1-weighted magnetic resonance images demonstrating a left lateral ventricular lesion (*arrow*). (From Albright AL, Pollack IF, Adelson PD, eds. Principles and Practice of Pediatric Neurosurgery. New York, NY: Thieme; 1999. Reprinted by permission.)

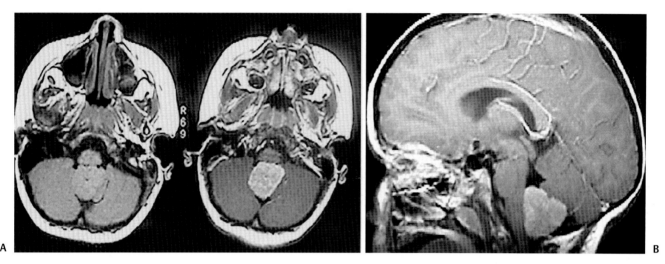

Fig. 3.78 Choroid plexus papilloma. (**A**) Axial nonenhanced and enhanced and (**B**) sagittal enhanced T1-weighted magnetic resonance images demonstrate a fourth ventricular enhancing mass (more common in the left lateral ventricle in children and the fourth ventricle in adults).

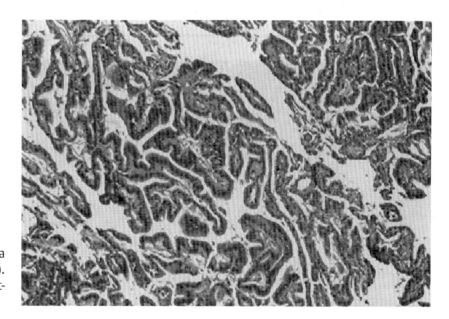

Fig. 3.79 Choroid plexus papilloma (hematoxylin and eosin [H&E] stain). Fairly well-ordered columnar cells resting on a delicate fibrovascular stroma.

d. Immunohistochemistry is positive for transthyretin, vimentin, keratin, S100, and GFAP. They may rarely invade the underlying brain even with benign pathologic findings and may seed the CSF.

e. Symptoms are usually from hydrocephalus because of increased CSF production or more likely due to blockage of CSF flow from hemorrhages or direct obstruction. The prognosis does not correlate with the pathologic findings because even benign-appearing tumors may act aggressively.

f. Surgical resection usually has a good outcome, although there may be recurrence. There are rare malignant transformations. Both intraventricular meningiomas and choroid plexus papillomas are more frequently on the left.

g. The normal choroid is formed from the tela choroidea (the zone of ependymal–pial apposition associated with a fibrovascular stroma) along the choroid fissure at the floors of the lateral ventricles, the roof of the third ventricle, and the lateral recesses of the fourth ventricle. The tela choroidea is composed of vascular tufts covered by choroid epithelium from the ependyma. The choroid plexus may contain benign cysts or xanthogranulomas.

h. Choroid plexus carcinoma — accounts for 15% of choroid plexus tumors. They usually occur before 10 years of age, median age is 2 years; they are rare in adults (consider metastasis, especially if they are positive for EMA and negative for S100 and vimentin). Most are located in the lateral ventricles and locally invade the parenchyma, as well as spread throughout CSF pathways. The pathologic findings are less organized, with piled-up epithelium, anaplasia, and necrosis. Treatment is with surgery and radiation with or without chemotherapy. The prognosis is poor (**Fig. 3.80**).

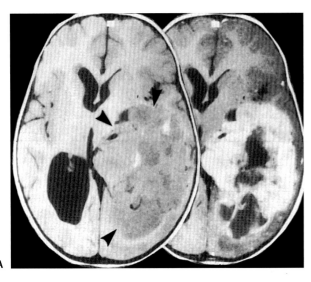
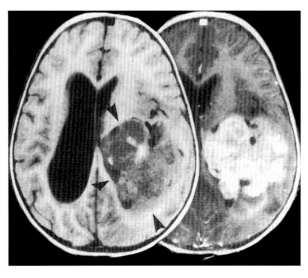

Fig. 3.80 Choroid plexus carcinoma. (**A,B**) Axial nonenhanced and enhanced T1-weighted magnetic resonance images demonstrating a large enhancing left intraventricular lesion with parenchymal extension. (From Albright AL, Pollack IF, Adelson PD, eds. Principles and Practice of Pediatric Neurosurgery. New York, NY: Thieme; 1999. Reprinted by permission.)

C. Mixed neuronal and glial tumors (usually a good prognosis)

1. Ganglioglioma — contains both neoplastic neurons and glial cells. 70% occur before 30 years of age. It is usually in the temporal lobe and most commonly presents with seizures. It is well circumscribed, cystic, firm, and often has a calcified nodule. It may enhance. Pathologic examination demonstrates perivascular inflammatory cells, reticulin, glia, and binucleate neurons with rare mitoses. Immunohistochemistry is positive for neurofilament, synaptophysin, neurosecretory granules, and GFAP (**Fig. 3.81** and **Fig. 3.82**).

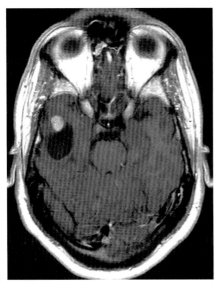
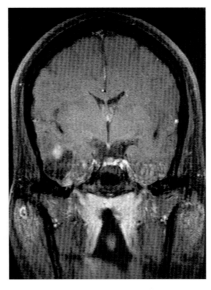

Fig. 3.81 Ganglioglioma. (**A**) Axial T1-weighted and (**B**) coronal enhanced magnetic resonance images demonstrate a right temporal cystic mass with mural nodular enhancement.

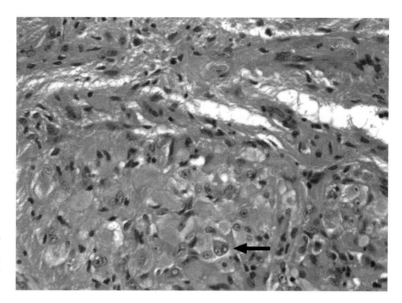

Fig. 3.82 Ganglioglioma (hematoxylin and eosin [H&E] stain). Clusters of abnormal appearing neurons (some are binucleate, *arrow*) in a background of neoplastic glial tissue.

2. Gangliocytoma — neoplastic neurons without neoplastic glia. They may be simply dysplastic brain.

3. Desmoplastic infantile ganglioglioma — rare and usually occur before 18 months. They are massive, frontal, cystic lesions adherent to the dura with a desmoplastic reaction. The tumor enhances. It is differentiated from meningioma because it is GFAP positive and EMA negative (**Fig. 3.83**).

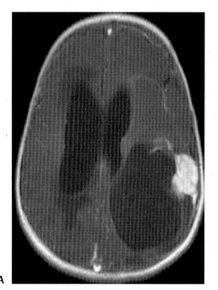
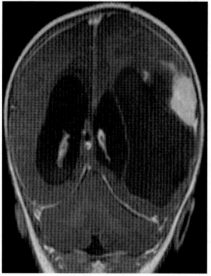

Fig. 3.83 Desmoplastic infantile ganglioglioma. (**A**) Axial T1-weighted and (**B**) coronal enhanced magnetic resonance images demonstrating a large left-sided posterior frontal-parietal cystic mass with mural nodular enhancement in a child.

4. Dysembryoplastic neuroepithelial tumor (DNET) — usually in people 1–19 years of age, presents with seizures and is located in the temporal lobe. It is circumscribed, cystic, multinodular, superficial, and cortical. It contains normal neurons with abnormal oligodendrocytes and astrocytes (a ganglioglioma has abnormal neurons, is in the white matter, and lacks nodularity). It is associated with cortical dysplasia. Surgical resection is usually curative, and radiation is not needed (**Fig. 3.84**).

5. Central neurocytoma — occurs in young adults, usually originates at the septum pellucidum, and occurs in the lateral and third ventricles near the foramen of Monro. It is circumscribed, lobulated, enhancing,

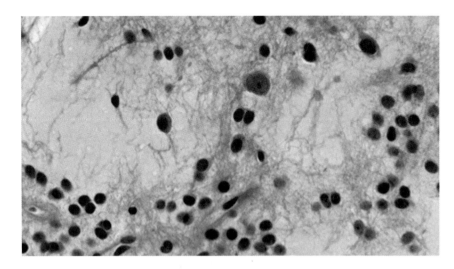

Fig. 3.84 Dysembryoplastic neuroepithelial tumor (hematoxylin and eosin [H&E] stain). Oligodendroglioma-like cells with axon bundles surrounding microcystic spaces in which large ganglion cells lie (i.e., "floating neurons").

noninfiltrative, and usually contains calcifications. Pathologic examination demonstrates monotonous hypercellularity similar to oligodendrogliomas with rare mitoses, frequent cysts, and occasionally hemorrhages. Immunohistochemistry is positive for synaptophysin (**Fig. 3.85** and **Fig. 3.86**).

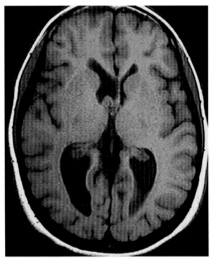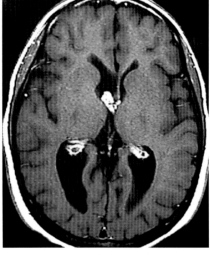

A   B

Fig. 3.85 Central neurocytoma. (**A**) Axial T1-weighted nonenhanced and (**B**) enhanced magnetic resonance images demonstrate an enhancing mass near the septum pellucidum and foramen of Monro.

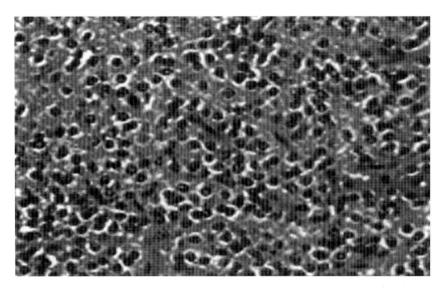

Fig. 3.86 Central neurocytoma (hematoxylin and eosin [H&E] stain). Closely packed uniform cells with small blue nuclei and perinuclear halos. The histologic findings are similar to oligodendrogliomas, but central neurocytomas stain with synaptophysin and neuron-specific enolase.

D. Primitive neuroectodermal tumors (PNETs)

1. Medulloblast — a term originally coined by Bailey and Cushing in 1925 to describe bipotential cells capable of differentiating into glia or neurons. These cells have features similar to the totipotent neural tube cells. It is postulated that they are derived from the external granular layer of the cerebellum or from dysplastic cell rests in the anterior and posterior medullary velum. The term *PNET* was introduced by Hart and Earle in 1973.

2. PNET varieties

    a. Medulloblastoma — 50% occur before 10 years and 75% before 15 years, and there is a second peak at 28 years (**Fig. 3.87** and **Fig. 3.88**). There is a male predominance, and they are more frequently off the midline in adults. They account for 20% of CNS tumors in children and one third of the posterior fossa tumors in children. The most common genetic abnormality is isochromosome 17q. It may be associated with Gorlin (basal cell nevus) syndrome that is due to a mutation of the PTCH gene on chromosome 9q. WHO grade IV.

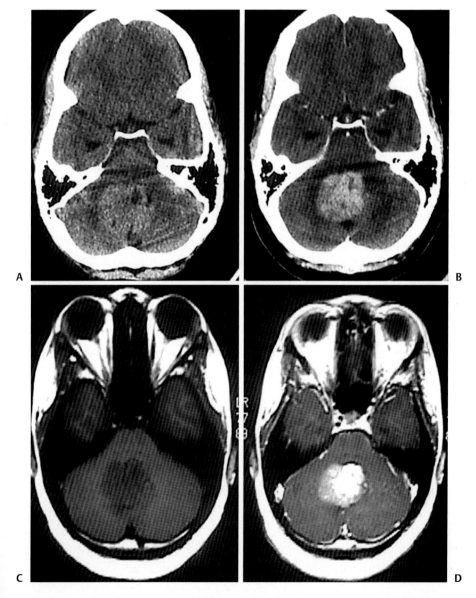

Fig. 3.87 Medulloblastoma. (**A**) Axial computed tomographic nonenhanced and (**B**) enhanced scans and (**C**) axial T1-weighted magnetic resonance imaging nonenhanced and (**D**) enhanced scans demonstrating a slightly hyperdense and hypointense enhancing mass in the posterior fossa.

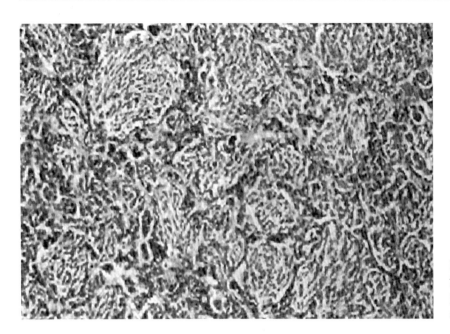

Fig. 3.88 Medulloblastoma (hematoxylin and eosin [H&E] stain). Closely packed undifferentiated cells with no discernable cytoplasm (small blue cells).

b. Retinoblastoma — the most common extracranial malignant solid tumor in children and 80% occur before 5 years. It is derived from a neural crest precursor of the sympathetic ganglia. There is a genetic predisposition by loss of a suppressor gene. It is treated with surgery and radiation. Retinoblastomas contain Flexner-Wintersteiner and Homer Wright rosettes. Trilateral retinoblastoma is bilateral retinoblastoma with pineoblastoma.

c. Pineoblastoma (see section I on Pineal Tumors) WHO grade IV

d. Ependymoblastoma — WHO grade IV

e. Atypical teratoid/rhabdoid tumor — densely cellular blue cell tumors mixed with rhabdoid cells. Rhabdoid cells have eosinophilic rounded, rhabdoid cytoplasmic inclusions. They occur mostly in infants and young children. They are associated with deletions of chromosome 22 containing the *INI1/hSNF5* gene; WHO grade IV.

f. Central neuroblastoma — usually supratentorial, hemispheric, and circumscribed. It usually occurs before 5 years. It may be hemorrhagic, necrotic, and cystic. The 5-year survival rate is 30%. Neuroblastoma is the third most common tumor in children after leukemia and brain tumor. 2% involve the brain. It is frequently congenital and makes up 18% of tumors in patients <2 months old. Peripheral neuroblastoma develops in the adrenal gland in children and may have spinal epidural metastases.

g. Medulloepithelioma — derived from ventricular matrix cells, is the most primitive of the PNETs, and affects very young children; WHO grade IV

3. PNET features

a. Locations (in descending order of frequency) — vermis, cerebellar hemispheres (older children), pineal, cerebrum, spinal cord, and brainstem

b. PNETs are hyperdense on CT, hypointense on T1-weighted MRI and enhancing (**Fig. 3.87**).

c. They are pink-brown in color and may be soft or firm. They occasionally hemorrhage, are rarely calcified, and are frequently cystic (80%). They have no capsule, are occasionally circumscribed, and frequently disseminate in the CSF. PNETs are densely cellular, contain small round cells with large nuclei and scant cytoplasm, have a variable number of mitoses and occasional necrosis (**Fig. 3.88**). There are Homer Wright rosettes (around central granulofibrillar material with radially arranged nuclei), pseudorosettes (around blood vessels), ependymal canals (especially with ependymoblastoma), and Flexner–Wintersteiner rosettes (columnar cells with a small lumen seen with retinoblastomas and also pineoblastomas) (**Figs. 3.89–3.91**). There may be a linear array of cells (Indian file) and round islands of cells. There are occasional astrocytes and oligodendrocytes. Neurons can be stained with silver, PTAH, etc. There rarely may be smooth or striated muscle cells or melanocytes.

d. 50% of these tumors metastasize (two thirds in the CNS and one third to bone), and 20–50% are disseminated at the time of diagnosis. The survival rate is >50% at 5 years with surgery, chemotherapy, and radiation therapy. Complete resection provides 75% 5-year and 25% 10-year survival rates.

E. Meningiomas — account for 15% of primary intracranial tumors. Peak age is 40–60 years. Females are more commonly affected. 72% of tumors have monosomy 22.

1. Meningioma incidence is increased by radiation and NF2.

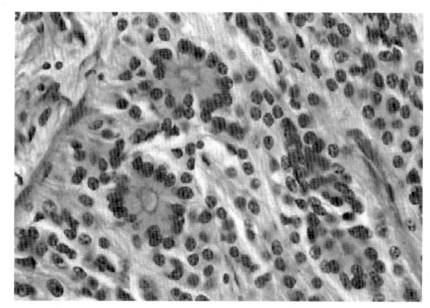

Fig. 3.89 True "ependymal" rosette (hematoxylin and eosin [H&E] stain). Polar ependymal cells with basal bodies of cilia (blepharoplasts) lining a central lumen; most commonly in ependymoma. (See **Fig. 3.29**)

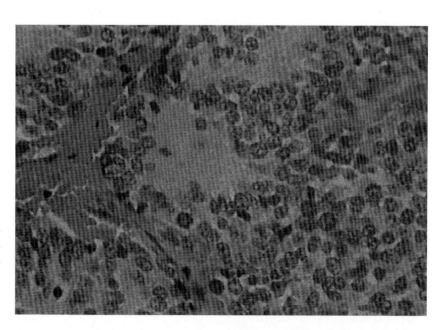

Fig. 3.90 Homer Wright rosette (hematoxylin and eosin [H&E] stain). Central fibrillar material (processes of tumor cells) ringed by radially arranged cell nuclei; most commonly seen with medulloblastoma and neuroblastoma.

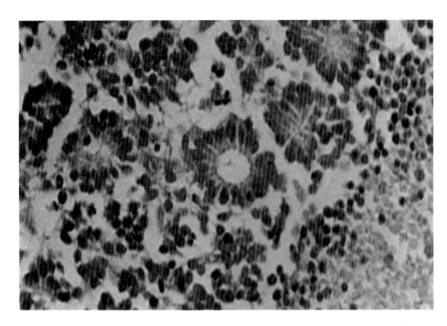

Fig. 3.91 Flexner-Wintersteiner rosette (hematoxylin and eosin [H&E] stain). Columnar cells that resemble cone-type photoreceptor cells, which form rosettes with small central lumens; most commonly in pineal tumors and also retinoblastoma.

2. Meningiomas have receptors for progesterone, estrogen, peptides, amines, androgen, glucocorticoids, somatostatin, and cholecystokinin. They may grow with pregnancy and breast cancer.

3. The blood supply is from external carotid artery branches such as the middle meningeal and anterior falcine arteries. They may parasitize pial vessels (from the ICA) and develop a dual supply. They invade dura and bone. Bony changes are hyperostotic more frequently than lytic. The hyperostotic bone usually is invaded by tumor.

4. Meningiomas rarely metastasize. They originate from the arachnoid cap cells (these also form whorls and psammoma bodies) that are most frequently located at the arachnoid granulations (near the superior sagittal sinus under the suture confluence) and the tela choroidea (intraventricular).

5. Locations — cranial (90%), spinal (9%), and ectopic (1%, intraosseous skull, orbit, neck, scalp, sinus, and parotid). Cranial locations in descending order are parasagittal (middle of the superior sagittal sinus), convexity (near the coronal suture), sphenoid ridge, tuberculum, olfactory groove, falcine, foramen magnum, optic nerve, tentorial, choroid (left lateral ventricle), and thoracic. The parasagittal and convexity groups account for 50% (**Figs. 3.92–3.97**).

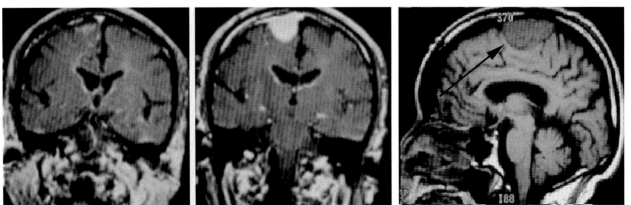

A–C

Fig. 3.92 Parasagittal meningioma. (**A**) Nonenhanced and (**B**) enhanced coronal and (**C**) nonenhanced sagittal T1-weighted magnetic resonance imaging scans demonstrating a homogeneously enhancing circumscribed isointense lesion arising from the medial dura and invading the wall of the superior sagittal sinus.

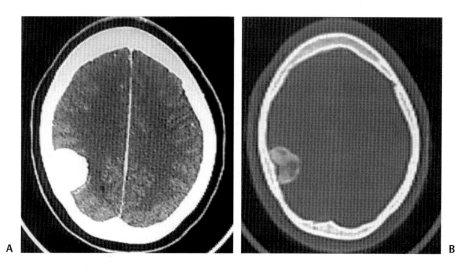

Fig. 3.93 Convexity meningioma. (**A**) Axial enhanced and (**B**) bone window computed tomographic scans demonstrating a homogeneously enhancing, circumscribed, calcified lesion arising from the convexity.

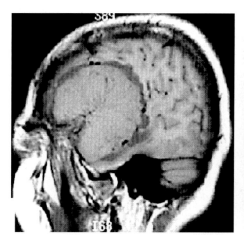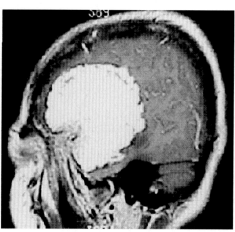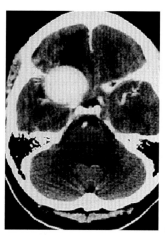

Fig. 3.94 Sphenoid wing meningioma. (**A**) Sagittal nonenhanced and (**B**) enhanced T1-weighted magnetic resonance imaging scans and (**C**) axial enhanced computed tomographic scan demonstrating a homogeneously enhancing circumscribed lesion arising from the sphenoid ridge.

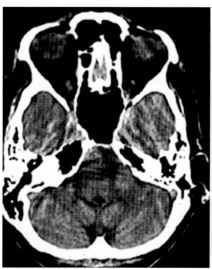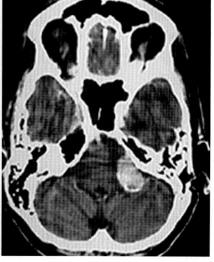

Fig. 3.95 Cerebellopontine angle meningioma. (**A**) Axial nonenhanced and (**B**) enhanced computed tomographic scans demonstrating the dural-based enhancing left-sided mass.

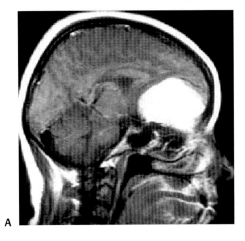
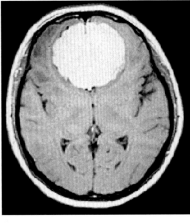

A

B

Fig. 3.96 Olfactory groove meningioma. (**A**) Enhanced sagittal and (**B**) axial T1-weighted magnetic resonance images demonstrating a homogeneously enhancing circumscribed lesion arising from the floor of the anterior fossa.

6. They are multiple in 9% of cases. Metastatic neoplasms have been reported inside of meningiomas.

7. Pathologically, they are well demarcated and usually firm and rubbery. The shape may be globular or en plaque. Radiographically, 10% are cystic, 25% have calcifications, 90% enhance, 75% are hyperdense on CT, and 25% are isodense on CT.

8. There is a sunburst pattern of dural feeders on angiography, basophilic psammoma bodies, and whorls (**Fig. 3.98** and **Fig. 3.99**). Immunohistochemistry is of mesenchymal and epithelial cells, positive for both vimentin and EMA.

9. Variants include (1) meningothelial or syncytial with whorls, lobules, but few psammoma bodies; (2) fibroblastic with sheets of cells; (3) transitional (the most common type) containing elements of both the syncytial and fibroblastic types; (4) psammomatous; and (5) angiomatous. These variants do not affect the prognosis, and nuclear atypia is common. 92% of meningiomas are "typical or grade I."

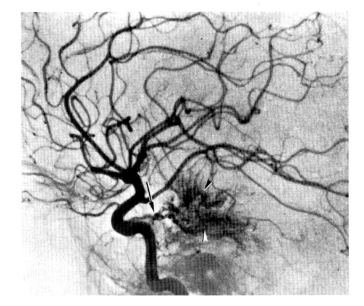

Fig. 3.97 Tentorial meningioma. Angiogram (lateral view) demonstrates the tumor blush of the meningioma with supply by an enlarged tentorial artery of Bernasconi-Cassinari. (From Huber P, Krayenbühl H, Yasargil MG. Cerebral Angiography. 2nd ed. New York, NY: Thieme; 1982. Reprinted by permission.)

10. The atypical group, grade II, (6%) has at least two of the following: hypercellularity, frequent mitoses, and necrosis. There is brain invasion. They have a 30% 5-year survival rate, 50% recur in 1.5 years, and 5% metastasize.

11. The anaplastic or malignant group, grade III, (2%) also invades the brain, can metastasize, has necrosis and a higher rate of mitosis than atypical meningiomas. 70% of these recur and 30% metastasize.

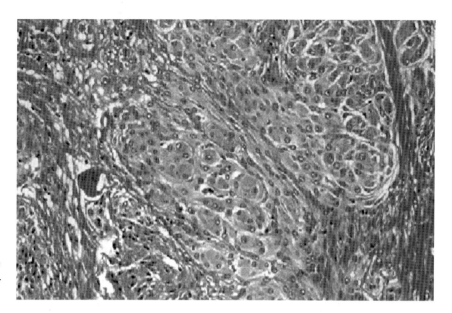

Fig. 3.98 Meningioma (hematoxylin and eosin [H&E] stain); syncytial pattern and a psammoma body.

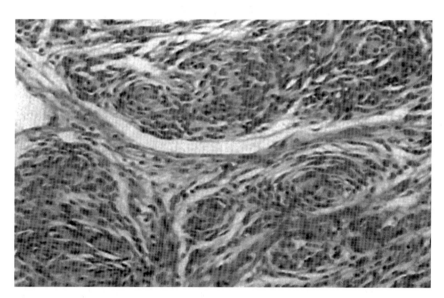

Fig. 3.99 Meningioma (hematoxylin and eosin [H&E] stain); whorls.

    12. Foster–Kennedy syndrome — optic atrophy in one eye and papilledema in the other with anosmia, seen occasionally with olfactory groove meningiomas (**Fig. 3.100** and **Fig. 3.101**).

F. Hemangiopericytoma — It used to be considered a type of meningioma but is now a distinct entity. Mean age is 40–50 years with a male predominance.

    1. They are usually supratentorial.

    2. The 5-, 10-, and 15-year survival rates are 63%, 37%, and 21%, respectively. Recurrence rate is 70%. 10–30% metastasize, especially to lung and bone. They respond poorly to radiation and chemotherapy.

    3. They are postulated to originate from pericytes that contract and surround capillaries. They are dural based, well demarcated, firm, and vascular (**Fig. 3.102**).

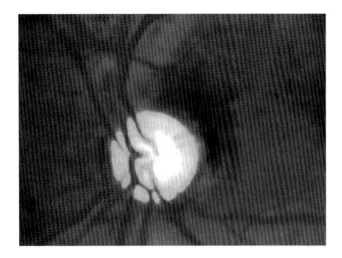

Fig. 3.100   Optic atrophy; severe optic disk pallor.

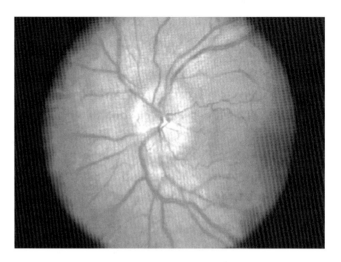

Fig. 3.101   Papilledema; obscured optic disk margins.

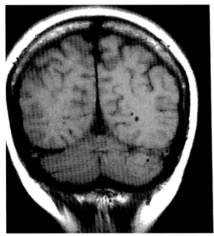 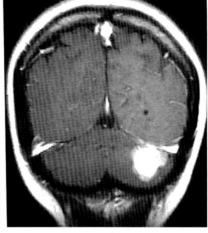

A   B

Fig. 3.102 Hemangiopericytoma. (**A**) T1-weighted coronal nonenhanced and (**B**) enhanced magnetic resonance images demonstrating an enhancing circumscribed mass inferior to the tentorium.

4. The blood supply is usually from the ICA or vertebrobasilar systems.

5. Pathologic findings are dense cellularity with frequent mitoses, increased reticulin, lobules around "staghorn" vascular channels, and the absence of whorls or psammoma bodies. Immunohistochemistry is positive for vimentin and CD34, but not to EMA (EMA is positive in meningiomas) (**Fig. 3.103**).

G. Hemangioblastoma — It accounts for 2% of intracranial tumors and 10% of posterior fossa tumors. Mean age is 20–40 years with a male predominance.

1. The most common locations are cerebellar hemispheres or vermis (80%), cervical spinal cord (10%), and brainstem (3%).

2. 60% are cystic with an enhancing mural nodule abutting the pia and 40% are solid (**Fig. 3.104**). In the spinal cord, they are frequently associated with a syrinx. They tend to be circular, yellow (secondary to lipid content), and contain capillaries with hyperplastic endothelial cells and pericytes surrounded by stromal cells with vacuoles and lipids (**Fig. 3.105**).

3. Hemangioblastomas are rich in reticulin, have no mitoses, and rarely have calcifications, hemorrhage, or necrosis.

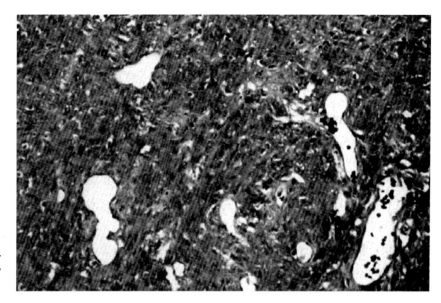

Fig. 3.103 Hemangiopericytoma (hematoxylin and eosin [H&E] stain). Densely cellular with "staghorn" vascular spaces.

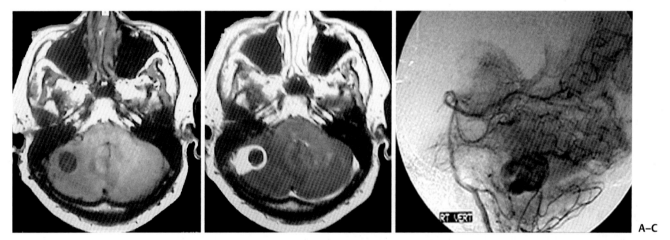

A–C

Fig. 3.104 Hemangioblastoma. (**A**) Nonenhanced and (**B**) enhanced axial T1-weighted magnetic resonance images demonstrating a cystic lesion with enhancement of rim and mural nodule and (**C**) lateral basilar artery angiogram with filling of a different hemangioblastoma.

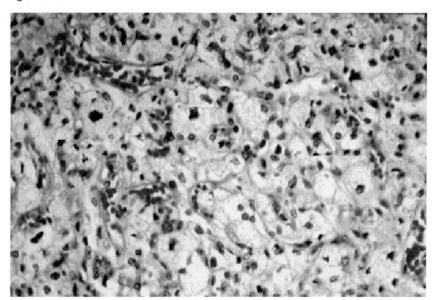

Fig. 3.105 Hemangioblastoma (hematoxylin and eosin [H&E] stain). Abundant thin-walled vascular channels interspersed with enlarged vacuolated stromal cells.

4. They can be differentiated from metastatic renal cell carcinoma because immunohistochemistry is positive for vimentin and negative for EMA.

5. There is occasional polycythemia caused by erythropoietin secreted from the tumor.

6. Surgery is usually curative, although the recurrence rate is 25%. 80% are sporadic and 20% are associated with von Hippel–Lindau disease (VHL).

H. Craniopharyngioma — it accounts for 2–5% of primary tumors. There is no sex predominance. Peak age is 0–20 years with a second peak at 50 years. 70% are suprasellar and intrasellar and they are rarely exclusively sellar, CPA, pineal, or nasopharyngeal.

1. The tumor is benign, but it invades into vital structures. It is derived from squamous cells from the Rathke cleft. They may be cystic with a nodule filled with "machine oil" fluid and cholesterol crystals that can elicit a granulomatous reaction.

2. Contains calcifications in 90% (100% in children and 50% in adults), usually enhances, and has sharp irregular margins with surrounding gliosis (**Fig. 3.106**).

3. Pathologic examination demonstrates an adamantinomatous pattern with rests of epithelial cells surrounded by a layer of columnar basal cells separated by a myxoid stroma of loose stellate cells, whorls of cells, and keratinized nodules of wet keratin (**Figs. 3.107–3.109**).

4. They may contain teeth, as found in jaw tumors. A papillary variant is usually present in adults, located in the third ventricle, solid, without calcifications, and contains papillae of well-differentiated squamous epithelium. This tumor has a better prognosis.

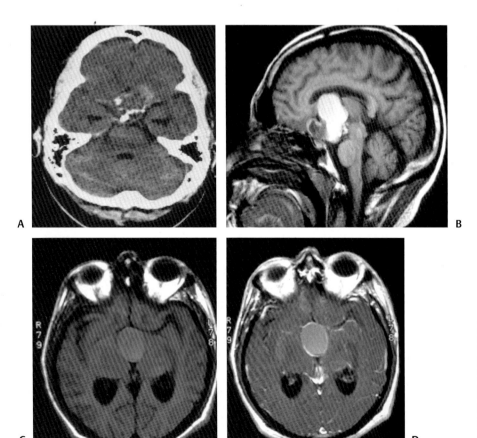

Fig. 3.106 Craniopharyngioma. (**A**) Nonenhanced axial computed tomographic scan demonstrating calcifications, (**B**) sagittal T1-weighted with hyperintense cyst, and (**C**) T1-weighted magnetic resonance images nonenhanced and (**D**) enhanced with rim enhancement.

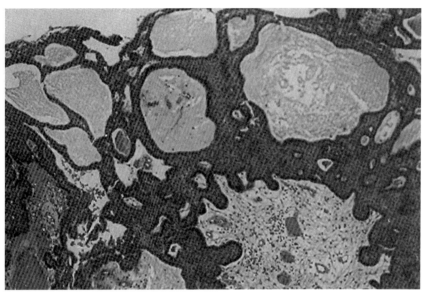

Fig. 3.107 Craniopharyngioma (hematoxylin and eosin [H&E] stain). "Adamantinomatous" pattern with basaloid layer of cells separated by loosely arranged stellate cells.

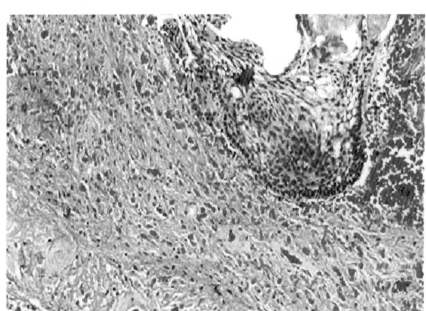

Fig. 3.108 Craniopharyngioma (hematoxylin and eosin [H&E] stain). "Adamantinomatous" pattern with basaloid layer of cells separated by loosely arranged stellate cells. Higher power view.

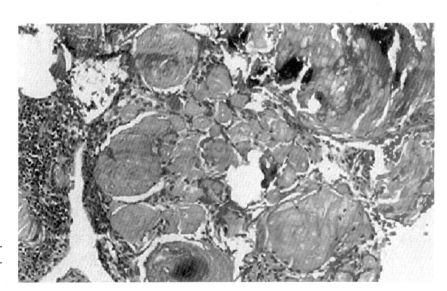

Fig. 3.109 Craniopharyngioma (hematoxylin and eosin [H&E] stain). Billowed "wet" keratin and calcifications.

I. Pineal tumors

1. General information
    a. The pineal gland contains pinealocytes (derived from APUD cells) and astrocytes. It is usually calcified by age 16 years. In reptiles, it functions as a photoreceptor to change skin color in response to light. In humans, it is involved with hormone secretion for circadian rhythms.
    b. It is innervated by sympathetic nerves from the superior cervical ganglion that release norepinephrine (NE) to increase the pineal gland's melatonin secretion. The pineal gland inhibits gonadal development and regulates menstruation, adrenal function, and thyroid function. The pineal gland secretes NE, serotonin (5-HT), and melatonin.
    c. Pineal tumors account for 1% of intracranial tumors in the United States and 6% in Japan. Pineal tumors may be derived from pineal cells (20%; includes pineocytoma and pineoblastoma), interstitial cells (rare; usually well-differentiated astrocytes), and germ cells (the most frequent pineal tumor).
    d. Trilateral retinoblastoma is bilateral retinoblastomas with a pineoblastoma. Pineal masses may compress the tectum and cause Parinaud syndrome with poor upgaze, pupillary dilation, lid retraction, nystagmus retractorius, and dissociated near-light response (reaction to near but not light).

2. Pineocytoma—peak age is 30 years and there is no sex predominance. It is well circumscribed, contained within the gland, with medium-sized round cells, and Homer Wright rosettes with central fibrillar material. There is a better outcome if there is some neuronal and/or astrocytic differentiation. There is rarely metastasis and CSF dissemination (**Fig. 3.110** and **Fig. 3.111**).

3. Pineoblastoma—a member of the PNET group with peak age <20 years. It infiltrates surrounding structures, disseminates in the CSF, and metastasizes to bone, lung, and lymph nodes. It enhances well. It is hypercellular and has small cells, mitoses, and necrosis. The mean survival is <2 years (**Fig. 3.112**)

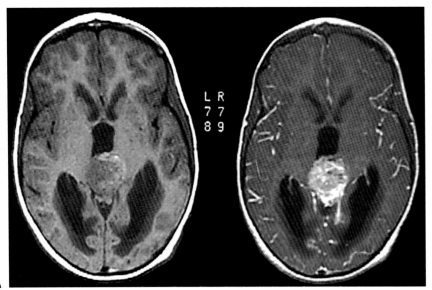

L R
7 7
8 9

A

B

Fig. 3.110 Pineocytoma. (**A**) Axial nonenhanced and (**B**) enhanced T1-weighted magnetic resonance imaging scans demonstrating enhancing, demarcated, posterior third ventricular mass.

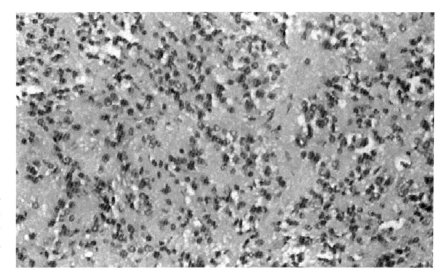

Fig. 3.111 Pineocytoma (hematoxylin and eosin [H&E] stain). Rosette-like clusters of nuclei surrounding fibrillary neuropil-like matrix recapitulating normal pineal parenchyma.

4. Pineal cyst – benign, nonneoplastic cyst located at the pineal gland, differentiated from neoplasm by lack of symptoms, hydrocephalus, and growth on serial imaging. No intervention required (**Fig. 3.113**).

J. Germ cell tumors (**Table 3.1**)

1. General information
   a. Mean age is 10–20 years (at the onset of puberty in males).
   b. These cells originate in the yolk sac endoderm and migrate throughout the embryo.
   c. The most frequent locations include pineal, suprasellar (especially in females), third ventricular, posterior fossa, and the midline mediastinum and retroperitoneum.

2. Germinoma — the most common pineal tumor (40%) and accounts for two thirds of germ cell tumors. Peak age is 10–30 years and there is a male predominance.
   a. It is usually in the pineal region, although the second most common site is suprasellar and intrasellar. 10% are both in the pineal and suprasellar regions.
   b. It is soft with large polygonal cells with clear cytoplasm and lacks necrosis or hemorrhage. There are interspersed lymphocytic infiltrates present (**Fig. 3.114**).
   c. It is isointense on T1-weighted MRI, hypointense on T2-weighted MRI, and hyperdense on CT. It enhances well (**Fig. 3.115**).

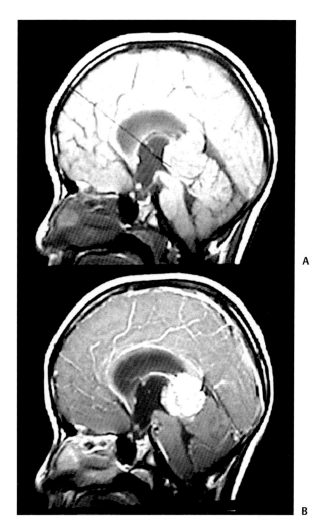

Fig. 3.112 Pineoblastoma. (**A**) Nonenhanced and (**B**) enhanced sagittal T1-weighted magnetic resonance images demonstrating a fairly circumscribed, enhancing pineal region mass.

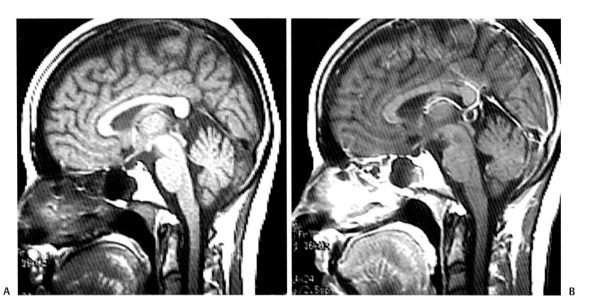

A   B

Fig. 3.113   Pineal cyst. Sagittal T1-weighted (**A**) nonenhanced and (**B**) enhanced magnetic resonance images demonstrating a cystic expansion of the pineal gland.

Table 3.1   Germ Cell Tumor Deviation

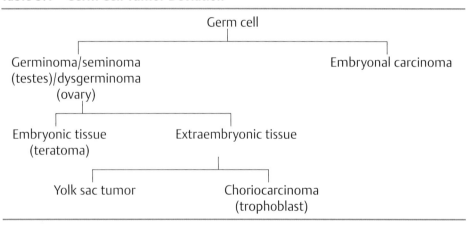

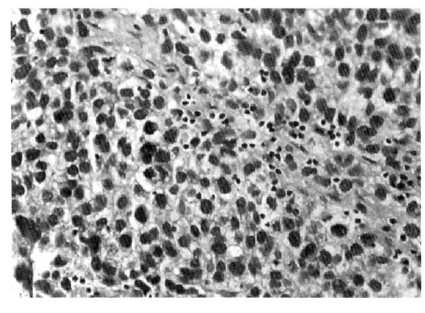

Fig. 3.114   Germinoma (hematoxylin and eosin [H&E] stain). Large polygonal cells with large nuclei and prominent nucleoli and T cell infiltrates.

d. 15% are associated with an increase in serum beta HCG. In males, choriocarcinoma can be associated with precocious puberty.

e. Positive for placental alkaline phosphatase on tumor staining

f. The tumor is highly radiosensitive, and treatment is with radiation to the entire neuraxis.

3. Embryonal carcinoma — rare, contains necrosis and hemorrhage, and has elevated serum AFP and beta HCG.

4. Yolk sac tumor (endodermal sinus tumor) — rare, occurs in young children, and has elevated serum AFP and Schiller–Duval bodies

5. Choriocarcinoma — may be primary or metastatic. Primary usually occurs in the first decade of life. It has a high propensity to hemorrhage because of thin-walled vessels. Serum is positive for beta HCG. Prognosis is poor.

6. Teratoma — the second most common pineal germ cell tumor (15%). It usually affects young males. It contains tissues from all three layers: skin, nerve, cartilage, bone, fat, muscle, respiratory glands, and GI glands. There may be elevated serum CEA (**Fig. 3.116**).

7. AFP — secreted by mucous glands of the GI tract and elevated with yolk sac tumors and hepatic carcinomas

8. Beta HCG—synthesized by the placenta and elevated with choriocarcinoma

K. Pituitary tumors

1. They account for 15% of intracranial tumors. Mean age is 20–50 years. There is a female predominance with prolactin (PRL)- and adrenocorticotropic hormone (ACTH)-secreting tumors and a male predominance with GH-secreting tumors. 25% of these tumors do not secrete hormones (nonfunctioning pituitary adenomas).

2. Microadenomas are <1 cm and are much more common than macroadenomas. Pituitary tumors are associated with multiple endocrine neoplasia (MEN) type 1. Less than 1% are malignant, and metastases are more frequent than primary malignancies in the sella.

3. H&E staining reveals acidophils (40%; PRL, growth hormone [GH], and follicle stimulating [FSH]/luteinizing hormone [LH]), basophils (10%; ACTH, and thyrotroph stimulating hormone [T]), and null cells (50%) (**Fig. 3.117**).

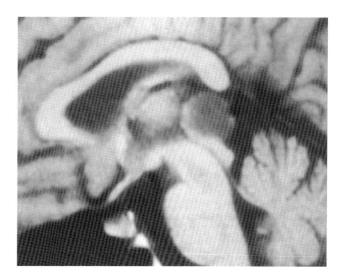

Fig. 3.115 Pineal region germinoma. Sagittal non-enhanced T1-weighted magnetic resonance image with low-intensity demarcated pineal mass.

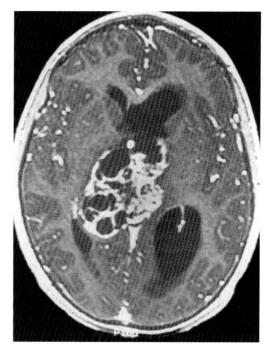

Fig. 3.116 Pineal teratoma. Axial T1-weighted enhanced magnetic resonance image demonstrating a lobulated cystic pineal mass with irregular enhancement. (From Albright AL, Pollack IF, Adelson PD, eds. Principles and Practice of Pediatric Neurosurgery. New York, NY: Thieme;1999. Reprinted by permission.)

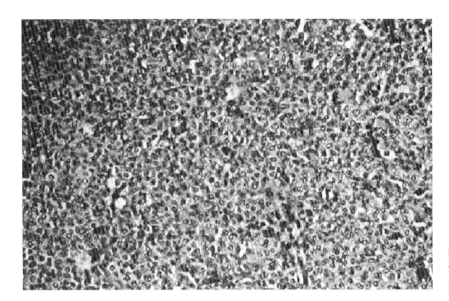

Fig. 3.117 Pituitary adenoma (hematoxylin and eosin [H&E] stain). Diffuse pattern of monotonous polygonal cells.

4. CT and T1-weighted MRI are isodense/isointense with decreased enhancement of the tumor compared with the normal pituitary gland. The T2-weighted MRI may be hypointense. Angiogram may demonstrate an enlarged meningohypophyseal trunk, and 4–7% of pituitary tumors are associated with intracranial aneurysms (**Fig. 3.118** and **Fig. 3.119**).

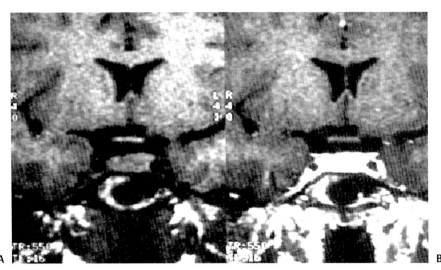

Fig. 3.118 Pituitary microadenoma. (**A**) Nonenhanced and (**B**) enhanced coronal T1-weighted magnetic resonance images demonstrating the left-sided nonenhancing lesion.

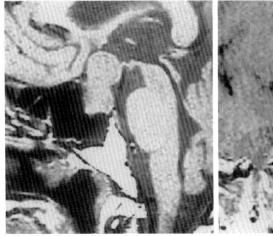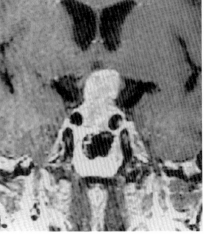

Fig. 3.119 Pituitary macroadenoma. (**A**) Nonenhanced sagittal and (**B**) enhanced coronal T1-weighted magnetic resonance images demonstrating an enhancing lesion filling the sella and suprasellar space, displacing the optic tracts, and invading into the cavernous sinus.

5. 40% have local invasion at the time of diagnosis. Recurrence after surgery is 16% at 8 years and 35% at 20 years.

6. PRL-secreting tumor is the most common pituitary tumor (30%). Symptoms include amenorrhea/galactorrhea in women and decreased libido or impotence in men. The tumors tend to be larger and patients older in men. Serum PRL level is >150 and is proportional to tumor size. These tumors respond well to bromocriptine, pergolide, or cabergoline (dopamine [DA] agonists) and usually decrease in size with treatment. The PRL may be elevated because of decreased DA (PRL inhibitory factor) from compression on the pituitary stalk from a nonprolactinoma ("stalk effect").

7. GH-secreting tumor is the second most common pituitary hormone–secreting tumor (13%). It causes acromegaly in adults and gigantism in children. 40% also have increased serum PRL and TSH. Treatment is surgical or with octreotide (somatostatin analog) (**Fig. 3.120** and **Fig. 3.121**).

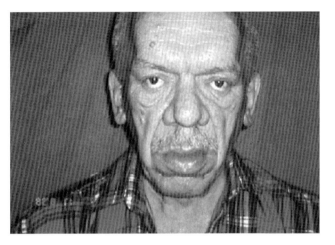

Fig. 3.120 Acromegaly; coarse facial features.

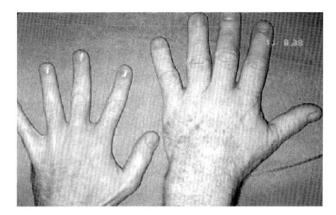

Fig. 3.121 Acromegaly; normal hand (left) and enlargement of hand in acromegaly (right).

8. ACTH-secreting tumor accounts for 10% of pituitary tumors. It is more common in females and produces Cushing disease. Treatment is surgical. Nelson syndrome occurs when there is pituitary enlargement after adrenalectomy (that was performed mistakenly for hypercortisolism thought to be peripherally mediated or as treatment for known Cushing disease). This tumor is characterized by Crooke hyaline change in the pituitary gland (accumulation of intermediate filaments in the nontumoral corticotrophs in the presence of elevated steroid levels). In Nelson syndrome, patients are hyperpigmented because of excess α-melanocyte stimulating hormone production.

9. FSH/LH-secreting tumor accounts for 9% of pituitary tumors and have no sex predominance. Most common in the elderly and cause compressive symptoms, although occasionally infertility in women.

10. TSH-secreting tumor accounts for 1% of pituitary tumors.

11. Null cell tumor (oncocytoma) accounts for 26% of pituitary tumors and is the second most common after PRL.

12. Pituitary apoplexy — hemorrhagic necrosis of a pituitary adenoma. It usually occurs with null cell macroadenomas. It is detected in 1% of pituitary adenomas while patients are alive, but in 10% of tumors at autopsy. Treatment is with surgery and steroid replacement.

13. Lymphocytic hypophysitis — pituitary insufficiency in peripartum females caused by an autoimmune mechanism with humoral and cellular components (B and T cells involved). There may also be inflammation in the ovaries and thyroid. Treatment is by surgical decompression if necessary and hormone replacement (**Fig. 3.122** and **Fig. 3.123**).

14. Giant cell pituitary granuloma — characterized by noncaseating granulomas, no sex predominance. It occurs in adults and is not associated with pregnancy.

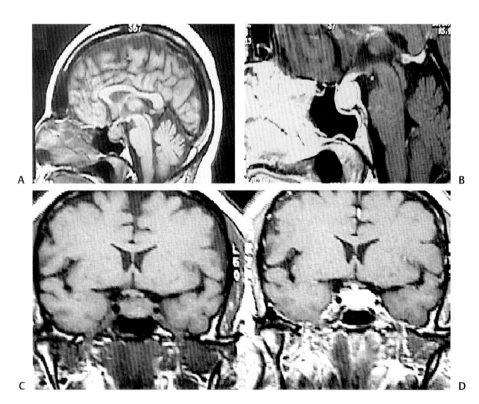

Fig. 3.122 Lymphocytic hypophysitis. (**A**) Sagittal nonenhanced and (**B**) enhanced and (**C**) coronal nonenhanced and (**D**) enhanced T1-weighted magnetic resonance images demonstrating irregular enhancement and diffuse enlargement of the pituitary gland and infundibulum.

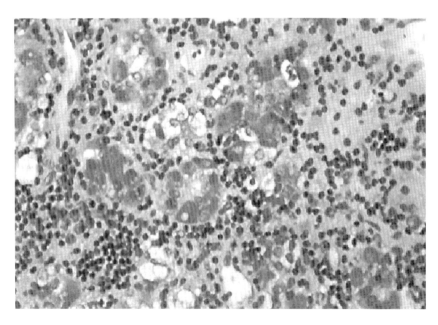

Fig. 3.123 Lymphocytic hypophysitis (hematoxylin and eosin [H&E] stain). Lymphocytes infiltrating into the pituitary gland.

15. Empty sella syndrome — primary is from the incomplete development of the diaphragma sella. The arachnoid bulges into the sella and may compress the pituitary gland. There may be an enlarged sella. Secondary occurs after radiation, surgery, stroke, or intrapartum shock with ischemic necrosis of the anterior pituitary gland (Sheehan syndrome).

16. Rathke cleft cyst — it usually occurs in women ages 30–40 years. It is a remnant of the craniopharyngeal duct that develops when the proximal part closes early and the distal cleft remains open between the pars distalis and pars nervosa. 70% are both suprasellar and intrasellar. It is usually >1 cm. Symptoms include visual changes and increased PR. The CT is hypodense and the T1-weighted MRI is homogeneously either hypo- or hyperintense. 50% have rim enhancement. There are no calcifications. It contains watery mucous fluid lined with goblet ciliated cells and columnar/cuboidal epithelial cells (**Fig. 3.124**).

L. Epidermoid cyst/tumor

1. It accounts for 1% of primary tumors. Peak age is 30–50 years and there is no sex predominance.

2. Intracranial locations in descending order of frequency include CPA (50%), suprasellar, intraventricular, and thalamic. 10% are extradural–intradiploic. It is the third most common CPA lesion after vestibular schwannomas and meningiomas.

3. On MRI, signal intensity is similar to CSF except for on FLAIR and DWI where the tumor is hyperintense to CSF. Generally, there is no enhancement (**Fig. 3.125**).

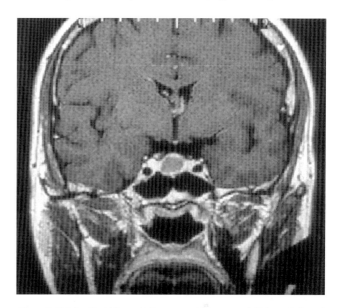

Fig. 3.124 Rathke cleft cyst. Enhanced T1-weighted coronal magnetic resonance image demonstrating a low-intensity cystic lesion in the sella.

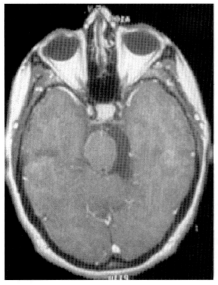
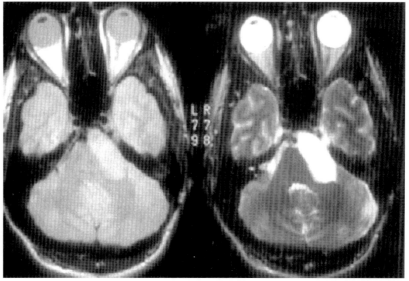

A–C

Fig. 3.125 Epidermoid cyst. (**A**) Enhanced T1-weighted, (**B**) proton density, and (**C**) T2-weighted axial magnetic resonance images demonstrating a low-intensity lesion in the cistern along the left side of the brainstem.

4. It is smooth, encapsulated, has a pearly sheen, and contains dry, flaky keratin and stratified cuboidal squamous epithelium (**Fig. 3.126** and **Fig. 3.127**). The progressive desquamation of the cyst wall causes a linear growth rate. 15% have calcifications. It rarely ruptures and frequently recurs after surgery.

5. An epidermoid tumor insinuates along the basal cisterns. An arachnoid cyst can be ruled out by DWI MRI that shows the epidermoid to be hyperintense to CSF.

6. It develops from ectoderm elements that become trapped intracranially. Epidermoids may form in the lumbosacral spine after lumbar puncture, especially if the stylet of the needle is not in place allowing skin elements to be deposited into deep layers.

7. Mollaret meningitis is recurrent aseptic meningitis with large cells in the CSF. It occurs in some patients with epidermoid tumors.

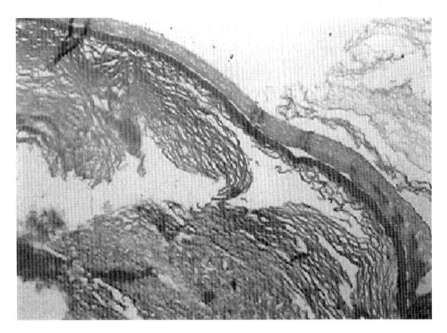

Fig. 3.126 Epidermoid cyst (hematoxylin and eosin [H&E] stain); thin "dry" keratin.

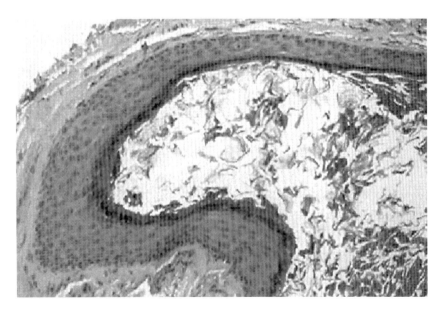

Fig. 3.127 Epidermoid cyst (hematoxylin and eosin [H&E] stain). Stratified squamous epithelium around thin "dry" keratin.

M. Dermoid cyst/tumor

1. It accounts for 0.1% of primary tumors. There is no sex predominance, and mean age in the spine is 10 years and in the head is 20 years. It tends to be located in the midline: parasellar, fourth ventricular, or interhemispheric.

2. It appears similar to fat on MRI and has frequent calcifications (**Fig. 3.128**). It is filled with oily fluid and cholesterol that causes chemical meningitis when it leaks, and this may lead to vasospasm and death. It contains cheesy material, pilosebaceous units with hair shafts and sebaceous glands, sweat glands, and occasionally teeth (**Fig. 3.129**). It grows by both desquamation and gland secretion and frequently ruptures.

3. Dermoid tumors may be congenital or acquired through trauma or lumbar puncture.

4. Dermoids (and epidermoids) rarely undergo malignant change to squamous cell carcinoma. There may be a fistula to the skin with recurrent bouts of bacterial meningitis.

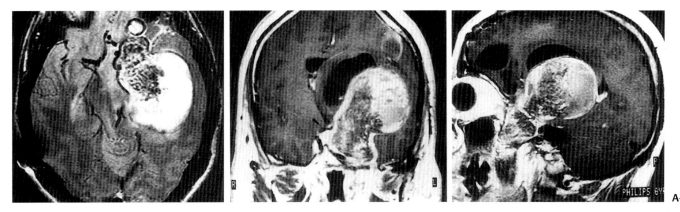

A–C

Fig. 3.128   Dermoid cyst. (**A**) T2-weighted axial and (**B**) T1-weighted nonenhanced coronal and (**C**) sagittal magnetic resonance images demonstrating the left-sided high intensity parasellar mass. (From Yasargil MG. Microneurosurgery IV B. New York, NY: Thieme; 1996. Reprinted by permission.)

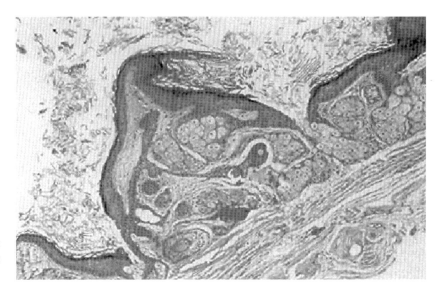

Fig. 3.129   Dermoid cyst (hematoxylin and eosin [H&E] stain). Epidermis with sebaceous cysts and hair follicles.

N. Lipoma

1. It accounts for 0.2% of intracranial tumors. It presents at any age and has no sex predominance. It is usually in the midline (90%): above the corpus callosum, at the quadrigeminal plate, in the third ventricle, CPA, or sylvian fissure.

2. It is composed of mature fatty tissue (**Fig. 3.130**). There may be peripheral calcifications, and it rarely contains bone, cartilage, or muscle. 50% are associated with brain malformations.

3. Lipomas are thought to occur from maldifferentiation of the meninx primitiva, a mesenchyme derivative of the neural crest with both ectodermal and mesodermal tissue that forms the dura, arachnoid, and arachnoid cisterns.

4. Variants are (1) tubulonodular — usually anterior over the corpus callosum and associated with corpus callosal dysgenesis, cephaloceles, and frontal lobe abnormalities; and (2) curvilinear — usually around the splenium, and the corpus callosum tends to be normal (**Fig. 3.131** and **Fig. 3.132**).

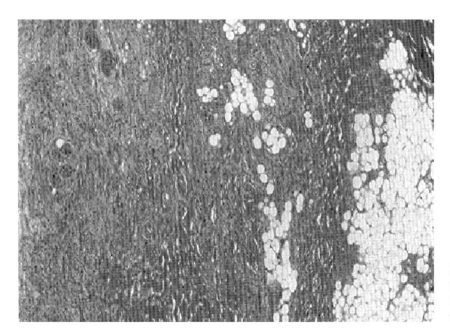

Fig. 3.130 Intradural spinal lipoma (hematoxylin and eosin [H&E] stain). Adipose tissue and collagenous connective tissue infiltrating cord parenchyma.

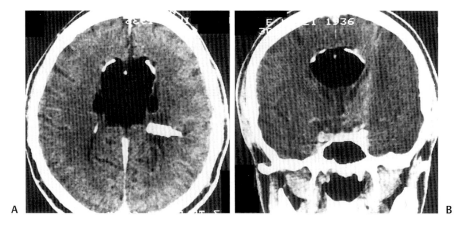

Fig. 3.131 Corpus callosum lipoma. (**A**) Nonenhanced axial and (**B**) coronal computed tomographic scans demonstrating a low-density lesion above the corpus callosum with a rim of calcification. (From Microneurosurgery IV B. Yasargil MG. New York, NY: Thieme; 1996. Reprinted by permission.)

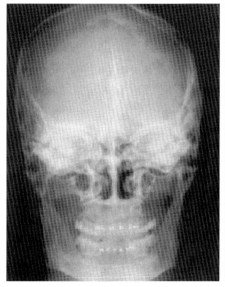 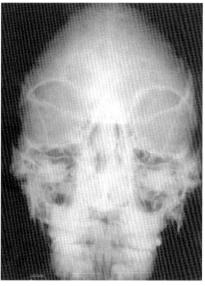

A   B

Fig. 3.132 Corpus callosum lipoma. Anteroposterior skull x-ray films demonstrate (**A**) curvilinear and (**B**) globular types of corpus callosum lipomas with calcifications.

O. Chordoma

1. Mean age is 20–60 years and there is a male predominance. 40% occur in the clivus and 60% in the sacrum (rarely in other parts of the spine) (**Fig. 3.133** and **Fig. 3.134**). They are derived from notochord remnants (as is the nucleus pulposus) at the extremes of the axial skeleton.

2. It is "benign," but locally aggressive, destroys surrounding bone, and is malignant by location (usually very difficult to remove). It tends to be painful. Chordomas metastasize (25–40%) and may change to sarcoma.

3. Pathologically, it is lobulated, gray, soft, with sheets or cords of large vacuolated cells (physaliphorous or bubble-bearing cells) surrounded by mucin. Immunohistochemistry is similar to the notochord with characteristics of both mesenchyme and epithelium: positive for cytokeratin and EMA (epithelial) and S100 (mesenchymal, neural crest) (**Fig. 3.135**).

4. Chondroid chordoma—a variant that contains cartilage and has a better prognosis. Low-grade chondrosarcoma is negative for cytokeratin and EMA, but positive for S100.

5. Treatment is surgical resection and radiation. Survival is usually 5–7 years.

P. Glomus jugulare tumor (paraganglioma)

1. It occurs in middle age with female predominance.

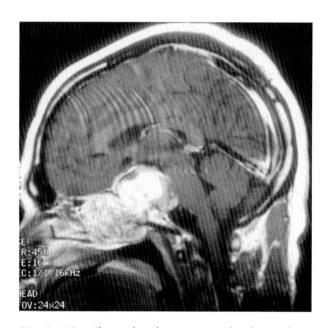

Fig. 3.133 Clivus chordoma. Sagittal enhanced T1-weighted magnetic resonance image demonstrating an enhancing mass eroding the clivus and filling the sella and suprasellar space. (From Sekhar LN, de Oliveira E. Cranial Microsurgery. New York, NY: Thieme; 1998. Reprinted by permission.)

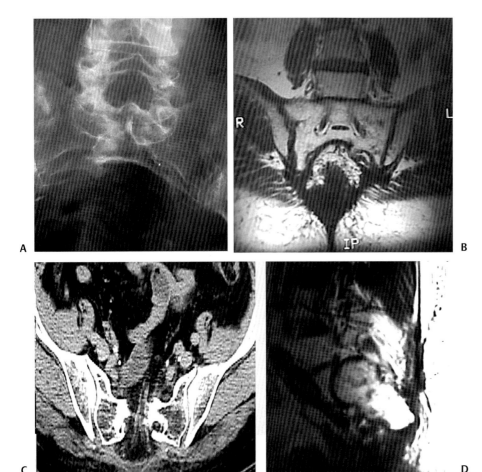

Fig. 3.134 Sacral chordoma. (**A**) Anteroposterior x-ray film, (**B**) coronal T1-weighted magnetic resonance image (MRI) scan, (**C**) coronal computed tomography scan, and (**D**) sagittal enhanced T1-weighted MRI scan demonstrating an erosive lower sacral mass.

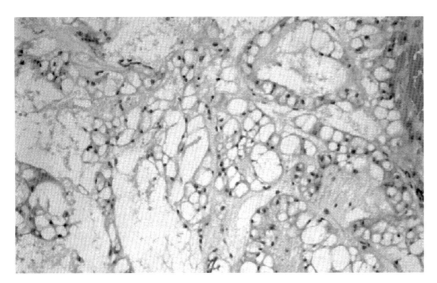

Fig. 3.135 Chordoma (hematoxylin and eosin [H&E] stain). "Physaliphorous" or bubble-bearing cells in a mucoid-rich stroma.

2. It originates from paraganglion tissue in the adventitia of the dome of the jugular bulb and may produce catecholamines.

3. Treatment is with mastoidectomy and resection followed by radiation. They are extremely vascular and consideration should be given to preoperative embolization (**Fig. 3.136**).

Q. Carotid body tumor (chemodectoma)

1. It occurs at the carotid bifurcation and forms a painless mass below the angle of the jaw (similar to a salivary gland tumor or a branchial cleft cyst). CNs IX–XII may be involved.

2. It has neurosecretory granules similar to those in the carotid body and may produce catecholamines.

3. 5% are bilateral and 5% are malignant. There is a familial tendency.

4. Treatment is with surgery and/or radiation.

R. Esthesioneuroblastoma

1. It arises in the high nasal cavity from neurosecretory receptor cells or basal cells (**Fig. 3.137**).

2. It may metastasize to the CNS.

3. Patients are usually >50 years.

S. Metastatic tumors to the nervous system

1. Skull — breast, lung, and prostate carcinoma and multiple myeloma

2. Epidural (mainly thoracic spine) — breast, lung, and prostate carcinoma; less frequently lymphoma, melanoma, renal cell carcinoma, multiple myeloma, and sarcoma.

3. Dural (found in 10% of diffuse metastatic case autopsies) — breast, lung, lymphoma, leukemia, melanoma, and GI tumors.

4. Leptomeningeal (found in 10% of CNS metastatic cases) — breast, lung, melanoma, and gastric carcinoma. Leptomeningeal carcinomatosis is diffuse seeding of the leptomeninges by tumor causing cranial neuropathies and CSF obstruction. The CSF has increased protein and tumor cells, decreased glucose, and no inflammatory cells (**Fig. 3.138**).

5. Parenchymal — lung (35%), breast (20%), kidney (10%), melanoma (10%), and GI (5%). They are multiple in 75%. They usually oc-

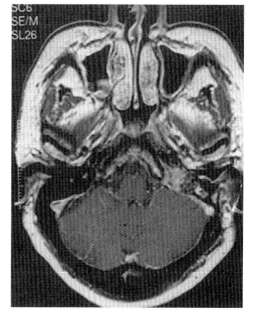

Fig. 3.136 Glomus jugulare tumor. Enhanced T1-weighted axial magnetic resonance image demonstrating a left-sided enhancing mass in the jugular foramen. (From Alleyne Jr. CH. Neurosurgery Board Review. New York, NY: Thieme;1997. Reprinted by permission.)

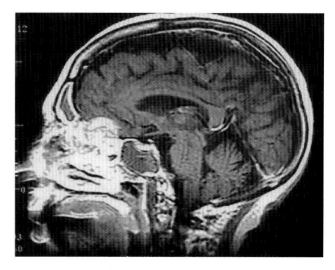

Fig. 3.137 Esthesioneuroblastoma. Enhanced sagittal T1-weighted magnetic resonance image demonstrating an enhancing mass invading through the floor of the anterior fossa.

cur at the gray/white matter junction and are round and well circumscribed. Hemorrhage is especially common with melanoma, renal cell carcinoma, and choriocarcinoma. Metastases to the spinal cord parenchyma are very rare but are usually caused by lung carcinoma and to a lesser extent breast, renal cell, and melanoma (**Figs. 3.139–3.142**).

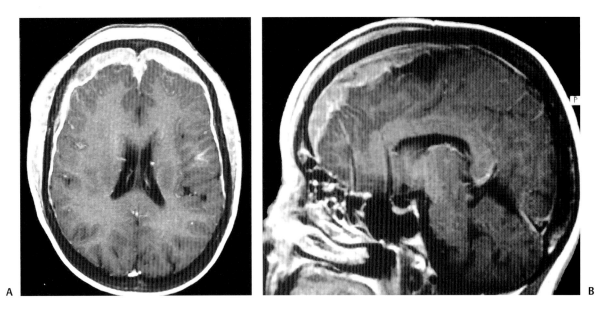

Fig. 3.138 Leptomeningeal carcinomatosis. (**A**) Axial and (**B**) sagittal enhanced T1-weighted magnetic resonance images demonstrating diffuse meningeal enhancement.

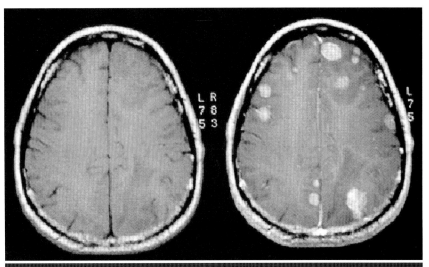

Fig. 3.139 Multiple brain metastases. (**A**) Axial nonenhanced and (**B**) enhanced T1-weighted magnetic resonance images demonstrating the multiple enhancing lesions.

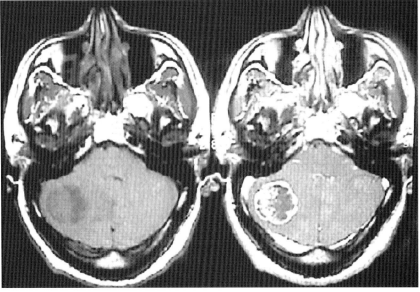

Fig. 3.140 Cystic brain metastasis. (**A**) Axial nonenhanced and (**B**) enhanced T1-weighted magnetic resonance images demonstrating a lesion with irregular rim enhancement.

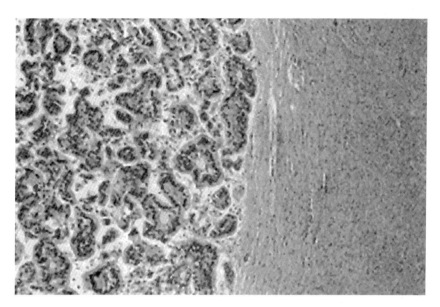

Fig. 3.141 Metastatic carcinoma (hematoxylin and eosin [H&E] stain); circumscribed glandular tumor.

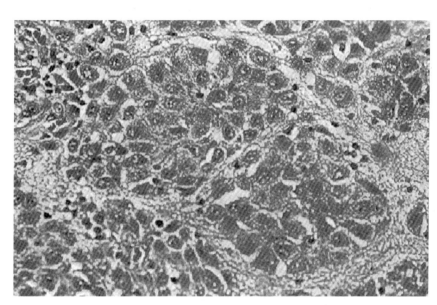

Fig. 3.142 Melanoma (hematoxylin and eosin [H&E] stain); epithelioid cells with melanin inclusions.

T. Tumors of blood cell origin

1. Non-Hodgkin lymphoma — usually B cell and diffuse. Pathologic examination demonstrates mixed small and large cells of intermediate or high grade. There are concentric reticulin rings around blood vessels. It is radiosensitive.
    a. Primary CNS lymphoma — usually parenchymal, subependymal, and subpial. It is most common in men 60 years of age who are immunocompetent and men 30 years of age who are immunosuppressed. Risk increases with Wiskott–Aldrich syndrome, transplant patients, AIDS, collagen vascular disease, and cancer. It may be associated with disease caused by Epstein–Barr virus infection. They may be hyperdense on CT and usually enhance brightly. 30% are multiple. Survival without treatment is <1 year and with chemotherapy, steroids, and radiation is up to 3.5 years (**Fig. 3.143** and **Fig. 3.144**). 98% are B cell derived, while 2% are T cell derived.
    b. Secondary (metastatic) CNS lymphoma — usually intracranial meningeal or spinal epidural. Treat with radiation. Intravascular lymphoma is spread of lymphoma inside blood vessels, causing strokes and dementia.

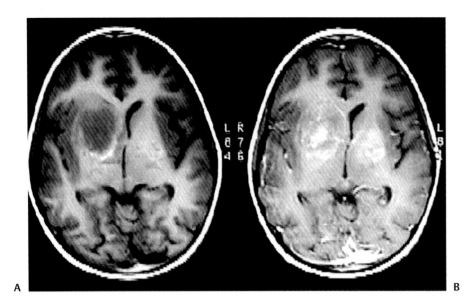

Fig. 3.143 Primary central nervous system lymphoma. (**A**) Axial nonenhanced and (**B**) enhanced T1-weighted magnetic resonance imaging scans demonstrating bilateral periventricular enhancing lesions.

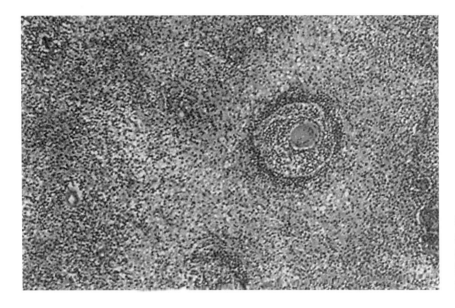

Fig. 3.144 Lymphoma (hematoxylin and eosin [H&E] stain). Diffuse perivascular infiltrate with small blue cells filling the Virchow–Robin space around the vessel.

2. Hodgkin lymphoma — has characteristic Reed–Sternberg binucleated cells. Varieties include lymphocyte predominant, mixed cellular, lymphocyte depleted, and nodular sclerosis. 20% develop neurologic complications, usually involving the skull or meninges.

U. Plasma cell disorders

1. Plasmacytoma (single location) and multiple myeloma (more than one location) — locations include vertebral bodies (fractures), ribs, and skull (70% of multiple myeloma, the inner table appears punched out). Pathologic examination demonstrates mixed small and large cells of intermediate or high grade. There is concentric reticulin and Russell bodies (eosinophilic intracytoplasmic inclusions filled with immunoglobulins).

2. Waldenstrom macroglobulinemia — plasma cells accumulate in the bone marrow, liver, spleen, and lymph nodes. There are no lytic lesions. 25% of cases develop neurologic complications, including peripheral neuropathy, stroke, and SAH.

3. Heavy chain disease

4. Primary amyloidosis—accumulation of light chains

V. Histiocytosis X (Langerhans cell histiocytosis) — usually involves bone. Extraskeletal sites are involved in 20%. Of these, 90% are intracranial. Symptoms include diabetes insipidus. Pathologically characterized by multinucleated giant cells. Electron microscopy demonstrates cytoplasmic Birbeck bodies that look like tennis rackets.

1. Letterer–Siwe disease — acute fulminant disseminated histiocytosis. Occurs in children ages 2–4 years. Death usually ensues within 2 years. It involves multiple organs.

2. Eosinophilic granuloma — unifocal Langerhans histiocytosis. It is benign and affects children and young adults. It is a painful, solitary, lytic bone lesion with clear margins (no sclerotic rim). Lesions involve the full thickness of the skull and may occasionally be located in the brain, spinal cord, or dura. Work-up should include a skeletal survey and treatment is with excision or radiation. It can present as vertebrae plana.

3. Multifocal histiocytosis — chronic, recurrent, and disseminated. Onset is before 5 years. It causes respiratory infections and infiltrates lymph nodes, liver, spleen, bones, orbit, pituitary, and hypothalamus. Hand–Schüller–Christian disease — lytic bone lesions, exophthalmos, and diabetes insipidus.

W. Leukemia — may be diffuse or focal (solid green mass called a chloroma). It hemorrhages frequently, and this results in 50% of the deaths. It usually involves the leptomeninges (especially acute lymphocytic leukemia). It is protected from chemotherapy in the CNS by the BBB. Evaluation should include a lumbar puncture, which, if positive, should be followed by prophylactic radiation and intrathecal chemotherapy with methotrexate. Necrotizing leukoencephalopathy may develop in patients <5 years and is due to methotrexate injury to the myelin after the radiation has broken down the BBB.

X. Nontumoral cysts

1. Colloid cyst
   a. Mean age is 20–40 years and there is no sex predominance.
   b. It is normally in the anterior roof of the third ventricle between the columns of the fornices and is frequently attached to the stroma of the choroid.
   c. It is believed to be of endodermal origin from a vestigial third ventricular structure (the paraphysis) and is rarely associated with craniopharyngioma. The cyst may be pendulous and cause intermittent CSF obstruction with a ball-valve mechanism.
   d. It is filled with mucus (mucopolysaccharides) that on CT may be either hyperdense (two thirds) or hypodense (one third). On MRI, it is hyperintense on T1-weighted images and hypointense on T2-weighted images (**Fig. 3.145**).
   e. There are no calcifications and there is usually enhancement of the cyst wall. The fibrous capsule is lined by a single pseudostratified layer of columnar cells with occasional cilia and PAS-positive goblet cells. The smallest documented cyst causing death is 1 cm (**Fig. 3.146**).
   f. Consider surgery if the cyst is >7 mm because resection is curative.

2. Arachnoid cyst—congenital, male predominance, usually in children (75%), and becomes symptomatic in 70% of cases. Locations are middle fossa (60%), suprasellar (10%), quadrigeminal cistern (10%), posterior fossa (10%, CPA and cisterna magna), and convexity (5%). It is associated with SDH because of tearing of the bridging veins that traverse the cyst (**Fig. 3.147**).

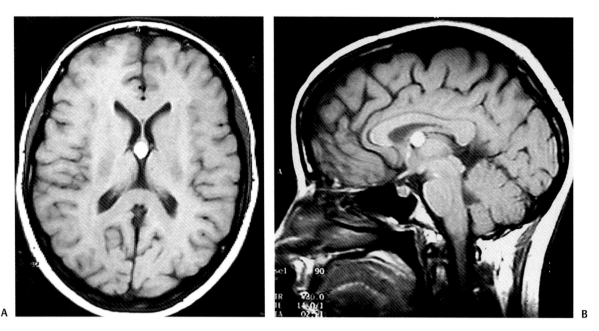

Fig. 3.145   Colloid cyst. (**A**) Axial and (**B**) sagittal T1-weighted nonenhanced magnetic resonance images demonstrate a hyperintense cyst in the roof of the third ventricle.

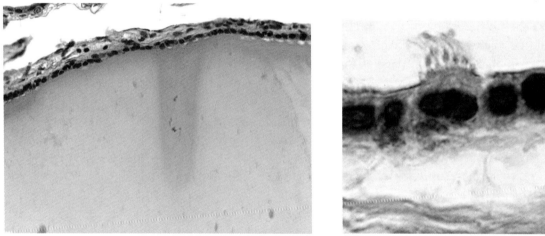
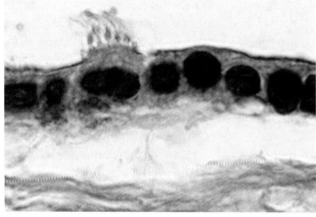

Fig. 3.146   Colloid cyst (hematoxylin and eosin [H&E] stain). (**A**) Colloid cyst in the third ventricle filled with mucin, and (**B**) high power view of the single layer of columnar cells lining the cyst with occasional cilia.

3. Neuroepithelial cyst—caused by the infolding of developing neuroectoderm. They may be located in the ependyma, choroid plexus, and choroidal fissure.

4. Enterogenous (neurenteric) cyst—filled with endoderm of GI or respiratory mucosa. They have a single layer of cuboidal/columnar cells with interspersed goblet cells. Locations are spine (80%), intracranial (15%), CPA, and craniocervical junction. There is a male predominance. They may be due to notochord-gut fusion.

5. Cavum septum pellucidum — at the level of the caudate head. CSF is in between the sheets of the septum pellucidum in the lateral ventricles.

6. Cavum vergae — a posterior continuation of the cavum septum pellucidum

7. Cavum velum interpositum—in the third ventricle because of failure of fusion of the tela choroidea

Y. Peripheral nerve sheath tumors

1. Traumatic neuroma — consists of a tangle of axons, Schwann cells, and fibroblasts in a collagen matrix. They are usually painful and rubbery.

2. Schwannoma
   a. 7% of intracranial tumors. 5% are multiple, usually with NF2. It is benign, has no sex predominance, and the mean age is 40–50 years (although onset is by 20 years with NF2). It grows slowly and almost never undergoes malignant change. Schwann cells are derived from the neural crest cells.
   b. Schwannomas occur intracranially and along the spinal cord at the root entry zone of sensory nerves, in the head and neck, posterior mediastinum, retroperitoneum, and the flexor surface of the extremities.
   c. Intracranially, the most common site is on the superior vestibular nerve where it originates in the internal acoustic meatus at the root entry zone. The second most common site is the trigeminal nerve (5%), and these are located in the middle fossa (50%), both middle and posterior fossa (dumbbell, 25%), and posterior fossa (25%).
   d. Rarely, they are intraaxial in the brain or spinal cord when they form on perivascular nerves. Spinal schwannomas form on sensory nerve roots, account for 30% of spinal tumors, and may be intraspinal or dumbbell shaped.
   e. Schwannomas are firm and encapsulated. They are initially fusiform when intraneural, but then enlarge and become eccentric with epineurium as a capsule. They contain no axons. There is a biphasic pattern of compact Antoni A (fusiform cells, reticulin, and collagen) and loose Antoni B (stellate round cells in stroma) areas (**Fig. 3.148**).

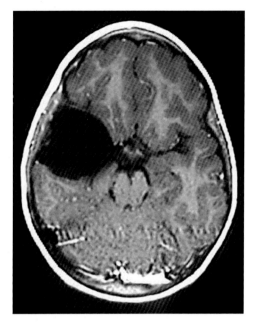

Fig. 3.147 Arachnoid cyst. Enhanced T1-weighted magnetic resonance image demonstrates a nonenhancing middle fossa extraaxial cyst.

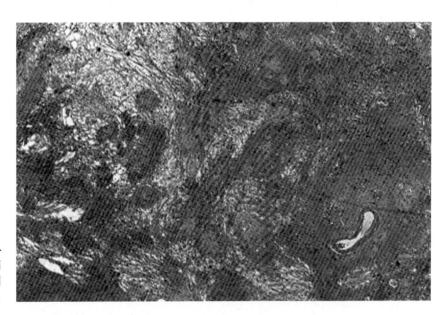

Fig. 3.148 Schwannoma (hematoxylin and eosin [H&E] stain). Dense Antoni A areas with compact spindle cells, and looser Antoni B areas with stellate cells.

f. There are multiple different planes of fascicle groups of spindle cells that look like schools of fish swimming in different directions. There are Verocay bodies, anuclear material with palisading cells in Antoni A areas. They are frequently cystic, hemorrhagic, and may contain fat (**Fig. 3.149** and **Fig. 3.150**). Mitotic figures do not change prognosis. Immunohistochemistry is S100 positive (**Figs. 3.151–3.153**).

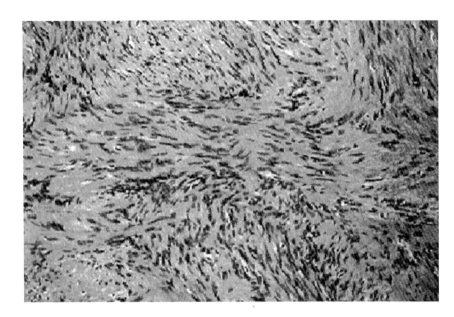

Fig. 3.149 Schwannoma (hematoxylin and eosin [H&E] stain). "Schools of fish" swimming in multiple different directions.

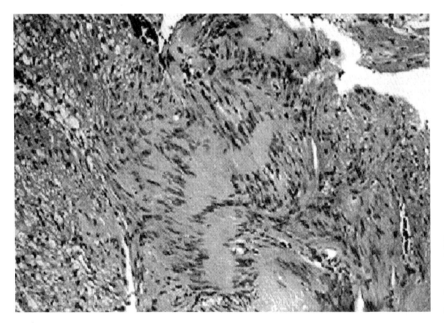

Fig. 3.150 Schwannoma (hematoxylin and eosin [H&E] stain). Verocay bodies with nuclear palisading around anuclear fibrillary material (occurs in Antoni A areas).

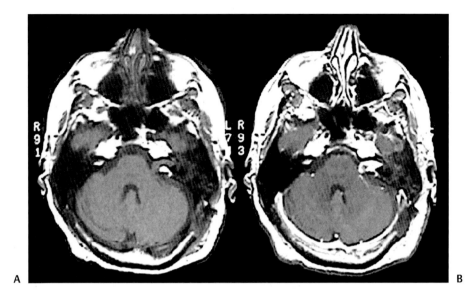

Fig. 3.151 Vestibular schwannoma. (**A**) Nonenhanced and (**B**) enhanced axial T1-weighted magnetic resonance images demonstrating an enhancing and thickened left vestibulocochlear nerve.

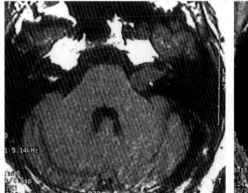 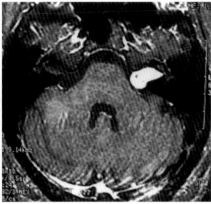 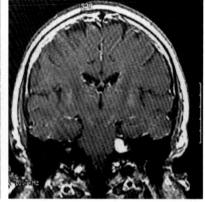

Fig. 3.152 Vestibular schwannoma. (**A**) Nonenhanced and (**B**) enhanced axial and (**C**) enhanced coronal T1-weighted magnetic resonance images demonstrating an enhancing mass emanating from the left internal acoustic meatus.

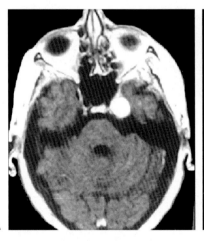 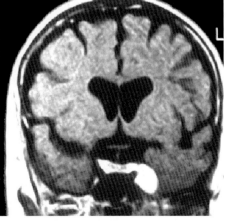

Fig. 3.153 Trigeminal schwannoma. (**A**) Axial and (**B**) coronal enhanced T1-weighted magnetic resonance images demonstrating a smooth, circumscribed, enhancing mass in the Meckel cave.

g. Schwannomas are isointense to hypointense on T1-weighted MRI, enhance, and are rarely calcified.

h. Variants are cellular (middle-aged women), ancient (hypocellular with cysts, calcifications, and old hemorrhage), plexiform (multinodular, not associated with NF), and melanotic (a few are malignant).

3. Neurofibroma

a. Develops at any age and has no sex predominance. They do not occur intracranially, but usually involve the posterior ganglia. They contain Schwann cells, fibroblasts, collagen, and reticulin. They are fusiform, unencapsulated, infiltrate nerves, and rarely have cystic, fatty, or hemorrhagic changes. Five to 13% undergo malignant change. Most are solitary cutaneous nodules coming from small terminal nerves. NF is associated with neurofibromas on larger nerve trunks and with malignant transformation (**Fig. 3.154**).

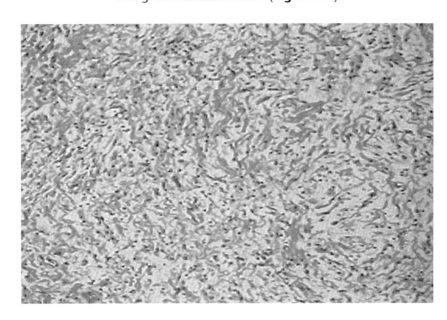

Fig. 3.154 Neurofibroma (hematoxylin and eosin [H&E] stain). Elongated Schwann cells with wavy nuclei in a loose mucopolysaccharide matrix.

b. Cutaneous neurofibroma — dermal or subcutaneous, painless, unencapsulated (so may infiltrate surrounding nerves), and soft. Multiple lesions are associated with NF1. They rarely undergo malignant transformation. Most are solitary and contain loose wavy nuclei in a matrix with axons (detected by silver stain). Immunohistochemistry is positive for vimentin, Leu7, S100, and occasionally GFAP.

c. Intraneural neurofibroma — involves large nerve trunks, has a higher potential for malignant transformation, and is associated with NF1. The plexiform neurofibroma (pathognomonic of NF1) appears like an enlarged bag of worms and it may involve an entire extremity, causing elephantiasis neuromatosa. 5% of plexiform neurofibromas undergo malignant change (**Fig. 3.155** and **Fig. 3.156**).

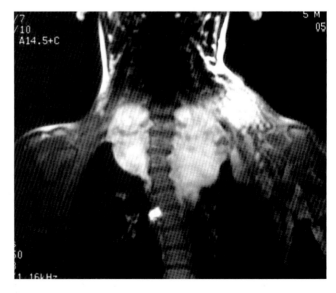

Fig. 3.155 Plexiform neurofibroma.

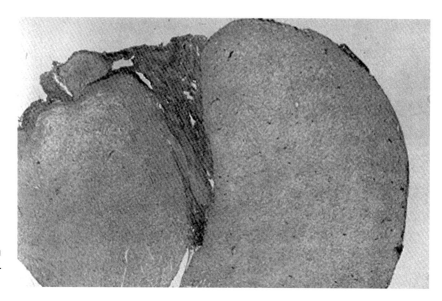

Fig. 3.156 Plexiform neurofibroma (hematoxylin and eosin [H&E] stain). Diffuse enlargement of adjacent nerves.

4. Perineuroma — Rare, occurs in adolescents, involves the distal extremity, and causes a motor mononeuropathy. Pathologically, it forms an onion bulb, is made of perineural cells, and is EMA positive and S100 negative.

5. Malignant peripheral nerve sheath tumor — involves proximal nerves, is very painful, and has increased cellularity and mitoses with necrosis. 50% have NF1. It very rarely develops from schwannomas. 10% have had prior radiation. 75% recur and cause death. Prognosis is worse if the tumor is >5 cm, has necrosis, or is associated with NF. 5–13% of neurofibromas in NF1 become malignant. The most common intracranial malignant peripheral nerve sheath tumor involves the trigeminal nerve (**Fig. 3.157**).

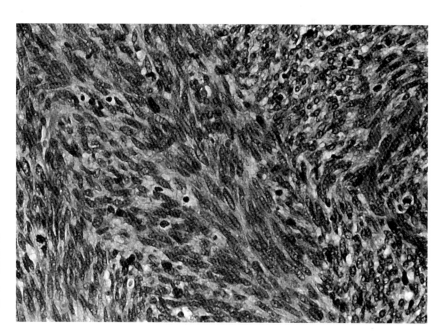

Fig. 3.157 Malignant peripheral nerve sheath tumor (hematoxylin and eosin [H&E] stain). Hypercellular spindle cell neoplasm. (From Bernstein M, Berger MS. Neuro-Oncology: The Essentials. New York, NY: Thieme; 2000. Reprinted by permission.)

XI. Differential Diagnosis by Location

A. Pineal region — includes the suprapineal recess of the third ventricle, the velum interpositum (the anterior extension of the quadrigeminal cistern above the pineal gland and extending under the fornices; may be "cavum" or filled with CSF), and the posterior commissure between the pineal gland and the colliculi. This region contains 1–3% of tumors and 3–8% of childhood tumors.

1. Germ cell tumors — the most common tumors here (66%) with a peak age of 15 years. Germinomas (66%) are more frequent than teratomas (15%), and 5% of germinomas have a concomitant pituitary germ cell tumor (**Fig. 3.115**).

2. Pineal parenchymal tumors — account for <15% (**Figs. 3.110–3.112**).

3. Pineal cysts — 40% of autopsy pineal masses, but only 1–5% of MRI pineal masses (**Fig. 3.113**).

4. Others — astrocytoma (**Fig. 3.158**), meningioma, metastatic tumor, and vascular malformation

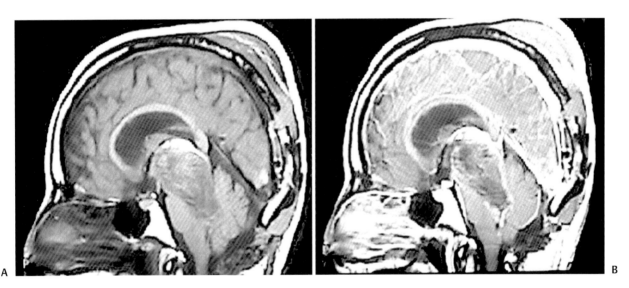

A   B

Fig. 3.158   Pineal region glioblastoma multiforme. (**A**) Nonenhanced and (**B**) enhanced sagittal T1-weighted magnetic resonance images demonstrating a diffuse, infiltrating, nonenhancing pineal region mass.

B. Posterior third ventricle — meningioma, choroid plexus papilloma, and metastatic tumor

C. Tectum — low-grade astrocytoma (detected by the fact that the inferior colliculus is always larger than the superior colliculus)

D. Intraventricular — the septum pellucidum extends from the fornix to the corpus callosum. An absent septum pellucidum is associated with holoprosencephaly, septooptic dysplasia, and callosal agenesis. Cavum septum pellucidum is present in 80% of neonates and 3% of adults. Cavum vergae is present in 30% of neonates and 3% of adults. These two are due to the persistence of normal fetal cavities. Vergae is a posterior extension of the cavum septum pellucidum and never occurs without one. It is located below the corpus callosum, between the fornices, and on the next higher cut than the cavum septum pellucidum (**Fig. 3.159**).

1. Primary septal tumor — astrocytoma, lymphoma, and germinoma

2. Frontal horn/septum pellucidum tumor — central neurocytoma, giant cell astrocytoma, and subependymoma

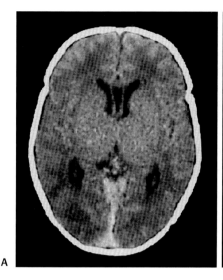 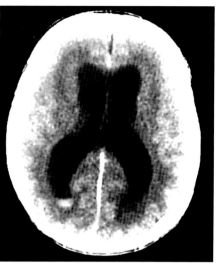

Fig. 3.159 (**A**) Nonenhanced computed tomographic scans of cavum septum pellucidum and (**B**) cavum vergae.

3. Children
    a. Frontal horn — low-grade astrocytoma and giant cell astrocytoma
    b. Body — PNET and astrocytoma
    c. Atrium — choroid plexus papilloma, ependymoma, and astrocytoma
    d. Occipital and temporal horns — meningioma (rare)
    e. Foramen of Monro — giant cell astrocytoma, colloid cyst, craniopharyngioma
    f. Anterior third ventricle — astrocytoma, histiocytosis (hypothalamic/infundibular), germinoma, and craniopharyngioma (extrinsic)
    g. Fourth ventricle — pilocytic astrocytoma, medulloblastoma, ependymoma, and exophytic brain stem glioma

4. Adults
    a. Frontal horn — high-grade astrocytoma, giant cell astrocytoma, central neurocytoma, and subependymoma
    b. Body — astrocytoma, central neurocytoma, oligodendroglioma, and subependymoma
    c. Atrium — meningioma, metastatic tumor, and lymphoma
    d. Occipital and temporal horns — meningioma
    e. Foramen of Monro — high-grade astrocytoma, central neurocytoma, oligodendroglioma, subependymoma, and colloid cyst
    f. Anterior third ventricle — colloid cyst, suprasellar extension of pituitary tumor, aneurysm, glioma, sarcoid, and germinoma
    g. Fourth ventricle — metastatic tumor, hemangioblastoma, exophytic brainstem glioma, subependymoma, and choroid plexus papilloma

5. Rarely, there are choroid plexus cysts and xanthogranulomas.

E. Cerebellopontine angle (CPA) tumors — usually occur where the flocculus projects into the CPA.

1. Vestibular schwannoma (acoustic neuroma) — 75%

2. Meningioma — 10%

3. Epidermoid — 5%

4. Others — vascular lesions such as dolichoectasia of the basilar artery, aneurysm, AVM (2–5%), and metastatic tumors (1–2%)

5. Internal auditory canal masses — vestibular schwannoma, postoperative fibrosis, and neuritis (Bell palsy and Ramsay–Hunt zoster otitis)

6. Temporal bone lesions involving the CPA — Gradenigo syndrome (osteomyelitis of the petrous apex with CN VI palsy, otorrhea, and retroorbital pain), malignant external otitis, cholesteatoma (hyperintense on T1-weighted and T2-weighted MRI), and paraganglioma (slow growing, hypervascular, from the neural crest, in the cochlear promontory, and called a glomus tympanicum tumor)

F. Foramen magnum — cervicomedullary low-grade astrocytoma, anterior intradural meningioma or schwannoma, chordoma, chondroma, chondrosarcoma, and metastatic tumor. The classic presentation of a foramen magnum mass is progressive weakness of the ipsilateral upper limb followed in order by the ipsilateral lower limb, contralateral lower limb, and then the contralateral upper limb.

G. Sella

1. Intrasellar masses — pituitary hyperplasia (seen with puberty, pregnancy, postpartum, and end organ failure), microadenoma (<1 cm), and nonneoplastic cyst (20% at autopsy, from the pars intermedia or Rathke cleft). Less common are craniopharyngioma (5–10% are intrasellar), breast metastases, epidermoid, dermoid, and aneurysm. The pituitary gland normally enhances.

2. Suprasellar masses (**Mnemonic: SATCHMO**) — "**s**arcoid, pituitary **a**denoma, **a**neurysm, **t**eratoma, **c**raniopharyngioma, **h**ypothalamic glioma or hamartoma, **m**eningioma, and **o**ptic glioma." In descending order of frequency: pituitary adenoma, meningioma, craniopharyngioma, hypothalamic/chiasm glioma (20–50% associated with NF1, enhances, hypointense on T1-weighted MRI, and usually pilocytic), and aneurysm. Less common are arachnoid cyst (10% suprasellar), Rathke cleft cyst (rarely purely suprasellar), hypothalamic hamartoma (associated with precocious puberty, partial complex seizures, and psychologic changes, and does not enhance or grow with time), sarcoid, and lymphocytic hypophysitis (anterior lobe, enhances, in peripartum women) (**Figs. 3.30** and **3.160**).

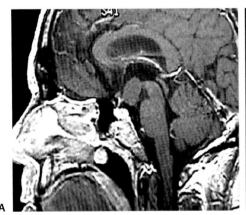 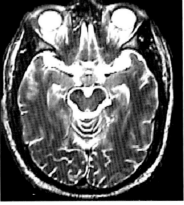

A   B

Fig. 3.160 Hypothalamic hamartoma. (**A**) Sagittal T1-weighted enhanced and (**B**) axial T2-weighted magnetic resonance images demonstrating a nonenhancing mass posterior to the optic chiasm.

3. Suprasellar "hot spot" (hyperintense on T1-weighted MRI) — Rathke cleft cyst, craniopharyngioma, subacute blood (thrombosed aneurysm, hemorrhagic tumor, and postoperatively), lipoma, dermoid, ectopic neurohypophysis, sarcoid, and histiocytosis

4. Infundibulum — normally enhances because there is no BBB
    a. Children — Langerhans cell histiocytosis (absent posterior pituitary bright spot and thickened stalk), germinoma, and meningitis .
    b. Adults — sarcoid, germinoma, and metastatic tumors

H. Skull base

1. Anterior skull base — mucocele (forms in the sinus with obstruction of flow), inverted papilloma, osteoma (frontal sinus), rhabdomyosarcoma (most common soft tissue sarcoma in children, especially in the head and neck), squamous cell carcinoma (80% of the malignant tumors in adults), adenocarcinoma (20%), esthesioneuroblastoma (from bipolar sensory receptor cells in the olfactory mucosa, of neural crest origin, peak ages are 10 years and 40 years), encephalocele, and nasal glioma. Intrinsic lesions include fibrous dysplasia, Paget disease, and osteopetrosis.

2. Central skull base — includes the clivus, sella, cavernous sinus, and sphenoid alae. Pituitary tumors, meningiomas, trigeminal schwannomas, juvenile angiofibroma (vascular, invasive, originates near the sphenopalatine foramen of adolescent males, most common benign nasopharyngeal tumor, and spreads along the foramen into the pterygopalatine fossa, orbit, sinus, etc.), chordoma, enchondroma (most common benign cartilaginous tumor of the skull), nasopharyngeal carcinoma, rhabdomyosarcoma, osteosarcoma (older patients, involves the maxilla or mandible, skull base involvement is rare, associated with Paget disease and radiation), multiple myeloma, chondrosarcoma, and metastatic tumors (prostate, lung, and breast) (**Fig. 3.161**)

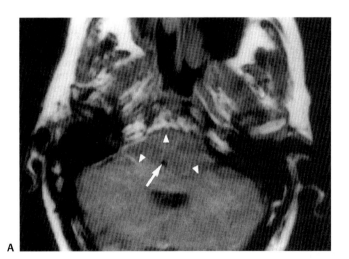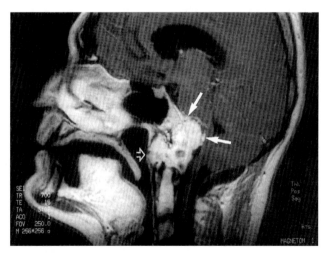

Fig. 3.161   Clivus chondrosarcoma. (**A**) T1-weighted nonenhanced and (**B**) enhanced sagittal magnetic resonance images demonstrating an enhancing destructive clival mass (A: basilar artery [arrow] and tumor margins [arrowheads]. B: enhancing dura pushed posterior to the tumor [arrows] and erosion into the nasopharynx [open arrow]). (From Vogl TJ, Balzer J, Mack M, Steger S. Differential Diagnosis in Head and Neck Imaging. New York, NY: Thieme, 1999. Reprinted by permission.)

3. Posterior skull base — includes the clivus below the sphenooccipital synchondrosis and the petrous temporal bone. Differential includes a clivus chordoma or metastatic tumors. A mass in the jugular foramen may be an enlarged jugular bulb, jugular vein thrombosis, paraganglioma (in the jugular bulb adventitia with frequent bony invasion, includes carotid body tumor, glomus jugulare, and glomus tympanicum), nasopharyngeal carcinoma metastases, schwannoma, neurofibroma, and epidermoid.

I.   Diffuse skull base lesions

1.   Fibrous dysplasia — presents in young adulthood. May be either monoostotic (70% of cases and 25% involve the skull/face) or polyostotic (30% of cases and 50% involve the skull/face). It expands and replaces normal bony medullary spaces with vascular fibrocellular tissue producing "woven bone." CT demonstrates thickened sclerotic bone with "ground-glass" expanded diploë. It is hypointense on T1-weighted images and enhances. There are sclerotic orbits and skull bases (facial, frontal, ethmoid, and sphenoid bones) causing lion-like facies. Narrowing of the optic foramen may cause visual loss (**Figs. 3.162–3.164**).

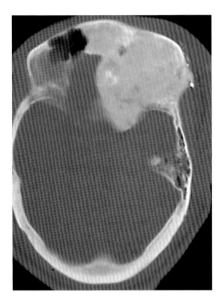

Fig. 3.162   Fibrous dysplasia; axial computed tomographic scan with expansion of diploë.

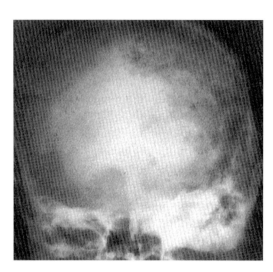

Fig. 3.163   Fibrous dysplasia. Thickened sclerotic left orbit. (From Alleyne Jr. CH. Neurosurgery Board Review. New York, NY: Thieme;1997. Reprinted by permission.)

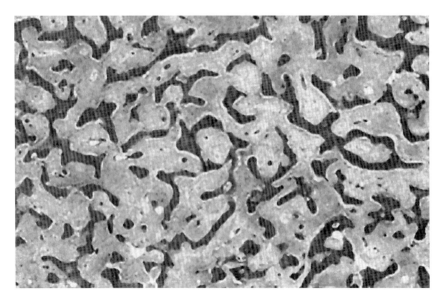

Fig. 3.164   Fibrous dysplasia (hematoxylin and eosin [H&E] stain); woven bone.

2. McCune–Albright syndrome — characterized by polyostotic fibrous dysplasia, pigmented skin lesions, and endocrine abnormalities such as precocious puberty or GH secreting pituitary tumors

3. Paget disease—onset is usually after 40 years, male predominance, and it may be monoostotic or polyostotic. Early in the course, it causes destruction, whereas late in the course it causes sclerosis. There is bony expansion that causes symptoms by cranial nerve compression, basilar invagination, and hydrocephalus. There may be a sarcomatous degeneration, especially to osteosarcoma.

4. Langerhans cell histiocytosis — monostotic (eosinophilic granuloma, 5–15 years, involves the skull) or diffuse (in young to middle age).

J. General calvarial thickening — normal variant, phenytoin (Dilantin; Pfizer Pharmaceuticals, New York, NY), shunted hydrocephalus, acromegaly, Paget disease, fibrous dysplasia, sickle cell disease, and iron deficiency

K. Regional/focal calvarial thickening—hyperostosis frontalis interna (frontal bone, elderly women, spares the superior sagittal sinus), Paget disease, fibrous dysplasia, metastatic tumors (prostate and breast), neuroblastoma ("hair-on-end" appearance), and meningioma (**Fig. 3.165**).

L. Generalized thinning — normal variant, hydrocephalus, osteogenesis imperfecta, Down syndrome, lacunar skull (associated with Chiari II malformation), Cushing disease, hyperparathyroidism, and hypophosphatemia. Craniolacunia (Lückenschädel) is a honeycomb pattern that is congenital and associated with spinal meningocele and myelomeningocele. It may be due to increased intracranial pressure (ICP) in utero.

M. Focal thinning — parietal foramina (bilateral, inner and outer tables meet, no clinical significance), venous lakes, pacchionian granulations, leptomeningeal cyst, arachnoid cyst, and tumor (**Fig. 3.166**).

N. Holes in the skull — cephalocele, dermoid, cleidocranial dysostosis, intradiploic arachnoid cyst, NF1 (absent sphenoid wing and lambdoid suture defects), hemangioma (spoke-wheel pattern and well circumscribed), epidermoid (sclerotic rim, scalloped margins, lucent, hypointense on T1-weighted and hyperintense on T2-weighted MRI), eosinophilic granuloma (nonsclerotic and has beveled edges with uneven involvement of the inner and outer tables), Paget disease lytic phase, multiple myeloma, and growing skull fracture (**Figs. 3.167–3.174**).

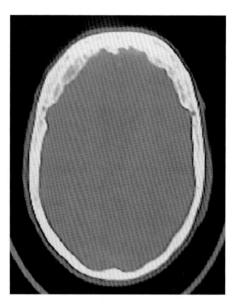

Fig. 3.165 Hyperostosis frontalis interna. Axial computed tomographic scan bone window demonstrates irregular thickening of the inner table of the frontal bone.

O. Meninges — The outer layer of dura (the periosteal layer) contains fibroblasts and blood vessels, and it does not extend caudal to the foramen magnum. The inner layer contains epithelial cells and is continuous with the spinal dura (one layer). The dura enhances a little because it has no BBB. The enhancement is patchy, smooth, thin, and most prominent near the vertex. The pia has an outer layer of collagen and inner layer of elastic fibers. Virchow–Robin spaces are made by the pia and CSF that follows vessels. Osteochondroma and osteosarcoma may arise from the dura. Dural enhancement is associated with leptomeningeal tumors, meningiomas, mucopolysaccharidosis, amyloidosis, CSF shunting, intracranial hypotension and sometimes after lumbar puncture or intracranial surgery.

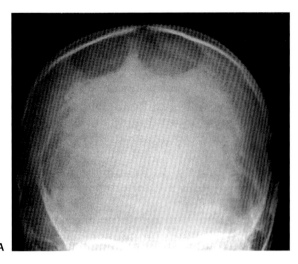
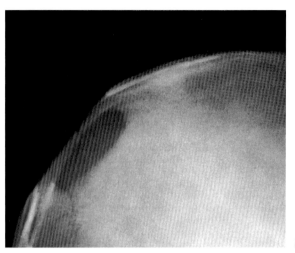

A   B

Fig. 3.166 Parietal foramina. (**A**) Anteropostrior and (**B**) lateral x-rays demonstrate the bilateral smooth-edged foramen. (From Albright AL, Pollack IF, Adelson PD, eds. Principles and Practice of Pediatric Neurosurgery. New York, NY: Thieme; 1999. Reprinted by permission.)

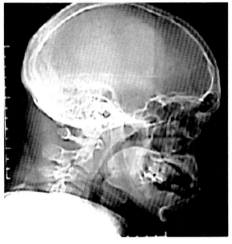
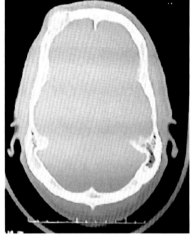

A   B

Fig. 3.167 Hemangioma. (**A**) Lateral skull x-ray film and (**B**) axial computed tomographic scan bone window demonstrate the "sunburst" pattern of the lesion.

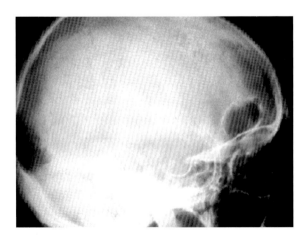
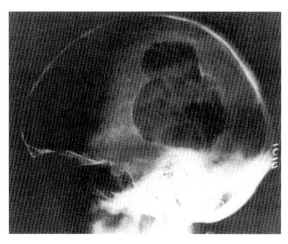

Fig. 3.168 Epidermoid. Lateral skull x-ray film demonstrates the sclerotic margins and scalloped bone edges.

Fig. 3.169 Skull epidermoid. Lateral skull x-ray with scalloped bone edges. (From Alleyne Jr. CH. Neurosurgery Board Review. New York, NY: Thieme; 1997. Reprinted by permission.)

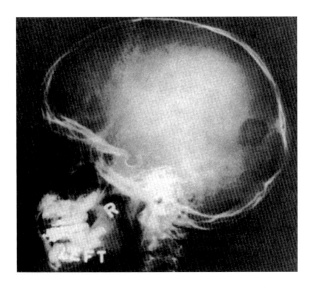

Fig. 3.170 Eosinophilic granuloma. Lateral x-ray demonstrates a single punched-out lesion without sclerotic margins. (From Alleyne Jr. CH. Neurosurgery Board Review. New York, NY: Thieme; 1997. Reprinted by permission.)

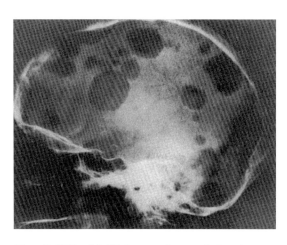

Fig. 3.171 Multiple myeloma. Lateral x-ray demonstrates multiple lytic lesions. (From Alleyne Jr. CH. Neurosurgery Board Review. New York, NY: Thieme; 1997. Reprinted by permission.)

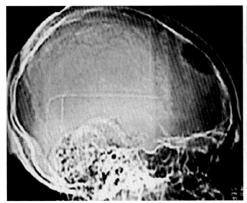
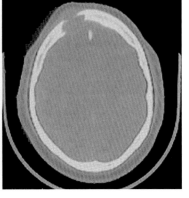

Fig. 3.172 Metastatic tumor. (**A**) Lateral skull x-ray and (**B**) axial computed tomographic scan bone window demonstrate the erosive lesion.

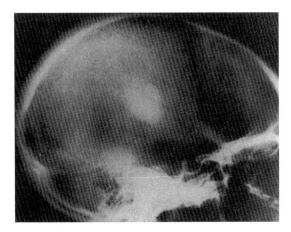

Fig. 3.173 Osteoma. Lateral x-ray demonstrates a single round radiopaque lesion. (From Alleyne Jr. CH. Neurosurgery Board Review. New York, NY: Thieme; 1997. Reprinted by permission.)

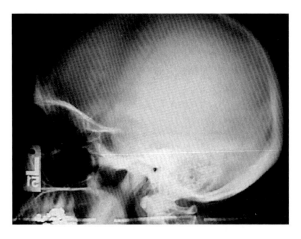

Fig. 3.174 Sellar erosion. Lateral skull x-ray film demonstrates sellar enlargement with absence of the posterior wall of the sella.

P. Bilateral basal ganglia lucencies — caused by stroke, hypoxia, toxicity (cyanide, methanol, manganese, and carbon monoxide), toxoplasmosis, *Cryptococcus,* Leigh disease, Wilson disease (copper deposition), Alexander disease, Canavan disease, metachromatic leukodystrophy, and Hallervorden–Spatz disease (iron deposition) (**Fig. 3.175** and **Fig. 3.176**).

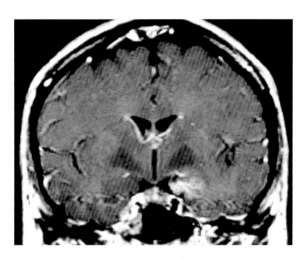

Fig. 3.175 Carbon monoxide toxicity. Coronal T1-weighted magnetic resonance image with bilateral hypointensities in the globus pallidus.

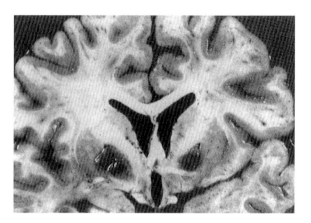

Fig. 3.176 Carbon monoxide poisoning. Gross specimen demonstrating bilateral hemorrhagic necrosis of the globus pallidus. (From Alleyne Jr. CH. Neurosurgery Board Review. New York, NY: Thieme; 1997. Reprinted by permission.)

Q. Bilateral basal ganglia calcifications — caused by Fahr disease, infections, tuberous sclerosis, Down syndrome, NF1, and postanoxic injury

R. Brain aging — associated with increased unidentified bright objects (seen on T2-weighted MRI, also seen with hypertension, diabetes, hypercholesterolemia, and heart disease) and increased iron deposition in the basal ganglia (hypointense on T1-weighted and T2-weighted MRI)

S. Ring enhancing lesions — abscess, metastasis, resolving hematoma, and stroke

T. Brain calcifications — normally occur in the basal ganglia, choroid plexus, pineal gland, habenula, and dentate nucleus

U. Scalp masses

    1. Children — dermoid, eosinophilic granuloma, hamartoma, hemangioma, neurofibroma, and cephalocele

    2. Adults — lipoma, cutis gyrata (redundant scalp tissue), neurofibroma, basal cell carcinoma, meningioma, and metastatic tumors

    3. Orbital lesions — cavernous hemangioma (the most common adult lesion), melanoma (the most common tumor), and retinoblastoma (the most common childhood lesion) (**Fig. 3.177**)

    4. Thick optic nerves — meningioma, pseudotumor, and glioma (**Fig. 3.178**, also see **Figs. 3.66–3.68**)

    5. Small round blue cells in childhood tumors — neuroblastoma, chondrosarcoma, rhabdomyosarcoma, lymphoma, and Ewing tumor

XII. Phakomatoses (Neurocutaneous Diseases)

A. Phakomatoses — a combination of malformative, dysplastic, and neoplastic lesions of the skin and nervous system. They may be hereditary or occur sporadically. All the more common varieties have dominant transmission except Sturge–Weber disease. There are ~20 types. A phakoma is a tumor-like retinal lesion.

B. Neurofibromatosis type I (NF1)

1. Von Recklinghausen NF accounts for 90% of NF, occurs in 1 in 3000 births, autosomal dominant transmission with 100% penetrance, but variable expressivity, and located on chromosome 17. The NF1 gene encodes for neurofibromin. 50% occur by spontaneous mutation without a family history. It usually has an early onset and affects mainly Caucasians. 20% of cases develop CNS lesions. 30% have mental retardation. It is cosmetically disfiguring. 5% develop malignant peripheral nerve sheath tumors, usually after 10 years.

2. Inclusion criteria are at least two of the following: six café au lait spots, two neurofibromas, one plexiform neurofibroma, axillary or inguinal freckling, an osseous lesion (sphenoid dysplasia or thinning of long bones or cortex), an optic glioma, two or more Lisch nodules (iris hamartomas, only seen with NF1) (**Fig. 3.179**), and a relative with NF1.

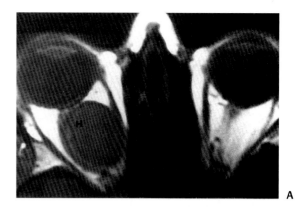

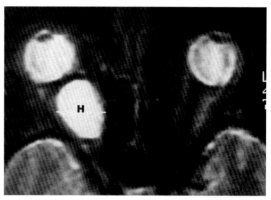

Fig. 3.177 Orbital cavernous hemangioma. (**A**) Axial T1-weighted and (**B**) T2-weighted magnetic resonance images demonstrate cystic orbital mass. (From Valvassori GE, Mafee MF, Carter BL. Imaging of the Head and Neck. New York, NY: Thieme; 1995. Reprinted by permission.)

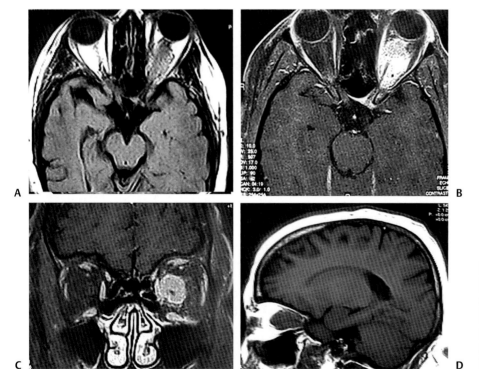

Fig. 3.178 Optic nerve meningioma. (**A**) T1-weighted axial nonenhanced and (**B**) enhanced, (**C**) coronal enhanced and (**D**) sagittal nonenhanced magnetic resonance images demonstrating enhancing mass with central hypointensity.

3. Associated tumors — optic gliomas (20% may be aggressive and they may spread along the optic radiations), low-grade astrocytomas, ependymomas, hamartomas (in the white matter and basal ganglia, no enhancement, no mass effect, and decreases with age), rare unilateral vestibular neuromas and meningiomas, and rare spinal hamartomas and astrocytomas. Malignancies (2–5%) include malignant peripheral nerve sheath tumor, pheochromocytoma, and leukemia.

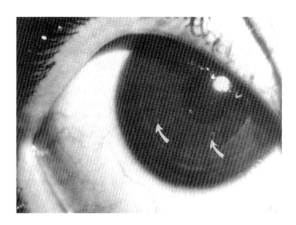

Fig. 3.179   Lisch nodules (*arrows*).

4. Neurofibromas develop on the posterior nerve roots and may be completely intradural (20%) or dumbbell (15%).

5. Other associated conditions — scoliosis, widened spinal canal, posterior vertebral body scalloping (by dural ectasias), patulous dura, meningocele, renal artery stenosis, aqueductal stenosis (by ependymal granulations), seizures, microphthalmia, retinal phakomas, moyamoya-type arterial occlusions, aneurysms, AVMs, mental retardation (5%), and learning disability (40%) (**Fig. 3.180**)

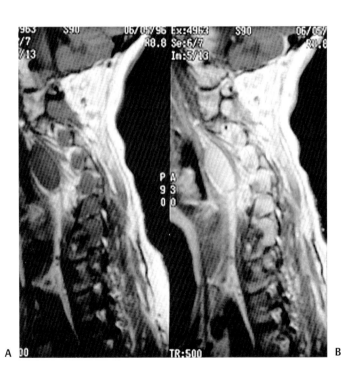

Fig. 3.180   Neurofibromatosis type I. (**A**) Sagittal T1-weighted nonenhanced and (**B**) enhanced magnetic resonance images with multiple enhancing thickened nerve roots. (From Albright AL, Pollack IF, Adelson PD, eds. Principles and Practice of Pediatric Neurosurgery. New York, NY: Thieme; 1999. Reprinted by permission.)

C. Neurofibromatosis type 2 (NF2)

1. Occurs in 1 in 50,000 births, autosomal dominant transmission, located on chromosome 22, and the gene involved is Merlin

2. Associated tumors — bilateral vestibular schwannomas, meningiomas, astrocytomas, hamartomas, spinal ependymomas (spinal astrocytomas are more common in NF1), and nerve root schwannomas. There are less café au lait spots and cutaneous neurofibromas. There are no plexiform neurofibromas or Lisch nodules.

3. Inclusion criteria — bilateral vestibular schwannoma or a relative with NF2 and one vestibular schwannoma or two of the following: neurofibroma, meningioma, glioma, schwannoma, or postcapsular cataract at a young age. 20% have spinal nerve schwannomas (70% are intradural extramedullary, 15% are extradural, and 15% are dumbbell). Two to 10% of people with a vestibular schwannoma have NF2. The osseous changes are caused by tumors, not dural ectasias (**Fig. 3.181**).

D. Tuberous sclerosis complex (TSC)

1. Bourneville disease, autosomal dominant transmission, usually sporadic (there are frequent forme-frustes), located on chromosomes 9 (TSC1, hamartin) and 16 (TSC2, tuberin), and occurs in 1 in 10,000–100,000 births. It may be diagnosed by a facial angiofibroma, periungual and subungual fibromas, or fibrous plaque of the forehead or scalp. The classic triad occurs in <50% of cases and includes mental retardation (two thirds), seizures, and adenoma sebaceum (angiofibromas).

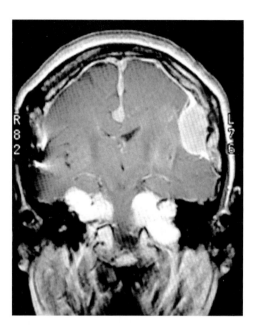

Fig. 3.181 Neurofibromatosis type 2. Enhanced coronal T1-weighted magnetic resonance image with bilateral vestibular schwannomas and meningiomas.

2. Associated tumors
   a. Tubers (seen in 95% of cases) — multiple firm lesions that are hamartomas with large dysplastic neurons and astrocytes in the thalamostriate sulcus, cortex, and subependymal region. These cause candle guttering in the floor of the lateral ventricle, frequently calcify, and occasionally enhance.
   b. Subependymal giant cell astrocytoma (15% of cases) — located near the foramen of Monro, rarely undergoes malignant change, grows slowly, and enhances.
   c. Cardiac rhabdomyoma (30% of cases)
   d. Renal angiomyolipoma (60% of cases)
   e. Cysts in the lung, liver, and spleen
   f. Pancreatic adenoma
   g. Retinal hamartoma (>50% of cases) — rarely affects vision

3. Associated conditions — hydrocephalus (25%), moyamoya changes of cerebral vessels, thoracoabdominal aortic aneurysm, ash-leaf hypopigmented macules, shagreen patches (subepidermal orange peel fibrosis of the lower trunk), and cystic metacarpals. The first symptoms may be "salaam" spasms of flexion myoclonus that can be treated with ACTH; 90% develop skin lesions (usually ash-leaf spots) by 10 years of age. There are frequent behavioral problems (hyperkinetic or aggressive) (**Fig. 3.182** and **Fig. 3.183**).

E. Von Hippel–Lindau disease (VHL)

1. Autosomal dominant transmission and occurs in 1 in 40,000 births. The disease results from mutation of the VHL gene, a classical tumor suppressor gene on chromosome 3. Its gene product, pVHL, is normally involved in the regulation of hypoxia-inducible genes; for example, vascular endothelial, platelet-derived and transforming growth factors. VHL syndrome rarely presents before 20 years and renal cell carcinoma usually occurs near 40 years of age. 20% of hemangioblastomas are in patients with VHL. The

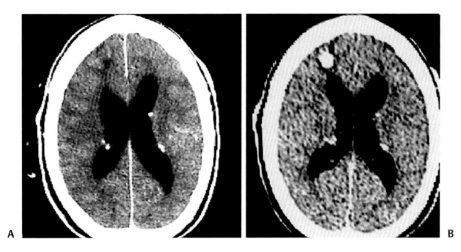

Fig. 3.182 Tuberous sclerosis. (**A**) Nonenhanced and (**B**) enhanced axial computed tomography scans demonstrate multiple calcified tubers lining the lateral ventricles ("candle guttering") and an enhancing right frontal tuber.

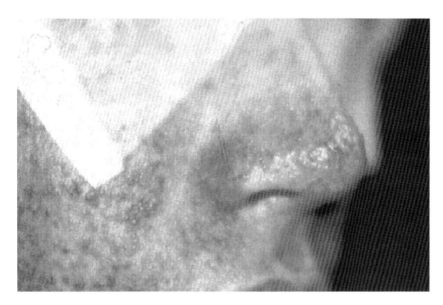

Fig. 3.183 Adenoma sebaceum. Facial lesion with tuberous sclerosis.

cerebellar hemangioblastoma is Lindau tumor. A cerebellar hemangioblastoma with an extra CNS lesion is Lindau disease. A retinal hemangioblastoma is von Hippel tumor. May be associated with polycythemia vera.

2. Associated tumors
   a. Hemangioblastomas (seen in 60% of cases) — cerebellum (65%), brainstem (20%), and spinal cord (15%)
   b. Retinal hemangioblastoma (50% of cases)
   c. Renal cell carcinoma (30% of cases) and angiomatosis
   d. Pheochromocytoma (10% of cases)
   e. Cysts (60% of cases) — liver, pancreas, and kidney
   f. Epididymal cystadenoma

3. Diagnosis—based on multiple CNS hemangioblastomas or one CNS hemangioblastoma and one visceral lesion with a first-order relative with VHL (**Fig. 3.184** and **Fig. 3.185**).

F. Sturge–Weber disease — sporadic transmission. It is characterized by a port-wine stain (facial nevus flammeus, often in the distribution of the first division of the trigeminal nerve) and ipsilateral venous malformation of the leptomeninges (enhances), choroid of the eye, or choroid plexus. There are ipsilateral cortical (especially

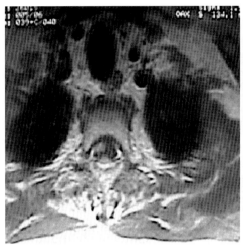

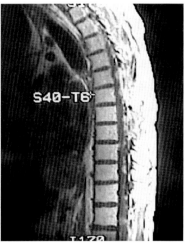

Fig. 3.184 Von Hippel–Lindau syndrome. Enhanced axial (**A**) and sagittal (**B**) T1-weighted thoracic magnetic resonance images demonstrating multiple superficial parenchymal enhancing lesions.

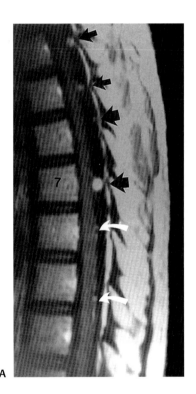

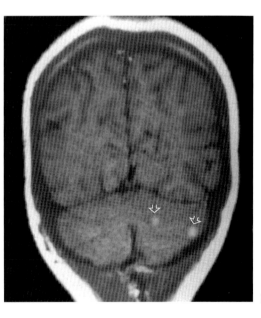

Fig. 3.185 Von Hippel-Lindau disease. (**A**) Enhanced sagittal T1-weighted magnetic resonance image of the thoracic spine demonstrating multiple enhancing dorsal masses. (**B**) Coronal T1-weighted enhanced MRI of the brain demonstrating two enhancing cerebellar hemangioblastomas. (From Ramsey RG. Teaching Atlas of Spine Imaging. New York, NY: Thieme; 1999. Reprinted by permission.)

parietooccipital) tram-track calcifications. Other findings include glaucoma (30–60%), mental retardation, and atrophy of the ipsilateral hemisphere with contralateral seizures, hemiparesis, hemisensory loss, and homonymous hemianopsia. There may be ipsilateral calvarial thickening and a large frontal sinus. The congestion in the cortical draining veins is believed to cause stasis, hypoxia, progressive atrophy, and dystrophic calcifications in the middle layers of the cortical gray matter (**Fig. 3.186**).

G. Osler–Weber–Rendu syndrome — hereditary hemorrhagic telangiectasia (HHT), autosomal dominant transmission with highly variable expressivity and age-dependent penetrance. At a genetic level, mutations in two genes involved in tumor growth factor beta (TGF-β) signal transduction pathways, HHT1 (endoglin, chromosome 9) and HHT2 (ALK1, chromosome 12), result in clinically indistinguishable disease. Haploinsufficiency is thought to cause a deficiency in angiogenesis. Disease is characterized by multiple mucocutaneous telangiectasias (in the skin, GI, and GU tracts), visceral vascular malformations (AVMs of the liver, lung, brain, and spinal cord), and rarely aneurysms. 50% of brain symptoms are due to pulmonary arteriovenous (AV)-fistulas

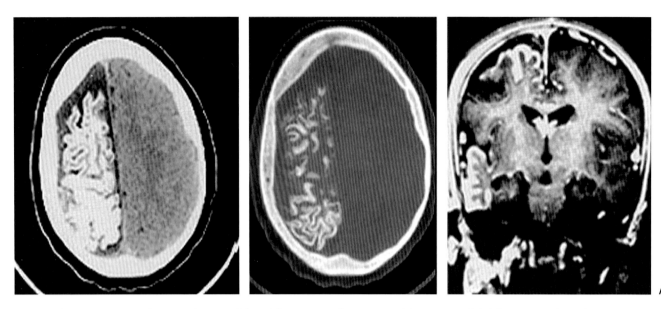

Fig. 3.186 Sturge–Weber syndrome. (**A**) Axial computed tomographic scan and (**B**) bone window demonstrate the "tram track" cortical calcifications and hemispheric atrophy, and (**C**) coronal enhanced T1-weighted magnetic resonance image with enhancing cortical venous malformations and hemiatrophy.

with paradoxical emboli and abscesses. There is increased risk of thrombosis because of polycythemia. Other symptoms include hepatic encephalopathy, GI or GU hemorrhage, and epistaxis (85%). The fragile vessels bleed easily and the red spider-like lesions blanch with pressure. One-third of patients with multiple AVMs have HHT or Wyburn–Mason syndrome.

H. Wyburn–Mason syndrome — unilateral cutaneous vascular nevi of the face and trunk with retinal, optic nerve, visual pathway, and midbrain AVMs. Retinal AVMs are known as racemose angiomas.

I. Ataxia–telangiectasia — oculocutaneous telangiectasias and cerebellar ataxia (caused by anterior vermian atrophy). There is a defect in DNA repair, transmission is autosomal recessive, and symptoms begin in childhood. It is associated with an increase in infections and cancer, and death usually occurs by 20 years.

J. Klippel–Trenaunay–Weber syndrome — angioosteohypertrophy (overgrowth of vessels and bones). One limb is usually enlarged. It is associated with leptomeningeal AVMs (some spinal) and dermatomal cutaneous hemangiomas.

K. Epidermal nevus syndrome — ipsilateral nevus and bone thickening associated with mental retardation, seizures, hemiparesis, and gyral malformations

XIII. Intoxications and Drugs

A. Carbon monoxide — hemoglobin binds carbon monoxide 250 times more avidly than it does O_2. Carbon monoxide also impedes oxygen release. When the hemoglobin is 25% saturated with carbon monoxide (carboxyhemoglobin), the patient may develop headaches, at 45% confusion, at 55% seizures and coma, and > 70% death from dysrhythmia. A cherry-red brain develops with bilateral necrosis of the medial segment of the GP (**Fig. 3.175** and **Fig. 3.176**).

B. Cyanide — binds cytochrome oxidase and halts cellular respiration. This leads to cerebral edema, SAH, respiratory failure, seizures, and death.

C. Ethanol (ETOH)

1. Chronic use — associated with infection, peripheral neuropathy, stroke, cerebral atrophy (especially white matter), and ventricular enlargement. The changes may be caused by a direct toxic effect or by associated nutritional deficits (possibly thiamine). ETOH cerebellar degeneration involves the superior vermis and causes leg ataxia with a wide-based gait. ETOH use is associated with central pontine myelinolysis (CPM), Wernicke–Korsakoff syndrome (see section XVI), cardiomyopathy, myopathy, and Marchiafava–Bignami disease.

2. A serum ETOH level >450 mg/dL is usually lethal unless there is substantial tolerance.

3. ETOH withdrawal — tremulousness (1–2 days), hallucinations/illusions (1–2 days), seizures (24 hours), and delirium tremens (2–4 days, 5–15% fatal, confusion, delusions, hallucinations, tremor, sleeplessness, and autonomic overactivity with tachycardia, hyperthermia, increased sweating, and mydriasis). Treat withdrawal with chlordiazepoxide or benzodiazepines such as diazepam.

D. Fetal ETOH syndrome

1. The world's leading cause of mental retardation and birth defects. The fetus is most susceptible shortly after conception, and high levels in the first 2 months may be teratogenic.

2. Manifestations
   a. CNS dysfunction — mental retardation, seizures, decreased white matter, periventricular heterotopias, hypotonicity, and cerebellar dysfunction
   b. Craniofacial deformities — short palpebral fissures, epicanthal folds, low nasal bridge, short up-turned nose, cleft palate, hypoplastic upper lip, and microcephaly
   c. Short body and decreased postnatal growth

E. Methanol — a potential contaminant in homemade liquor such as "moonshine." It is converted by ETOH dehydrogenase to formaldehyde and formic acid (blocks cellular respiration). It causes necrosis of the lateral putamen and claustrum, optic disk swelling (caused by ischemia at the border zone between the CNS and the optic blood supply), edema, anion-gap metabolic acidosis, nausea, and vomiting. Blindness may develop after ingestion of 4 mL and death after ingestion of 100 mL.

F. Ethylene glycol — antifreeze. It is converted to glycoaldehyde and glycolic acid, and causes edema, Ca^{2+} oxalate crystal deposition in the blood vessels, and anion-gap metabolic acidosis. Ingestion of 100 mL may be lethal.

G. Isopropyl alcohol — rubbing alcohol, does not cause acidosis. Ingestion of 250 mL is lethal.

H. Hexachlorophene — germicide. It is absorbed through the skin and when exposure is excessive causes spongiform degeneration of white matter.

I. Dilantin — causes atrophy of the Purkinje and granular cell layers of the cerebellum. It also causes congenital fetal hydantoin syndrome with growth retardation, mental retardation, craniofacial deformities, limb deformities, microcephaly, hydrocephalus, and neural tube defects. It may also lead to gingival hyperplasia and calvarial thickening.

J. Opiates — cause hypothermia, decreased respiration, miosis, constipation, urinary retention, pruritus, and sphincter of Oddi spasm (pancreatitis). Treat overdose with naloxone. Withdrawal may occur after 16 hours with rhinorrhea, lacrimation, sweating, insomnia, mydriasis, twitches, and cold/hot flashes, after 36 hours with diarrhea, and peaks at 72 hours. It is usually only potentially fatal in infants. Withdrawal can be treated with methadone, a narcotic with less euphoria and less production of desire for more narcotics.

K. Barbiturates

1. They bind GABA A receptors at the α and β subunits, are metabolized in the liver, and are excreted from the kidney.

2. They cause decreased mental status, respiratory rate, blood pressure, temperature, deep tendon reflexes, and pupillary reactivity. Chronic use causes dysarthria, nystagmus, and incoordination. Severe intoxication causes slow and shallow respirations, coma, pulmonary edema, retention of mild pupillary reflexes, decreased brainstem reflexes, and a flat EEG.

3. Clearance is proportional to urine output and may be increased by fluid boluses. Bicarbonate increases excretion of phenobarbital only. Dialysis may be necessary.

4. Withdrawal may occur in 12–72 hours with insomnia, hypotension, tremor, seizures, rapid eye movement sleep rebound, and death. Treat with phenobarbital and attempt to wean over 14–21 days.

L. Benzodiazepines — safer, less addictive, less respiratory suppression, less hypotension, and less hypnotic than barbiturates. They bind GABA A receptors at the gamma subunit to increase Cl⁻ influx for postsynaptic inhibition, and affect the cortex (decreases seizures) and the limbic system (decreases anxiety).

M. Antipsychotic medications — neuroleptics and psychotropics. They block postsynaptic dopaminergic D1 and D2 receptors. The D2 receptors are in the frontal cortex, hippocampus, and limbic system. The D1 receptors are in the striatum, and blockage causes Parkinson-like side effects and increased PRL.

1. Phenothiazines — chlorpromazine and prochlorperazine have antiemetic, antihistamine, and antischizophrenic activities. Side effects include
   a. Parkinsonian side effects that develop within 3 weeks. Treatment is with anticholinergics.
   b. Dystonia of the face and tongue, torticollis, and dyskinesia (tonic spasm of limbs) that develops early. Treatment is with diphenhydramine or amantadine.
   c. Akathisia/restlessness treated with propranolol.
   d. Tardive dyskinesia (dystonic movements of the limbs and trunk) that develops late. It occurs by hypersensitivity to DA in the basal ganglia or decreased GABA.
   e. Neuroleptic malignant syndrome — hyperthermia, increased serum creatine kinase (CK), autonomic instability, rigidity, stupor, and catatonia. It is most common with haloperidol and fluphenazine. Mortality is 20%. It occurs from blockage of DA receptors in the basal ganglia and hypothalamus. Treatment is with dantrolene or bromocriptine.
   f. Cholestatic jaundice, agranulocytosis, seizures, orthostatic hypotension, and mental status changes

2. Butyrophenones — Haloperidol has similar side effects to phenothiazines, but without any antiadrenergic action and is also used to treat Tourette syndrome and Huntington disease.

N. Marchiafava–Bignami disease — rare, demyelination, and necrosis of the genu and body of the corpus callosum. It was first described in Italian men drinking inexpensive red wine. Symptoms include dementia, depression, apathy, and delusions.

O. Central pontine myelinolysis (CPM) — occurs with rapid correction of hyponatremia. It is probably an osmotic injury to the vascular endothelium that disrupts the BBB and causes edema. It affects oligodendrocytes where gray matter is interspersed with white matter (mainly in the pons). Pathologic examination reveals demyelination and necrosis with preserved axons and neurons and absence of inflammatory cells. Symptoms include quadriparesis, hyperreflexia, seizures, coma, and pseudobulbar palsy. It may lead to death in severe cases (**Fig. 3.187** and **Fig. 3.188**).

P. Antidepressants

   1. Monoamine oxidase inhibitors — increase NE, 5-HT, and epinephrine levels and increase NE release. They increase heart rate and blood pressure. Side effects include hypertension, especially with phenothiazines, stimulants, tricyclic antidepressants, tyramine, cheese, red wine, and beer.

   2. Tricyclic antidepressants — decrease the reuptake of amines and thus increase the levels of NE and 5-HT, and decrease acetylcholine (ACh; urinary retention and orthostatic hypotension). Side effects include insomnia and agitation that can be treated with phenothiazine at night. These should not be taken with monamine oxidase inhibitors.

   3. Lithium — used to treat bipolar disease. Side effects include nephrogenic diabetes insipidus and asterixis; overdose causes ataxia, nystagmus, and coma with levels >3.5. It should be dosed carefully with renal insufficiency or thiazides.

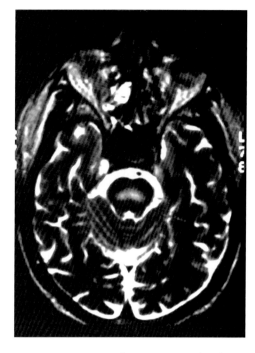

Fig. 3.187 Central pontine myelinolysis. Axial T2-weighted magnetic resonance image with central pontine hyperintensity.

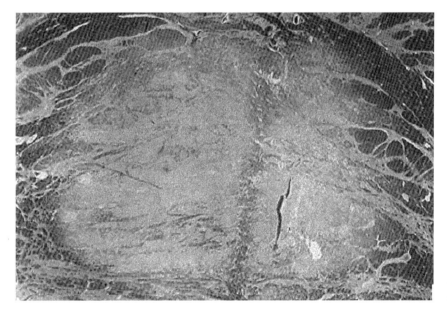

Fig. 3.188 Central pontine myelinolysis (Luxol fast blue stain). Central demyelination with rim of preserved myelin.

Q. Stimulants

   1. Amphetamines (analeptics) — increase respiratory rate and blood pressure and decrease appetite. They are used to treat children with attention deficit disorder, fatigue, obesity, and narcolepsy. Intoxication causes hallucinations, SAH, and vasculitis.

   2. Methylphenidate — used to treat narcolepsy and children with attention deficit disorder

   3. Caffeine — causes hyperglycemia, diuresis, and cardiac stimulation

XIV. Chemotherapy

A. Methotrexate — folic acid antagonist. It can cause meningitis, encephalitis, transverse myelitis, stroke, sub-acute necrotizing leukoencephalitis (with coagulation necrosis, lipid-laden macrophages, absence of inflammatory cells, mineralizing angiopathy of the gray matter, and mainly affects astrocytes) that is seen when used with radiation (**Fig. 3.189**).

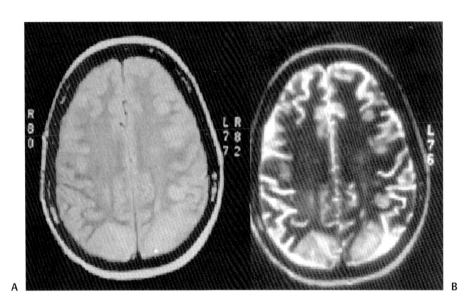

A   B

Fig. 3.189 Methotrexate toxicity. (**A**) Axial proton density and (**B**) T2-weighted magnetic resonance images demonstrate the bilateral symmetric demyelinating lesions.

B. Cisplatin — causes neurosensory hearing loss, visual loss, leukoencephalopathy, and sensory and autonomic neuropathy involving axons and myelin

C. Vincristine — used to treat lymphoma and leukemia, impairs microtubule formation, and causes axonal degeneration with peripheral neuropathy. The BBB spares CNS of vincristine's effects, but it is lethal by respiratory failure if injected intrathecally; may have decreased antidiuretic hormone (ADH) secretion.

D. Nitrosurea (BCNU) — associated with necrotizing encephalomyelopathy with arterial obliteration and axonal swelling if given arterially; directly implanted in the tumor bed to treat GBM

E. Procarbazine — used to treat malignant gliomas, pulmonary carcinoma, and Hodgkin disease; causes mood changes

F. Temozolomide — myelosuppression with neutropenia and thrombocytopenia

XV. Metal Toxicities

A. Arsenic — from insecticides. It causes encephalopathy, peripheral neuropathy, abdominal pain, nausea and vomiting, diarrhea, and shock. Chronic exposure causes malaise, transverse white lines (Mees lines) on the fingernails, and increased pigment and hyperkeratosis on the palms and soles. It can be detected in hair and urine. Treatment is with 2,3-dimercaptopropanol (BAL).

B. Lead (plumbism) — causes encephalitis in children (pica from paint ingestion) that manifests as irritability, seizures, abdominal pain, ataxia, coma, and increased ICP. In adults, it causes pure motor demyelinating peripheral neuropathy (especially the radial nerve with wrist drop), anemia, and a gingival lead line. Diagnosis is by erythrocyte basophilic stippling, long bone metaphyseal lead lines, increased serum lead levels, and increased urinary coproporphyrin and delta-aminolevulinic acid. Treatment is with ethylenediaminetetraacetic acid (EDTA), BAL, and penicillamine.

C. Mercury — from contaminated fish ingestion and exposure to felt hat dyes. It causes psychologic dysfunction ("mad as a hatter"), tremor, movement disorders, peripheral neuropathy, cerebellar signs, GI dysfunction, and renal tubular necrosis. Treatment is with penicillamine. BAL actually increases mercury levels in the brain.

D. Manganese — occurs in miners. It causes parkinsonian symptoms, psychologic disorders, and headache. There is neuronal loss and gliosis in the pallidum and striatum. The symptoms are improved with l-DOPA. Chelator medications do not help.

XVI. Vitamin Deficiencies

A. Thiamine deficiency

1. It is common with chronic alcoholics, GI tumors, dialysis, IV feedings, and gastric plication. Thiamine is needed as a cofactor for some enzymes, especially those involved in carbohydrate metabolism. The mamillary bodies, which are frequently affected, have the highest transketolase activity in the normal brain. There may be abnormal release of excitatory neurotransmitters in Wernicke encephalopathy and decreased 5-HT in Korsakoff psychosis. Deficiency is more frequent in Europe because of hereditary thiamine binding to transketolase.

2. Wernicke encephalopathy
   a. It causes conjugate gaze and lateral rectus palsies, nystagmus, gait ataxia, and confusion. Rarely, it may lead to coma, hypotension, and hypothermia.
   b. It affects the mamillary bodies, mediodorsal nucleus of the thalamus, periaqueductal gray, floor of the fourth ventricle (dorsal motor nuclei of X and the vestibular nuclei), and superior cerebellar vermis. The gaze palsies are related to CNs III and VI nuclei lesions, nystagmus to vestibular nuclei lesions, and ataxia to superior cerebellar vermian lesions.
   c. It involves both the gray and white matter, causing a brown-gray discoloration, edema, hemorrhage, demyelination, necrosis, loss of Purkinje cells, and reactive astrocytosis.
   d. Laboratory findings include increased pyruvate and thymidine triphosphate, and decreased transketolase.
   e. Mortality is 17% and is usually due to infection or associated cirrhosis. Treatment is with thiamine 50 mg IV and then 50 mg intramuscularly daily, until normal diet is resumed. Ocular movements recover first, and horizontal nystagmus and ataxia tend to persist longer.

3. Korsakoff psychosis — a more chronic disorder characterized by deterioration in retrograde and anterograde memory. There is frequently unintentional confabulation by poor memory of recent events. It is usually associated with Wernicke encephalopathy. Lesions are in the dorsomedial thalamus. HSV or tumors involving the inferomedial temporal lobe may also cause a similar syndrome. Complete recovery occurs in 20% of patients.

4. Beriberi — most common in rice eaters. It causes peripheral neuropathy with axonal degeneration and demyelination, autonomic dysfunction (orthostatic hypotension), and rarely heart disease.

B. Niacin — most common in corn eaters by deficiency of tryptophan that it is used to synthesize niacin. The deficiency causes pellagra resulting in the "3Ds": dermatitis, diarrhea, and dementia.

C. Vitamin B$_{12}$ (cobalamin)

1. Deficiency is usually caused by decreased intrinsic factor production from pernicious anemia (autoimmune attack on gastric cells), tumors, infection, parasites, and surgery.

2. Vitamin B_{12} binds intrinsic factor (made by the gastric parietal cells) and is absorbed in the ileum.

3. Deficiency causes megaloblastic anemia (mean corpuscular volume >100), hypersegmented polymorphonuclear leucocytes (PMN), glossitis, anorexia, and diarrhea. Subacute combined degeneration of the spinal cord involves the lower cervical and upper thoracic posterior and lateral columns and causes spongiform demyelination, impaired vibration, proprioception sensation, and paraplegia. The posterior columns are affected first. It may also cause visual deterioration, mental deterioration, and symmetric peripheral neuropathy.

4. Nitrous oxide from inhalation anesthesia inactivates vitamin B_{12} and may increase symptoms.

5. Diagnosis is made by hypersegmented PMNs on a peripheral blood smear, megaloblastic anemia, and vitamin B_{12} assay. The most reliable indication of decreased intracellular cobalamin is increased serum methylmalonic acid and homocysteine.

6. Treatment is with B_{12} injections. If treatment is with folic acid, the anemia may be corrected, but the neurologic symptoms may worsen (**Fig. 3.190**).

D. Pyridoxine (vitamin B_6) — deficiency is seen with isoniazid and hydralazine treatment and causes lower limb paresthesias, pain, and weakness.

E. Vitamin A — deficiency causes decreased vision. Increased levels have been associated with pseudotumor and increased ICP.

F. Vitamin D — deficiency causes rickets with decreased parathyroid hormone and decreased bone strength.

G. Vitamin E — deficiency is associated with biliary atresia and cystic fibrosis (impaired fat absorption) and causes thick dystrophic axons in the posterior columns with polyneuropathy. Patients may develop ataxia and ophthalmoplegia.

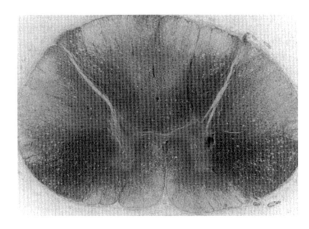

Fig. 3.190 Subacute combined degeneration (Luxol fast blue stain). Spongy degeneration of predominantly the posterior and lateral columns. (From Alleyne Jr. CH. Neurosurgery Board Review. New York, NY: Thieme; 1997. Reprinted by permission.)

XVII. Acquired Metabolic Diseases and Bacterial Toxins

A. Serum osmolarity = $2(Na^+ + K^+) + BUN/28 + Glucose/18$

B. Hypercarbia causes asterixis, papilledema, and elevated ICP.

C. Hypoglycemia <30 mg/dL causes symptoms and <10 mg/dL causes coma.

D. Hepatic encephalopathy

1. It causes asterixis, mental status changes, and EEG slow waves. The serum ammonia is usually >200 mg/dL.

2. Alzheimer type II protoplasmic astrocytes form in the deep cortex, basal ganglia, thalamus, SN, cerebellum, and pontine nuclei.

3. The increased ammonia that is not converted to urea in the liver may cause increased GABA.

4. Symptoms are worse with constipation, increased protein intake, and GI hemorrhage.

5. Treatment is by decreasing protein intake, ingesting lactulose, and neomycin orally to control colon flora.

E. Reye syndrome — nonicteric hepatic encephalopathy that develops in children with influenza B or varicella and often who have received acetylsalicylic acid. The brain swells and the liver becomes fatty. Mortality is 10%.

F. Uremic encephalopathy — no edema is present. The mechanism is unknown. A postdialysis headache lasts for 8–48 hours. Uremia also produces a peripheral polyneuropathy.

G. Syndrome of inappropriate secretion of ADH (SIADH) — caused by trauma, infection, stroke, medications, and tumors

H. Hypokalemia — causes muscle weakness, constipation, propensity to cardiac arrhythmias, and occasionally mental status changes

I. Hyperkalemia — causes muscle weakness and cardiac arrest

J. Central pontine myelinolysis (CPM) — there is no inflammation. There is myelin loss in the pons and occasionally in other sites. It is associated with rapid correction of hyponatremia in patients with ETOH abuse, malnutrition, renal failure, and burns. Symptoms may include quadriparesis, locked-in syndrome, and pseudobulbar palsy. See section XI.

K. Hypoparathyroidism — causes hypocalcemia with tetany, cramps, and seizures. Ca^{2+} deposits may form in the basal ganglia, dentate nucleus, and cortex and cause choreoathetosis, rigidity, and ataxia.

L. Hyperthyroidism — causes tremor

M. Hypothyroidism — causes apathy and neuropathy. If it occurs early in life, it causes cretinism with jaundice, mottled skin, wide posterior fontanel, mental retardation, spasticity, and deafness. If it occurs later, it causes myxedema.

N. Tetanus

1. Caused by *Clostridium tetani*. The exotoxin may enter through a cut and move to the CNS by means of the peripheral nerves.

2. It produces presynaptic excitation of agonist and antagonist muscles (especially the masseter causing lockjaw or trismus) by inhibiting the neurotransmitter release of glycine from inhibitory interneurons such as Renshaw cells in the spinal cord. Tetanus toxin specifically cleaves synaptobrevin.

3. Local tetanus occurs with wounds on the extremities, causes tightness and spasms, and disappears over a few weeks. Cephalic tetanus occurs with facial wounds. Generalized tetanus is the most common and causes diffuse spasms, trismus, and apnea. It has a 50% mortality.

4. The clinical picture is similar to strychnine poisoning, black widow spider bite, and stiff-man syndrome.

5. Electromyography (EMG) reveals a loss of the silent period after contraction with continuous discharge of normal motor units.

6. Treatment is with antitoxin, penicillin, and wound debridement. Diazepam, pharmacological neuromuscular blockade, and intubation/tracheostomy may be needed. Active immunization with a booster should be obtained every 10 years.

O. Diphtheria — from *Corynebacterium diphtheriae* and causes throat and tracheal inflammatory exudate with exotoxins that affect the heart and nerves, causing ascending paralysis and cardiomyopathy. It is distinguished by early bulbar and ciliary dysfunction and delayed symmetric sensorimotor peripheral neuropathy with demyelination. Treatment is with antitoxin.

P. Botulism — from *Clostridia botulinum*, obtained by contamination in home-canned vegetables or from wound infections. The exotoxin causes presynaptic inhibition at the neuromuscular junction by decreasing ACh release (similar to Eaton–Lambert syndrome). It cleaves target synaptosome associated protein (SNAP) and N-ethylmaleimide-sensitive factor (NSF) attachment receptors (t-SNAREs) and vesicles SNAREs (v-SNAREs). Symptoms include blurred vision, unreactive pupils, diplopia, bulbar paralysis, and then respiratory suppression and quadriparesis in a descending pattern that evolves over 2–4 days. There are no sensory changes. Diagnose by EMG that may have an incremental response like Eaton–Lambert syndrome. Extraocular muscles recover first. Treatment is with antiserum, guanidine, and supportive respiratory care.

Q. Black widow spider venom — depletes the presynaptic ACh stores into the neuromuscular junction, causing cramps and spasms followed by weakness. Treatment is with Ca^{2+} gluconate and $MgSO_4$.

XVIII. Congenital Metabolic Diseases

A. Many of these diseases affect neonates and thus a good neonatal neurologic examination is necessary. Assess for diencephalic function (alertness and responsivity), brainstem, and cerebellar function (automatisms such as sucking, rooting, swallowing, and grasping), reticulospinal/cerebellar/spinal function (posture and movements), midbrain and pons function (eye movements), upper brainstem and spinal function with cortical facilitation (Moro/startle and placing reactions), and hypothalamic function (respiration, thirst, and temperature). Monitor food intake to detect failure to thrive.

B. Aminoacidopathies — there are 48 types and they cause mental retardation by 2 years.

1. Phenylketonuria — the most frequent type. Deficiency of phenylalanine hydroxylase in the liver that is needed to convert phenylalanine to tyrosine. Phenylalanine accumulates and causes defective myelination. Inheritance is autosomal recessive on chromosome 12. Diagnose by increased urine phenylpyruvic acid and serum phenylalanine. Typically, it affects fair-skinned children with blue eyes and causes a musty odor. Treatment is by limiting intake of l-phenylalanine to decrease mental retardation.

2. Homocystinuria — causes a defect in methionine metabolism. There is decreased collagen and elastin in vessels. There is increased homocysteine in the blood, urine, and CSF. Inheritance is autosomal recessive with a deficiency of cystathionine β-synthase on chromosome 21. It is physically similar to Marfan syndrome (tall and thin), but with mental retardation and increased incidence of stroke, lens dislocations, and arachnodactyly.

3. Maple syrup urine disease — causes decreased branched-chain amino acid catabolism. Inheritance is autosomal recessive with a deficiency of branched-chain α-keto acid dehydrogenase. Death occurs by 4 weeks unless leucine, isoleucine, and valine intake is limited. Symptoms present in the first week of life as poor feeding, vomiting, failure to thrive; patients have a characteristic "burned sugar smell of the urine."

4. Hartnup disease — autosomal recessive disorder with a defect in neutral amino acid transport in the proximal tubule of the nephron with inability to reabsorb neutral amino acids. They develop niacin deficiency with pellagra-like symptoms.

C. Sphingolipidoses — lysosomal storage diseases caused by enzyme deficiency with accumulation in the lysosomes of various products from glycolytic or peptide degradation. There is accumulation of lipids including cholesterol, cerebrosides, and phospholipids. Sphingomyelin is a phospholipid with sphingosine. Ceramide is sphingosine with a long chain fatty acid. Sphingomyelin is ceramide and phosphocholine. Cerebroside is ceramide and a hexose. Ganglioside is ceramide and sialic acid. Gray matter has more gangliosides and less phospholipids than white matter. White matter is 60% lipid, whereas gray matter is 35%. Accumulation of these products damages neurons and myelin sheaths (**Table 3.2**).

Table 3.2 Sphingolipidoses

Disease	Genetics	Enzyme Deficiency	Histology	Clinical Presentation
Gaucher	AR	Glucocerebrosidase	Foamy histiocytes	MR, spasticity, HSM, CRS
Niemann–Pick	AR	Sphingomyelinase	Foam cells	CRS, motor decline, HSM
Fabry	XR	α-Galactosidase		Pain, dysesthesias, strokes
Tay-Sachs	AR	Hexosaminidase A	GM_2 gangliosides	CRS, hypotonia, seizures
Sandhoff	AR	Hexosaminidase A & Hexosaminidase B	GM_2 gangliosides	Like Tay-Sachs but have organomegaly

Abbreviations: AR, autosomal recessive; XR, x-linked recessive; MR, mental retardation; HSM, hepatosplenomegaly; CRS, cherry red spot.

1. Niemann-Pick disease — caused by a deficiency of sphingomyelinase with accumulation of sphingomyelin and cholesterol. Inheritance is autosomal recessive with chromosomal abnormalities on 11 and 18. It occurs usually in infants 3 to 9 months with death in 2 years. There is a predilection for Ashkenazi Jews. It can cause a cherry-red spot (50%), supranuclear paresis of vertical gaze, psychomotor retardation, hepatosplenomegaly, and normal head size. (Cherry red spots develop as the retinal ganglion cells enlarge and finally burst from intracellular accumulation of lipids; thus, the red choroid is seen through the retina upon funduscopic examination). Niemann–Pick cells or "foam cells" are large vacuolated histiocytes and lymphocytes. Accumulation occurs in the brainstem, cerebellum, spinal cord, and visceral organs.

2. Gaucher disease — the most frequent sphingolipidosis. There is a deficiency of glucocerebrosidase with accumulation of glucocerebrosides. Inheritance is autosomal recessive. It usually develops in late childhood and is usually nonneuropathic with accumulation in the liver, spleen, marrow, and lung with symptomatic hypersplenism with anemia and thrombocytopenia. There are rare infantile and juvenile forms affecting neurons and causing death by 2 years. There is a predilection for Ashkenazi Jews. Gaucher cells have wrinkled tissue paper appearance from stored glucocerebroside. Patient may develop cherry red spots.

3. Fabry disease — caused by a deficiency of α-galactosidase with accumulation of ceramides. Inheritance is X-linked recessive with onset in adolescence. It causes painful dysesthesias. Deposits accumulate in blood vessel walls, cornea, kidneys, cardiac muscle fibers, and noncortical neurons. Symptoms include hypertension, renal failure, congestive heart failure (CHF), and death by myocardial infarction or stroke usually in the sixth decade.

4. Tay–Sachs disease — caused by a deficiency of hexosaminidase A with accumulation of GM_2 gangliosides. Inheritance is autosomal recessive with onset by 6 months and death by 4 years. There is a predilection for Ashkenazi Jews. It causes cherry-red spots with macrocephaly without visceromegaly. Accumulation occurs in the gray matter.

5. Sandhoff disease — caused by a deficiency of hexosaminidase A and B with accumulation of GM_2 gangliosides. There is no predilection for Jews. It has a similar clinical picture to Tay–Sachs disease, but has visceral storage in the liver, spleen, kidney, and heart.

6. GM_1 gangliosidosis — caused by a deficiency of acid β-galactosidase with accumulation of GM_1 gangliosides. Inheritance is autosomal recessive with onset in 3 months and death in 2 years. There is both CNS and visceral involvement with dysmorphic face, cherry-red maculae, hepatosplenomegaly, bone abnormalities, and contractures.

D. Mucopolysaccharidoses — enzyme deficiencies of mucopolysaccharide degradation producing lipid accumulation in the lysosomes of the gray matter (causing neuronal death) and polysaccharide accumulation in the connective tissue (**Table 3.3**).

Table 3.3 Mucopolysaccharidoses

Syndrome	Genetics	Enzyme Deficiency	Urine Sulfate Metabolites	Clinical Presentation
Hurler	AR	α-L-iduronidase	Heparan and dermatan	MR, corneal opacification, gargoyle facie, dwarfism
Scheie	AR	α-L-iduronidase	Heparan and dermatan	Milder form of Hurler; skin pebbling
Hunter	XR	Iduronidase sulfatase	Heparan and dermatan	CTS
Sanfilippo	AR	Sulfamidase	Heparan	MR, ataxia, dysostosis multiplex, seizures
Morquio	AR	β-Galactosidase	Keratin	Atlantoaxial subluxation, dens hypoplasia
Maroteaux–Lamy	AR	Sulfatase B	Dermatan	CTS
Sly	AR	β-Glucuronidase	Heparan and Dermatan	MR, dwarfism, HCP

Abbreviations: AR, autosomal recessive; CTS, carpal tunnel syndrome; HCP, hydrocephalus; MR, mental retardation; XR, x-linked recessive.

1. Hurler disease — caused by a deficiency of α-l-iduronidase with accumulation of mucopolysaccharides (MPS). The urine contains heparin and dermatan sulfate. Inheritance is autosomal recessive with onset at 1 year and death by 5–10 years from cardiac or respiratory causes. Symptoms include gargoyle face, mental retardation, dwarfism, corneal opacities, conduction deafness, hepatosplenomegaly, cardiac dysfunction, skeletal abnormalities, and thick meninges that may cause spinal cord compression. Neurons are enlarged (**Fig. 3.191** and **Fig. 3.192**). On electron microscopy, can see Zebra bodies.

2. Scheie syndrome is a milder rare form of Hurler disease with autosomal recessive inheritance. There is no mental retardation or neuronal storage. It may produce spinal cord compression from thickened dura, corneal opacities, and carpal tunnel syndrome.

3. Hunter syndrome — caused by a deficiency of iduronate sulfatase. Inheritance is X-linked recessive. The urine contains heparin and dermatan sulfate. Presentation is similar to Hurler disease but milder, with no mental retardation, less corneal clouding, and slower progression. There is a characteristic skin pebbling and peripheral nerve entrapment. Patients may survive to adulthood.

4. Sanfilippo syndrome — caused by deficiencies of heparin sulfate pathways, for example, sulfamidase. The urine contains heparin sulfate. Inheritance is autosomal recessive. It produces mental retardation, ataxia, dysostosis multiplex, and seizures but less corneal clouding and dwarfism.

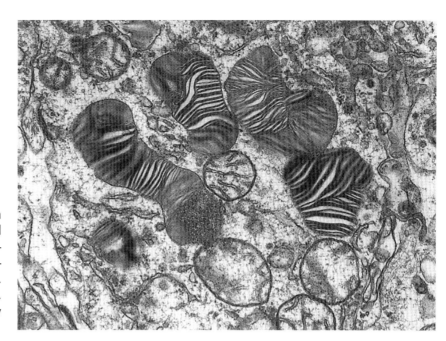

Fig. 3.191 Hurler disease (electron micrograph). "Zebra bodies" of stored gangliosides. (From Schochet SS Jr. Intoxications and disease of the central nervous system. In Nelson JS, Parisi JE, Schochet SS Jr, eds. Principles and Practice of Neuropathology. St. Louis, MO: Mosby; 1993:334. Reprinted by permission.)

5. Morquio syndrome — caused by a deficiency of galactose 6-sulfatase and β-galactosidase. The urine contains keratan sulfate. Inheritance is autosomal recessive. There is no mental retardation, but severe skeletal deformities with ligamentous laxities, odontoid hypoplasia, and thick cervical dura with cervical myelopathy, dwarfism, and osteoporosis.

6. Maroteaux–Lamy disease — caused by a deficiency of sulfatase B. The urine contains dermatan sulfate. Inheritance is autosomal recessive. There is no mental retardation, but there may be carpal tunnel syndrome and valvular heart disease.

7. Sly syndrome — caused by a deficiency of β-glucuronidase. The urine contains dermatan sulfate, heparan sulfate, and chondroitin sulfate. Inheritance is autosomal recessive. There is moderate mental retardation, corneal clouding, hydrocephalus, hepatosplenomegaly, and bony changes.

E. Leukodystrophies — caused by enzyme deficiencies with abnormal formation, destruction, or maintenance of myelin. They mainly affect white matter (**Table 3.4**).

1. Krabbe disease (globoid cell leukodystrophy) — caused by a deficiency of galactocerebroside β-galactosidase on chromosome 14 with accumulation of galactocerebroside from myelin sheaths in lysosomes. Inheritance is autosomal recessive with onset 3–6 months and death by 2 years. It causes psychomotor delay and microcephaly.

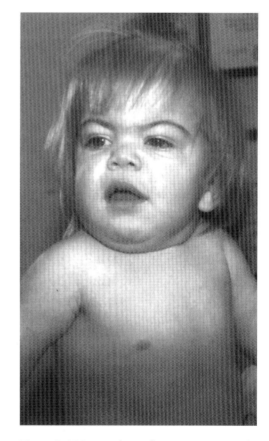

Fig. 3.192 Hurler disease. "Gargoyle face." (From Matalon RK: Disorders of mucopolysaccharide metabolism. In Nelson WE, senior ed., Behrman RE, Kliegman RM, Avrin AM, eds. Nelson Textbook of Pediatrics. 15th ed. Philadelphia, PA: WB Saunders; 1996:398. Reprinted by permission.)

Table 3.4 Leukodystrophies

Disease	Genetics	Enzyme Deficiency	Histology	Clinical Presentation
Krabbe	AR	β-Galactosidase	Globoid macrophages; psychosine build-up	Spasms, motor loss
Metachromatic leukodystrophy	AR	Arylsulfatase A	PAS+ macrophages	Ataxia, motor loss
Adrenoleukodystrophy	XR	ABCD1	Perivascular inflammation	Cognitive decline, adrenal insufficiency
Pelizaeus– Merzbacher	XR	PLP-1	CNS demyelination	Ataxia, nystagmus
Canavan	AR	Aspartoacylase	Spongy WM U fibers affected. Alz type II astrocytes	Blindness, motor loss, megaencephaly
Alexander	Unknown	GFAP mutation	Rosenthal fibers	Seizures, MR
Refsum	AR	Phytanic acid α-hydroxylase	Onion-bulbs in PNS	Motor and sensory loss, blindness, ataxia

Abbreviations: ABCD1, ATP binding cassette, subfamily D (ALD), member 1 gene; Alz, Alzheimer; AR, autosomal recessive; CNS, central nervous system; GFAP, glial fibrillary acidic protein; MR, mental retardation; PAS, periodic acid Schiff reaction; PLP-1, proteolipid protein-1; PNS, peripheral nervous system; WM, white matter; XR, x-linked recessive.

There is cavitation of the white matter, with sparing of the subcortical U-fibers. The basal ganglia and thalamus appear hyperdense on CT. Globoid cells are large macrophages around blood vessels. Psychosine accumulation kills oligodendrocytes.

2. Metachromatic leukodystrophy — the most common leukodystrophy. There is a deficiency of arylsulfatase A with accumulation of sulfatides in lysosomes. Inheritance is autosomal recessive on chromosome 22 with usually late infantile onset at 1–4 years with death in 3 years. It causes psychomotor deterioration. There is cavitation of the white matter with sparing of the subcortical U-fibers and degeneration of PNS myelin. It also damages the liver, spleen, and kidneys. The Hirsh–Peiffer reaction is with acidic cresyl-violet aniline dye causing cells with sulfatides to change to a brown color instead of purple (**Fig. 3.193**).

3. Adrenoleukodystrophy — caused by a deficiency of lipid oxidation in peroxisomes with accumulation of long chain fatty acids. It involves the ATP binding cassette, subfamily D (ALD), member 1 (ABCD1 gene). Inheritance is X-linked recessive so it affects males. Onset is 3–10 years with death in 3–5 years.

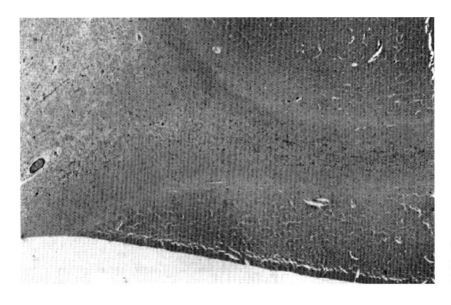

Fig. 3.193 Metachromatic leukodystrophy (hematoxylin and eosin [H&E] stain). Demyelination with U-fiber sparing.

Symptoms start with behavioral and intellectual deterioration followed by visual, auditory, and motor decline and adrenal insufficiency with bronze skin. There is cavitation of the parietooccipital white matter. Disease is generally fatal but may be treated with Lorenzo oil and a diet low in long chain fatty acids.

4. Pelizaeus–Merzbacher disease — caused by defective synthesis of proteolipid protein, a myelin protein, required for oligodendrocyte differentiation and survival. Inheritance is X-linked recessive so it usually affects males. Onset is in infancy with death in young adulthood. It produces an atrophic brain with demyelination that spares perivascular white matter. There is a tigroid pattern on MRI from intact and degenerating myelin. Symptoms include abnormal eye movements, spasticity, ataxia, and mental retardation. It is the only leukodystrophy with 100% incidence of nystagmus.

5. Canavan disease — caused by a deficiency of N-acetyl-aspartoacylase. There is increased urine N-acetylaspartic acid. Inheritance is autosomal recessive with a predilection for Ashkenazi Jews. Onset is in infancy with death by 5 years. There is spongy white matter degeneration with vacuoles that preferentially affects subcortical U-fibers. Also present are Alzheimer type II astrocytes. The brain actually increases in size; psychomotor regression, blindness, and spasticity.

6. Alexander disease — sporadic inheritance with a defect in the GFAP gene. Onset is in infancy with death by 3 years. There is hemispheric demyelination with macrocephaly and mitochondrial dysfunction. It mainly affects the frontal lobe with white matter demyelination. Rosenthal fibers (eosinophilic hyalin bodies that are likely glial degeneration products) form especially periventricular, perivascular, and subpial in location. Symptoms include psychomotor retardation and seizures.

7. Refsum disease — autosomal recessive disease caused by a mutation in the gene encoding phytanic acid α-hydroxylase. Symptoms include motor and sensory loss, ataxia, blindness, cardiac abnormalities, and deafness.

F. Mitochondrial disorders

1. MELAS (mitochondrial encephalopathy, lactic acidosis, and stroke-like syndrome) — transmission from maternal mitochondrial DNA. Patients have encephalopathy, elevated serum and CSF lactic acid levels, stroke-like episodes with cortical blindness, or hemianopia.

2. MERRF (myoclonic epilepsy with ragged red fibers) — transmission from maternal mitochondrial DNA with onset in early childhood. Patients have myoclonic epilepsy and ragged red fibers on muscle biopsy.

3. Kearns–Sayre syndrome — transmission from maternal mitochondrial DNA with onset before the age of 20. Patients have pigmentary retinopathy, cardiac abnormalities with heart block or cardiomyopathy, and progressive ophthalmoplegia. They also have ragged red fibers on muscle biopsy.

4. Leber hereditary optic neuropathy — transmission from maternal mitochondrial DNA with onset in adulthood. Patients develop a progressive painless loss of central vision.

G. Other metabolic disorders

1. Menke kinky hair disease — caused by a defect in copper absorption in the GI tract (opposite of Wilson disease). Inheritance is X-linked recessive with death before 2 years. Defect is in the copper transporting ATPase (ATP7a). There is decreased serum copper and serum ceruloplasmin. There is diffuse loss of all neurons, tortuous cerebral and systemic vessels, and metaphyseal spurring. Secondary hair growth is brittle, twisted, and colorless (pili torti). Symptoms include seizures and mental retardation.

2. Leigh disease (subacute necrotic encephalomyelopathy) — mitochondrial dysfunction by multiple metabolic defects. There may be a deficiency of cytochrome C oxidase. Inheritance is autosomal recessive with onset before 1 year. There is bilateral symmetric spongiform degeneration and necrosis of the thalamus, basal ganglia, brainstem, and spinal cord with peripheral nerve demyelination. Symptoms include decreased muscle tone and head control, seizures, myoclonus, ophthalmoplegia, and respiratory and swallowing problems.

3. Lowe syndrome (oculo–cerebro–renal syndrome) — an X-linked recessive disease causing bilateral cataracts, large eyes, nystagmus, psychomotor retardation, and death by renal failure

4. Ataxia-telangiectasia — caused by defective DNA repair with autosomal recessive inheritance. Death occurs by 20 years of age from infection or lymphoma. There is degeneration of CNS and decreased antibodies.

5. Lesch–Nyhan disease — X-linked recessive inheritance with deficiency of hypoxanthine-guanine phosphoribosyltransferase (HGPRT) enzyme. There is accumulation of uric acid with self-mutilation and choreoathetosis.

6. Zellweger syndrome (cerebrohepatorenal syndrome) — autosomal recessive inheritance with defects in the peroxin genes with death in a few months. There are decreased liver peroxisomes and accumulation of long-chain fatty acids. There is cortical dysgenesis and white matter degeneration with hepatorenal dysfunction. Patients may have hepatomegaly and renal cysts.

XIX. Degenerative Diseases

A. They usually occur in older patients. The CSF protein is usually slightly elevated, but with a normal cell count. Usually slow deterioration over many years, but may appear to have sudden onset when a system's neuronal loss exceeds its "safety factor." Degenerative diseases are usually bilaterally symmetric with certain systems involved as a result of selective vulnerability (i.e., Purkinje cells to hyperthermia, cerebellar granular layer to mercury, and hippocampus to hypoxia).

B. Alzheimer disease

1. It is the most frequent cause of dementia. Onset is generally after 45 years and it affects 10% of the population over 65 years old. There is no sex predilection. Inheritance is usually sporadic but is occasionally dominant with multiple chromosomal associations. Risk is increased with family history, age, less education, trauma, myocardial infarction, and Down syndrome.

2. There is diffuse atrophy with decreased neurons and synapses in the neocortex and hippocampus. There are neurofibrillary tangles (intracytoplasmic, paired helical filaments, immunoreactive for tau protein–stain with silver; most frequent in hippocampus and adjacent temporal lobe) and neuritic plaques (extracellular aggregates of Aβ [amyloid] protein–stain with silver). These both occur normally with aging but are increased in Alzheimer disease. There are Hirano bodies (rod-shaped eosin inclusions made of actin); decreased neurotransmitters (especially ACh with decreased neurons in the nucleus basalis of Meynert) and granulovacuolar degeneration of neurons (especially in the hippocampus) (**Fig. 3.194**).

3. Symptoms start with forgetfulness and then lead to confusion, ideomotor apraxia, visuospatial disorientation, dysnomia, and akinetic mutism. There are usually no major cortical deficits such as hemiplegia, sensory loss, or visual deterioration. 10% of patients may develop seizures. The temporoparietal area is usually affected first.

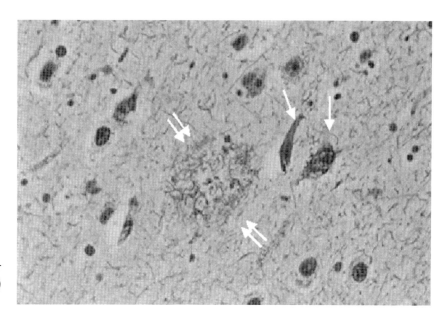

Fig. 3.194 Alzheimer disease (silver stain). A neuritic plaque (*double arrows*) and neurofibrillary tangles (*single arrows*).

4. Diagnosis is made by history, examination, CT, or MRI (that demonstrates atrophy and enlarged ventricles), and by ruling out treatable causes of dementia.

5. Treatment is geared toward cholinergic pathways including donepezil and Tacrine.

C. Pick disease (frontotemporal dementia) — onset is at 40–60 years with female predominance. Inheritance is sporadic but occasionally dominant. Symptoms are similar to Alzheimer disease but with increased frontal lobe dysfunction (impaired social restraint, etc.) and aphasias. There is frontotemporal atrophy without pathologic changes of Alzheimer disease. It spares the superior posterior temporal gyrus. Pick bodies (intracytoplasmic eosinophilic inclusions made of tau protein) form especially in hippocampal neurons. It affects gray and white matter. Death occurs in 2–5 years.

D. Huntington disease — onset in the 30s, with survival 15–30 years more. Inheritance is autosomal dominant on chromosome 4 with no sex predilection. It is a trinucleotide repeat disorder of CAG. Symptoms begin with personality changes followed by subcortical dementia (no aphasia, agnosia, or apraxia) and choreiform movements (affects hands and face first). There is atrophy mostly of the caudate (with boxcar ventricles) more than the putamen, GP, and cortex. Medium spiny type 1 neurons are affected first and aspiny neurons are spared. There is decreased GABA and ACh and increased NE and somatostatin. Haloperidol 2–10 mg/day may be used to treat the athetosis, with low doses and frequent drug holidays to decrease the risk of tardive dyskinesia (**Fig. 3.195**).

E. Wilson disease (hepatolenticular degeneration) — autosomal recessive inheritance on chromosome 13 with male predominance. There is accumulation of copper in the brain with decreased serum ceruloplasmin but increased serum free copper with increased urinary copper excretion. CT shows hypodense basal ganglia. Kayser–Fleischer rings form in the deepest corneal layer around the iris. There is neurologic and psychologic deterioration with tremor, dysarthria, and rigidity; spongy red degeneration and cavitation of the putamen and GP with occasional atrophy of the superior and middle frontal gyri. Alzheimer II astrocytes with large vesicular nuclei form in the gray matter of the cerebrum, cerebellum, and brainstem. Opalski cells (microglia) form in the GP. Onset is 10–30 years and liver disease starts before 20 years and leads to cirrhosis and splenomegaly. Treat by limiting foods high in copper (i.e., liver and chocolate) and chelate copper with d-penicillamine. With treatment, there may be disappearance of Kayser–Fleischer rings and improvement of liver function tests.

F. Fahr disease (idiopathic basal ganglia calcification) — primary basal ganglia and cerebellar blood vessel calcification associated with renal disease or decreased parathyroid hormone. It may also involve the dentate nuclei.

G. Progressive supranuclear palsy — onset of 50–60 years and death within 1–12 years with male predominance. Symptoms include deterioration of intellect, vision, speech, and gait, with vertical gaze palsy, loss of voluntary eye movements and opticokinetic nystagmus, decreased oculocephalic reflexes, pseudobulbar palsy, and axial rigidity without tremor. Patients have a history of multiple falls and a poor response to l-dopa therapy. There is atrophy of the midbrain, superior colliculus, and subthalamic nuclei with ventricular dilation and decreased neurons in the GP, SN, and various brainstem nuclei. The neurofibrillary tangles are different than the Alzheimer type (i.e., globose versus flame-shaped).

H. Striatonigral degeneration — onset around 50 years. Symptoms include rigidity and akinesia (Parkinson-like

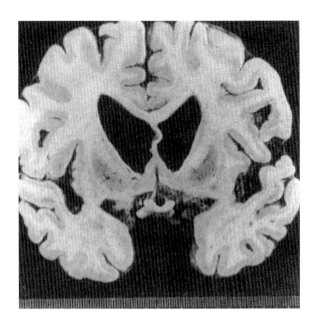

Fig. 3.195 Huntington disease. Gross specimen with atrophic caudates and "box-car" ventricles. (From Alleyne Jr. CH. Neurosurgery Board Review. New York, NY: Thieme; 1997. Reprinted by permission.)

symptoms) with syncope. There are atrophic and brown putamen and depigmented SN as well as decreased neurons in the putamen, caudate, and SN. There are no Lewy bodies or neurofibrillary tangles.

I. Hallervorden–Spatz disease — onset in late childhood with death in early adulthood. The disease is progressive over 20 years. It has autosomal recessive inheritance. Symptoms include extrapyramidal and corticospinal dysfunction with dementia. CT has hypodense basal ganglia. There are brown atrophic GP and SN secondary to iron deposition.

J. Acquired hepatocerebral degeneration — occurs with chronic liver disease and is increased with elevated ammonia levels. It is associated with long-term total parenteral nutrition (by manganese toxicity). T1-weighted MRI shows hyperintense basal ganglia. There is pseudolaminar necrosis with gray/white matter junction changes.

K. Parkinson disease (paralysis agitans)

1. Onset is 40–50 years with male predominance. It affects 1% of the population older than 50 years.

2. Bradykinesia (slow to initiate and execute movements), resting pill-rolling tremor, rigidity, abnormal gait, and dementia (30%).

3. Pathology — decreased neuromelanin and neurons in the pars compacta of the SN, locus ceruleus, and dorsal motor nucleus of the vagus. There are neuronal intracytoplasmic Lewy bodies (eosinophilic deposits of α-synuclein, βA-crystallin, ubiquitin, and neurofilaments) and decreased DA in the caudate and putamen. It may be idiopathic or secondary to encephalitis (after von Economo viral encephalitis in the early 20th century, with no Lewy bodies), manganese, carbon monoxide, and 1-methyl-4-phenyl-1,2,3,6-tetrahydropyridine (MPTP) toxicity. Parkinson-plus is multisystem atrophy (**Fig. 3.196**).

4. Diffuse Lewy body disease — occurs in cortical neurons and may be a variant

5. The rate-limiting enzyme in DA production is tyrosine β-hydroxylase.

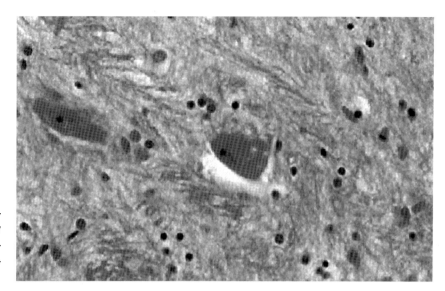

Fig. 3.196 Parkinson disease (hematoxylin and eosin [H&E] stain). Lewy bodies (neuronal intracytoplasmic inclusion with an eosinophilic core surrounded by a clear halo).

6. Treatment — (a) carbidopa (L-DOPA and carbidopa, a decarboxylase inhibitor), (b) amantadine (increases DA release, anticholinergic), (c) benztropine or trihexylphenidyl (anticholinergics, may cause slow mentation and constipation), (d) bromocriptine, pergolide or cabergoline (stimulate D2 receptors), and (e) selegiline (monoamine oxidase-b inhibitor, decreases degradation of DA and slows disease progression). Try to limit protein intake because amino acids antagonize L-DOPA; initial therapy is with selegiline amantadine, benztropine, or propranolol (for tremor); therapy for more severe disease is with carbidopa.

7. Surgical options — subthalamic deep brain stimulation is best for contralateral bradykinesia and tremor. Survival rate is 80% at 10 years with two thirds disabled in 5 years.

L. Multisystem atrophy — 25% of patients with Parkinson symptoms have poor response to DA. Consider Parkinson-plus syndrome with multisystem atrophy including Shy–Drager syndrome, striatonigral degeneration, progressive supranuclear palsy, and olivopontocerebellar degeneration with autonomic dysfunction (decreased sweating, impotence, incontinence, and orthostatic hypotension).

1. Shy–Drager syndrome — multiple system atrophy (MSA) with predominant autonomic dysfunction, onset at 50–60 years and death within 7 years. There is no sex predilection and inheritance is sporadic. There are Parkinson symptoms without Lewy bodies and with autonomic dysfunction (orthostatic hypotension, urinary incontinence, and impotence). There is loss of cells in the intermediolateral column of the spinal cord and putamen.

2. Olivopontocerebellar atrophy — onset is at 15 years with sporadic, recessive, and dominant inheritance. Ataxia of the lower limbs occurs first. There is atrophy of the pons, middle cerebellar peduncle, inferior olive, and cerebellar cortex. It is associated with Parkinson syndrome.

M. Dementia with Lewy bodies — dementia with increased frontal atrophy, parkinsonian features, and eosinophilic intracytoplasmic Lewy bodies in the cerebral cortex and brainstem.

N. Friedreich ataxia — the most frequent hereditary ataxia. It is the only autosomal recessive trinucleotide repeat disease. It affects the frataxin gene on chromosome 9. Onset is before 20 years with death in mid-30s and inability to walk 5 years after onset. It is associated with cardiomyopathy and diabetes. There is degeneration of axons and myelin in the posterior columns and corticospinal tracts, more prominent distally. It also affects the spinocerebellar tracts, cerebellum (decreased Purkinje cells in the superior vermis), inferior olive, brainstem nuclei (CNs VIII, X, and XII), and DRG. It spares motor neurons and mainly affects large peripheral myelinated fibers. Symptoms begin with gait ataxia followed by loss of proprioception and vibratory sense, and upper motor neuron signs.

O. Familial myoclonic epilepsy

1. Lafora body disease — onset in the mid-teens and autosomal recessive inheritance. Symptoms include myoclonic seizures and dementia. There is brain atrophy and diffuse neuronal Lafora bodies (round basophilic polyglucosans) also found in the heart, muscle, and liver.

2. Baltic myoclonus — onset is before 11 years and autosomal recessive inheritance. There are myoclonic seizures and Purkinje cell atrophy.

P. Motor neuron disease

1. Spinal muscular atrophy (SMA) — degeneration of the anterior horn and hypoglossal nuclei with sparing of the corticospinal tracts and bulbar nuclei
   a. Werdnig–Hoffman disease (SMA type 1, infantile) — onset from 0 to 6 months and death within 1.5 years from pneumonia. It is the most common spinal muscle atrophy. It has autosomal recessive inheritance on chromosome 5q. Atrophy is most severe in the proximal extensors and trunk. The extraocular muscles are spared; no mental retardation. Causes "floppy infant syndrome."
   b. Wohlfart–Kugelberg–Welander disease (SMA type 2) — onset usually before 5 years (although it may be up to 17 years) with death usually by 5–10 years. There is male predominance, and different forms have autosomal recessive, dominant, and X-linked inheritance (on chromosome 5). Symptoms are bilateral and symmetric with proximal limbs affected first.
   c. SMA type 3 — adult onset with multiple forms with sporadic, dominant, recessive, and X-linked inheritance. It is slowly progressive.

2. ALS — the most frequent adult-onset progressive motor neuron disease. Onset is around 55 years with death 50% in 3 years and 90% in 6 years. There is a slight male predominance with sporadic inheritance, but 10% are dominant on chromosome 21 with a mutation in the superoxide dismutase gene. There is degeneration of motor neurons (including Betz cells) and the corticospinal tracts. There are upper and lower motor neuron signs with fasciculations in all extremities and diffuse hyperreflexia. Symptoms usually begin in the hands and there is progressive bulbar palsy with face and tongue weakness. Bladder control is maintained. There are no sensory changes. Bunina bodies (intracytoplasmic, anterior horn cells) form. Amyotrophy is deinnervation atrophy of muscle. There may be antibodies to gangliosides. EMG demonstrates fasciculations and fibrillations (**Fig. 3.197**).

Q. Memory aid

1. X-linked metabolic diseases — Fabry, Hunter, adrenoleukodystrophy, Pelizaeus–Merzbacher, Menke kinky hair, Lowe, and Lesch–Nyhan. Most others are recessive with a few indeterminate.

2. Autosomal dominant diseases — Wohlfart–Kugelberg–Welander disease and Huntington chorea

3. Adolescent regression of intellect and behavioral changes — Wilson, Hallervorden–Spatz, Lafora body, Gaucher, mucopolysaccharidosis, metachromatic leukodystrophy, and GM2 gangliosidosis

4. Metabolic diseases that may have adult onset — metachromatic adrenoleukodystrophy, Krabbe disease, GM2 gangliosidosis, Wilson disease, Leigh disease, Niemann–Pick disease, Gaucher disease, mucopolysaccharidosis, Refsum disease, and porphyria.

5. Strokes in children — Fabry disease, homocystinuria

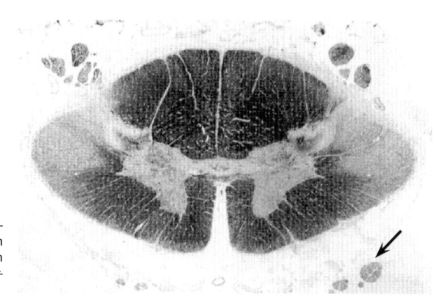

Fig. 3.197 Amyotrophic lateral sclerosis (Luxol fast blue stain). Degeneration of the lateral corticospinal tracts with atrophic demyelinated ventral roots (*arrow*) compared with the dorsal roots.

6. Parkinson symptoms in adolescents — Wilson disease, Hallervorden–Spatz disease

7. Cerebellar degeneration — ethanol, phenytoin (Dilantin), paraneoplastic syndromes, Down syndrome, and Friedreich ataxia

8. Mitochondrial DNA diseases — Kearns–Sayre syndrome, Leber hereditary optic atrophy, MELAS, and MERRF

XX. Demyelinating Diseases

A. Myelin

1. CNS myelin–associated proteins are myelin basic protein (MBP) and proteolipid protein-1. Peripheral nervous system myelin — associated proteins are MBP, P2, and P0.

2. The CNS and peripheral nervous system myelin have different protein and lipid components and different periodicity of lamellae. The CNS myelin does not regenerate well.

3. Primary demyelination is by processes that affect myelin or myelin-forming cells. Segmental demyelination is myelin loss with preserved axons.

B. Peripheral demyelination

1. Toxic — Diphtheria (toxin inhibits Schwann cell myelin synthesis mainly in the DRG and ventral and dorsal roots, where the blood–nerve barrier is leaky, and causes segmental demyelination), lead, and hexachlorophene.

2. Immune mediated
   a. Guillain–Barré (idiopathic polyneuritis) — rapid onset, and occurs with trauma, surgery, infection, immunization, and neoplasm. It is usually monophasic but occasionally relapsing. It involves the peripheral nerves. It affects mainly motor and autonomic function. There are perivascular mononuclear infiltrates and segmental demyelination. The CSF reveals normal pressure, acellularity (albuminocytologic dissociation), and a protein peak around 5 weeks. Treatment is mainly supportive. Steroids have not been shown to help.

b. Experimental allergic neuritis — caused by T cell attack of the P2 protein by cell-mediated immunity

3. Metabolic — diabetes mellitus, uremia, and hypothyroidism

C. Hypertrophic (onion bulb) neuropathies — caused by repeated demyelination-remyelination and seen with Dejerine–Sottas, Charcot–Marie–Tooth, and Refsum diseases. Schwann cell processes and collagen layers surround the axons and myelin.

D. Central demyelination

   1. Immune mediated

      a. Multiple sclerosis (MS)

         (1) Peak age is at 20–40 years, with female predominance. The highest incidence is in Northern Europe. The risk is related to one geographic location before age 15 years. Influences are considered to be latitude (distance from the equator), familial (15% have an affected relative), infectious, and autoimmune. The findings are visual (optic neuritis 25%, most improve in 2 weeks, and one-third recover completely), autonomic, and sensorimotor (50%).

         (2) Associated genetic factors include HLA DR2 and DR4 alleles.

         (3) Lhermitte sign is common. Charcot triad is nystagmus, scanning speech, and intention tremor. Bilateral intranuclear ophthalmoplegia is almost pathognomonic. Trigeminal neuralgia and bladder spasticity also occur. 50% of patients that have optic neuritis will get MS.

         (4) It is usually relapsing/remitting (Charcot type) and 10% of cases are progressive. The 25-year survival rate is 74% compared with 86% of the rest of the population in a study from Rochester, Minnesota. Pregnancy does not increase the relapse rate. Diagnosis is made by MRI (85% sensitive), CSF oligoclonal bands, and visual evoked potentials (abnormal in 80%, brainstem and somatosensory evoked potentials may also be abnormal) (**Fig. 3.198**).

         (5) CSF has increased protein but seldom >100 mg/dL, increased macrophages, IgG index (CSF/serum IgG, CSF/serum albumin) is >1.7, and oligoclonal bands (also seen with SSPE and syphilis). There may be increased CSF MBP during an exacerbation. Gross pathologic examination reveals plaques (acute are pink and older are gray) that are gelatinous, firm, ovoid, perpendicular to the ventricles, and in the superolateral periventricular white matter (where the subependymal veins line the ventricles), corpus callosum, subcortical white matter, optic nerves/chiasm/and tracts (90%), brainstem, and spinal cord (especially subpial where veins are near white matter).

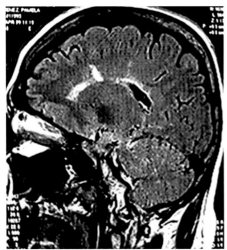 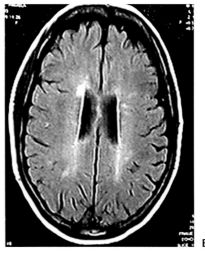

A   B

Fig. 3.198 Multiple sclerosis. (**A**) Sagittal and (**B**) axial enhanced T1-weighted magnetic resonance images demonstrate periventricular white matter enhancement and perivenular extension (Dawson finger).

(6) Dawson fingers are periventricular extensions of inflammation into the deep white matter. The plaques do not extend past the root entry zone into the peripheral nerves. The posterior fossa is more commonly affected in children. Microscopic examination of an active plaque demonstrates decreased myelin, macrophages, destruction or proliferation of oligodendrocytes, axonal sparing, perivascular lymphocytes (T > B cells), parenchymal T4 cells, perivascular T8 cells and B cells, reactive astrocytosis, and edema (**Fig. 3.199**).

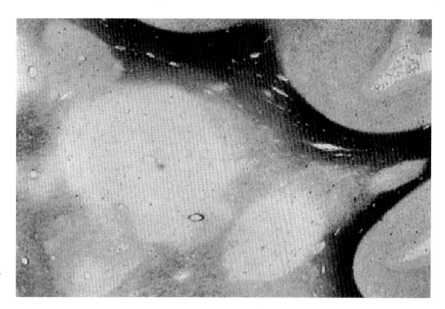

Fig. 3.199 Multiple sclerosis (Luxol fast blue stain). Multiple white matter demyelinated plaques.

(7) Remyelination may occur at the periphery as shadow plaques. Inactive plaques have few cells, sharp margins, no oligodendrocytes, and naked axons and astrocytes. MS is similar to experimental allergic encephalomyelitis and is transferable by T cells. MS may be caused by a postviral autoimmune reaction to MBP or antibodies to oligodendrocytes. Decreased Ts:Th ratio is associated with flare-ups.

(8) Treatment is with steroids (help to decrease attack duration, but not with optic neuritis), and β-interferon (decreases attack rate). Copaxone reduces frequency of relapses.

(9) Acute MS or Marburg-variant — Monophasic, diffuse, larger plaques, may be rapidly fatal.

(10) Neuromyelitis optica (Devic disease) — a variant of acute MS in adults, primarily affects optic nerves (unilateral or bilateral optic neuritis with blindness) and spinal cord (acute necrotizing transverse myelitis), often rapidly progressive, occasionally fatal, and is more common in Japan.

(11) Baló concentric sclerosis — acute MS in young adults, fatal, and has a concentric loss of myelin.

(12) Schilder disease — affects children, not familial like the leukodystrophies, aggressive bilateral acute MS-type demyelination, hemispheric involvement, may also affect axons, and is usually fatal.

b. Acute disseminated encephalomyelitis — postinfectious, monophasic, occurs after a viral illness or vaccination (smallpox or rabies), occasionally fatal but most recover. There is perivenous demyelination with axonal sparing and mononuclear infiltration. It is an autoimmune response to a CNS antigen possibly from the virus and is likely a T cell response to MBP like experimental allergic encephalomyelitis.

     c. Acute hemorrhagic leukoencephalitis (Weston–Hurst disease) — monophasic, rapid progression, fatal, occurs after a respiratory infection, drugs, or immunizations, and causes white matter edema and hemorrhages.

     d. Experimental allergic encephalomyelitis — an experimental allergic disseminated encephalomyelitis model, although the chronic relapsing model is used to study MS. It is caused by a T cell–mediated immune response to MBP.

2. Infectious — PML, SSPE, rubella (like SSPE but without intranuclear inclusions), and HIV

3. Ischemic — Binswanger encephalopathy, carbon monoxide (may initially survive and then develop symptoms days later due to white matter degeneration), and chronic edema (spares subcortical U-fibers)

4. Metabolic demyelination (leukodystrophy) — widespread confluent myelin loss, astrocytosis, minimal inflammation (except adrenoleukodystrophy with perivascular lymphocytes), and sparing of subcortical U-fibers (except Canavan disease)

5. Iatrogenic — CPM

XXI. Ischemia and Hypoxia

A. The brain receives 15% of the cardiac output, uses 20% of the blood's O_2, and uses 15% of the blood's glucose. Effects of ischemia depend on the level of flow, duration, collateral flow, location, temperature, age, and serum glucose level (increased lactate formation by the glia causes acidosis that may worsen ischemic damage). The ischemic neurons accumulate Ca^{2+}, Na^+, Cl^-, and water. Anaerobic glycolysis causes acidosis and increased extracellular glutamate and free radicals.

B. Early changes at the cellular level

1. 6 hours — neuronal changes and edema, microvacuolation (by dilated mitochondria), shrunken hyperchromatic cells, shrunken cells with incrustations on the surface and cytoplasmic bulging, and homogeneous cell changes seen at 6 to 12 hours after injury. These changes may be due to decreased energy or the abnormal release of excitatory neurotransmitters causing a metabolic cascade.

2. 24 hours — PMNs accumulate.

3. 48 hours — PMNs peak.

4. 3–5 days — Some macrophages arrive.

5. 2 weeks — Vessels start to form around the periphery and enhancement begins.

C. The astrocytes swell and accumulate glycogen and filaments. The oligodendrocytes swell and the microglia form rod cells and ingest debris. All the mechanisms of cell death are associated with increased intracellular Ca^{2+}. Delayed neuronal death (maturation phenomenon, may be apoptosis) is caused by reperfusion with altered ionic homeostasis, lactate accumulation, increased excitatory neurotransmitters, free radicals, and prostaglandins (causing vasoconstriction).

D. Ischemic penumbra — the zone of isoelectric silence where the CBF is 8–23 mL/100 g per minute. The low blood flow prevents neuronal depolarization, but does not yet cause ionic changes leading to cell death. The neurons do not function but are still salvageable. Normal CBF is 50–55 mL/100 g per minute. At a level <8, there is ionic pump failure and rapid cell death. The blood vessels in the brain respond to decreased flow first by vasodilating to increase the CBF and then by increasing the O_2 extraction. They are unable to compensate when the CBF is <20.

CBF (mL/100 g/min)	0	10	15	18
Time until death (min)	<4	40	80	infinite

Or you could just say that the time for neuronal death depends on CBF and is <4 minutes at a CBF of 0, 40 minutes at a CBF of 10, 80 minutes at a CBF of 15, and infinite at a CBF of 18 mL/100g/min.

E. Selective vulnerability — all neurons have different vulnerabilities to ischemia that may be related to local changes in vascular supply or cellular differences such as differences in zinc or lactate dehydrogenase concentrations. The most vulnerable cells are in the hippocampus, cortex (parietooccipital deep sulci third, fifth, and sixth layers), basal ganglia (caudate and putamen), and cerebellum (Purkinje cells). In the hippocampus, the CA1 (Sommer area) and CA3 (endplate) areas are most susceptible, and the CA2 area is the resistant sector. The white matter U-fibers, the extreme and external capsules, and the claustrum are fairly resistant because they receive dual blood supplies. With ischemia, premature babies have periventricular leukomalacia with spastic diplegia because the germinal matrix is in a borderzone. In full-term babies, there is loss of cortex and subcortical white matter. In children and adults, there is loss of the deep gray structures, hippocampus, brainstem, and cerebellum. The borderzone areas are between the ACA/MCA and MCA/PCA distributions.

F. Hypoxic-ischemic encephalopathy — due to global hypoperfusion or hypoxia. Symptoms are the "man in a barrel" syndrome with weakness mainly in the proximal upper limbs, and the stroke usually forms at the border zones in the parietooccipital area (at the junction of the ACA and MCA/PCA). There may also be laminar necrosis of cortical layers 3, 5, and 6 and the putamen.

G. Symptoms of global ischemia range from light-headedness and syncope to coma and death. Hippocampal damage may result in long-term memory deficits.

H. Excitatory neurotransmitters — glutamate and aspartate. The N-methyl-D-aspartate receptor binds glutamate, causes an influx of Ca^{2+}, and has been implicated in cellular necrosis after ischemia. Glutamate levels are increased by ischemia. Experimental blockage of these receptors during ischemia increases hippocampal neuronal survival.

I. After ischemia, blood vessels may become obstructed by large, stiff PMNs that adhere to the endothelial cells. Adhesion is mediated by intercellular adhesion molecule 1 and 2 surface markers on endothelial cells and interleukins on white blood cells. Expression of endothelial cell adhesion molecules is increased by tumor necrosis factor, interferon, and interleukin-1. The serum levels of these cytokines are increased with ischemia. They enter the circulation 30 minutes after occlusion and reach peak levels in 12 hours. There is increased binding of laminin and fibronectin by PMNs after stroke. New ischemia therapies may be directed toward blocking these factors.

XXII. Vascular Diseases

A. Atherosclerosis

1. Plaques consist of eccentric fibrofatty deposits and intimal thickening. The plaques are most common at the ICA origin and the distal basilar artery. They form most likely as a reaction to injury. A subtle intimal injury causes platelet aggregation, and endothelial injury increases the permeability to lipoproteins.

2. Macrophages and smooth muscle cells proliferate, accumulate fatty esters, and form lipid-filled foam cells that die and form cholesterol deposits. Initially, the fatty streak develops and then a fibrotic cap

forms over it. Underlying inflammatory changes ensue with neovascularity, and this is followed by hemorrhage, rupture, and ulceration forming a nidus for thrombi and emboli.

3. In evaluating with Doppler ultrasonography, convention is that flow toward the probe is red, away is blue, and nonlaminar flow distal to the stenosis is mixed color. There is normally flow reversal in the distal carotid bulb.

4. Ultrasonography tends to overestimate stenosis and may have difficulty differentiating high-grade stenosis from occlusion.

5. Angiography assesses the degree of stenosis and evaluates for tandem lesions in the carotid siphon and intracranially and for associated vascular lesions such as aneurysms. It helps to determine whether the collateral circulation is adequate to determine whether a shunt will be needed during surgery. Only 20% of the population has a complete circle of Willis. If both the ACA and anterior communicating artery (ACommA) fill, or the PCA fills, usually a shunt is not needed. 2% of patients have tandem lesions such as distal stenoses, most frequently in the carotid siphon, but also in the first segment of the MCA. These lesions may require angioplasty (**Fig. 3.200**).

6. There may be atherosclerosis in the aortic arch, proximal subclavian artery, brachiocephalic artery, or vertebral artery.

7. The North American Symptomatic Carotid Endarterectomy Trial (NASCET) determined that surgery is beneficial if there are symptomatic lesions with 70 to 99% stenosis. The percent stenosis is determined by measuring the distal normal ICA diameter and the stenotic diameter: (Distal–stenotic/distal) x 100.

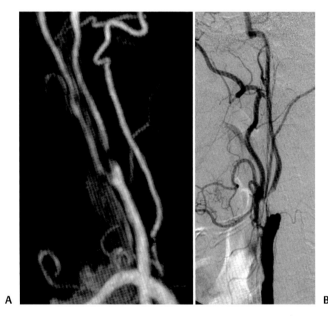

Fig. 3.200 Carotid artery stenosis. (**A**) Magnetic resonance and (**B**) catheter angiograms demonstrate examples of proximal internal carotid artery plaques causing carotid stenosis.

B. Transient ischemic attack (TIA) — sudden onset of a focal neurologic deficit lasting less than 24 hours and caused by a vascular lesion. Usually caused by a platelet-fibrin embolus from an ulcerative atherosclerotic plaque.

C. Reversible ischemic neurologic deficit — lasts 24 hours–1 week

D. Cerebrovascular accident or stroke

1. Stroke — sudden onset of neurologic deficit caused by hemorrhage or ischemia from thrombus, emboli, or hemodynamic alterations

2. Most strokes are caused by atherosclerosis.

3. Most emboli are either from mural thrombi or valve vegetations. The most common distribution is MCA (75%), followed by PCA, and rarely ACA (0.6%).

4. Death in these patients is most frequently caused by myocardial infarction because of the systemic nature of vascular disease.

5. Angiography after stroke may demonstrate the cause of the stroke. Findings of an infarct are hyperemia or vascular blush in the penumbra from venous luxury perfusion and arteriovenous shunting with early draining veins.

6. CT findings (**Fig. 3.201**)
   a. Hyperacute phase (<12 hours) — normal CT (50%), hyperdense MCA with luminal clot (25–50%), and obscured lentiform nuclei
   b. Acute phase (12–24 hours) — decreased density of the basal ganglia and decreased gray/white matter differentiation at the insula (insular ribbon sign) and cortex
   c. 1–3 days — mass effect, wedge-shaped low density of the gray and white matter, and possibly hemorrhage
   d. 4–7 days — gyral enhancement and edema
   e. 1–8 weeks — enhancement, decreased mass effect, and calcification in children
   f. Months — calcifications and encephalomalacia

7. MRI findings
   a. Immediate — absence of flow void and intravascular enhancement
   b. Hyperacute (<12 hours) — hypointense on T1-weighted and hyperintense on T2-weighted MRI
   c. Acute (12–24 hours) — hyperintense on T2-weighted MRI, enhancing meninges adjacent to the stroke, and mass effect
   d. 1–3 days — parenchymal enhancement and hemorrhage
   e. 4–7 days — hemorrhage (25%), increased enhancement, and decreased mass effect

8. Stroke pathology
   a. After 1 hour — axonal changes
   b. 12–24 hours — neuronal necrosis, eosinophilic neurons, neuronal pyknosis
   c. 24 hours — well-circumscribed necrosis in an arterial territory
   d. 1–2 days — PMNs accumulate.
   e. 2–5 days — BBB breakdown, edema, and axon retraction balls at the edge
   f. 5–7 days — Gitter cells (lipid-laden macrophages) and neovascularization
   g. 10–20 days — astrocytosis around infarct, rim of gemistocytes
   h. >3 months — cystic space with fibrillary astrocytes. A 1-cm stroke takes 3 months to become cystic. A stroke tends to preserve the outermost cortical layers, unlike a contusion, which usually extends to the pia and affects the crests of the gyri.

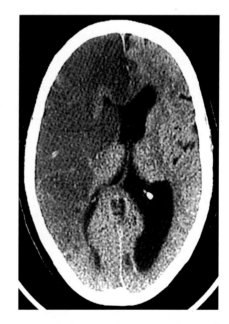

Fig. 3.201 Stroke. Nonenhanced computed tomographic scan demonstrates right internal carotid artery hemispheric hypodensity.

E. Pseudolaminar cortical necrosis — caused by generalized hypoxia, not focal. The middle cortical layers are affected (layers 3, 5, and 6), and there is frequent gyriform hemorrhage.

F. Hemorrhagic stroke — 10% of ischemic strokes hemorrhage as a result of reperfusion into areas of brain with damaged blood vessels. Hemorrhage is more common with emboli than with thrombi. It usually occurs 24 to 48 hours after a stroke. The incidence is higher in large strokes (25%). There is an increased risk of hemorrhage if a hypodensity is detected within 4 hours of a stroke.

G. Lacunar stroke — <1.5 cm, occurs in the basal ganglia, thalamus, and white matter and accounts for 20% of strokes. They are usually caused by hypertension and less commonly by atherosclerosis and thromboemboli. The small arteries are affected by lipohyalinosis. The CT is usually negative early on, although the lesion is hypointense on T1-weighted MRI.

H. Venous stroke

1. It is more often hemorrhagic and more frequently involves the white matter instead of the gray (unlike an arterial stroke). It is frequently secondary to a dural sinus thrombosis.

2. The risk is increased with dehydration, pregnancy, infection, oral contraceptives, surgery, hypercoagulable state (factor V Leiden, deficiencies of protein C and S or antithrombin 3), trauma, drugs, paroxysmal nocturnal hemoglobinuria, lupus anticoagulant, Behçet syndrome, and inflammatory bowel disease. No cause is identified in 25% of cases.

3. The most frequent sinuses involved in descending order are superior sagittal sinus, transverse sinus, sigmoid sinus, and cavernous sinus. Internal cerebral and deep venous occlusion is rare and causes bilateral deep gray and diencephalic ischemia.

4. Angiography demonstrates parasagittal collateral venous channels surrounding an empty channel.

5. The CT is hyperdense and may demonstrate an empty-delta sign caused by a clot in the sinus (the dural veins become engorged and enhance; the inside of the sinus does not enhance) (**Fig. 3.202**).

6. Magnetic resonance venography (MRV) and/or angiography (MRA) is the best test for diagnosis.

7. Mortality is 20–30%.

I. Pediatric/young adult stroke

1. Accounts for 3% of strokes and is usually caused by congenital heart disease with an embolism. It may also be caused by dissection, infection (syphilis), drugs, oral contraceptives, migraine, coagulation disorder (usually venous stroke, protein C and S, antithrombin III deficiency or factor 5 Leiden), Fabry disease, homocystinuria, fibromuscular dysplasia (FMD), Marfan syndrome, collagen vascular disease, ulcerative colitis/Crohn disease, moyamoya disease, NF1, tuberous sclerosis, vasculitis, radiation, and tumors.

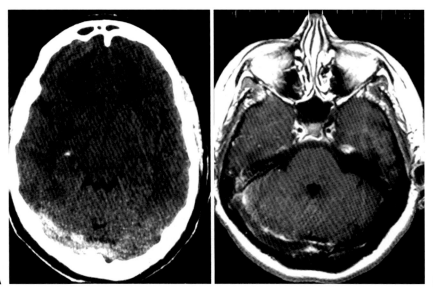

Fig. 3.202 Venous sinus thrombosis. (**A**) Nonenhanced computed tomographic scan and (**B**) T1-weighted magnetic resonance image demonstrate a thrombosed right transverse sinus.

A   B

2. There is congenital vascular stenosis associated with NF1 and tuberous sclerosis.

3. The risk with oral contraceptives is higher if the age is >35 years or there is tobacco use, hypertension, or migraines. Oral contraceptives also increase the risk of heart disease and SAH. Pregnancy is associated with hemorrhagic stroke secondary to eclampsia, hemolysis, elevated liver enzymes, and low platelet count (HELLP) syndrome, and venous thrombosis.

J. Stroke syndromes

1. Multiinfarct dementia — distinguish from vasculitis, intravascular lymphoma, hypertensive encephalopathy, and emboli

2. Locked-in syndrome — the only voluntary motor function preserved is vertical eye movement (in the classic form). It is caused by a large ventral pontine stroke from an occluded basilar artery branch.

3. Weber syndrome — from a lesion in the midbrain caused by vascular occlusion, tumor, or aneurysm. Findings are oculomotor palsy with crossed hemiplegia. It involves CN III and the corticospinal tract.

4. Benedikt syndrome — from a lesion in the tegmentum of the midbrain caused by ischemia, hemorrhage, TB, or tumor. Findings are oculomotor palsy with contralateral hemiplegia and cerebellar ataxia and tremor. It involves CN III, the red nucleus, corticospinal tract, and brachium conjunctivum.

5. Millard-Gubler syndrome — from a lesion in the pons. Findings are facial and abducens palsies with contralateral hemiplegia. It is caused by ischemia or tumor and involves CNs VI, VII, and the corticospinal tract.

6. Wallenberg syndrome (lateral medullary syndrome) — from a lesion in the lateral tegmentum of the medulla. Findings are ipsilateral palsies of CN V (loss of facial sensation of pain and temperature), IX (decreased gag and taste), X (dysphagia and hoarseness), Horner syndrome, cerebellar ataxia, and contralateral loss of pain and temperature sense in the body. It is caused by vertebral artery (more common) or posterior inferior cerebellar artery (PICA) occlusion, usually by thrombosis of the artery secondary to an atherosclerotic plaque, but occasionally by embolism or dissection. It involves the spinal nucleus and tract of CN V, CNs IX and X; lateral spinothalamic tract; the descending sympathetic fibers; and the inferior cerebellar peduncle (spinocerebellar and olivocerebellar tracts) (**Fig. 3.203**).

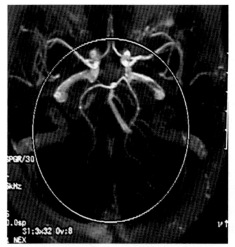 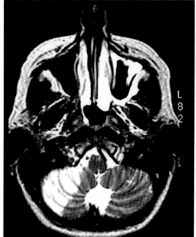 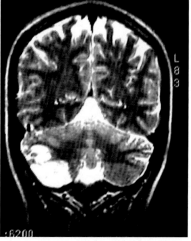

Fig. 3.203 Stroke. Magnetic resonance angiogram (**A**) demonstrating absence of right vertebral artery flow and (**B**) axial and (**C**) coronal T2-weighted magnetic resonance images demonstrating right posterior inferior cerebellar artery distribution stroke (from vertebral artery occlusion).

7. Medial medullary syndrome — from a lesion in the medial medulla. Findings are ipsilateral tongue paralysis, and contralateral paralysis of upper and lower extremities (spares face) and decreased body touch and proprioception. It is caused by vertebral artery or anterior spinal artery occlusion. It involves CN XII, pyramidal tract, and medial lemniscus.

8. Subclavian steal — proximal subclavian artery stenosis (proximal to the origin of the vertebral artery) with reversal of flow in the vertebral artery to the upper limb. There is a noticeable pulse difference between the two upper limbs (**Fig. 3.204**).

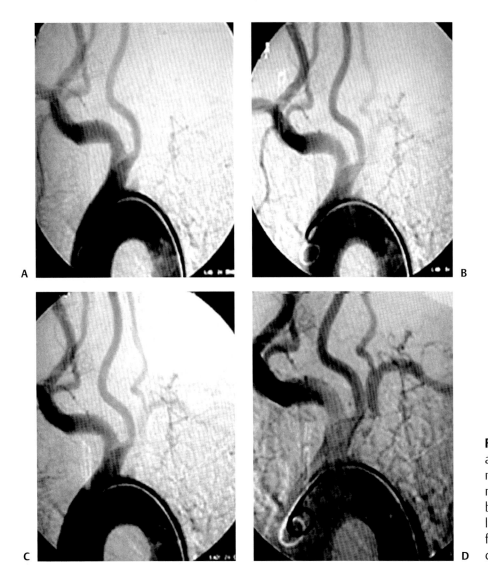

Fig. 3.204 Subclavian steal. Serial angiograms (**A–D**) demonstrate proximal subclavian artery stenosis with retrograde filling from the left vertebral artery. A bovine variant with the left internal carotid artery originating from the brachiocephalic trunk is also demonstrated.

K. Stroke-related diseases

1. Moyamoya disease
   a. Idiopathic progressive arteriopathy of childhood, with unknown cause. It is more frequent in Japan. It causes progressive stenosis or occlusion of the distal ICA and proximal ACA and MCA.
   b. Multiple parenchymal, leptomeningeal, and transdural collaterals develop.
   c. Angiogram demonstrates enlarged lenticulostriate, thalamoperforate, and collateral vessels forming a "puff of smoke." 80% of patients develop stroke and 50% have atrophy, especially in

the anterior circulation (**Fig. 3.205**). A similar vascular pattern may be seen with any progressive occlusive vascular disease (radiation, atherosclerosis, and sickle cell disease).

    d. In children, it presents with ischemia and transient weakness and in adults with hemorrhage.

    e. Pathologic examination demonstrates intimal thickening and fibrotic changes. Moyamoya disease is associated with Down syndrome.

2. Sickle cell anemia — 6–9% of patients have strokes that are usually ischemic. There are occlusions of small and large vessels and multiple aneurysms in unusual locations. There is endothelial injury caused by adhesions of sickle cells followed by vascular degeneration and sometimes aneurysm formation.

3. Marfan syndrome and homocystinuria — cause large vessel vasculopathy, coagulopathy, and subluxation of lenses

4. Ehlers–Danlos syndrome — vascular fragility associated with carotid-cavernous fistulas and arterial narrowing.

5. NFI — associated with aortic, celiac, mesenteric, and renal vascular stenosis, and cerebrovascular stenosis, aneurysms, AVMs, and moyamoya disease. There are no vascular abnormalities associated with NF2.

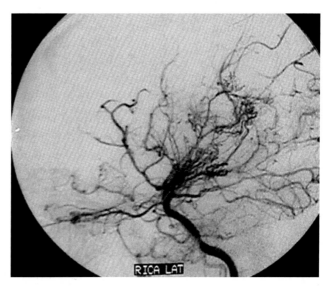

Fig. 3.205 Moyamoya disease. Angiogram demonstrates distal internal carotid artery occlusion with prominent leptomeningeal collaterals ("puff of smoke").

6. Tuberous sclerosis — associated with stenoses and aneurysms (especially the thoracic abdominal aorta)

7. Klippel–Trenaunay–Weber syndrome — associated with spinal AVMs and carotid aplasia

8. Menke kinky hair disease — associated with tortuous abdominal, visceral, and intracranial arteries

9. Fibromuscular disease (FMD) — a segmental noninflammatory narrowing of blood vessels by intimal or medial proliferation. It most commonly affects the cervical ICA (75%), vertebral artery (25%), and renal arteries. 75% are bilateral. There is a female predominance and it develops before 50 years. Angiogram has a "string of beads" appearance. 20% are associated with an intracranial aneurysm and they are also associated with dissection, embolic stroke, and possibly aneurysms and AVMs. It is believed to be caused by degeneration of elastic tissue with loss of muscle and accumulation of fibrous tissue. The segmental dilations are caused by atrophy of the vessel wall. Treatment if there is a stroke may be with endovascular dilation or excision of an affected segment with reconstruction (**Fig. 3.206**).

10. Radiation vasculopathy — causes gradual narrowing and occlusion that occurs usually after 18 months.

11. CADASIL (cerebral autosomal dominant inherited arteriopathy with subcortical infarcts and leukoencephalopathy) — is a genetic disorder with a mutation of the Notch 3 gene on chromosome 19. Patients develop recurrent infarcts with subsequent dementia and demonstrate leukoencephalopathy with U fiber sparing. Pathologic examination of the cerebral vasculature demonstrates arteriopathy with granular osmiophilic material deposition.

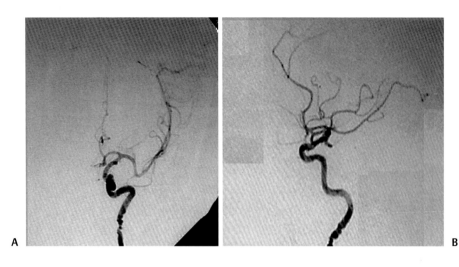

Fig. 3.206 Anterior choroidal artery aneurysm. (**A**) Anteroposterior and (**B**) lateral angiograms. There is also fibromuscular dysplasia in the cervical internal carotid artery.

12. Dissection of the ICA
    a. It may cause a sudden onset of nonthrobbing ipsilateral head and neck pain, Horner syndrome, peripheral neuropathy of CNs X, XI, or XII (by occlusion of arterial feeders), and focal ischemic symptoms.
    b. Risk is increased with trauma, FMD, cystic medial necrosis, hypertension, migraine, drugs, oral contraceptives, pharyngeal infections, vasculopathy, Marfan syndrome, and homocystinuria.
    c. Evaluation is with MRI/MRA and angiogram that demonstrates a string sign or occlusion (**Fig. 3.207**).

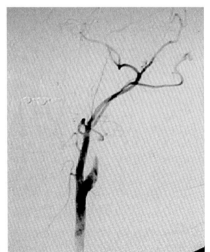
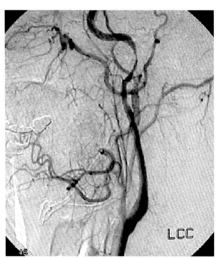

Fig. 3.207 Carotid artery dissection. Angiograms demonstrate (**A**) cervical internal carotid artery (ICA) and (**B**) petrous ICA tapered narrowings.

    d. The dissection typically spares the carotid bulb and starts 2 cm above the carotid bifurcation. It less frequently involves the supraclinoid ICA and the proximal ACA or MCA.
    e. Treatment is with antiplatelet or anticoagulant drugs. Without stroke, 85% do well. With stroke, 25% mortality is present and 50% are permanently impaired.

13. Dissection of the vertebral artery — usually occurs at the segment between C2 and the occiput. See Chapter 5 for more detail on dissections (**Fig. 3.208**).

14. Extrinsic compressive lesions — tumor, osteophytes, fibrous bands, and infection

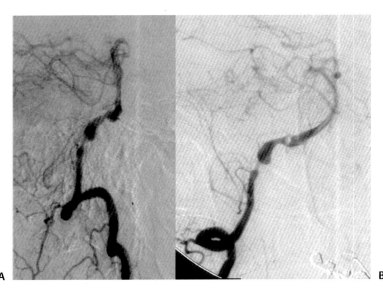

Fig. 3.208 Vertebral artery dissection. (**A**) Lateral and (**B**) oblique catheter angiograms demonstrate left distal vertebral artery narrowing and then dilation characteristic of vertebral artery dissection.

15. Raeder syndrome — unilateral headache and face pain of the V1 and V2 distributions and Horner syndrome. The ICA may be narrowed by sinusitis, arteritis, or dissection.

L. Vasculitis / Vasculopathy

1. Infectious vasculitis — caused by *H. influenzae* (common cause of stroke in children), TB, *Actinomyces* (directly invades vessel wall), herpes encephalitis, and syphilis (MCA distribution gummas and diffuse involvement of cortical arteries and veins). There is inflammation in the vessel wall with necrosis, occlusion, stroke, or hemorrhage. Endocarditis has a 5–10% risk of SAH as a result of infectious aneurysms, stroke, or focal vasculitis. Encephalitis is rarely hemorrhagic, except with HSV-2.

2. Immune complex vasculitis
    a. Polyarteritis nodosa — the most common necrotic vasculitis with CNS lesions. It affects small and medium-sized arteries throughout the body. It causes polyneuropathy that may be symmetric or asymmetric (mononeuropathy multiplex) by obliteration of the vasa nervosum, and is associated with microaneurysms (70%), stenosis, and thrombosis. It also causes skin purpura and renal dysfunction.
    b. SLE — an autoimmune disease caused by antinuclear antibodies. 75% of cases involve the CNS. 50% of cases develop stroke mainly caused by antiphospholipid antibodies, coagulopathy (with hemorrhage), and cardiac valve disease (Libman–Sacks endocarditis). Vasculitis is rare. It may also cause myelopathy or peripheral neuropathy. There is frequently a malar butterfly rash. Treatment is with steroids (**Fig. 3.209**).
    c. Others — allergic angiitis, serum sickness, and other collagen vascular diseases

3. Cell-mediated vasculitis
    a. Temporal arteritis
        (1) A subacute granulomatous inflammation with giant cells. Peak age is 70 years. It affects extracranial vessels (especially the temporal branches of the external carotid artery). Remember as a cause of visual loss to differentiate from carotid stenosis.

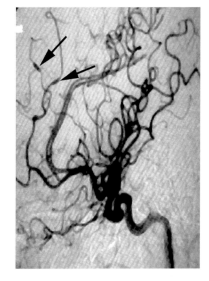

Fig. 3.209 Lupus vasculitis. Angiogram demonstrates multiple distal anterior cerebral artery fusiform dilations (*arrows*) and narrowings.

(2) It is an autoimmune disease with mononuclear cell inflammation of all three layers with multinucleated giant cells and resorption of the internal elastic lamina. There may be antibodies to the external elastic lamina.

(3) Skip lesions are common so that segments of abnormal artery are interspersed with unaffected segments.

(4) Symptoms include low-grade fever, weight loss, headache, local tenderness, elevated erythrocyte sedimentation rate (ESR), and C-reactive protein, and occasionally polymyalgia rheumatica with proximal muscle pain. The ophthalmic artery may be involved, but never intracranial vessels.

(5) Treatment is with low-dose steroids to decrease the risk of blindness.

b. Takayasu arteritis — occlusive thromboaortopathy with giant cell arteritis affecting the aorta and its branches and the pulmonary arteries causing stenosis and aneurysms. It most commonly occurs in young Asian females. Symptoms include fever, weight loss, elevated ESR, and decreased peripheral pulses (pulseless disease). There may be visual loss. Treatment is with steroids and revascularization.

c. Wegener granulomatosis — occurs in adults with male predominance. It involves respiratory, renal, and CNS vessels and causes peripheral and cranial neuropathies. It is due to antineutrophil antibodies and is treated with cyclophosphamide.

4. Chemical vasculitis — caused by ergots, pseudoephedrine, amphetamine, and oral contraceptives (especially with tobacco use)

5. Other causes of vasculitis and vasculopathy
   a. Sarcoid
   b. Kawasaki disease (mucocutaneous lymph node syndrome) — fusiform ectasia and aneurysms
   c. Buerger disease (thromboangiitis obliterans) — affects small and medium-sized arteries and veins and is associated with tobacco use
   d. Behçet disease — a recurrent inflammatory disease with male predominance that affects arteries and veins. It is most common in Japan and the Mediterranean. It is associated with oral and genital ulcers, uveitis, ulcerative colitis, erythema nodosum, polyarthritis, arterial occlusions, aneurysms, and thrombophlebitis. There may be brainstem, meningoencephalitic, or organic confusional syndromes. The CNS is involved in 10–45% of patients. Treatment is with steroids.
   e. Thrombotic thrombocytopenic purpura is not a vasculitis, but rather a thrombotic microangiopathy. Patients typically present with the clinical triad of severe thrombocytopenia, microangiopathic hemolytic anemia, and neurologic dysfunction. Fever and renal failure complete the classical pentad originally ascribed to the condition. Without the immediate institution of daily plasma exchange, the disease is almost universally fatal. Histopathologically, platelet- and von Willebrand factor-rich thrombi are seen in small arterioles. Perivascular inflammation is conspicuously absent. Neurologic sequelae involve predominantly stroke and seizures. It is caused by deficiency of the von Willebrand factor-protease, ADAMTS13.

M. Hypertension

1. Acute hypertension — causes increased pinocytosis in the cerebral capillaries and arterioles with BBB breakdown, fibrin deposition around blood vessels, brain swelling and edema, and increased ICP

2. Chronic hypertension
   a. It causes serum proteins to accumulate in the basement membrane and causes collagen deposition, medial hyalinization, loss of muscularis layer, vessel dilation or stenosis, and occasionally fatty macrophage accumulation (lipohyalinosis) in small muscular arteries.

b. It most commonly affects the basal ganglia, pons, centrum semiovale, and cerebellum.

c. Charcot-Bouchard aneurysms form on the lenticulostriate arteries. There are dilated perivascular spaces, état lacunaire (in the centrum semiovale), and état criblé (in the basal ganglia), which form lacunae with gliosis but no symptoms.

d. Hemorrhage may be caused by rupture of Charcot–Bouchard aneurysms or by occlusion and secondary rupture of small penetrating arteries.

3. Hypertensive encephalopathy
   a. Extreme hypertension causes loss of autoregulation with vasospasm, dilation, BBB breakdown, and edema.
   b. Lesions form in the external capsule, basal ganglia, gray–white matter junction, and occipital lobe (more in the posterior circulation because there is less sympathetic input).
   c. Symptoms include headaches, seizures, obtundation, and focal deficits, as well as manifestations of other end organ damage such as renal and cardiac disease.
   d. Hypertensive encephalopathy usually occurs with toxemia, preeclampsia/eclampsia, chronic renal failure, thrombotic thrombocytopenic purpura, hemolytic uremic syndrome, SLE, or renovascular hypertension.

4. Binswanger disease — causes hypertension and dementia with lacunae or demyelination in the centrum semiovale with arteriolar sclerosis.

5. Preeclampsia — hypertension and proteinuria that develop after 24 weeks of pregnancy. It occurs in 5–10% of pregnancies. Eclampsia is present when seizures or coma develop. It occurs in 0.1% of pregnancies, is fatal in 13%, and is associated with deep hemorrhages and white matter changes on MRI.

N. Intraparenchymal hemorrhage (IPH)

1. Etiologies — hypertension, amyloid angiopathy, tumor, AVMs, coagulopathy, venous thrombosis, and aneurysms

2. CT appearance
   a. Acute — the clot is hyperdense because of increased hemoglobin (Hb) and proteins. It may be hypodense if there is unretracted liquid clot, active bleeding, a coagulation disorder, or a hematocrit <30.
   b. Subacute (1–6 weeks) — isodense
   c. Chronic — hypodense
   d. Residua — hypodense (37%), slit lesion (25%), calcification (10%), or no abnormality (27%)

3. MRI appearance (**Table 3.5**)
   a. Hyperacute (4–6 hours) — contains oxyHb, isointense (iso-) T1, and hyperintense (hyper-) T2
   b. Acute (6 hours–3 days) — contains deoxyhemoglobin (deoxyHb), hypointense- (hypo-) or iso-T1, and hypo-T2
   c. Subacute (days to months) — contains methemoglobin (metHb), intracellular (3–6 days) hyper-T1 and hypo-T2, and extracellular (6 days–2 months) hyper-T1 and -T2
   d. Chronic (2 months to years) — contains ferritin and hemosiderin, transition to hypointense on T1- and T2-weighted MRIs with changes appearing first as hypointense rim on T1- and T2-weighted MRIs
   e. Nonparamagnetic heme — hypo-T1 and hyper-T2
   f. Rim of hemosiderin — hypointense on T1 and T2
   g. The clot interior is hypoxic, and this may delay the Hb denaturation.

Table 3.5 **Magnetic Resonance Imaging Characteristics of Intraparenchymal Hemorrhage**

Age of IPH	T1-Weighted Image	T2-Weighted Image	Comments
Hyperacute phase (4–6 h)	Iso	Hyper	OxyHb
Acute phase (6 h–3 d)	Iso / Hypo	Hypo	DeoxyHb
Early subacute phase (3–6 d)	Hyper	Hypo	MetHb (intracellular)
Late subacute phase (6 d–2 mo)	Hyper	Hyper	MetHb (extracellular)
Early chronic phase (2–4 mo)	Hyper with rim of hypointensity	Hyper with rim of hypointensity	Infiltration of macrophages
Late chronic phase (months to years)	Hypo	Hypo	Ferritin, hemosiderin

Abbreviations: DeoxyHb, deoxyhemoglobin; hyper, hyperintense; hypo, hypointense; iso, isointense; MetHb, methemoglobin; oxyHb, oxyhemoglobin.

4. Hypertensive IPH
   a. The most common cause of nontraumatic intracranial hemorrhage. Average age is younger than the thrombotic stroke group. There is no sex predominance, and in the United States, African Americans are affected more than Caucasians.
   b. It is due to Charcot-Bouchard aneurysms or lipohyalinosis of the penetrating arterioles of the brain. Locations are putamen (60%), thalamus (20%), pons (10%), cerebellum (near the dentate, 5%), and subcortical white matter (2%). The clot extends to the ventricle in 50% of cases, and this carries a worse prognosis (**Fig. 3.210**).
   c. Overall mortality is 25% and is related mainly to the size of the hemorrhage.
   d. Lobar hemorrhages are more likely due to amyloid angiopathy in the elderly. Putamen hemorrhages cause weakness by compression of the internal capsule and eye deviation toward the lesion. Thalamic hemorrhages cause weakness, sensory loss, and ocular dysfunction (persistent downgaze). Cerebellar hemorrhages cause eye deviation away from the lesion, and ocular bobbing although the latter sign is much more common with destructive pontine lesions. Pontine lesions cause fixed pinpoint pupils and ocular bobbing.
   e. Surgery may be beneficial for lesions >3 cm in the cerebellum but has not proven helpful for putamen or thalamus hemorrhages.

5. Amyloid angiopathy (congophilic)
   a. It usually occurs after 70 years of age and is the most common cause of intracranial hemorrhage in the normotensive elderly. It occasionally occurs in younger patients in the familial variety (in the Netherlands and Iceland).
   b. The contractile elements in the media of the arteries and arterioles of the leptomeningeal and superficial cortical vessels are replaced by noncontractile amyloid β-protein with a β-pleated sheet configuration. Blood vessels become dilated with thick walls containing pink amorphous material. They may form aneurysms.
   c. The amyloid is yellow-green with dichromism/birefringence when stained with Congo red dye and viewed under polarized light (**Fig. 3.211**).
   d. The major protein is amyloid β peptide (although it is the cystatin C variant in the hereditary type).

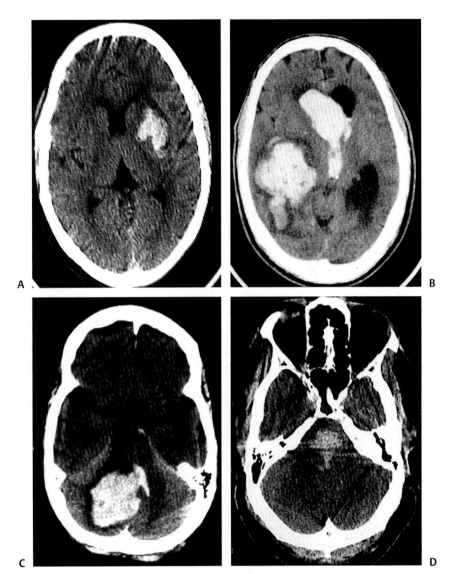

Fig. 3.210 Hypertensive intraparenchymal hemorrhage. Nonenhanced computed tomographic scans demonstrate (**A**) putamen, (**B**) thalamus, (**C**) cerebellum, and (**D**) pons hemorrhages.

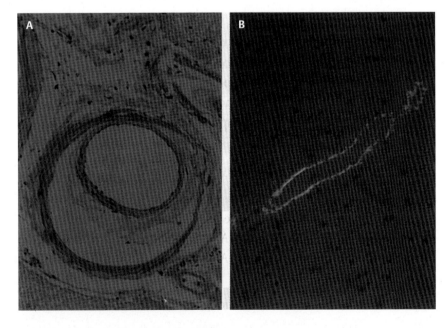

Fig. 3.211 Amyloid angiopathy. (**A**) Hematoxylin and eosin (H&E) stain demonstrating amyloid deposition within the vessel wall; (**B**) Congo red stain demonstrating negative birefringence in polarized light.

e. Amyloid angiopathy causes multiple lobar hemorrhages in the centrum semiovale that often extend to the subarachnoid space. These vessel changes also are seen with Down syndrome, Alzheimer disease, spongiform encephalitis, radiation necrosis, and vasculitis.

6. Drugs — 50% of drug-related hemorrhages are spontaneous, and 50% are associated with an AVM or aneurysm. Manifestations may include stroke, venous occlusion, abscess, vasculitis, and infectious aneurysms. Cocaine enhances platelet aggregation and spasm and may cause ischemic strokes. Amphetamines directly irritate the vessel wall and may cause vasculitis.

7. Blood dyscrasias — 15% of nontraumatic nonaneurysmal intracranial hemorrhages are caused by anticoagulant therapy. 1% of patients with myocardial infarction treated with thrombolytics develop intracranial hemorrhage. This complication carries a 60% mortality rate.

8. Germinal matrix hemorrhages
   a. They occur in premature infants.
   b. The germinal matrix consists of thin-walled vessels and proliferating cells in the subependymal zone, and it normally involutes at 36 weeks' gestational age.
   c. The blood supply is from the lenticulostriate arteries, choroidal arteries, and the artery of Heubner. It typically hemorrhages a few days after a premature birth because of hypoxia/ischemia in the deep borderzone zone that supplies the germinal matrix.
   d. In fullterm births, the most common location of intracranial hemorrhage is IVH from the choroid plexus.
   e. Germinal matrix hemorrhage grades
      (1) Grade 1 — limited to the germinal matrix
      (2) Grade 2 — blood in the ventricles, but no increase in ventricular size
      (3) Grade 3 — blood in the ventricles with hydrocephalus
      (4) Grade 4 — intraparenchymal extension of the hemorrhage

9. Hemorrhage with malignancies
   a. There is increased incidence with coagulopathy and chemotherapy.
   b. The cause may be neovascularization, necrosis, plasminogen activators, or direct vessel invasion. It occurs in 1–15% of tumors.
   c. The most commonly hemorrhagic primary tumors are high-grade astrocytoma, oligodendroglioma, pituitary adenoma, hemangioblastoma, lymphoma, sarcoma, ependymoma, schwannoma, epidermoid, PNET, choroid plexus papilloma, and teratoma.
   d. The most commonly hemorrhagic metastatic tumors are melanoma, renal cell carcinoma, and choriocarcinoma. Hemorrhage is detected in 15% of metastatic brain tumors.
   e. Arachnoid cysts may hemorrhage and are associated with SDH.

O. Aneurysms

1. The rupture of cerebral aneurysms accounts for 75% of nontraumatic SAH (15% benign perimesencephalic, and the remainder include AVM, arterial dissection, and unknown causes). 90% of the blood is cleared from the CSF in 1 week. MRI is better than CT for detecting subacute and chronic SAH. Repeated SAH or IVH may cause hemosiderin and ferritin to deposit over the leptomeninges and brain (superficial siderosis) and manifest with cerebellar dysfunction, long tract signs, and impaired hearing.

2. Saccular aneurysms
   a. The most common type of aneurysm. Peak age at rupture is 40–60 years with a female predominance.

b. They usually occur at the arterial bifurcations at the base of the brain. 90% are in the anterior circulation (posterior communicating artery [PcommA] 30%, anterior communicating artery [AcommA] 30%, MCA 20%, and ICA), and 10% are in the posterior circulation (basilar apex 5%, superior cerebellar artery, vertebrobasilar junction, PICA, and rarely anterior inferior cerebellar artery [AICA]) (**Figs. 3.206** and **3.212–3.228**).

c. The risk of rupture is related to size and location. In multiple aneurysm cases, the site of the ruptured aneurysm can be predicted by aneurysm location, irregular shape, daughter loculus, surrounding clot, more proximal location, and focal spasm. Aneurysms are multiple in 20% of cases.

d. Risk factors include female sex, age, hypertension, atherosclerosis, FMD (20–50% have aneurysms), Marfan syndrome, Ehlers–Danlos syndrome, polycystic kidney disease, coarctation of the aorta, high flow state (AVM), and familial.

e. They were originally thought to be congenital and caused by medial defects of the elastic lamina at the vessel bifurcations but now are thought to be acquired from hemodynamically induced vascular injury because they rarely are seen before 20 years of age.

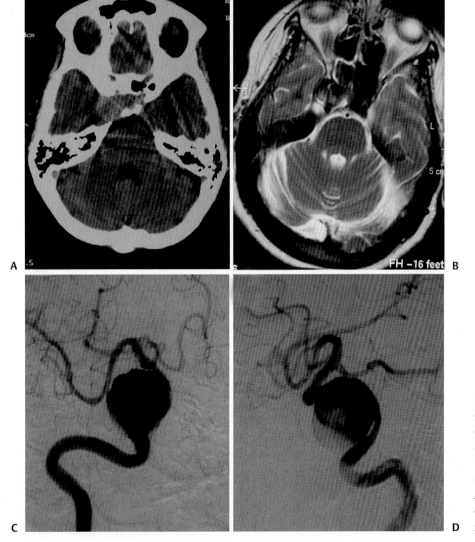

Fig. 3.212 Cavernous internal carotid artery aneurysm. (**A**) Plain computed tomographic scan shows a mass in the cavernous sinus that is (**B**) hypointense on T2-weighted magnetic resonance imaging. (**C**) Anteroposterior and (**D**) lateral angiograms show a large cavernous sinus aneurysm.

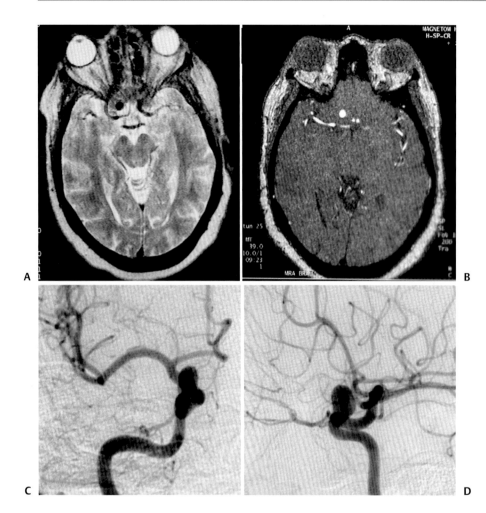

Fig. 3.213 Ophthalmic internal carotid artery aneurysm. (**A**) Axial T2- and (**B**) T1-weighted magnetic resonance images with gadolinium and (**C**) anteroposterior and (**D**) lateral angiograms showing aneurysm.

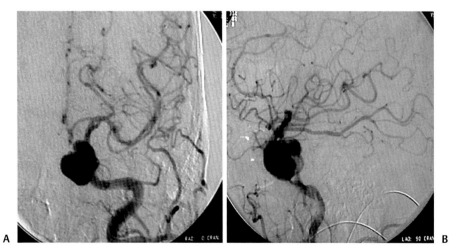

Fig. 3.214 Giant ophthalmic internal carotid artery aneurysm. (**A**) Anteroposterior and (**B**) lateral angiograms.

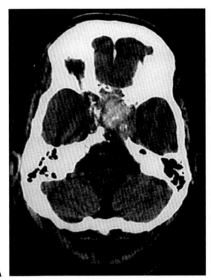
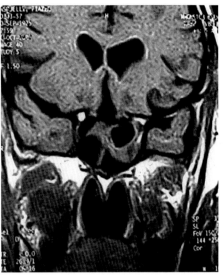

A   B

Fig. 3.215 Giant ophthalmic internal carotid artery aneurysm. (**A**) Axial computed tomographic scan and (**B**) coronal T1-weighted magnetic resonance image demonstrate erosive mass with partial thrombus and flow void.

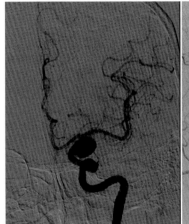
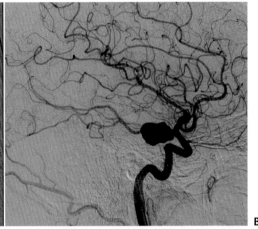

A   B

Fig. 3.216 Posterior communicating artery aneurysm. (**A**) Anteroposterior and (**B**) lateral angiograms.

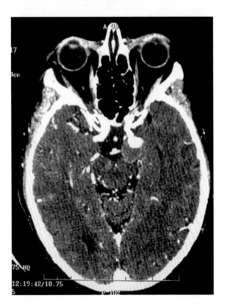

Fig. 3.217 Posterior communicating artery aneurysm. Enhanced axial computed tomographic scan demonstrates left-sided mass.

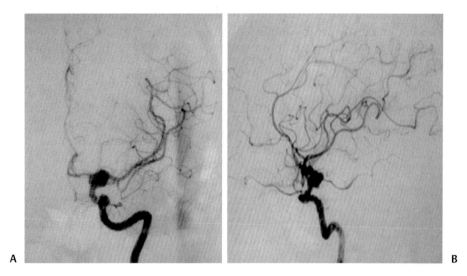

Fig. 3.218 Internal carotid artery bifurcation aneurysm. (**A**) Anteroposterior and (**B**) lateral angiograms.

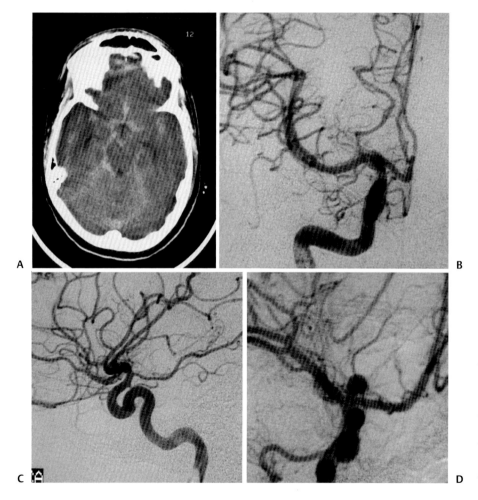

Fig. 3.219 Internal carotid artery bifurcation aneurysm. (**A**) Computed tomographic scan shows subarachnoid hemorrhage. (**B**) Anteroposterior (AP) and (**C**) lateral angiograms do not clearly show the aneurysm. Note the double density at the bifurcation on the AP view. (**D**) A submental-vertex view demonstrates the aneurysm.

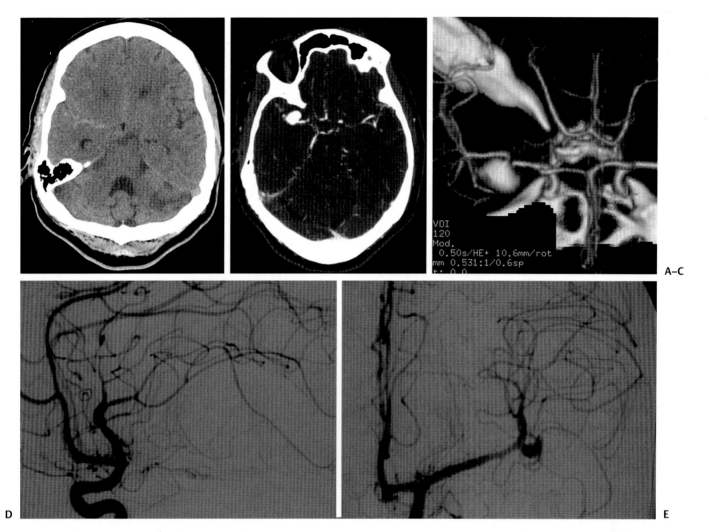

Fig. 3.220 Middle cerebral artery (MCA) aneurysm. (**A**) Top row shows subarachnoid hemorrhage in the right sylvian fissure and (**B**) MCA aneurysm on axial source computed tomographic (CT) angiogram and (**C**) CT reconstruction. (**D**) Bottom row shows lateral and (**E**) anteroposterior angiograms showing left MCA aneurysm with mass effect from a temporal lobe hematoma.

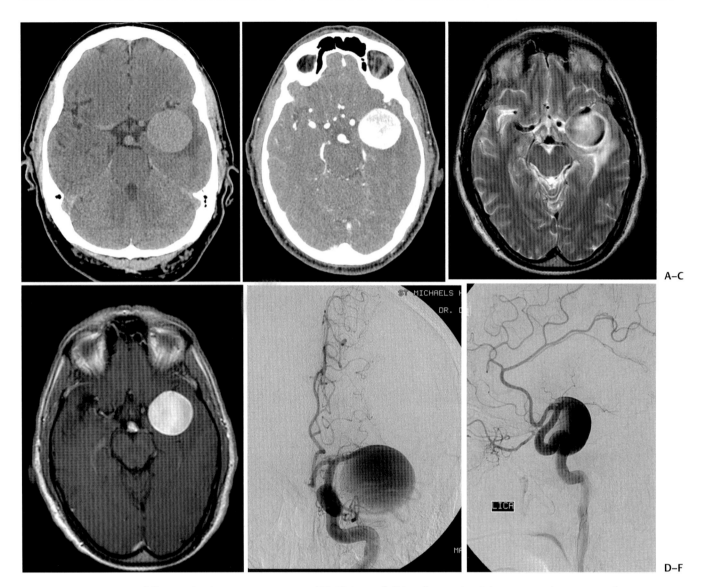

Fig. 3.221 Giant middle cerebral artery aneurysm. (**A**) Plain and (**B**) enhanced axial computed tomographic scans and (**C**) axial T2-weighted and (**D**) T1-weighted with gadolinium magnetic resonance images demonstrating left-sided aneurysm. (**E**) Anteroposterior and (**F**) lateral angiograms show the aneurysm.

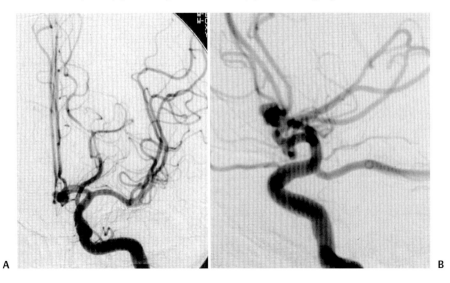

Fig. 3.222 Anterior communicating artery aneurysm. (**A**) Anteroposterior and (**B**) lateral angiograms.

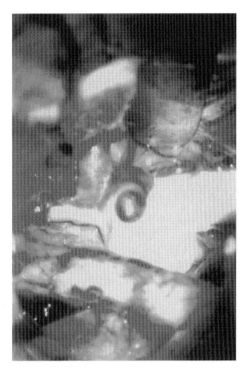

Fig. 3.223 Anterior communicating artery aneurysm. Aneurysm pointing anteriorly.

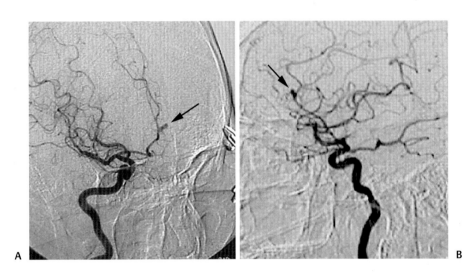

A

B

Fig. 3.224 Distal anterior cerebral artery aneurysm (*arrows*). (**A**) Antero-posterior and (**B**) lateral angiograms.

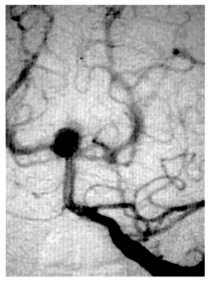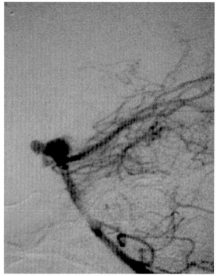

Fig. 3.225 Basilar artery apex aneurysm. (**A**) Anteroposterior and (**B**) lateral angiograms.

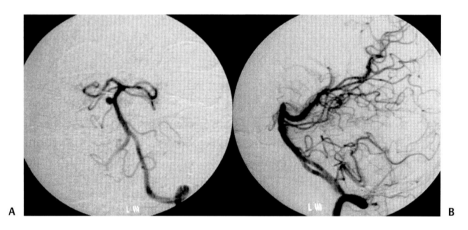

Fig. 3.226 Anterior inferior cerebellar artery aneurysm. (**A**) Anteroposterior and (**B**) lateral angiograms. (From Sekhar LN, de Oliveira E. Cranial Microsurgery. New York, NY: Thieme; 1998. Reprinted by permission.)

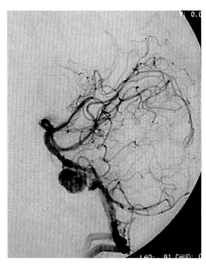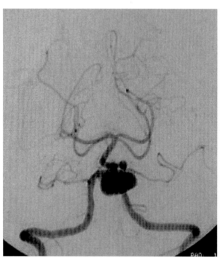

Fig. 3.227 Vertebrobasilar junction aneurysm. (**A**) Lateral and (**B**) anteroposterior angiograms.

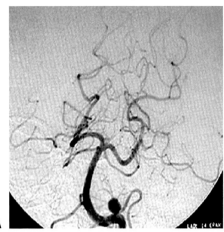
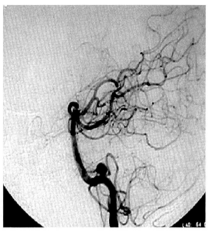

Fig. 3.228 Posterior inferior cerebellar artery aneurysm. (**A**) Anteroposterior and (**B**) lateral angiograms.

   f. Pathologic examination reveals deterioration of the internal elastic lamina and muscularis at the junction of the vessel and the aneurysm.

   g. In children, they are rare, more common in boys, larger, in unusual locations, and frequently associated with trauma and infection.

   h. Rehemorrhage rate is highest in the first 24 hours, 20% in 2 weeks, 50% in 6 months, and 3% per year after that. The hemorrhage risk is 1–2% per year if unruptured (see Chapter 6).

   i. The long-term outcome after hemorrhage in patients who survive to reach the hospital is death (25%), impairment (15%), and normal (60%).

   j. Angiography — used to assess spasm, collateral supply, filling vessels, and the relationship of the aneurysm to the parent vessel and perforators

   k. Giant aneurysms (>2.5 cm) — They usually contain multilayered clots, and have a thick fibrous wall. They frequently cause symptoms by mass effect, but also are at high risk of rupture.

   l. Classical SAH locations — frontal horn (anterior choroidal), interhemispheric fissure (AcommA), sylvian fissure (MCA), and fourth ventricle (posterior circulation) (**Fig. 3.229**)

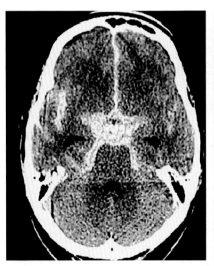
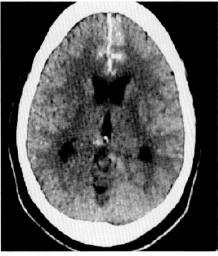
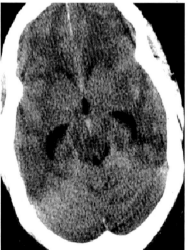

Fig. 3.229 Subarachnoid hemorrhage. (**A**) Nonenhanced axial computed tomographic scans of suprasellar cistern hemorrhage from a ruptured posterior communicating artery aneurysm, (**B**) interhemispheric hemorrhage from a ruptured anterior communicating artery aneurysm, and (**C**) interpeduncular cistern hemorrhage from a ruptured basilar apex aneurysm.

m. Complications of aneurysmal SAH — vasospasm (angiographic in 70% and symptomatic in 30%; 50% of these patients die or suffer permanent deficits; peak time is 4–14 days), rehemorrhage (20% in 2 weeks if not treated, occurs in 8–12% of patients, most frequently immediately after SAH and declines with time), hydrocephalus, and stroke (**Fig. 3.230**)

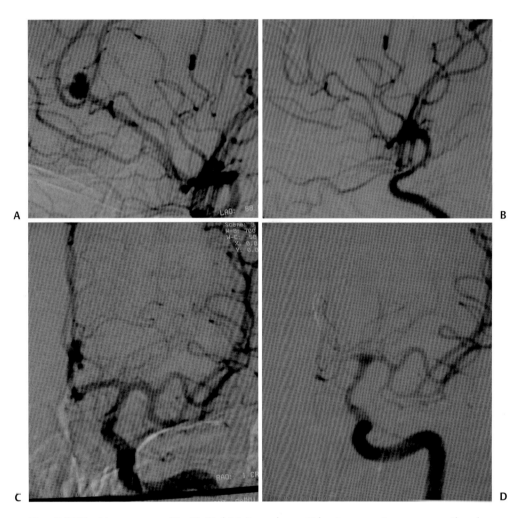

Fig. 3.230 Vasospasm. (**A, C**) Right internal carotid artery angiograms on the day of subarachnoid hemorrhage and (**B, D**) 7 days later show narrowing of the proximal and distal anterior cerebral artery and of the internal carotid artery and middle cerebral artery.

n. Aneurysmal SAH is associated with fever, ECG changes (possibly by hypothalamic ischemia with sympathetic dysfunction), and retinal hemorrhages (Terson syndrome).

o. In 15% of SAH, no aneurysm is demonstrated. If the angiogram is repeated in 2 weeks, some of these reveal an aneurysm, usually in the anterior circulation, the detection rate depending on the quality of the initial angiogram.

p. Treatment options are surgical clipping or endovascular coiling. Partial treatments like wrapping are of uncertain value. Operative mortality is 3%.

q. If the aneurysm is unruptured and <7 mm, consider repeat imaging every year. Consider intervention if it enlarges.

r. Infundibulum — a funnel-shaped dilation at the origin of a vessel, <3–4 mm wide, with a vessel exiting from the apex of the funnel. It probably is caused by incomplete regression of the vessel during fetal development. They are most common at the origin of the PcommA from the ICA, but occasionally occur on other arteries (**See Fig. 1.7**).

s. Benign perimesencephalic SAH — located in the interpeduncular, prepontine, and ambient cisterns, seldom rehemorrhages, has a good prognosis, and is postulated to be caused by the rupture of small pontine and perimesencephalic veins (**Fig. 3.231**)

3. Fusiform aneurysms — caused by atherosclerosis, infection (syphilis), and possibly dissection or vasculitis. They form when damage to the media causes the artery to elongate and dilate. They are most common in older patients and in the posterior circulation. Symptoms are caused by stroke, thrombus with mass effect, or hemorrhage (**Fig. 3.232**).

4. Infectious aneurysms — caused by an infected embolism to the intima or vasa vasorum and account for 2–3% of aneurysms. The thoracic aorta is the most frequent site, and the most common intracranial location is the distal MCA territory. They are usually multiple and are caused by bacteria or fungi. 10% of patients with SBE will develop an infectious aneurysm (**Fig. 3.233**).

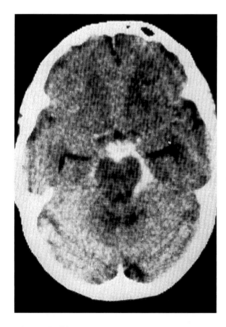

Fig. 3.231 Benign perimesencephalic hemorrhage. Computed tomographic scan demonstrates typical subarachnoid hemorrhage in the interpeduncular cistern extending into the left ambient cistern (angiogram was normal).

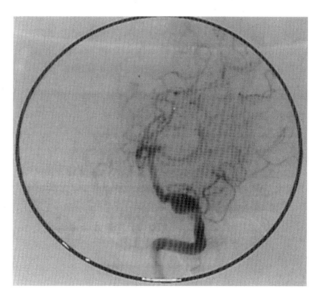

Fig. 3.232 Fusiform aneurysm. Oblique vertebral artery angiogram with left distal vertebral fusiform aneurysm

5. Dissecting aneurysms—more commonly extracranial and tend to spare the CCA and carotid bulb. They usually involve the mid-cervical and petrous ICA, and in the vertebral artery occur from C2 to the occiput. They are caused by trauma, cystic medial necrosis, FMD, iatrogenic after angiography, and rarely infection. Blood accumulates in the vessel wall by means of a tear in the intima and internal elastic lamina. Subintimal accumulation may cause occlusion, whereas subadventitial accumulation, which typically occurs with intradural vertebral artery dissections, causes an aneurysm and SAH.

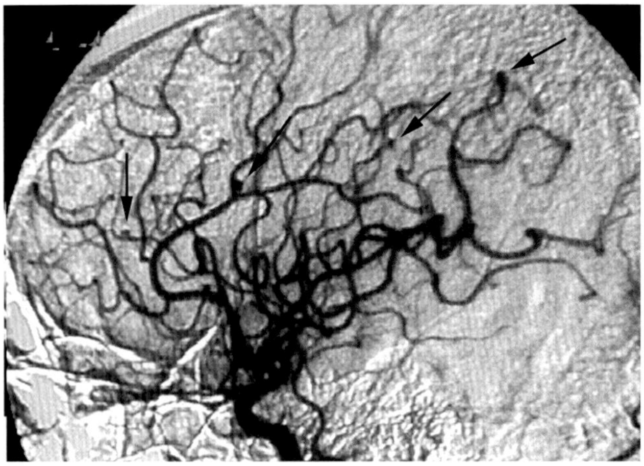

Fig. 3.233   Infectious aneurysms. Angiogram demonstrates multiple distal anterior circulation aneurysms (*arrows*).

6. Traumatic aneurysms — occur with 50% of gunshot wounds to the head and are usually pseudoaneurysms. With nonpenetrating trauma, they are usually on the distal ACA. Suspicion should be raised if there is abundant SAH in head injury, after penetrating head injury, or with late bleeding after head injury.

7. Oncotic aneurysms — occur with left atrial myxoma and choriocarcinoma.

8. Flow-related aneurysms — occur with AVMs (2.7–30%) and are usually located on the proximal or distal feeding vessels. There is no increased hemorrhage risk with proximal arterial feeder aneurysms, although the risk is increased with a nidus aneurysm (10% hemorrhage). They are thin-walled, have arterial pressure, and frequently hemorrhage.

9. True aneurysms — classic terminology is that they involve all three layers (intima, media, and adventitia). False aneurysms have no media or internal elastic lamina so lack some layers of the arterial wall. Pseudoaneurysms are recanalized blood clots and have no wall besides the clot. Cerebral aneurysms are usually false.

P. Vascular malformations

1. They are probably congenital and arise in the fetus during vessel development. Only AVMs and cavernous malformations have a clinically important hemorrhage risk.

2. Arteriovenous malformation (AVM)
   a. Peak age at presentation is 20–40 years and there is no gender predilection. 25% occur before 15 years and they are one-tenth as common as aneurysms.
   b. They are composed of thin-walled and thick-walled channels connecting arteries to veins without intervening capillary beds. 90% are hemispheric and 15% are in the posterior fossa. They are frequently cone-shaped, extending from the subpial surface with the apex at the ventricle because they receive ependymal feeder vessels. There usually is no intervening normal brain.
   c. CT — demonstrates serpiginous vessels and calcifications (30%). MRI demonstrates flow voids with characteristic vascular appearance.
   d. Angiogram — demonstrates early draining veins (also seen with stroke, luxury perfusion, tumors, contusions, postictal, and infection). An aneurysm is found on the feeding vessel or nidus in 8–12% of cases (**Figs. 3.234–3.236**).
   e. "Cryptic" AVMs — not detected by angiogram, in some cases because the feeding vessels are occluded by thrombus.

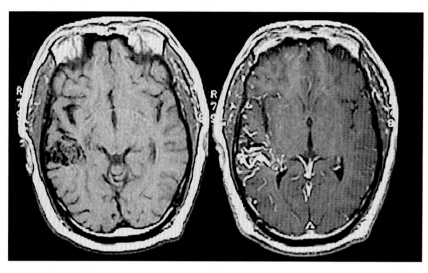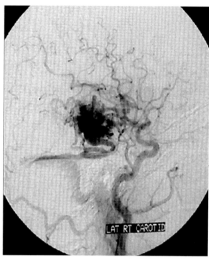

A–C

Fig. 3.234 Arteriovenous malformation (AVM). Axial T1-weighted magnetic resonance images (**A**) nonenhanced and (**B**) enhanced demonstrating serpentine vessels and (**C**) angiogram demonstrating early draining veins and AVM nidus.

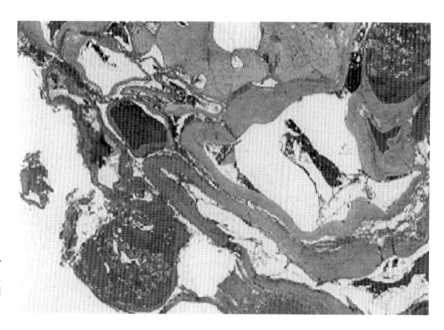

Fig. 3.235 Arteriovenous malformation (hematoxylin and eosin [H&E] stain). Multiple irregular thick and thin-walled vessels.

    f. Vascular steal rarely causes local ischemia and atrophy. The adjacent brain has ischemic changes, surrounding gliosis, hemosiderin-laden macrophages, and calcifications.

    g. They are developmental but may increase, decrease, or not change in size spontaneously over time.

    h. Symptoms — hemorrhage (50%, typically parenchymal with IVH and less commonly SAH), seizures (25%), headaches (20%), and focal symptoms (15%). A bruit may be heard, especially in dural AVMs.

    i. Hemorrhage risk — 2–4% per year. Rehemorrhage risk is 6% for the first year and then 3% per year. Each hemorrhage carries a 10% mortality and 25% morbidity. There is increased risk of hemorrhage if they are small, have deep drainage, are periventricular, have bled before, or have an intranidal aneurysm. 98% are solitary, and if multiple consider Wyburn–Mason and HHT.

j. Surgery. See Section VI — mortality of 1% and morbidity of 8%, but depends highly on case selection

k. Stereotactic radiosurgery — an option if the AVM diameter is <3 cm (85% rate of obliteration at 3–4 years)

l. Endovascular embolization — helpful surgical adjuvant, but is seldom effective by itself in the long term, except for small AVMs that can be completely obliterated by glue embolization

3. Vein of Galen aneurysm/malformation

a. Presentations — in the neonate with cyanotic heart disease, in the infant with hydrocephalus and seizures, and in children with SAH

b. Type 1 — the most common, is present at birth and is associated with high-output heart failure and hydrocephalus. It is an arteriovenous fistula (AVF) of the anterior and posterior choroidal arteries to the median venous sac (embryonal precursor of the vein of Galen).

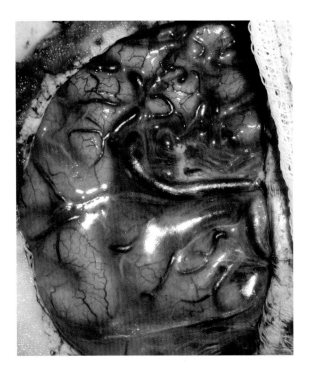

Fig. 3.236 Arteriovenous malformation. Arterialized cortical veins.

c. Type 2 — occurs in older infants, causes developmental delay and ocular symptoms, and is a parenchymal AVM in the thalamus/midbrain with thalamoperforate feeders draining into the vein of Galen. Occasionally, there is thrombosis of the venous sac (**Fig. 3.237**).

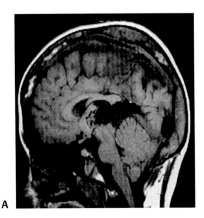
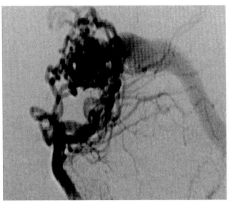

Fig. 3.237 Vein of Galen malformation. (**A**) Sagittal T1-weighted magnetic resonance image with diencephalic serpentine vessels and an enlarged vein of Galen, and (**B**) lateral basilar artery angiogram with early filling of vein of Galen system.

A

B

4. Dural AVMs

a. There is no discrete nidus, and the feeding vessels are usually in the wall of a dural venous sinus. They are acquired (not congenital) after dural thrombosis and recanalization with microfistula formation. The peak age at presentation is 40–60 years.

b. The transverse and sigmoid sinuses are the most common sites followed by the cavernous sinus and rarely the superior sagittal, straight, or other sinuses. 7% are multiple. They account for 10–15% of AVMs and up to 30% of posterior fossa AVMs.

c. Symptoms are bruit and headache (if sigmoid or transverse) and proptosis, chemosis, ophthalmoplegia, and bruit (if cavernous).

d. If the dural AVM drains forward into the sinus, it rarely hemorrhages (Borden type 1). If there is retrograde cortical venous drainage, there is a higher incidence of SAH and IPH (Borden types 2 and 3). They may also cause venous ischemia and communicating hydrocephalus from venous congestion.

e. Feeders usually are from the external carotid artery circulation (occipital or meningeal arteries) and occasionally from dural branches of the ICA and vertebral artery. There is frequent sinus occlusion.

f. Traumatic cavernous carotid fistula (CCF) usually due to tear in the ICA. Spontaneous CCF has multiple feeders from the ICA, the external carotid artery, or both and usually occurs in middle-aged women.

g. CT demonstrates a dilated superior ophthalmic vein in CCF. MRI demonstrates dilated cortical veins without a nidus with a dural AVM (**Figs. 3.238** and **3.239**).

h. Mixed pial and dural AVMs — 15–50% of pial AVMs have meningeal arterial supply.

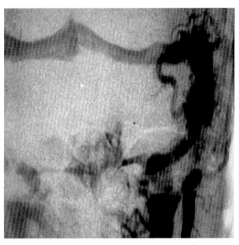 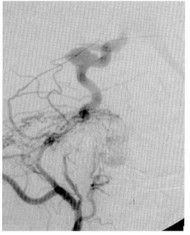

Fig. 3.238 Dural arteriovenous malformation. (**A**) Anteroposterior and (**B**) lateral external carotid artery (ECA) angiograms demonstrate supply from the ECA with early filling into the sigmoid sinus.

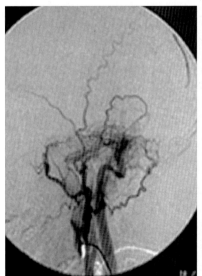 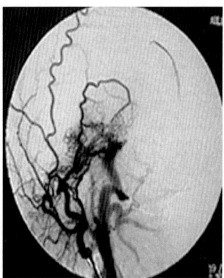 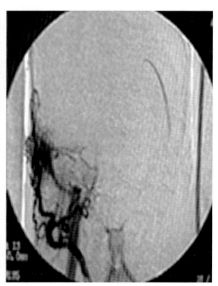

Fig. 3.239 Dural arteriovenous malformation. (**A**) Lateral, (**B**) oblique, and (**C**) anteroposterior angiograms with filling of the sigmoid sinus through the external carotid artery with a small dural nidus.

5. Cavernous malformations
   a. They are multilobulated berrylike structures full of blood of different ages. They are composed of closely approximated endothelial-lined sinusoidal spaces, large thin-walled vessels, no feeding artery, and no intervening brain. There are frequent calcifications and a surrounding hemosiderin ring. 80% are supratentorial, but they may also be in the cerebellum, pons, and spinal cord. 10% are multiple and 5% are familial. Identified genetic loci include (CCM1, Krev1 interaction trapped 1 [KRIT1], chromosome 7q), (CCM2, malcavernin [MGC4607], chromosome 7p), and PDCD10 (CCM3, chromosome 3q). The peak age of presentation is 20–40 years (**Fig. 3.240**).

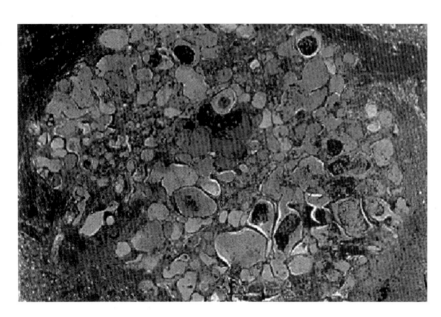

Fig. 3.240 Cavernous malformation (hematoxylin and eosin [H&E] stain). Multiple thin-walled vessels without intervening brain tissue.

   b. CT may demonstrate the calcifications, a hyperdense lesion, or a hematoma, sometimes with a fluid-fluid level.
   c. The angiogram is normal, and the MRI has a characteristic "popcorn" lesion that is hyperintense on T1-weighted MRI with a hypointense rim. They may or may not enhance (**Fig. 3.241**).
   d. Risk of hemorrhage is 0.5–1% per year, although it may be higher in the familial form in Hispanics.

6. Capillary telangiectasias — the second most common vascular malformation. They are small, multiple, clinically silent, firm capillary lesions, located in the white matter or classically the pons, and consist of multiple normal-sized and dilated thin vascular spaces without smooth muscle or elastic fibers. There is usually normal brain between lesions. Rarely there is evidence of old hemorrhage or gliosis. The angiogram is normal and the MRI reveals a lesion that is hypointense on T2-weighted images. In HHT, the mucocutaneous lesions are capillary telangiectasias, but the brain lesions are AVMs (**Fig. 3.242**).

7. Venous malformations — the most common vascular malformation. There is intervening normal brain. They consist of a large draining cortical vein receiving a collection of medullary veins (caput medusa) that usually occur near the angle of the ventricle. They rarely hemorrhage. They are caused by arrested development. 33% are associated with cavernous malformations. They are usually solitary, although they are multiple with blue rubber nevus syndrome. They rarely require treatment (**Figs. 3.243–3.245**).

8. Venous varix — a single tortuous draining vein that is a normal variant. It is associated with AVMs.

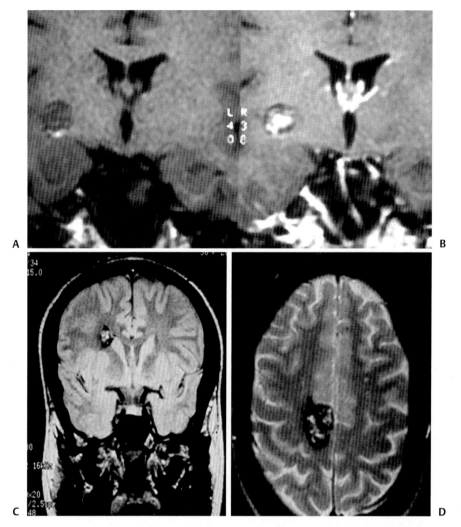

Fig. 3.241 Cavernous malformation. Coronal T1-weighted magnetic resonance imaging (MRI) scans (**A**) nonenhanced and (**B**) enhanced, and (**C**) coronal and (**D**) axial T2-weighted MRI scans demonstrating typical "popcorn" lesions with surrounding hemosiderin ring.

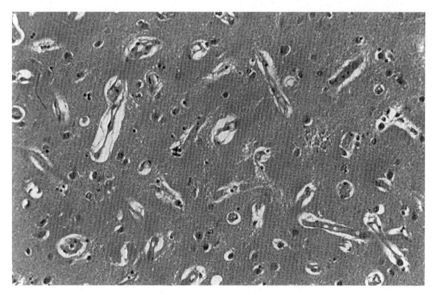

Fig. 3.242 Capillary telangiectasia (hematoxylin and eosin [H&E] stain). Multiple thin-walled vascular channels separated by normal brain parenchyma.

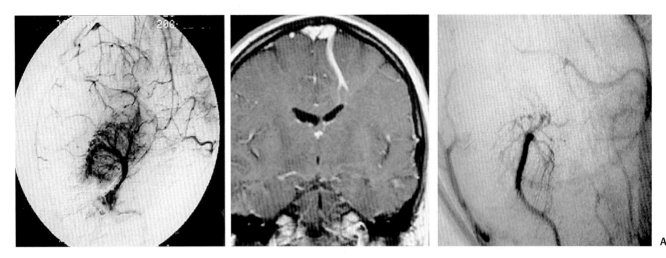

Fig. 3.243 Venous malformation. (**A,C**) Angiograms and (**B**) infused magnetic resonance image demonstrating a "caput medusae" of small veins draining into a large irregular vein.

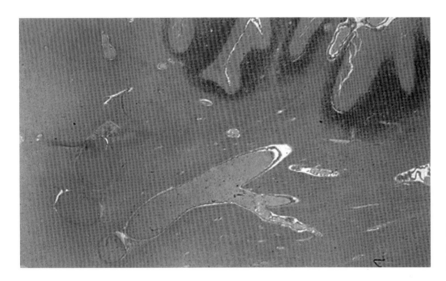

Fig. 3.244 Venous malformation (hematoxylin and eosin [H&E] stain). Ectatic, large diameter, thin-walled vessel.

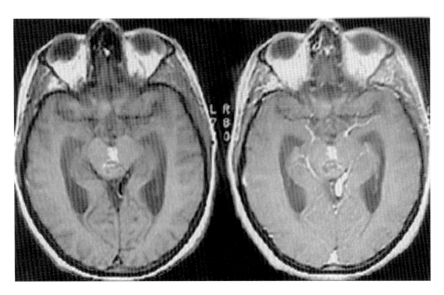

Fig. 3.245 Cavernous malformations with associated venous malformation. (**A**) Axial T1-weighted nonenhanced and (**B**) enhanced magnetic resonance images demonstrating a posterior midbrain cavernous malformation draining into a venous malformation. Hemorrhage is present in the medial anterior midbrain.

9. Sinus pericranii — a large communication between intracranial and extracranial veins. It may be congenital or caused by trauma. It is a soft mass that changes with head position. It is associated with other malformations.

XXIII. CNS Trauma

A. Before the age of 44 years, trauma is the leading cause of death, and 50% of the deaths are from head trauma.

B. Abrasion — a scraping injury where a layer of tissue is removed

C. Laceration — an injury creating a break in the tissues without tissue loss.

D. Contusion — a compressive injury to a tissue.

E. Ecchymosis — movement of blood from one extravascular site to another. Periorbital ecchymosis (raccoon's eye) is into the upper and lower eyelids from an orbital roof fracture. Mastoid ecchymosis (Battle's sign) is from a petrous temporal fracture.

F. Concussion — a reversible transitory neurologic deficit associated with trauma and caused by rotational shear stress. There is loss of consciousness for <24 hours by definition.

G. Fractures

1. Linear fracture — a line of fracture forms from the point of impact until the force is dissipated. 10% of adults with a linear skull fracture have a surgical lesion (mostly EDH). Linear fractures account for 75% of childhood skull fractures. Children <3 years old have a risk of a growing skull fracture developing where a leptomeningeal cyst progressively protrudes through a dural tear.

2. Depressed fracture — caused by force to a more narrow surface area and has a higher frequency of parenchymal injury (**Fig. 3.246**).

3. Comminuted fracture — caused by a stronger force to a wider surface area.

4. Diastatic fracture — occurs when the fracture extends to and opens a suture. These are more common in childhood because the sutures are not as adherent.

5. Compound (open) fracture — associated with open skin.

6. Basilar fracture — at the base of the skull. They may be linear, comminuted, or depressed (**Fig. 3.247** and **Fig. 3.248**).

7. Nonaccidental fracture — suspect if multiple, depressed, width >3 mm, growing fracture, more than one cranial bone involved, nonparietal, or with an associated injury. Work-up should include a skeletal survey and funduscopic examination for retinal hemorrhages.

H. Contusion

1. The second most common traumatic brain injury (after diffuse axonal injury [DAI]) and has a lower occurrence of initial loss of consciousness.

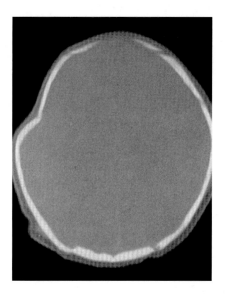

Fig. 3.246 Ping-pong skull fracture. Axial computed tomographic scan with right-sided depressed fracture involving mainly the outer table. Equivalent of orthopedic greenstick fracture.

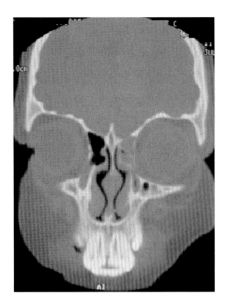

Fig. 3.247 Cribriform plate and skull fracture with cerebrospinal fluid leak. Coronal computed tomographic scan bone window demonstrates left side cribriform plate fracture with opacification of the ethmoid sinus.

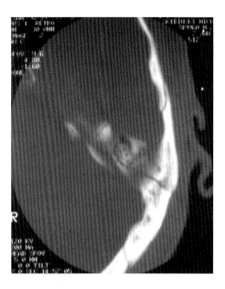

Fig. 3.248 Longitudinal petrous bone fracture. Axial computed tomographic scan demonstrating fracture.

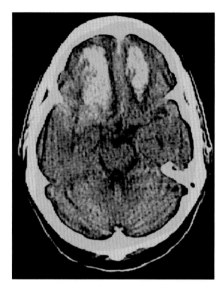

Fig. 3.249 Parenchymal contusion. Nonenhanced computed tomographic scan demonstrates bilateral frontal contusions.

2. Locations — temporal (50%), frontal (30%), and parasagittal/convexity (25%)

3. Definition — bruise of the cortical surface with hemorrhage from a torn vessel into the cortex. It affects the superficial layers, unlike stroke.

4. Contre-coup injury — caused by rotational shear. The anterior and middle skull bases have rigid sphenoid wings and petrous ridges. Rotation causes the frontal and temporal cortices to sweep across these structures and slow down, shearing the axons and vessels (**Fig. 3.249**).

5. Coup contusions — impact through the skull to the underlying brain. They occur at the convexities, are less common, and less severe. The bones are usually intact.

6. It is less common to have contusions in children because they have a softer, unmyelinated brain with smoother skull bases and more pliable skulls. 20% of contusions develop delayed hemorrhages.

I. Diffuse axonal injury (DAI) — the most common traumatic brain injury (50%). There is immediate loss of consciousness. Petechiae are found in the gray–white matter junction (66%), corpus callosum (20%), dorsolateral rostral brainstem, and superior cerebellar peduncle. Axon retraction balls form first, followed by Wallerian degeneration. The injury may be due to shearing of axons but also to impaired transport and organelle accumulation with the axons separating after the edema resolves. DAI is best identified with MRI where lesions are hyperintense on T2-weighted MRI (**Fig. 3.250**).

J. Gunshot wounds — 50% are associated with major vascular injuries. The wounding capacity depends on the energy of the missile. Low-velocity missiles travel at <2000 ft/s (civilian bullets) and the damage is caused by the tract and a cavity 4 times the size of the bullet. High-velocity missiles travel at >2000 ft/s (military bullets) and the cavity created is 30 times the size of the bullet because of high-energy shock waves.

K. Epidural hematoma (EDH)

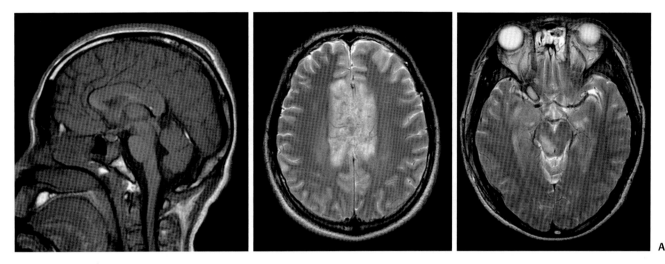

Fig. 3.250 Diffuse axonal injury. (**A**) Sagittal T1-weighted magnetic resonance image (MRI) demonstrates low-intensity lesion with some high-intensity (hemorrhage) in the corpus callosum as well as (**B**) hyperintensity in the corpus callosum and (**C**) superior colliculus on T2-weighted MRI.

1. They have a characteristic lentiform biconvex shape, do not cross suture lines, may cross dural attachments, and are most frequently in the temporoparietal region (**Fig. 3.251**).

2. They are seen in 3% of head injuries; peak age is 10–30 years. They are rare before 2 years or after 60 years because at the extremes of age the dura is more adherent to the bone.

3. One third of EDHs have the characteristic lucid interval before deterioration. The hemorrhage is from the middle meningeal artery, a dural sinus, or a diploic vein.

4. 85% are associated with a skull fracture, 43–75% with other brain lesions, and 13% with SDH. 5% are bilateral, and 5% are in the posterior fossa. Delayed formation occurs in 20%, and delayed enlargement at 48 hours occurs in 20%.

5. The overall mortality is 5%, but it is less if the patient is awake on arrival.

L. Subdural hematoma (SDH)

1. They are crescent shaped, cross suture lines but not dural attachments, and occur in 10–35% of severe head injuries. 50% of patients present flaccid or decerebrate, and the mortality is 40–70%. 8% have a complete recovery (**Figs. 3.252** and **3.22**).

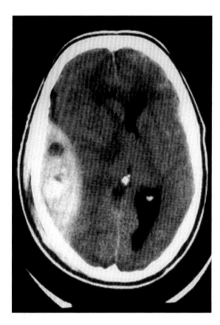

Fig. 3.251 Epidural hematoma. Nonenhanced computed tomographic scan demonstrates low-density unclotted hyperacute hemorrhage within the high-density biconvex (lentiform) clot.

2. The hemorrhage is caused by tearing of a bridging vein by angular acceleration.

3. 50% are associated with skull fractures. There is frequent SAH and DAI. 5% occur in the posterior fossa and 15% are bilateral.

4. Subacute SDH is 1–2 weeks old and chronic SDH is >3 weeks old.

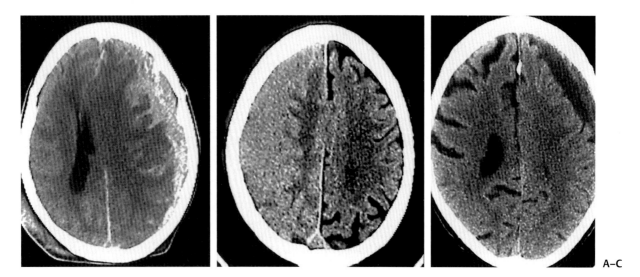

Fig. 3.252   Subdural hematoma (SDH). Nonenhanced computed tomographic scans demonstrate (**A**) acute left SDH with concave (crescent-shaped) high-density blood and associated subarachnoid hemorrhage, (**B**) subacute right SDH with isodense blood, and (**C**) chronic left SDH with low-density blood.

5. Chronic SDH may rebleed (10–30%) because of stretching of bridging veins or by neomembrane formation over the calvarial surface's arachnoid with fibroblasts and fragile capillaries. The membranes enhance. 2% of SDHs calcify.

6. Child abuse is associated with bilateral interhemispheric SDHs.

M. Subarachnoid hemorrhage (SAH) — the most common traumatic hemorrhage

N. Intraventricular hemorrhage (IVH) — occurs in 1–5% of closed-head injuries and indicates severe trauma. It is also seen with hypertensive hemorrhages and ruptured AVMs.

O. Intraparenchymal hemorrhage (IPH) — associated with contusion or DAI

P. Edema — There may be cytotoxic edema (intracellular) caused by brain injury and/or vasogenic edema caused by hyperemia with breakdown of the BBB. Vasogenic edema (extracellular) is seen in 15% of severe brain injuries and is more common in children.

Q. Vascular complications — aneurysm, pseudoaneurysm, dissection, laceration, and AVF (at the skull base, usually CCF, and may or may not be associated with a fracture).

R. Arterial dissections — associated with trauma, hypertension, migraines, activity, FMD, Marfan disease, cocaine, oral contraceptives, pharyngeal infections, and syphilis. The cervical ICA is affected by hyperextension and lateral flexion stretching the ICA over the transverse processes. Extracranial ICA dissections spare the carotid bulb and usually begin 2 cm distal to the bifurcation. Less commonly, intracranial dissections occur at the midsupraclinoid ICA where it is more mobile. Vertebral artery dissections occur between C2 and the skull.

S. Secondary complications of trauma

1. Increased ICP — The most common cause of death in trauma and is usually related to edema and/or hemorrhage.

2. Hypoxic injury — secondary to increased ICP, hypotension, hypoxia, or vasospasm (5–10% of cases), and usually occurs at the ACA/MCA territory junction, hippocampus, basal ganglia, and cerebellum.

T. Sequelae of trauma — encephalomalacia, pneumocephalus, CSF leakage, cranial nerve palsies (especially the olfactory nerve), diabetes insipidus, cephalocele, leptomeningeal cyst, hydrocephalus, and long-term personality or cognitive changes (dementia)

U. Posttraumatic seizures — occur with 5% of closed-head injuries and 50% of penetrating injuries. Treat with 7 days of phenytoin (Dilantin) and then discontinue if no further seizures occur.

V. Postconcussive syndrome — characterized by headaches, lethargy, etc., in the weeks after major head trauma

W. Pediatric trauma — The infant's skull is malleable and thus tolerates much more deformity without a fracture developing. Child abuse/nonaccidental trauma is associated with multiple long bone fractures, chronic SDH, retinal hemorrhages, SDH of different ages, and multiple, complex, bilateral, and depressed skull fractures. Shaking an infant causes the hemispheres to rub along the falx, resulting in an interhemispheric SDH.

X. Diffuse cerebral swelling — occurs mainly in children after head trauma. It is caused by hyperemia with venous congestion and manifests with severe swelling and ICP elevation.

Y. Herniation syndromes

1. Subfalcine herniation — The cingulate gyrus moves under the free edge of the falx, and the ipsilateral foramen of Monro becomes trapped, causing an ipsilateral large lateral ventricle and contralateral small lateral ventricle. The ACA may also be compressed.

2. Transtentorial herniation — usually a descending herniation with the uncus and parahippocampal gyrus being pushed over the tentorial edge. There is obliteration of the suprasellar cistern and inferomedial displacement of the anterior choroidal artery, PcommA, and PCA. The PCA may be compressed causing occipital strokes. The anterior choroidal artery and perforators may be compressed causing midbrain Duret hemorrhages (these may also be caused by vessel stretching) and basal ganglia infarction. The contralateral brainstem is compressed against the Kernohan notch producing ipsilateral hemiparesis (false localizing sign). Ascending transtentorial herniation causes effacement of the superior vermian cistern, quadrigeminal cistern, and fourth ventricle (**Fig. 3.253**).

3. Transalar (transsphenoidal) herniation — The frontal lobe may descend against the greater sphenoid wing, or the temporal lobe may ascend against it.

4. Tonsillar herniation — The cerebellar tonsils descend through the foramen magnum.

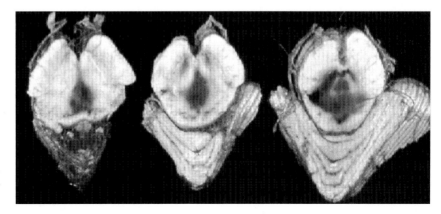

Fig. 3.253 Duret hemorrhages (gross). Midbrain hemorrhages caused by herniation.

XXIV. Skull Diseases

A. Fibrous dysplasia — presents in young adulthood. It may be either monostotic (70% of cases and 25% involve the skull/face) or polyostotic (30% of cases and 50% involve the skull/face). It expands and replaces normal bony medullary spaces with vascular fibrocellular tissue. CT demonstrates thickened sclerotic bone with "ground-glass" expanded diploë. It is hypointense on T1-weighted images and enhances. There may be sclerotic orbits and skull bases causing lion-like facies. McCune–Albright syndrome is unilateral polyostotic disease and endocrinopathy (**Figs. 3.162–3.164**).

B. Paget disease — seen in older adults and may be monostotic or polyostotic. Early in the course, it causes destruction and late it causes sclerosis. There is bony expansion that may cause basilar invagination.

C. Basilar impression/invagination — settling of the skull on the spine with the odontoid process 4–5 mm above the McGregor line or occipital condyles above the plane of the foramen magnum. Evaluation includes McRae line (foramen magnum diameter 35 ± 4 mm), Chamberlin line (diagonal line from the hard palate to the posterior foramen magnum, the odontoid should not have ⅓ of its length above it), and McGregor line (line from the hard palate to the most caudal portion of the occipital curve, odontoid tip should be <4 mm above the line). Symptoms include lower cranial nerve palsies, headache, and limb spasticity. It is associated with atlantoaxial fusion, osteogenesis imperfecta, rheumatoid arthritis, and Paget disease.

D. Platybasia — flattened skull base with an increased angle of the clivus to the spine or clivus to the anterior fossa >135 degrees. It is associated with basilar invagination or Chiari I malformation.

E. Wormian bones — small intrasutural bones, usually in the lambdoid suture. They are seen with cleidocranial dysostosis, cretinism, osteogenesis imperfecta, chronic hydrocephalus, and as a normal variant.

F. Hemangioma — may involve the frontal or parietal skull and has a honeycomb pattern with radiating spicules. See section XXIV B.

G. Foramen magnum lesions — may classically cause weakness of first the ipsilateral upper extremity (UE), followed by the ipsilateral lower extremity (LE), the contralateral LE, and then the contralateral UE.

H. Also see section IX.

XXV. Developmental Spinal Lesions

A. Spinal lipoma

  1. It is associated with occult spinal lesions and the most common cause of tethered cord.

  2. Lipomyelomeningocele — accounts for 84% of spinal lipomas and 20% of skin-covered masses. It has a female predominance. Symptoms include bladder dysfunction, decreased sensation, and orthopedic deformities. It is not associated with Chiari II malformations (**Fig. 3.254** and **Fig. 3.255**).

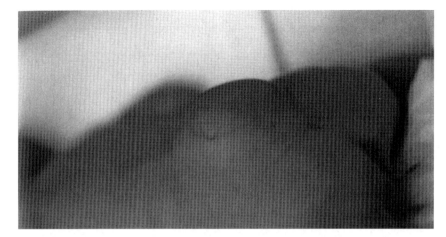

Fig. 3.254 Lipomyelomeningocele. Skin-covered lumbar hump.

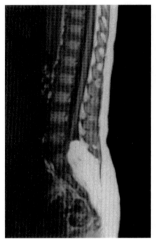
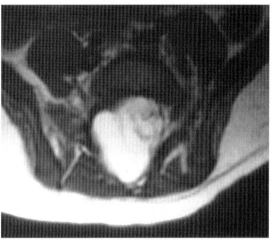

A

B

Fig. 3.255 Lipomyelomeningocele. (A) Sagittal and (B) axial T1-weighted nonenhanced magnetic resonance imaging scans demonstrating the spinal cord terminating in a dorsal lipoma that extends to the sacral surface.

3. Filum terminale fibrolipoma — accounts for 12% of spinal lipomas and is formed by faulty retrogressive differentiation. It is frequently asymptomatic.

4. Intradural lipoma — accounts for 4% of spinal lipomas. It occurs most commonly in the cervical and thoracic spines and the spinal cord is open posteriorly (**Fig. 3.256** and **Fig. 3.257**).

B. Tethered cord — when not associated with a lipoma, it may be caused by a thick filum terminale preventing the spinal cord from ascending in the spinal canal. The low-lying conus and a filum >1.5 mm in diameter are identified on MRI or CT. Tethered cord is also associated with a spinal lipoma (72%). It most commonly presents at 3–35 years of age with no sex predominance. Symptoms include spasticity, pain, decreased sensation, bladder dysfunction, recurrent urinary tract infections, and kyphoscoliosis (25%) (**Fig. 3.258**).

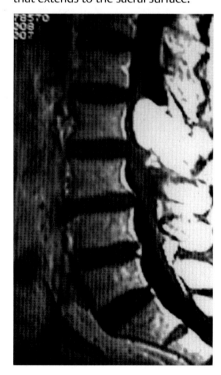

Fig. 3.256 Spinal lipoma. Sagittal T1-weighted magnetic resonance image demonstrates a high-intensity lipoma extending from the subcutaneous tissue to the spinal cord.

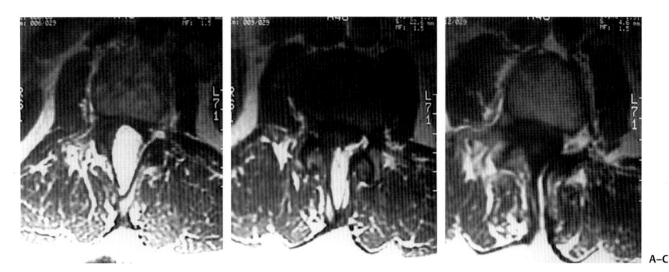

A–C

Fig. 3.257   Spinal lipoma. (**A–C**) Axial T1-weighted magnetic resonance imaging scans demonstrating a lipoma extending through a bifid spine to the middle of the spinal cord.

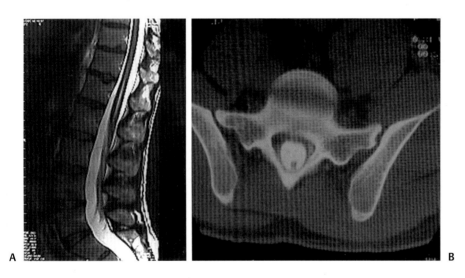

A   B

Fig. 3.258   Tethered cord. (**A**) T2-weighted sagittal magnetic resonance image and (**B**) axial computed tomographic myelogram demonstrate the conus extending to L3 with a small terminal syrinx and a thickened filum terminale.

C. Caudal spinal anomalies (malformations associated with GI or GU abnormalities)

1. Caudal regression syndrome — consists of lumbosacral agenesis, imperforate anus, genital malformations, renal dysplasia, and sirenomelia (fused legs). It may be mild or severe (**Fig. 3.259**).

2. Terminal myelocystocele — consists of posterior spina bifida or partial sacral agenesis with tethered cord and hydromyelia.

3. Anterior sacral meningocele — extends into the pelvis by an anterior defect. It may be a form of caudal regression syndrome and is associated with NF1 and Marfan syndrome.

4. Occult intrasacral meningocele — the arachnoid herniates through a sacral dural defect.

5. Sacrococcygeal teratoma — the most common presacral mass in children

D. Split notochord syndrome — A persistent connection exists between the gut and the dorsal ectoderm. It may be caused by an adhesion between the endoderm and ectoderm.

E. Diastematomyelia — split cord with a fibrous, bony (50%), or cartilaginous septum. It is a local split with a complete cord above and below. 50% have a single dural tube; 85% have vertebral body anomalies, 40% have thick filums, 50–75% have cutaneous stigmata (hair patch, nevi, lipoma, etc.), 50% have orthopedic problems (i.e., clubfoot), and 90% have nonspecific neurologic symptoms (pain, weakness, and bladder dysfunction). It is most common in the lumbar area (T9–S1: 85%). 20% of Chiari II malformations have an associated diastematomyelia. There is a female predominance (**Fig. 3.260**).

F. Enterogenous cyst — caused by failure of the notochord and foregut to separate. They are thin-walled, fluid-filled masses lined by columnar/cuboidal cells with some goblet cells. Peak age is 0–20 years with a male predominance. They usually form in the midline, are intradural extramedullary, and are most common in the thoracic spine (42%) and cervical spine (32%). Symptoms include pain, myelopathy, and septic or chemical meningitis. 43% have associated vertebral anomalies.

G. Hydromyelia — a fluid collection within the spinal cord lined by ependymal cells, and thus a dilation of the central canal. This contrasts with a syrinx cavity that is not lined by ependymal cells. 20% communicate with the fourth ventricle by way of the obex, and these are associated with hydrocephalus, SAH, meningitis, and cancer. 80% are noncommunicating and are associated with Chiari I and II malformations, trauma, tumor, and cord compression. Symptoms are a cape-like loss of pain and temperature, pain (<50%), and upper motor neuron findings in the lower limbs with lower motor findings in the upper limbs (80%) (**Fig. 3.11**).

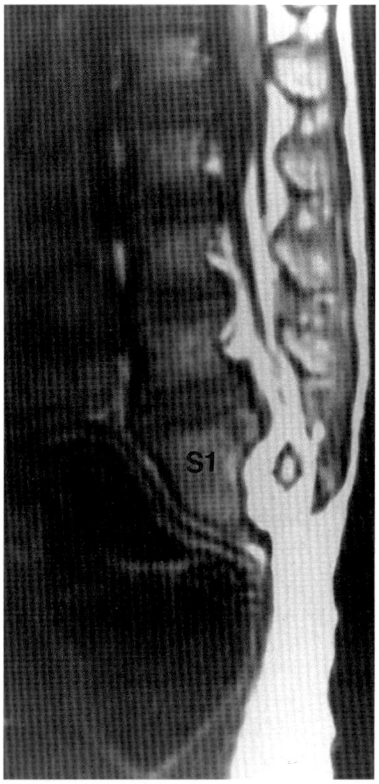

XXVI. Spinal Tumors

A. General — The spinal bone marrow contains more of the red marrow than the yellow variety before age 7 years and thus enhances. The dorsal root ganglia have less of a BBB and also may enhance. Spinal canal tumors may be intramedullary (5%, ependymoma and astrocytoma), intradural-extramedullary (40%, meningioma at any location or schwannoma mostly in the thoracic spine), or epidural (55%, metastatic).

Fig. 3.259 Sacral agenesis. Sagittal T1-weighted magnetic resonance image demonstrates agenesis of the sacrum below S1 with an associated lipoma. (From Ramsey RG. Teaching Atlas of Spine Imaging. New York, NY: Thieme; 1999. Reprinted by permission.)

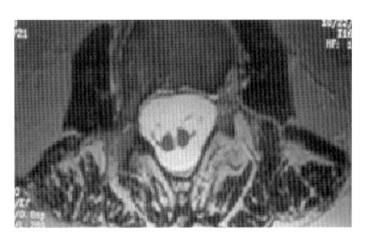

Fig. 3.260 Diastematomyelia. Axial T2-weighted magnetic resonance image demonstrates the dual spinal cords.

B. Bone tumors

1. Hemangioma — Peak age is 30–50 years, female predominance, benign, and found in 10% of autopsies. 75% are spinal (lower thoracic and lumbar) and they are usually in the vertebral body and rarely in the posterior elements (10%). 1% are extraosseous and 30% are multiple. CT demonstrates the "polka dot" lesion in the vertebral body. They may be vascular, fatty, and enhancing. Most are asymptomatic (60%), although they can expand and fracture the vertebral body causing cord compression. Symptoms include pain (20%) and neurologic deficit (20%, mainly after hemorrhage) (**Fig. 3.261**).

2. Osteoid osteoma — Peak age is 10–20 years with a male predominance. They are usually in the long bones of the lower limb and the spine is involved in 10% (lumbar neural arch, rarely the body). The CT reveals dense sclerosis around a lytic lesion with a central calcified nidus of osteoid and woven bone. They are usually <2 cm and if they are larger, they are likely to be osteoblastoma. They account for 6% of benign spinal tumors. Symptoms include scoliosis and pain that responds to acetylsalicylic acid (aspirin) (**Fig. 3.262**).

3. Osteoblastoma (giant osteoid osteoma) — >2 cm in size, peak age is 20 years, and have a male predominance. They occur in the posterior elements of the cervical spine and cause pain. 10% recur and they may grow aggressively.

4. Giant cell tumor — Peak age is 10–40 years with a female predominance. They are mainly in the ends of long bones and occasionally in the sacrum, but rarely elsewhere in the spine. They are lytic, expansile, and locally aggressive. They extend to the cortex but rarely beyond. They frequently hemorrhage and rarely metastasize. Symptoms include pain and neurologic deficits. They recur frequently, and 10% undergo malignant change.

5. Osteochondroma — Peak age is 20 years with a male predominance. 4% are spinal and usually are on the C2 spinous process or transverse processes at other levels. They are multiple in 12%. They arise from lateral displacement of the epiphyseal growth cartilage and have a bony projection with a medullary cavity contiguous with the parent bone and covered with cartilage.

6. Aneurysmal bone cyst
    a. Usually present before 20 years of age and have a female predominance

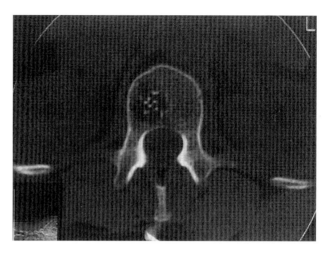

Fig. 3.261   Vertebral hemangioma. Axial computed tomographic scan demonstrating "polka dot" lesion in the vertebral body. (From Alleyne CH Jr. Neurosurgery Board Review. New York, NY: Thieme; 1997. Reprinted by permission.)

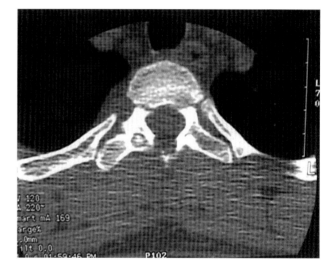

Fig. 3.262   Osteoid osteoma. Axial computed tomographic scan demonstrating lytic lesion with surrounding sclerosis and a central nidus in the right laminar base

b. They usually occur at the metaphyses of long bones, but 20% are spinal, usually in the cervical and thoracic posterior elements. They are nonneoplastic and of unknown cause. They may begin as a hemorrhage into some other type of lesion.

c. They are multiloculated, expansile, lytic, vascular, and surrounded by eggshell cortical bone and no calcifications.

d. Microscopic examination reveals thin-walled blood cavities without endothelium or elastic lamina and frequent multinucleated giant cells.

e. Symptoms include pain, swelling, fracture, and compression.

f. They frequently recur and are associated with chondroblastoma, giant cell tumor, osteoblastoma, and fibrous dysplasia (**Fig. 3.263**).

7. Eosinophilic granuloma — Peak age is 5–10 years; benign, nonneoplastic, and in the Langerhans cell histiocytosis group (see Chapter 4, section VII R). They are lytic without surrounding sclerosis and are a classic cause of a single collapsed vertebral body (vertebrae plana). They enhance and are hyperintense on T2-weighted MRI (**Fig. 3.170**).

8. Chordoma — Peak age is 50–60 years with male predominance. Located at the ends of the spinal axis: sacral (50%), clivus (35%), and less often in the vertebral bodies (15%). They are lytic soft tissue masses with vacuolated physaliphorous cells with mucin. They may contain calcifications (30–70%). Chordomas are derived from notochord remnants and are the most common primary sacral tumors. See section VIII O.

9. Lymphoma — Peak age is 40–65 years with a male predominance. Usually non-Hodgkin lymphoma. Median survival is 2 years. Treatment is with chemotherapy and radiation.

10. Ewing sarcoma — Peak age is 10–20 years with a male predominance. They are usually nonspinal and only involve the spine by metastasis.

11. Osteosarcoma — Peak age is 10–25 years with a male predominance. It is rarely spinal and is more common with Paget disease or radiation. CT reveals matrix calcifications with a sunburst pattern.

12. Chondrosarcoma — Peak age is 50–70 years with a male predominance. They may arise from a solitary osteochondroma (1%) or multiple exostoses (20%).

13. Fibrosarcomas — rare

14. Plasmacytoma — a solitary lesion of plasma cells (called multiple myeloma when multiple). Peak age is 50 years and the vertebral body is the most common location. It is lytic.

C. Epidural lesions — The most common lesions are degenerative, traumatic, or metastatic tumors.

1. Metastatic tumors — most frequently breast, lung, and prostate. In children, the most common are Ewing sarcoma and neuroblastoma. They are usually in the lower thoracic and lumbar spine, correlating with areas having the highest concentration of red marrow. Most are lytic except

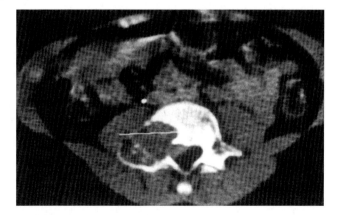

Fig. 3.263 Aneurysmal bone cyst. Nonenhanced axial computed tomographic scan demonstrates expansive lytic lesion surrounded by a thin rim of cortical bone. (From Albright AL, Pollack IF, Adelson PD, eds. Principles and Practice of Pediatric Neurosurgery. New York, NY: Thieme; 1999. Reprinted by permission.)

breast and prostate, which are sometimes sclerotic and blastic. They usually enter the spinal canal by way of the neural foramina and cause circumferential compression. Do not perform a lumbar puncture below the obstruction (**Fig. 3.264** and **Fig. 3.265**).

2. Epidural lipomatosis — fat accumulation in the epidural space with male predominance. It usually develops in the thoracic or lumbar spine and presents with pain and weakness; it is associated with obesity and steroid use. Treatment is by weight loss, discontinuation of steroids if being used, and decompressive surgery if necessary (**Fig. 3.266**).

3. Spinal angiolipoma — rare, peak age is <10 years, female predominance, and is usually in the dorsal epidural thoracic spine

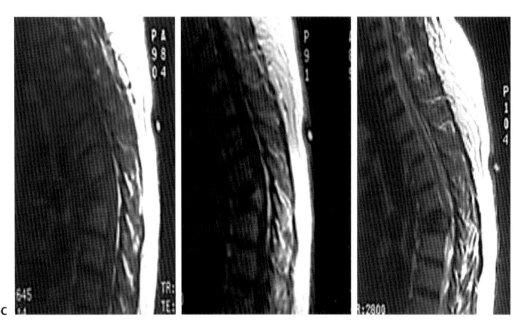

Fig. 3.264 Epidural/vertebral metastatic tumor. (**A**) Sagittal nonenhanced and (**B**) enhanced T1-weighted, and (**C**) T2-weighted magnetic resonance images demonstrating enhancing thoracic vertebral body lesion with extension into ventral epidural space.

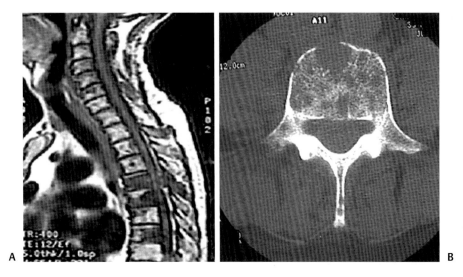

Fig. 3.265 Multiple myeloma. (**A**) Sagittal enhanced T1-weighted magnetic resonance image and (**B**) axial computed tomographic scan demonstrating diffuse bony involvement.

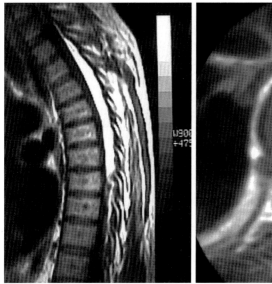
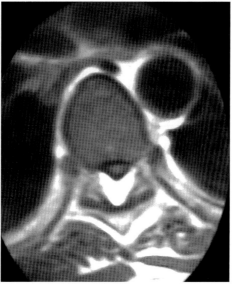

A   **B**

Fig. 3.266 Epidural lipomatosis. (**A**) Sagittal and (**B**) axial T1-weighted magnetic resonance images demonstrating dorsal high-intensity adipose tissue accumulation with cord compression.

  4. Extradural arachnoid cyst — usually thoracic, protrudes through a dural defect and may cause cord compression

D. Intradural/extramedullary lesions

  1. Nerve sheath tumors — the most common spinal tumors (30%). Schwannomas are more common than neurofibromas (unencapsulated, no cystic or hemorrhagic degeneration, nerves run through them, and fusiform-shaped). 40% of patients with nerve sheath tumors have NF. Locations are intradural/extramedullary (70%), extradural (15%), dumbbell (15%), and intramedullary (1%). Symptoms include pain, radiculopathy, and myelopathy. See Chapter 4 section VIII T (**Fig. 3.267** and **Fig. 3.268**).

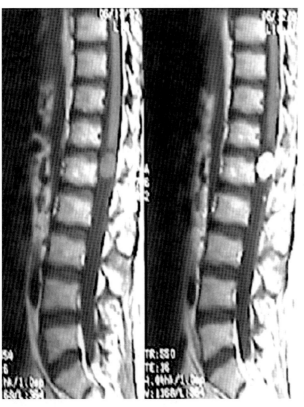

A   **B**

Fig. 3.267 Intradural extramedullary schwannoma. (**A**) Sagittal nonenhanced and (**B**) enhanced T1-weighted magnetic resonance images demonstrating a T12/L1 circumscribed enhancing lesion.

2. Meningioma — accounts for 25% of spinal tumors, peak age is 40–60 years and has a female predominance. It is usually in the thoracic spine, is occasionally multiple, and is intradural (90%), extradural (5%), and dumbbell (5%). Symptoms are motor and sensory deficits. Less than 10% recur. There are rarely bone erosions or calcifications (**Fig. 3.269**).

3. Paraganglioma — rare, usually in the cauda equina, from accessory organs of the peripheral nervous system (carotid body, glomus jugulare, paraaortic, mediastinal, and pheochromocytoma), encapsulated, hemorrhagic, and enhancing. They are GFAP negative.

4. Epidermoid—may be congenital or acquired.

5. Dermoid—congenital, accounts for 20% of intradural masses <1 year, 50% are intramedullary and 50% are extramedullary.

6. Neurenteric cyst — ventral to the thoracic spinal cord

7. Arachnoid cyst — usually dorsal to the thoracic spinal cord

8. Hypertrophic neuropathies — Dejerine–Sottas and Charcot–Marie–Tooth diseases. There may be intradural and extradural onion bulb formations.

9. Metastatic tumors — GBM, anaplastic astrocytoma, ependymoma, medulloblastoma, pineal tumors, germinoma, choroid plexus papilloma, lung carcinoma, breast carcinoma, melanoma, lymphoma, and leukemia. These malignancies carry an 80% mortality rate at 4 months.

E. Intramedullary tumors

1. Ependymoma
    a. It accounts for 60% of intramedullary tumors and is the most common intramedullary tumor in adults.

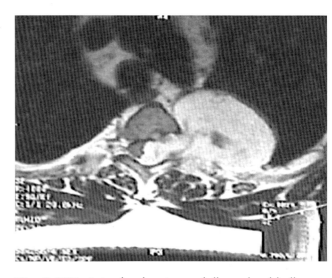

Fig. 3.268 Intradural extramedullary dumbbell neurofibroma. Enhanced axial T1-weighted magnetic resonance image demonstrating a large circumscribed enhancing tumor extending through the widened left intervertebral foramen.

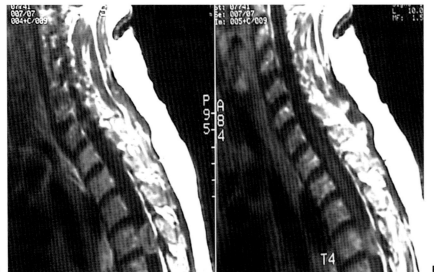

Fig. 3.269 Intradural extramedullary meningioma. (**A,B**) T1-weighted nonenhanced magnetic resonance images with dorsal lesion extending along dural base.

A

B

b. Cellular type — usually cervical, peak age is 43 years, female predominance, circumscribed, frequently cystic or hemorrhagic, and causes symmetric cord expansion and pain (**Fig. 3.270**)

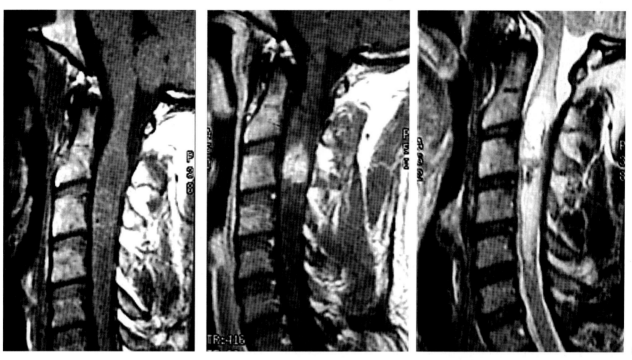

Fig. 3.270   Intramedullary ependymoma. (**A**) Sagittal T1-weighted nonenhanced and (**B**) enhanced and (**C**) T2-weighted magnetic resonance images demonstrating enhancing expansile lesion in the central cervical spinal cord.

c. Myxopapillary type — occurs at the conus or filum, peak age is 28 years, male predominance, slow growing, may metastasize to the lymph nodes, bone, or lung, and 20% destroy bone. Are GFAP positive (**Fig. 3.271**).

d. They are isointense on T1-weighted MRIs, hyperintense on T2-weighted MRIs, and enhancing.

2. Astrocytoma — accounts for 30% of intramedullary tumors and is the most common intramedullary tumor in children. They are usually cervical, peak age is 21 years, no sex predominance, low grade (75% in adults and 90% in children), frequently cause an eccentric cyst and syrinx, and are of the fibrillary type. They can cause scoliosis. Cervical astrocytomas usually enhance on CT and MRI (**Fig. 3.272** and **Fig. 3.273**).

3. Hemangioblastoma — accounts for 5% of intramedullary tumors, peak age is 30 years, 50% are thoracic, and 40% are cervical. 75% are intramedullary and 15% are intradural/extramedullary. 20% are multiple. 30% are associated with VHL. They are usually cystic with a vascular nodule and have dilated feeding vessels on angiography (**Fig. 3.184** and **Fig. 3.185**).

4. Others — Rarely there are oligodendrogliomas, ganglioglioma, schwannomas, and metastases.

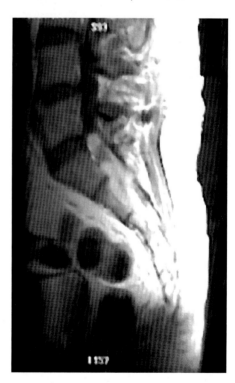

Fig. 3.271   Myxopapillary ependymoma. Sagittal enhanced T1-weighted magnetic resonance image demonstrates enhancing nodular mass filling the distal spinal canal.

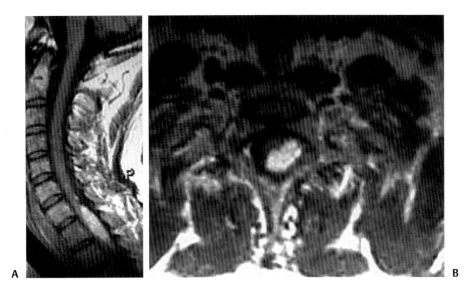

Fig. 3.272 Intramedullary astrocytoma. (**A**) Sagittal and (**B**) axial enhanced T1-weighted magnetic resonance images demonstrating left-sided eccentric cervical mass.

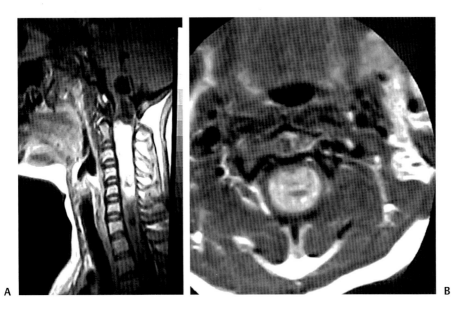

Fig. 3.273 Intramedullary juvenile pilocytic astrocytoma. (**A**) Sagittal and (**B**) axial enhanced T1-weighted magnetic resonance images demonstrate the enhancing tumor with the associated syrinx extending into the brainstem.

5. The most common symptom of intramedullary tumors is pain.

XXVII. Spinal Vascular Diseases

A. Intramedullary hemorrhages — usually due to a vascular malformation, tumor, trauma, or anticoagulation

B. Aneurysms — Peak age is 20 years with no sex predominance. 70% are on the anterior spinal artery, usually cervical or thoracic. They are usually associated with AVMs feeding arteries and do not occur at branch points. Presentation is SAH (85%) and neural compression (15%).

C. Spinal AVMs (an AVM has a true nidus and an AVF does not)

1. Type 1 — the most frequent spinal AVM (actually a dural AVF). Peak age is 40–70 years with a male predominance. It usually occurs in the dorsal lower thoracic or upper lumbar spine. It is usually acquired. There is a single transdural arterial feeder that goes to an intradural arterialized vein over multiple segments. There is rostral venous drainage. The nidus is in or adjacent to the dura around a nerve root.

Symptoms are progressive neurologic deterioration caused by venous hypertension. It has low flow. It is less likely to hemorrhage and is not associated with aneurysms. A good surgical outcome is obtained in 88% (**Fig. 3.274**).

2. Type 2 (glomus AVM) — intramedullary, has multiple feeders, drains into a venous plexus around the cord, usually dorsal cervicomedullary, affects younger people, and is congenital. It presents acutely with hemorrhage and has both high flow and high pressure.

3. Type 3 (juvenile AVM) — rare, congenital, large, intramedullary and extramedullary malformation with multiple extraspinal feeders. It has high pressure and high flow, more frequent hemorrhage and vascular steal symptoms, and is associated with arterial and venous aneurysms. It has bidirectional venous drainage. It involves the entire cross-section of the cord. A good surgical outcome is obtained in 49% of cases.

4. Type 4 — intradural/extramedullary AVF, anterior to the spinal cord, fed by the anterior spinal artery, usually near the conus. Peak age is 20–50 years. It is congenital and has low pressure, but high flow. It rarely hemorrhages, and symptoms are progressive by venous congestion.

5. Foix–Alajouanine syndrome — subacute necrotizing myelitis, especially in the gray matter, usually with a type 1 AVM, and caused by venous hypertension. It presents as spastic and then flaccid paraplegia with an ascending sensory loss and loss of sphincter control.

6. Klippel–Trenaunay–Weber syndrome — a spinal cord AVM with a cutaneous vascular nevus and an enlarged finger or upper limb (if cervical).

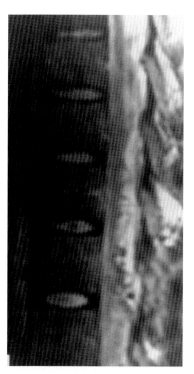 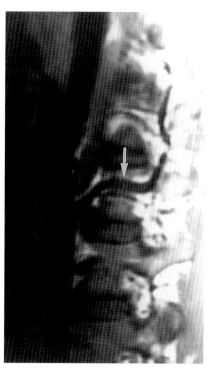 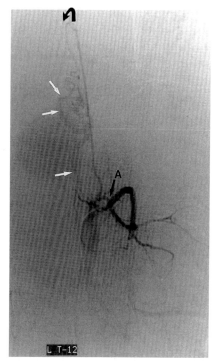

A–C

Fig. 3.274 Spinal arteriovenous fistula. (**A,B**) Sagittal T2-weighted magnetic resonance images and (**C**) angiogram demonstrate upper lumbar segment with vascular blush and enlarged draining veins. (From Ramsey RG. Teaching Atlas of Spine Imaging. New York, NY: Thieme; 1999. Reprinted by permission.)

D. Cavernous malformations — rare, peak age is 20–50 years, female predominance, usually thoracic, occasionally multiple, may hemorrhage, and angiogram is usually normal (**Fig. 3.275**).

E. Venous malformations — rare

F. Capillary telangiectasias — rarely identified during life, but occasionally found at autopsy

G. Spinal cord stroke

1. It usually occurs in patients with severe atherosclerosis, may be caused by hypotension, commonly affects the midthoracic portion, involves the ventral posterior horns and the dorsolateral anterior horns, and has relative white matter sparing.

2. Borderzones — anterior/posterior spinal arteries, central/peripheral blood supply, and at the upper/middle/lower segments. An aortic branch injury may reduce the thoracic blood supply.

3. Etiologies — cross clamping the aorta >18 minutes, syphilis, atherosclerosis, embolism, aortic dissection, and spondylosis (usually affects the anterior spinal artery and preserves the posterior columns). Very rarely there may be a fibrocartilage embolus from a disk to a vessel.

4. Venous thrombosis — may cause hemorrhage and may have sudden or slow onset of neurologic deficit

5. Anterior spinal artery syndrome — from similar causes as the preceding. It is characterized by weakness and dissociated sensory loss (loss of spinothalamic pain and temperature sensation with sparing of posterior column function).

H. Decompression sickness — intravascular accumulation of N_2 with vessel obstruction. It frequently causes spinal cord dysfunction in the posterior columns of the thoracic cord.

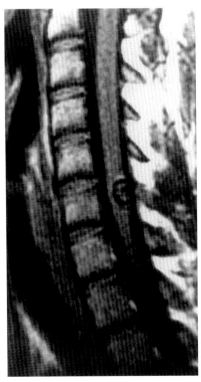
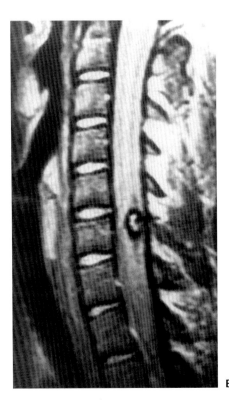

Fig. 3.275 Spinal cord cavernous malformation. (**A**) Sagittal T1- and (**B**) T2-weighted magnetic resonance images demonstrating the lesion with surrounding hemosiderin ring within the cervical spinal cord. (From Ramsey RG. Teaching Atlas of Spine Imaging. New York, NY: Thieme; 1999. Reprinted by permission.)

A

B

XXVIII. Spinal Infections

A. Pyogenic osteomyelitis

1. It is usually caused by *Staphylococcus aureus* (60%), and *Enterobacter* (30%).

2. The infection reaches the spine by (1) hematogenous spread (the most common route, comes from the skin, GU system, lungs, or Batson venous plexus), (2) contiguous spread, and (3) iatrogenic transmission.

3. In adults, the infection begins in the subchondral body and spreads to the disk space.

4. In children, the infection starts in the vascular disk space.

5. Peak age is 50–60 years with a male predominance.

6. The lumbar spine is affected most frequently followed by the thoracic spine.

7. Symptoms are pain, with or without fever, increased ESR, and leukocytosis.

8. X-ray is usually normal for 10 days and then demonstrates endplate erosion and disk space narrowing. MRI is hypointense on T1-weighted images, hyperintense on T2-weighted images, and enhancing (**Fig. 3.276** and **Fig. 3.277**).

9. Risk factors include IV drug abuse, diabetes, and immunocompromised states.

B. Granulomatous osteomyelitis — caused by TB and fungus. The spine is involved in 6% of TB cases (Pott disease). Peak age is 40 years with no sex predominance. It affects the lower thoracic and upper lumbar spine. 90% involve at least two bodies and 50% at least three bodies. Skip lesions are common. 55–95% have an associated paraspinal abscess. There is slow progression of the disease with wedging and gibbus formation. Most cases eventually fuse. The risk increases with debilitation, immunosuppression, alcoholism, and IV drug abuse.

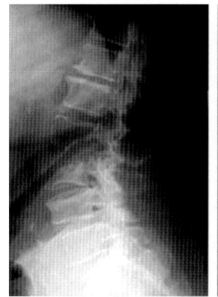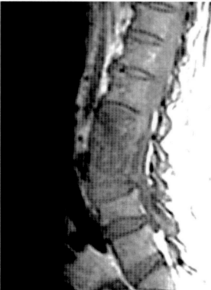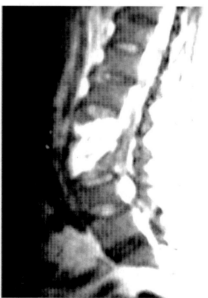

A–C

Fig. 3.276 Osteomyelitis. (**A**) Lateral x-ray film demonstrating L2/3 endplate erosion and (**B**) sagittal T1-weighted and (**C**) T2-weighted magnetic resonance images demonstrating the vertebral body signal changes extending across the L2/3 disk space.

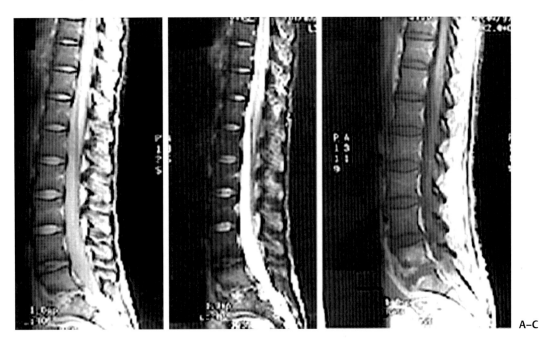

A–C

Fig. 3.277   Diskitis. (**A**) Proton density, (**B**) T2-weighted, and (**C**) enhanced T1-weighted magnetic resonance images demonstrating the L5/S1 enhancing disk inflammation.

C. Epidural abscess — usually caused by *Staphylococcus aureus* and peak age is 50 years with a male predominance. The infection is caused by bacterial seeding from the skin, lung, or bladder. It is associated with osteomyelitis and diskitis (80%) and is frequently multilevel. Symptoms include fever, pain, and neurologic deficit. Initially, a phlegmon forms followed by liquid pus. The risk increases with diabetes mellitus, IV drug abuse, and trauma. Symptoms may be due to direct neural compression or ischemia from venous compression or thrombosis (**Fig. 3.278**).

D. Subdural abscess — rare

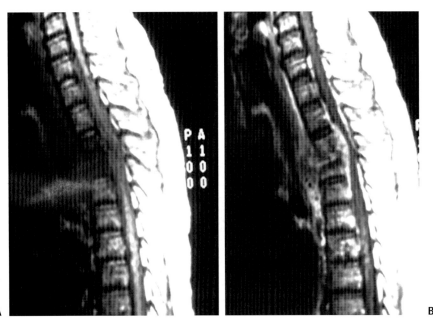

A

B

Fig. 3.278   Spinal epidural abscess. (**A**) Sagittal T1-weighted nonenhanced and (**B**) enhanced magnetic resonance images demonstrating thoracic osteomyelitis with a ventral enhancing epidural abscess.

E. Abscess — rare

F. Meningitis and myelitis — see Chapter 4 section VI

XXIX. Spinal Inflammatory Diseases

A. Acute transverse myelitis — affects all ages, no sex predominance, usually thoracic, and causes demyelination. The MRI is normal in 50% of patients in the acute stage. It is associated with acute infection, postinfection, postvaccination, autoimmune diseases, SLE, MS, and malignancies. The prognosis is variable, and there are frequently permanent deficits.

B. Necrotizing myelopathy

   1. Devic disease (neuromyelitis optica) — progressive fulminant demyelination of the optic nerve and spinal cord. It can result in blindness and paraplegia. It is associated with MS, varicella-zoster, mumps, rubeola, mononucleosis, TB, SLE, and tetanus booster. It tends to be more severe and monophasic than MS. See Chapter 4 section XVI (**Fig. 3.279**).

   2. Lupus myelitis — usually at or below the thoracic level and has a variable course

   3. Paraneoplastic necrotizing myelopathy — usually with lung or lymphoreticular cancers, subacute or rapid progression, and absence of inflammatory cells

   4. Idiopathic

C. Radiation myelopathy

   1. Usually, a chronic progressive myelopathy and most frequently occurs after radiation for nasopharyngeal carcinoma in the cervical spine.

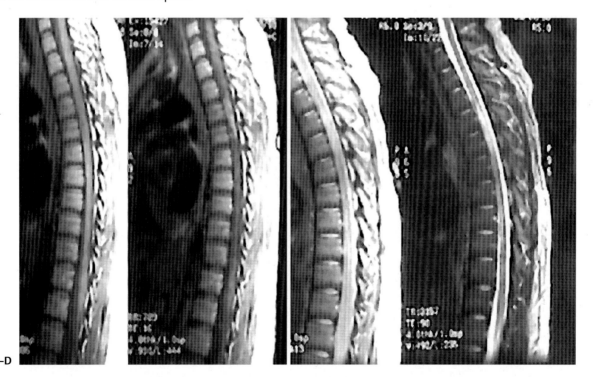

A–D

Fig. 3.279 Devic disease. (**A**) Sagittal unenhanced and (**B**) enhanced T1-weighted, (**C**) proton density, and (**D**) T2-weighted magnetic resonance images demonstrating upper thoracic inflammation extending over three levels.

2. Symptoms usually occur 12–15 months after radiation and include painless paresthesias and dysesthesias, with sensory loss more common than motor loss.

3. Pathologic examination demonstrates coagulative necrosis affecting the white matter more than the gray matter and thrombosed hyalinized vessels (**Fig. 3.280**).

4. Postradiation changes to the vertebral bodies include hyperintensity on T1-weighted images due to increased fat content in the marrow (**Fig. 3.49**).

5. There is no effective treatment; steroids are often tried.

6. The risk is decreased by keeping the total radiation dose <6000 rad, the weekly dose <900 rad, and the daily dose <200 rad.

D. ALS — see Chapter 4, section XV

E. Anterior horn diseases — poliomyelitis, ALS, Creutzfeldt–Jakob, Werdnig–Hoffmann disease, and Kugelberg–Welander syndrome

F. Myelopathy differential diagnosis — congenital degeneration (Friedreich ataxia), radiation, AIDS, viral, compression, vascular malformation, toxic (ethanol), and metabolic (B_{12}) (**Figs. 3.190, 3.197**, and **3.281–3.285**).

G. Vertebral inflammatory diseases

1. Ankylosing spondylitis (Marie–Strumpell disease) — presents at 10–30 years and affects 1.4% of the population at the entheses, a site where a ligament attaches to a bone. It is an autoimmune disease with an HLA-B27 association, causing sacroiliac and lumbar calcifications. X-ray films may demonstrate

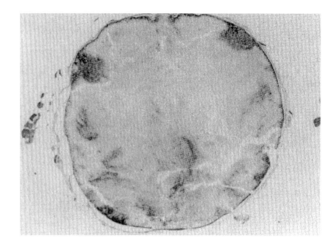

Fig. 3.280 Radiation myelopathy. Coagulation necrosis. (From Alleyne Jr. CH. Neurosurgery Board Review. New York, NY: Thieme; 1997. Reprinted by permission.)

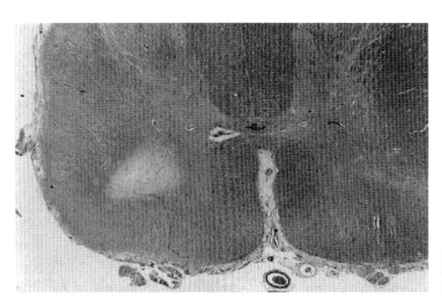

Fig. 3.281 Poliomyelitis (hematoxylin and eosin [H&E] stain). Cystic degeneration of the anterior horn.

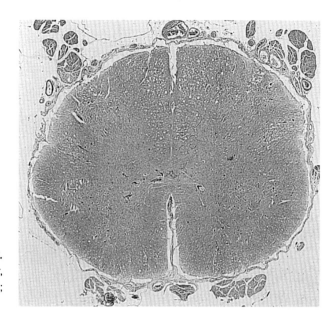

Fig. 3.282 Human immunodeficiency virus myelopathy. Vacuolar myelopathy. (From Nelson JS, Parisi JE, Schochet SS Jr, eds. Principles and Practice of Neuropathology. St. Louis, MO: Mosby; 1993:95. Reprinted by permission.)

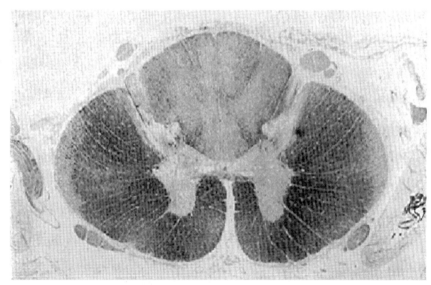

Fig. 3.283 Friedreich ataxia (Luxol fast blue stain). Degeneration of axons and myelin in the posterior columns and ventral spinocerebellar tracts (corticospinal tracts may also be involved).

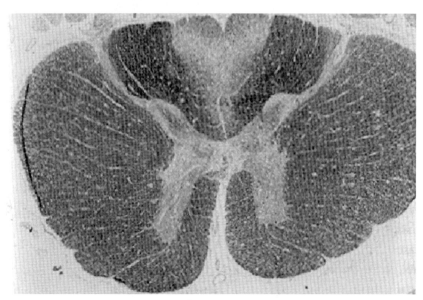

Fig. 3.284 Tabes dorsalis (Luxol fast blue stain). Posterior column demyelination.

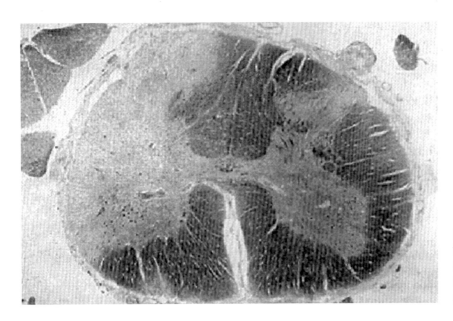

Fig. 3.285 Multiple sclerosis (Luxol fast blue stain). Demyelinative plaques extend across spinal cord tract boundaries involving lateral and dorsal columns and central gray.

"bamboo spine" from syndesmophytes and zygapophyseal joint fusion. It is associated with uveitis, conjunctivitis, epidural spinal hemorrhages, and spine fractures (**Fig. 3.286**).

2. Rheumatoid arthritis — an autoimmune disease causing neurologic symptoms by necrotizing parenchymal vasculitis, leptomeningeal rheumatoid nodules, pannus formation, atlantoaxial instability (by transverse atlantoaxial ligament weakness), subaxial subluxations, and cranial settling. 80% have spinal involvement. Also affects the metatarsophalangeal joints, metacarpophalangeal joints, and proximal interphalangeal joints (Bouchard nodes). Heberden nodes form at the distal interphalangeal joints with degenerative arthritis (**Fig. 3.287**).

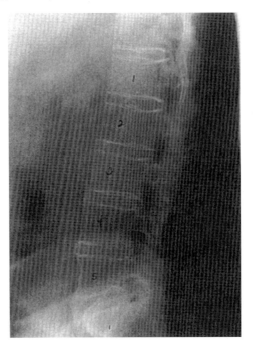

Fig. 3.286 Ankylosing spondylitis. Lateral x-ray demonstrates "Bamboo spine." (From Alleyne CH Jr. Neurosurgery Board Review. New York, NY: Thieme; 1997. Reprinted by permission.)

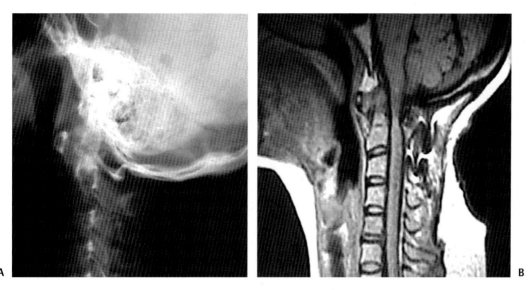

Fig. 3.287 Rheumatoid arthritis pannus. (**A**) Lateral x-ray film and (**B**) sagittal T1-weighted magnetic resonance images with a C1/2 pannus and anterior subluxation.

XXX. Spinal Degenerative Diseases

A. 80% of adults will have an episode of lower back pain at some time in their lives.

B. Intervertebral disk disease

    1. In the lumbar spine, 90% are at L5/S1 and L4/5; in the cervical spine, 70% are at C6/7 and 25% at C5/6.

    2. Most disk herniations are paracentral or central, 3% are foraminal, and 4% are far-lateral. Rarely a herniated disk may be intradural. Thoracic discs account for <1% of herniated disks, and 15% of these are asymptomatic (**Figs. 3.288–3.290**).

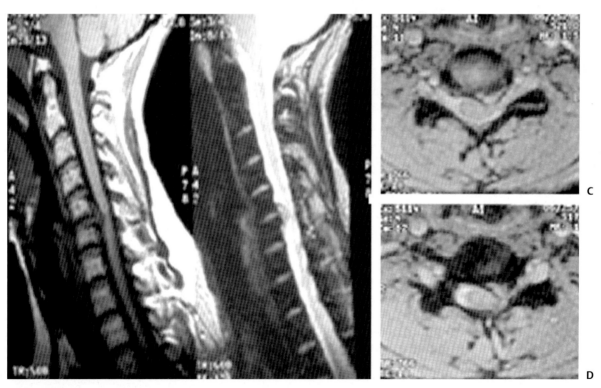

Fig. 3.288 Herniated cervical disk. (**A**) Sagittal T1 and (**B**) T2-weighted and (**C,D**) axial T2-weighted magnetic resonance images demonstrate the left paracentral C5/6 herniation.

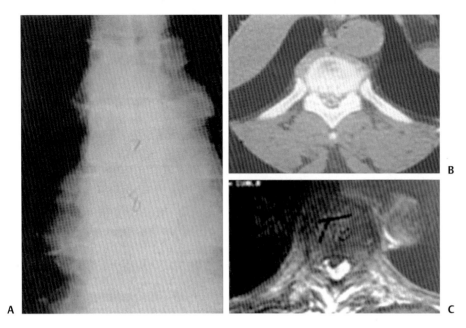

Fig. 3.289 Herniated thoracic disk. (**A**) Anteroposterior thoracic x-ray film and (**B**) axial computed tomographic scan demonstrate the calcified central T7/8 herniation. (**C**) An axial T2-weighted magnetic resonance image demonstrates a soft T10/11 herniation.

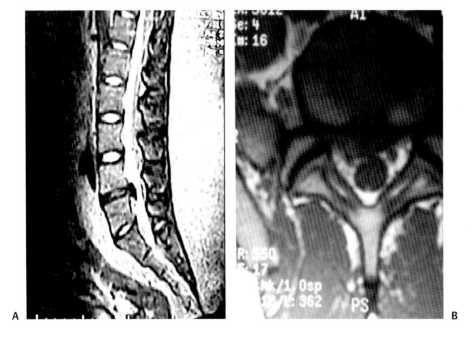

Fig. 3.290 Herniated lumbar disk. (**A**) Sagittal T2-weighted and (**B**) axial T1-weighted magnetic resonance images demonstrate the L4/5 herniation.

3. With aging, disks lose water and proteoglycans and accumulate collagen. Annular tears may be concentric, radial (most frequent), or transverse.

4. The disks are weakest posteriorly between the PLL fibers. A lumbar disk bulge is seen in 35% of the normal population 20–39 years and in almost all patients >60 years. Asymptomatic herniations are seen in 33% of people >60 years.

5. Herniated disks may have peripheral enhancement. Epidural postoperative fibrosis enhances diffusely. The DRG and posterior roots may enhance because there is no BBB.

6. A Schmorl node is a disk herniation through the endplate and is seen in 75% of the normal population.

7. A vacuum disk forms by nitrogen accumulation with degenerative disease.

8. Recurrent disks after surgery have rim enhancement on MRI with gadolinium, whereas fibrous scar tissue homogeneously enhances.

C. Spondylosis

1. It is most common after 50 years of age and affects 70% of the population >50 years old.

2. When the disks degenerate, the bones rub against each other and elicit spurring. It is especially common at C5/6 (25%) and C6/7 (70%) because of increased mobility at these levels. Osteophytes develop near Sharpey fibers where the annulus is connected to bone. Lumbar stenosis is usually due to hypertrophy of the superior articulating process (**Fig. 3.291**).

3. The normal cervical spine diameter is 18 mm, and symptoms usually develop when it is <10 mm.

4. Symptoms are caused by microtrauma to the spinal cord (sliding up and down with flexion/extension and compression) and ischemia.

D. Congenital spinal stenosis (short pedicle syndrome) — seen with achondroplasia and Morquio syndrome

E. Spondylolysis — caused by a pars defect and seen in 5% of the population

F. Spondylolisthesis — slippage of one vertebral body over another. It may be congenital, isthmic, pathologic, degenerative, or traumatic: 66% at L4/5 and 30% at L5/S1 (**Figs. 3.292–3.294**).

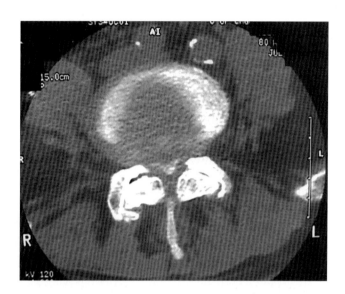

Fig. 3.291 Lumbar stenosis. Axial computed tomographic scan demonstrates hypertrophic facets and thickened ligamentum flavum causing thecal sac compression.

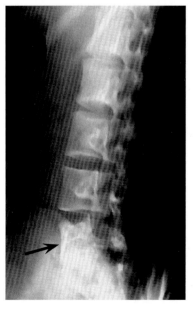

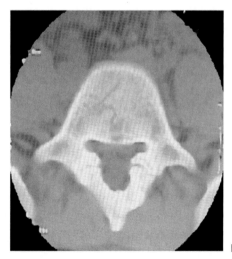

Fig. 3.292 Spondylolisthesis. (**A**) Oblique lumbar x-ray film demonstrating L5 "Scotty dog with broken neck" (*arrow*) and (**B**) axial computed tomographic scan demonstrating the sclerotic pars defect of lytic spondylolisthesis.

A

B

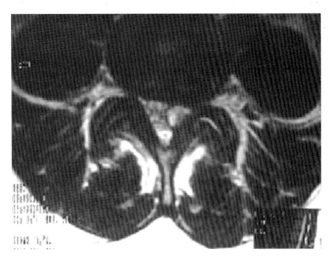

Fig. 3.293 Synovial cyst. Axial T2-weighted magnetic resonance image demonstrates a cyst emerging from the left facet joint.

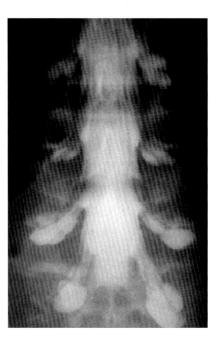

Fig. 3.294 Tarlov cyst. Anteroposterior myelogram demonstrates the multiple nerve sleeve dilations.

G. Ossified posterior longitudinal ligament — more common in Japan and usually affects C3–C5 and T4–T7. Ossified ligamentum flavum also occurs in Japan (**Fig. 3.295**).

H. Arachnoiditis — arachnoid collagen scar formation tethering nerve roots. It occurs after surgery, infection, intrathecal contrast, trauma, hemorrhage, and degenerative disease (**Fig. 3.296**).

I. Failed back syndrome — possible causes include arachnoiditis, epidural fibrosis, hematoma, disk disease, infection, facet arthrosis, and referred hip pain. Most authorities believe that it is not helped by scar resection. It is associated with enhancing roots after 6 months; the intradural roots normally do not enhance.

J. Syringomyelia

   1. 90% are associated with Chiari I malformation but they also occur with tumors, infections, and trauma.

   2. It is most commonly cervical. Onset is 35–45 years of age. It causes pain, lower motor neuron findings in the upper limbs, upper motor neuron findings in the lower limbs, and a cape-like loss of pain and temperature sensation (by damage to the spinothalamic fibers crossing in the anterior commissure).

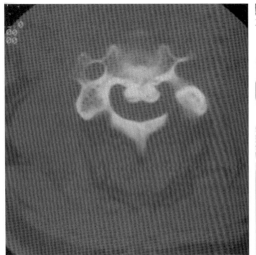

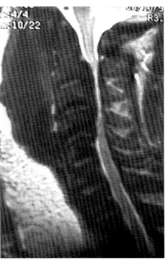

Fig. 3.295 Ossified posterior longitudinal ligament. (**A**) Axial computed tomographic scan bone window and (**B**) sagittal T2-weighted magnetic resonance image demonstrate C2–C5 posterior longitudinal ligament calcification with cord compression.

A   B

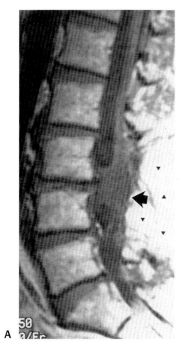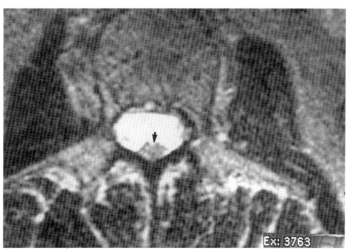

Fig. 3.296 Arachnoiditis. (**A**) Sagittal T1-weighted nonenhanced and (**B**) axial T2-weighted magnetic resonance images demonstrating clumped and scarred nerve roots. (From Ramsey RG. Teaching Atlas of Spine Imaging. New York, NY: Thieme; 1999. Reprinted by permission.)

       3. It is also associated with Charcot joints (neuropathic osteoarthropathy) with a lytic humeral head or hypertrophic hip. These are usually seen with diabetes (in the foot or knee), syphilis (tabes dorsalis), MS, and leprosy. A Charcot shoulder joint is highly suspicious for a cervical syrinx (**Figs. 3.11** and **3.297**).

K. Morquio syndrome — associated with a hypoplastic dens that may cause cord compression

L. Achondroplasia — associated with increased periosteal bone and short pedicles (especially thoracolumbar) with frequent stenosis. It is also associated with hydrocephalus.

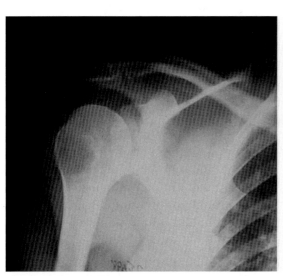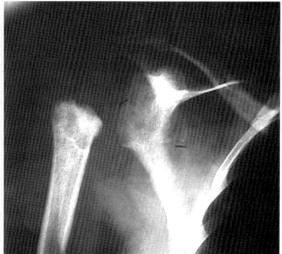

Fig. 3.297 Charcot joint. (**A**) Anteroposterior shoulder x-ray film is normal and (**B**) demonstrates complete erosion of the humeral head.

XXXI. Spinal Trauma

A. Spinal shock — see Chapter 2 section XI

B. Hyperreflexia may develop after spinal shock resolves and includes Babinski responses, triple flexion responses, and spasticity of the bowel and bladder. The mass reflex is a complete autonomic discharge that includes urination, defecation, etc. Autonomic dysreflexia may develop where a stimulus such as a distended bladder may cause the levels of NE and epinephrine to increase, causing hypertension, tachycardia, etc.

C. Anterior cord syndrome — due to severe flexion injury and causes hypesthesia (anterior spinothalamic tract), hypalgesia (lateral spinothalamic tract), and spastic paralysis (corticospinal tract). Posterior column function is retained.

D. Central cord syndrome — classically due to a hyperextension injury in a patient with a narrow cervical spinal canal. Symptoms and signs include decreased posterior column function, decreased sensation over the upper limbs and shoulders, and weakness greater in upper than lower limbs (the upper limbs are more medial in the corticospinal tract).

E. Brown–Séquard syndrome — decreased contralateral pain and temperature, decreased ipsilateral proprioception, and ipsilateral hemiplegia. It is usually caused by a penetrating injury.

F. Primary injury — caused by concussion (transient decreased function), contusion, laceration, and compression

G. Secondary injury — caused by ischemia, infection, hypoxia, hyperthermia, edema, hemorrhage, arachnoiditis, persistent compression, and syrinx. The syrinx is thought to form by progressive tearing from increased venous back pressure from Valsalva maneuver on the spinal cord that is no longer mobile because of adhesions. Patients with nonpenetrating spinal cord injury may be treated with methylprednisolone 30 mg/kg over 1 hour, followed by 5.4 mg/kg/h for 23 hours if started within 3 hours of the injury or for 47 hours if started between 3 and 8 hours of injury to help decrease secondary injury.

H. Common traumatic spinal injuries — fracture-dislocation, fracture, and dislocation (3:1:1)

I. Most frequent levels involved — C1/2, C4–C6, and T11–L2

J. Thoracic injuries — less common because of high facets and ribs (decrease motion) and more canal space (no cervical and lumbar enlargements)

K. Flexion injuries — wedge fractures and dislocations

L. Extension injuries — posterior element fractures

M. Axial loading — compression, burst, and pillar fractures

N. Rotational injuries — lateral mass fractures, unilateral facet subluxation, and uncovertebral fractures

O. C1 injuries

1. Atlantooccipital dislocation — frequently fatal. The dens–basion distance is >12 mm and the Power ratio >1. The Power ratio is defined as the distance of the basion (B) to the posterior arch of the atlas (C) divided by the distance of the anterior arch of the atlas (A) to the opisthion (O) to the (**Fig. 3.298**).

2. Jefferson fracture — bilateral burst fractures through the anterior and posterior neural arches. It is usually stable unless the transverse ligament is disrupted (**Fig. 3.299**).

3. Rotatory atlantoaxial subluxation — C1 is rotated over C2 >45 degrees and the facets are locked. It is associated with flexion injuries, rheumatoid arthritis, and tonsillitis/pharyngitis (Grisel syndrome) (**Fig. 3.300**).

4. Atlantoaxial dislocation — may be anterior, posterior, or longitudinal dislocation of C1 relative to C2

P. C2 injuries

1. Odontoid fracture type 1 — a fracture at the tip of the dens

2. Odontoid fracture type 2 — a fracture at the base of the dens. It is the least likely of the dens fractures to heal with external immobilization (**Figs. 3.301**).

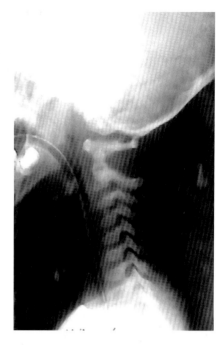

Fig. 3.298 Atlantooccipital and atlantoaxial dislocations. Lateral cervical spine x-ray demonstrates increased distance from the occiput to the atlas and the atlas to the axis.

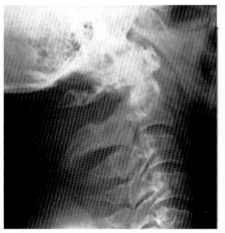
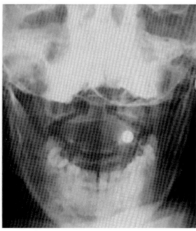
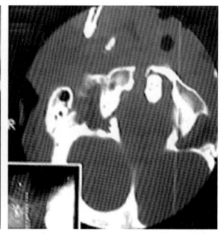

A–C

Fig. 3.299 Jefferson fracture. (**A**) Lateral and (**B**) open mouth x-ray films and (**C**) axial computed tomographic scan demonstrate anterior and posterior arch fractures with prominent right-sided overhang seen in (**B**).

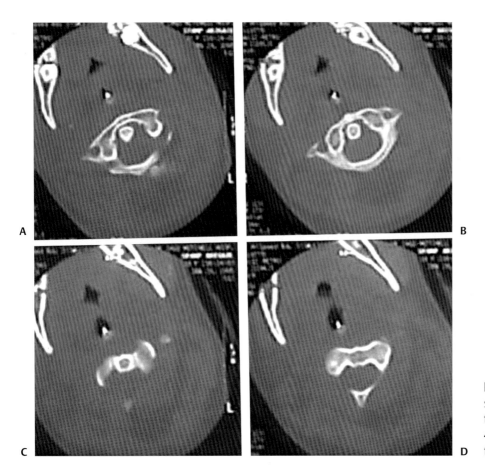

A

B

C

D

Fig. 3.300 Atlantoaxial rotatory subluxation. (**A–D**) Axial computed tomographic scans demonstrate the 45-degree rotation of the atlas on the axis.

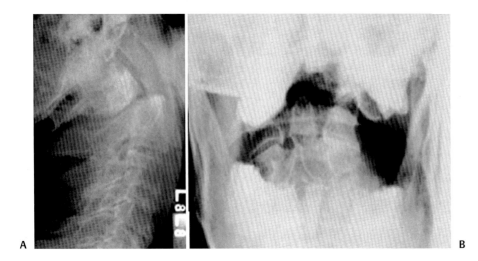

A

B

Fig. 3.301 Odontoid fracture (type 2). (**A**) Lateral and (**B**) open mouth cervical spine x-ray films demonstrate the fracture through the base of the dens with posterior dislocation.

3. Odontoid fracture type 3 — a fracture through the base of the axis body

4. Os odontoideum — represents a segment of the odontoid with smooth cortical bone that is not fused with the body of the dens and may mimic an odontoid fracture. It can be congenital or acquired from an old nonunion fracture (**Fig. 3.302**).

5. Hangman fracture — C2 traumatic spondylolisthesis with bilateral pars interarticularis fractures caused by hyperextension. It rarely causes cord injury (**Fig. 3.303**).

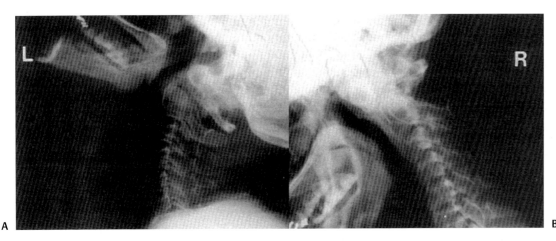

Fig. 3.302 Os odontoideum. (**A**) Lateral extension and (**B**) flexion x-rays demonstrating an old dens defect with instability. (From Albright AL, Pollack IF, Adelson PD, eds. Principles and Practice of Pediatric Neurosurgery. New York, NY: Thieme; 1999. Reprinted by permission.)

Q. C3–C7 injuries

   1. Flexion — wedge fracture (may disrupt interspinous and posterior longitudinal ligaments), facet fracture/dislocation, Clay shoveler fracture (C6–T1 spinous process), and tear drop fracture (**Figs. 3.304–3.307**).

   2. Extension — disrupts the anterior longitudinal ligament and causes an avulsion fracture of the anterior edge of the vertebral body and facet fracture

R. Thoracic injuries — compression or burst fractures. They are usually stable (**Fig. 3.308**).

S. Thoracolumbar junction injuries — 75% are compression injuries with anterior wedge fractures and intact posterior elements. 20% are fracture dislocations.

XXXII. Peripheral Nerve Disorders

A. Etiologies — **Mnemonic: DANG THE RAPIST. D**iabetes and drugs, **A**lcohol, **N**eoplasm and nutritional, **G**uillain–Barré disease, **T**rauma, **H**ereditary, **E**lectrolytes and endocrine, **R**enal, **A**myloid and AIDS, **P**orphyria, **I**mmune and ischemic, **S**arcoid, and **T**oxins

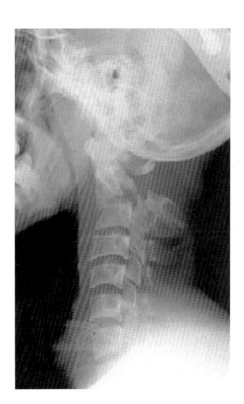

Fig. 3.303 Hangman's fracture. Lateral cervical spine x-ray film demonstrates the C2 traumatic spondylolisthesis with anterior angulation.

B. Sural nerve specimens are stained with H&E, trichrome (for connective tissue), and silver (for axons).

C. Peripheral nerves should contain 3 times more unmyelinated than myelinated fibers.

D. Amyloid affects the small fibers, whereas uremia affects the large fibers.

E. Wallerian degeneration — occurs distal to the site of damage after several days. The soma undergoes chromatolysis with increased protein synthesis. Retraction balls form from the build-up of transported material at the

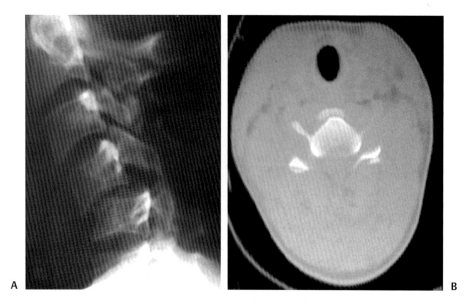

Fig. 3.304 Unilateral interfacetal dislocation. (**A**) Lateral cervical spine x-ray film and (**B**) axial computed tomographic scan demonstrate the rotation with the left superior articulating process of C5 now dorsal to the inferior articulating process of C4.

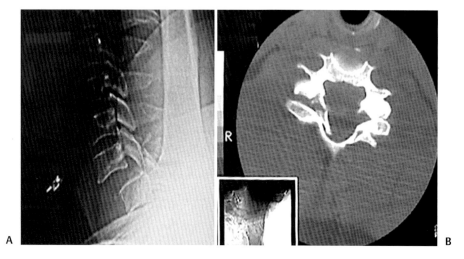

Fig. 3.305 Bilateral interfacetal dislocation. (**A**) Lateral cervical x-ray film and (**B**) axial computed tomographic scan demonstrates the C6/7 injury with bilateral jumped facets.

proximal and distal ends of cut nerves. All of the fascicles are at the same stage of degeneration/regeneration, and after regeneration, the nodes are at regular intervals.

F. Bands of Bungner — proliferation of Schwann cells under the old basal lamina of a nerve with axons growing inside.

G. Segmental demyelination — scattered demyelination with replacement by thinner myelin and shorter variable internodes (normally the nodes of Ranvier have a set internodal length). There is relative axonal sparing.

H. Secondary demyelination—only demyelination over certain axons (as with uremia) from axonal degeneration or Wallerian degeneration distal to an injury (starts after 3–4 days)

I. Toxic neuropathy

   1. Axonal transport — affected by diabetes (decreases turnaround transport), vincristine/vinblastine (microtubules), mercury (translation), actinomycin D (transcription), and dinitrophenol (oxidative phosphorylation)

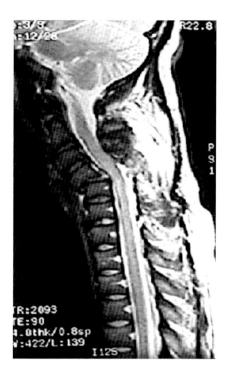

Fig. 3.306 Flexion dislocation. Sagittal T2-weighted magnetic resonance image demonstrates the C4/5 subluxation and angulation.

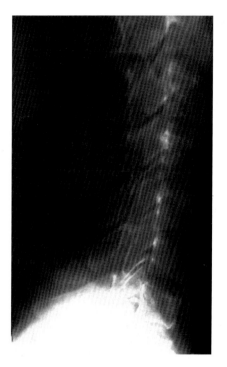

Fig. 3.307 Clay shoveler's fracture. Lateral cervical x-ray film demonstrating C6 spinous process fracture.

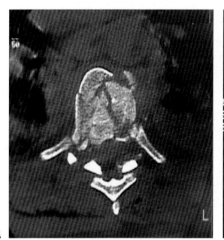

A

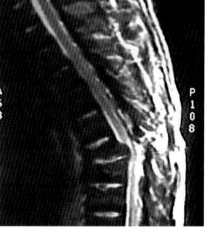

B

Fig. 3.308 Burst fracture. (**A**) Axial computed tomographic scan and (**B**) sagittal T2-weighted magnetic resonance image demonstrate angulation with retropulsion at T9.

    2. Schwann cells and myelin — affected by lead (bilateral wrist drop, see section XIII), diphtheria toxin (toxin inhibits Schwann cell myelin synthesis mainly in the DRG and ventral and dorsal roots where the blood–nerve barrier is normally absent, causes segmental demyelination without inflammation), and hexachlorophene.

J. Metabolic neuropathy

    1. Diabetes mellitus — most frequently causes a symmetric sensorimotor polyneuropathy with stocking-glove decreased sensation and loss of myelin and axons. The neuropathy has multiple causes including increased glucose transport into axons, decreased intracellular transport, and hypoxia/ischemia. It may also cause a focal mononeuropathy resulting from ischemia. Diabetes also affects the autonomic nervous system.

2. Amyloid — extracellular β-pleated sheets form from immunoglobulin light chains. With Congo red staining, there is green birefringence with polarized light. It causes axonal degeneration with myelin destruction. Symptoms involve mainly autonomic dysfunction and loss of pain and temperature.

3. Porphyria — rapid, severe, symmetric, motor > sensory loss, bilateral brachial weakness, and tachycardia, abdominal pain, psychiatric changes, and seizures. Autosomal dominant form is associated with acute intermittent porphyria, and the attack may resolve in a few weeks. Death is by cardiac or respiratory causes. Axons and myelin are damaged and there is no inflammation. The liver defect causes a buildup of δ-aminolevulinic acid and porphobilinogen and the urine turns dark as it oxidizes. Treatment is with vitamin B6, glucose, β-blockers, and hematin.

4. Others — uremia (painless, symmetric, sensorimotor, lower > upper limbs), leukodystrophy (metachromatic and Krabbe disease affect both central and peripheral myelin), Fabry disease, vitamin deficiencies, and hypothyroidism

K. Autoimmune neuropathy

1. Cell-mediated immunity
   a. Guillain–Barré (idiopathic polyneuritis) disease
      (1) It is one of the most frequent and most fatal neuropathies. It causes an acute inflammatory polyneuropathy with rapid onset. It affects all ages, has unknown cause, and is associated with trauma, surgery, infection, immunization, and neoplasm.
      (2) It is usually monophasic, peaking in 10–14 days, but occasionally relapsing.
      (3) It involves the DRG, ventral and dorsal nerve roots, and peripheral nerves, causing mainly motor and autonomic dysfunction with less marked sensory symptoms. Symmetric weakness starts in the lower limbs and moves cranially, progressing over 2 weeks.
      (4) Pathologic examination demonstrates perivascular mononuclear infiltrates and segmental demyelination. The CSF reveals normal pressure, acellularity (90%), and a protein peak around 5 weeks.
      (5) Nerve conduction study demonstrates decreased velocity and amplitude.
      (6) The mechanism may be due to cell-mediated immunity to MBP P2 in the peripheral myelin, humoral immunity, or a viral cause.
      (7) Differentiate from poliomyelitis (fever, asymmetric, no sensory findings), myasthenia gravis (fatigability and no sensory findings), and botulism (abnormal pupillary reflexes and decreased heart rate)
      (8) Most recover with supportive care. Mortality is 3% and is usually due to cardiac arrest or respiratory problems. 10% have severe permanent weakness. Improvement may occur for up to 2 years; 3% relapse.
      (9) Treatment may entail plasmapheresis in the first 3 weeks to lessen the attack duration and severity if ambulation or respiration is in jeopardy. It does not respond to steroids.
   b. Experimental allergic neuritis — caused by T cell-mediated attack of the P2 protein

2. Humoral immunity — multiple causes

L. Ischemic neuropathy (the vessel disease must be very severe because there are multiple anastomoses around nerves)

1. Polyarteritis nodosa (necrotizing panarteritis) — the most common necrotic vasculitis with CNS lesions. It affects small and medium-sized arteries throughout the body and causes polyneuropathy that may be symmetric or asymmetric (mononeuropathy multiplex) by obliteration of the vaso nervorum. It is associated with microaneurysms (70%), stenosis, and thrombosis. There is axonal degeneration and the

vessel walls have intimal proliferation and inflammation with PMNs, lymphocytes, plasma cells, and eosinophils. Nodosa means segmental inflammation. It also causes skin purpura and renal dysfunction.

2. Collagen vascular disease

3. Paraneoplastic syndrome — usually distal, sensorimotor, peaks in months, and remains 1–2 years until death. The anti-Hu antibody is associated with oat cell pulmonary carcinoma and causes a sensory neuropathy involving the DRG.

M. Infectious neuropathy — the perineurium usually protects the nerve from the infectious process, but the overlying feeding vessel is at risk. Causes include varicella-zoster (may cause hemorrhagic ganglioradiculitis and rarely myelopathy), HIV, and leprosy (large swollen nerves in the distal extremities where it is cooler, ulnar nerve at the elbow and peroneal nerve at the fibular head).

N. Hereditary/hypertrophic (onion bulb) neuropathy

1. It occurs after demyelination/remyelination and has interspersed layers of Schwann cell processes and collagen. Nerves may be palpably enlarged. The nerve conduction velocity is decreased (**Figs. 3.309–3.311**).

2. Charcot–Marie–Tooth disease — autosomal dominant inheritance with onset in adolescence. It causes peroneal muscle atrophy and also degeneration of anterior horn cells, posterior columns, DRG, axons, and myelin. Distal muscle atrophy occurs in the feet and then the hands (develop claw hand). There is sensory ataxia and weakness without autonomic dysfunction. The CSF is normal. Patients develop pes cavus and hammertoe deformities.

3. Dejerine–Sottas disease — autosomal recessive inheritance and occurs <10 years. It is slowly progressive with development of claw feet and hands, symmetric weakness, wasting of distal limbs, foot pain, and paresthesias, without autonomic dysfunction. There is axon loss and enlarged nontender ulnar, median, radial, and peroneal nerves.

4. Refsum disease — autosomal recessive inheritance with onset in late childhood–early adulthood. There is a deficiency of phytanic acid oxidase with accumulation of phytanic acid. There is distal symmetric sensorimotor loss in lower limbs, and is associated with retinitis pigmentosum, cardiomyopathy, and hearing loss.

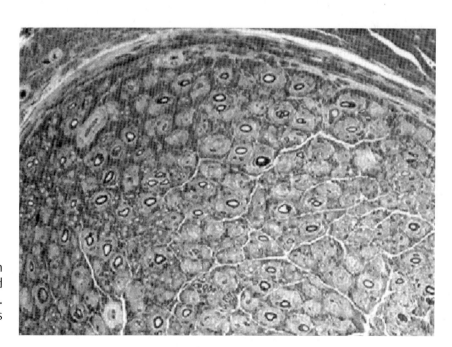

Fig. 3.309 Onion-bulb formation (semithin Epon section of osmicated sural nerve stained with toluene blue). Layers of Schwann cells and processes form around the axons.

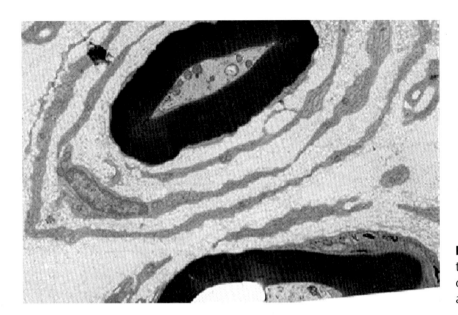

Fig. 3.310 Onion-bulb formation (electron micrograph). Layers of Schwann cells and processes form around the axons.

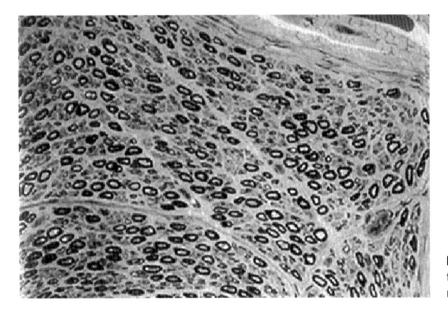

Fig. 3.311 Normal sural nerve (semithin Epon section of osmicated sural nerve stained with toluene blue).

5. Chronic inflammatory demyelinating polyradiculopathy — may be a chronic form of Guillain–Barré syndrome, but it responds to steroids

6. Others — lead, Krabbe disease, and metachromatic leukodystrophy

O. Traumatic neuropathy

1. Neuropraxia — there is functional but no structural damage (nerve concussion) with temporary loss of function that may last 6 to 8 weeks. Motor function is affected more than sensation.

2. Axonotmesis — interruption of axons and myelin with intact perineurium and epineurium. Spontaneous regeneration may occur at 1–2 mm/day.

3. Neurotmesis — complete transection of the nerve and nerve sheath. Axonal regeneration may lead to neuroma formation. Brachial plexus injury can avulse nerve roots from spinal cord, producing meningoceles (**Fig. 3.312**).

P. Motor deficits — by nutritional, metabolic, Guillain–Barré syndrome and toxic causes. It is usually symmetric in the distal lower limbs (affects the longest and largest nerves).

Q. Sensory deficits — by amyloid and toxic causes. It is usually symmetric distal limb lower > upper limbs and affects all modalities, but vibration is usually the most sensitive.

R. Paresthesias/dysesthesias — due to diabetes and ethanol. They are from ectopic impulse transmission in damaged nerves.

S. Autonomic deficits — secondary to amyloid, diabetes, Shy–Drager syndrome, and small fiber polyneuropathies

T. Toxins — tend to cause sensory > motor deficits, whereas Guillain-Barré tends to cause motor > sensory deficits

U. Evaluation of neuropathy

1. Mononeuropathy versus polyneuropathy versus mononeuropathy multiplex versus plexus injury.

2. Motor > sensory (Guillain–Barré syndrome, lead, diphtheria, porphyria, and uremia), sensory > motor (ethanol, arsenic, and isoniazid), or pure motor, sensory, or autonomic.

3. Time course — rapid (vascular, toxic, inflammation, immune), subacute (toxic, nutritional, systemic), and slow (hereditary, metabolic)

4. Axonal versus myelin degeneration

5. Diagnostic tests include EMG/nerve conduction velocities, CSF studies, nerve and muscle biopsies, and biochemical studies.

V. Mononeuritis multiplex (subacute asymmetric polyneuropathy)

1. Diabetes — acute ophthalmoplegia (CN III nerve palsy, sudden onset, spares pupil, lesion in center of nerve, usually painful, and often recovers well), acute ischemic femoral neuropathy (recovers well), progressive distal symmetric sensory loss (most common), symmetric or asymmetric motor with or without sensory loss, autonomic loss, and pain dysesthesia syndromes. The mechanism is ischemia of the vasa nervorum with segmental demyelination.

2. Ischemia and vasculitis

W. Morton neuroma — a traumatic neuroma that forms on the digital nerve between the toes

X. Neonates — may have a plexus injury involving C5 and C6 (Erb palsy, arms hang at side with a normal hand) or C7, C8, and T1 (Klumpke palsy, claw-hand with wasting, occasional Horner syndrome)

Y. Brachial plexitis — idiopathic onset of upper limb pain and weakness that usually resolves in 6 to 12 weeks. There is no fever, leukocytosis, or increased ESR. The cause is unclear (CMV, AIDS, unknown). Mononuclear cells may be seen in the nerve fascicles.

Z. Carpal tunnel syndrome — distal median neuropathy caused by compression at the wrist from the transverse carpal ligament. There is female predominance. 50% are bilateral. It usually is more severe in the dominant hand and causes wasting of the thenar eminence, weakness of the flexor pollicis brevis, opponens pollicis,

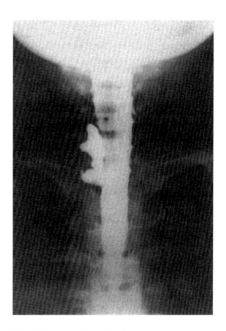

Fig. 3.312 Brachial plexus avulsion. (From Alleyne CH Jr. Neurosurgery Board Review. New York, NY: Thieme; 1997. Reprinted by permission.)

abductor pollicis brevis, sensory loss of the thumb and first finger, and nocturnal paresthesias. It is associated with multiple myeloma, amyloid, rheumatoid arthritis, acromegaly, mucopolysaccharidosis, hypothyroidism, and pregnancy. A pronator syndrome is caused by median nerve compression between the heads of the pronator teres.

AA. Ulnar neuropathy — may cause claw-hand with extension at the metacarpophalangeal joint and flexion at the interphalangeal joint of the fourth and fifth digits because of decreased function of the lumbricals. Lumbricals 1 and 2 are innervated by the median nerve. Cubital tunnel syndrome is caused by compression of the ulnar nerve under the two heads of the flexor carpi ulnaris.

BB. Posterior interosseous syndrome — weakness of the radial-innervated forearm and hand muscles (supinator, extensor digitorum, extensor carpi ulnaris, and abductor pollicis longus). No sensory loss. It causes a finger drop without a wrist drop because of sparing of the extensor carpi radialis longus.

CC. Anterior interosseous syndrome — pure weakness without sensory loss caused by compression of the anterior interosseous branch of the median nerve in the deep forearm. It involves the pronator quadratus, flexor pollicis longus, and flexor digitorum profundus 2 and 3 (FDP 4 and 5 are innervated by the ulnar nerve). Patients are unable to form the "okay" sign and demonstrate the "pinched" sign.

DD. Meralgia paresthetica — compression of the lateral femoral cutaneous nerve (L2, 3) under the inguinal ligament. It causes anterolateral thigh numbness and dysesthesia. It is associated with obesity, pregnancy, and diabetes.

EE. Tarsal tunnel syndrome — compression of the tibial nerve with paresthesias of the sole of the foot without motor changes

FF. Reflex sympathetic dystrophy — an abnormal response of the sympathetic nervous system that develops after trauma or an incomplete peripheral nerve injury. It is associated with vasomotor and trophic changes: causalgia (a persistent burning pain that is elicited by contact, pain, temperature changes, and emotion), limb cyanosis and coldness, and Sudek atrophy (atrophy of the bone, joints, muscle, and skin without nerve atrophy). The skin is smooth and shiny. Develops after a partial tear of a nerve and may be due to an abnormal connection of efferent and afferent sympathetic fibers. Treatment is with spinal cord stimulators, antisympathetic medications, or sympathectomy.

GG. Facial nerve diseases

1. Bell palsy — causes unilateral CN VII dysfunction with sudden onset. The cause is unknown though it is possibly viral. Weakness peaks in 2–5 days. There may also be decreased taste and sensation, and hyperacusis. 80% recover completely. Treatment is with steroids for 1 week, and prevention of corneal damage due to inability to close the eye and decreased lacrimation.

2. Ramsay Hunt syndrome — herpes zoster infection of the geniculate ganglion with CN VII dysfunction, possibly CN VIII dysfunction, and vesicular lesions of the ear

3. Bilateral CN VII nerve palsy — Guillain–Barré syndrome and Lyme disease

4. Supranuclear lesions — spare the upper face because of its bilateral innervation and may be associated with dissociation of emotional and voluntary lower face movements

5. Hemifacial spasm — intermittent spasms of the CN VII muscles. Onset is at 40–60 years with female predominance. Spasms start near the eye and move caudally. It is possibly caused by segmental demyelination with ephaptic transmission. Treatment is with microvascular decompression (the AICA is usually the artery that compresses CN VII), carbamazepine, or botulinum toxin injections.

6. Adie syndrome — degeneration of the ciliary ganglion and postganglionic parasympathetic fibers. There is female predominance. It causes paralysis of the pupillary sphincter with mydriasis. The pupil responds better to near than light (also with syphilis and Parinaud syndrome), and the pupil constricts with 0.1% pilocarpine (denervation hypersensitivity).

XXXIII. Neuromuscular Junction Diseases

A. Myasthenia gravis

1. It affects two populations: 30-year-old women (most common) and 60-year-old men with thymomas. 10% of cases have a thymoma, but 80% have thymic hyperplasia.

2. Symptoms begin with extraocular weakness and are worse with exertion and better with rest. Proximal muscles are affected more than distal, and it is remitting/relapsing. Symptoms include ptosis, expressionless facies, and dysphagia. There is rarely muscle atrophy. The pupillary response is normal. The symptoms are caused by antibodies to nicotinic ACh receptors (Ach-R) on the postsynaptic endplate, but 10–15% of cases do not have ACh-R antibodies.

3. There is a decremental EMG (strength deteriorates with use) and a positive Tensilon test (using edrophonium).

4. Associated with hyperthyroidism, rheumatoid arthritis, SLE, and polymyositis. Botulism may have a similar initial presentation but causes unreactive pupils. Aminoglycosides may worsen symptoms by decreasing Ca^{2+} influx at the neuromuscular junction.

5. Treatment is with anticholinesterase medications (neostigmine or pyridostigmine), steroids, thymectomy, plasmapheresis, and azathioprine (immunosuppressant). Initial treatment is with anticholinesterase medications. If the dose is too high, a "cholinergic crisis" may develop with muscle weakness, salivation, diarrhea, bradycardia, miosis, sweating, and nausea/vomiting. Assess by giving edrophonium: if the symptoms are worse or not improved, decrease the anticholinesterase dose. If the strength improves, increase the dose.

6. Consider thymectomy if a thymoma is seen on CT, although one third of patients improve after thymectomy even when no thymoma is detected. If there are only ocular symptoms for >1 year, there is no need for thymectomy because most patients do very well. Thymectomy should be performed between puberty and 60 years.

7. Steroids should be started after both anticholinesterases and thymectomy fail. Azathioprine may be used if prednisone is not tolerated. The final option is plasma exchange.

B. Eaton–Lambert syndrome—is usually caused by a paraneoplastic syndrome (oat-cell lung carcinoma in 60% of cases) that produces autoimmune antibodies against the presynaptic voltage-gated Ca^{2+} channels. Hence, there is decreased ACh quanta release because there is a reduction of Ca^{2+} ion entry into the presynaptic terminal. Seen with a male predominance. It causes proximal limb fatigue, has an incremental EMG (with strength improving at first with contractions), spares ocular and bulbar muscles, reduces reflexes, and impairs autonomic function. There is a poor response to anticholinesterase medications. Treatment is with removal of the tumor, plasmapheresis, steroids, and immunosuppression. Symptoms may be improved with guanidine.

C. Botox, aminoglycosides, increased Mg^{2+}, and decreased Ca^{2+} decrease the presynaptic ACh release.

XXXIV. Muscle Diseases

A. A muscle fiber contains multiple parallel myofibrils made up of sarcomeres (Z line to Z line). The nuclei are on the periphery of the cell, although they may be internal at the tendon junction or with myotonic dystrophy or centronuclear myopathy (Chapter 2).

   1. Type 1 muscle fibers (red muscle) — remember "IRS" with type I fibers being red and slow. Increased mitochondria, aerobic metabolism, slower, but more sustained action with less fatiguing and used for posture.

   2. Type 2 muscle fibers (white muscle) — less mitochondria, relies on anaerobic metabolism with glycolysis, quick action but fatiguable, more numerous than red muscle, and used for flight. Has some aerobic capacity.

   3. A band — myosin thick filaments and actin thin filaments

   4. I band — actin thin filaments

   5. H band — only myosin thick filaments

   6. With muscle contraction, the H and I bands shorten

   7. Muscle biopsy — demonstrates the number and size of fibers, storage diseases, segmental necrosis with regeneration (myositis), mosaic pattern changes (deinnervation), and the neuromuscular junction

   8. Type 1 fiber atrophy — myotonic dystrophy, congenital myopathy

   9. Type 2 fiber atrophy — myasthenia gravis, deinnervation, disuse, paraneoplastic syndrome, and steroids

   10. Nonselective atrophy — deinnervation (85% decrease in volume in 3 months)

   11. Nonselective hypertrophy — limb-girdle dystrophy, myotonia congenita, acromegaly

B. Congenital myopathies usually — cause a mild disability, are nonprogressive, and are more severe proximally. Includes central core disease, multicore disease, nemaline rod myopathy, and myotubular myopathy

C. Muscular dystrophy (MD)

   1. Hereditary diseases causing degeneration of muscle with symmetric weakness with normal neural function. They usually cause progressive proximal weakness. The most common varieties are myotonic dystrophy and Duchenne dystrophy. Evaluation should include serum CK, aldolase, and myoglobin, urine myoglobin, EMG, and muscle biopsy. In adults, the differential diagnosis includes polymyositis (more rapid course, higher CK than MD except Duchenne dystrophy, which is only in children, more fibrillation potentials on EMG, and improvement with steroids) and spinal-muscular atrophy (usually younger, and with abnormal conduction velocities). There is no treatment for MD, except for Duchenne dystrophy for which prednisone may help. Quinine may help decrease the hypertonicity in myotonic MD. Old contractures can be treated with fasciotomy and tendon lengthening.

   2. Congenital MD — autosomal recessive, weakness present at birth, more common in Japan, with or without mental retardation

   3. Duchenne MD — the most common type. It is X-linked recessive, but 30% are from spontaneous mutation. There is male predominance. It occurs in 1 in 3500 births, and peak age is 2–5 years. There is rapid progression. There is absent dystrophin that is needed to stabilize membranes. It causes atrophy of the shoulder and pelvic girdles and pseudohypertrophy of the calf with fatty and fibrous replace-

ment. It starts in the lower trunk and then spreads to the lower extremity and later the proximal upper extremity with sparing of the hands, face, and eyes. Patients use the Gower maneuver to stand, have a waddling gait (from bilateral gluteus medius weakness), occasionally have mental retardation, and are prone to CHF and respiratory infections. The serum CK levels are very elevated and peak at 3 years. Biopsy demonstrates muscle fiber necrosis and regeneration. Mortality is 75% by 25 years.

4. Becker MD — X-linked recessive inheritance with male predominance that occurs in 1 in 30,000 births. It has a later onset (11 years), is less severe than Duchenne MD, and there is rarely heart failure or mental retardation. There is abnormal dystrophin and pseudohypertrophy, but no fiber necrosis and regeneration. Patients are nonambulatory by 30 years and usually die by 50 years.

5. Facioscapulohumeral dystrophy — autosomal dominant inheritance. The defect is located on chromosome 4. It is mild and slowly progressive with peak age 10–20 years. It involves the face, shoulder, and upper arm and starts at the face and descends. There is preservation of the forearm muscle with a "Popeye" appearance. There is no pseudohypertrophy, mental retardation, or CHF. There is sensorineural hearing loss. It is the only MD with chronic inflammatory cells within the muscle. There is no fiber necrosis or regeneration, and the serum CK is normal. There is frequently absence of a muscle.

6. Limb-girdle syndrome — autosomal recessive or dominant inheritance with onset in childhood or early adulthood. There is slow progression with proximal axial weakness, frequent heart failure, but no mental retardation, and pseudohypertrophy in 33%.

7. Humeroperoneal dystrophy — X-linked recessive inheritance with biceps, triceps, and distal muscle weakness. Patients develop contractures and have cardiac conduction abnormalities.

8. Oculopharyngeal MD — autosomal dominant inheritance with peak age 45 years. The serum CK is normal. There is ptosis and dysphagia.

9. Myotonic MD — the most common MD in adults with autosomal dominant inheritance. The gene is located on chromosome 19, and it is a trinucleotide repeat disease. It occurs in 5 of 100,000 births, and peak age is 30 years. It initially affects the face and then the distal extremities with weakness or myotonus first. The muscles are unable to relax after contraction (myotonia). There are dysrhythmias, decreased intelligence, cataracts (90%), endocrine dysfunction (with testicular atrophy), temporalis and masseter atrophy, and frontal balding in both sexes. They are usually nonambulatory within 20 years of disease onset. The congenital form is inherited from the mother. The myotonia can be treated with quinine or procainamide (these may increase an atrioventricular block) or phenytoin (Dilantin).

D. Metabolic myopathies

1. They usually involve the proximal lower limb, rarely involve the face and eyes, and the serum CK is usually elevated.

2. Glycogen storage (in vacuoles)
   a. Acid maltase deficiency — autosomal recessive inheritance with glycogen storage in vacuoles. The infantile form is Pompe disease with onset at 1 month and death by 2 years, hepatomegaly, and a cardiorespiratory death. Glycogen accumulates in the liver, heart, skeletal muscle, and motor neurons.
   b. McArdle disease — autosomal recessive inheritance with myophosphorylase deficiency. Peak age at onset is 15 years. It is only symptomatic with increased activity and causes myalgia, increased CK, and myoglobinuria. They commonly complain of muscle cramps after activity.
   c. Phosphofructokinase deficiency — autosomal recessive inheritance with male predominance, and similar features to McArdle disease.

    d. Lafora disease — autosomal recessive inheritance with peak age 6–18 years. It is systemic, fatal, and causes seizures, decreased mentation, and focal deficits, and affects the heart, liver, skin, nerves, and muscles with accumulation of Lafora bodies (basophilic with dark center caused by the intracellular accumulation of polyglucosans).

3. Lipid storage (in vacuoles)
    a. Carnitine deficiency — inability to use long-chain fatty acids for metabolism. It may be systemic or muscular and causes mild weakness.
    b. Fabry disease — X-linked inheritance with deficiency of α-galactosidase and accumulation of ceramides. It causes peripheral nerve pain, decreased sweating, corneal opacities, renal insufficiency, and skin angiokeratomas. Patients are prone to cerebral infarctions.

4. Mitochondrial myopathy — ragged red muscle fibers caused by large subsarcolemmal mitochondria. It is associated with retinal, ocular, and cardiac abnormalities. It is inherited from maternal mitochondrial DNA. Variants are MELAS, MERRF, Kearns–Sayre syndrome, and Luft disease.

5. Malignant hyperthermia — autosomal dominant inheritance and occurs in 1 in 15,000 anesthetic procedures. The risk is increased with inhalation anesthetics (halothane) and succinylcholine in combination. The body temperature increases 1°C every 5 minutes and may reach 110°F. It is caused by increased muscle metabolism from sustained rigidity. There is increased O_2 use and lactate formation causing acidosis. Symptoms include tachycardia, dysrhythmia, hypertension or hypotension, hyperventilation, muscle rigidity, fever (50%), hyperkalemia, increased serum CK, myoglobinuria, and renal failure. There is a 70% mortality rate without treatment with dantrolene, 2.5 mg/kg IV every 15 minutes, then 2 mg/kg orally 4 times per day for 3 days. Dantrolene acts by reducing the Ca^{2+} release from the sarcoplasmic reticulum and reduces the mortality to 7%. Treatment also requires discontinuation of anesthesia, cooling, hydration, and IV sodium bicarbonate. The disease is related to a defect in a Ca^{2+} release channel (ryanodine receptor) with increased Ca^{2+} release from the sarcoplasmic reticulum. Patients at highest risk have a family history, increased serum CK, and central core disease. Diagnose high-risk patients by the contracture test; see muscle contraction in vitro with exposure to caffeine or halothane.

6. Thyroid myopathy — chronic thyrotoxic myopathy (affects middle-aged men, weakness and wasting of proximal muscles), exophthalmic ophthalmoplegia (associated with Grave disease, spares pupillary and ciliary function, painful, muscle is infiltrated with monocytes and lipocytes, inferior and medial rectus are most affected, impaired upgaze, and treatment is with steroids), thyrotoxic periodic paralysis (treat with β-blockers), and hypothyroidism (stiff, slow, and swollen muscles) (**Fig. 3.313**).

7. Others — steroids, Addison disease, and Cushing disease

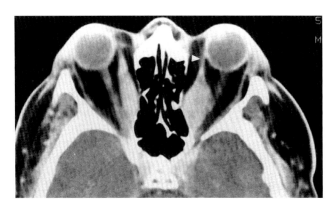

Fig. 3.313 Thyroid ophthalmopathy. Axial computed tomographic scan demonstrating enlarged medial rectus muscles. (From Valvassori GE, Mafee MF, Carter BL. Imaging of the Head and Neck. New York, NY: Thieme; 1995. Reprinted by permission.)

E. Inflammatory myopathy

1. Bacterial myositis — usually caused by *Staphylococcus aureus*. The risk is increased with closed injuries. It causes fever, leukocytosis, and tenderness.

2. Trichinosis myositis — involves the eye, face, and proximal limbs. It causes a puffy face, muscle tenderness, and eosinophilia. Both muscle fiber types are involved. Treatment is with thiabendazole and prednisone. Parasitic myositis is also caused by toxoplasmosis and cysticercosis.

3. Viral myositis — usually caused by influenza and Coxsackie viruses. It is seen in childhood epidemics. It is occasionally associated with rhabdomyolysis, acute tubular necrosis, and renal failure. It resolves in 1–2 weeks. Viral myositis is also caused by HIV and HTLV.

4. Polymyositis — the most frequent acquired inflammatory myopathy in adults with peak age 30–50 years and female predominance. It causes subacute, painless, symmetric, proximal more than distal, limb and trunk weakness with dysphagia, rare fever, malaise, and myalgia. It has a relapsing course with increased serum ESR and CK and urine myoglobinuria. More than 50% of cases have antinuclear antibodies and are EMG positive. There are T cells in the muscle fibers with macrophages. Treatment is with steroids and physical therapy to prevent contractures. 10% are associated with cancer. The active phase of the disease lasts around 2 years, most people improve, 20% recover, and there is a 15% mortality rate. Histopathology reveals inflammation in the endomysium. EMG demonstrates fibrillation and positive sharp waves.

5. Dermatomyositis — There is a female predominance and it occurs in children and adults. The initial symptom is a maculopapular skin rash: butterfly lesion over the face or on the eyelid with periorbital edema (heliotrope or lilac colored), or skin lesions on the neck, shoulders, and extensors of the extremities. The weakness is proximal and there is an angiopathy affecting skin, muscle, peripheral nerve, and intestines (causing ulcerations). The inflammation is humoral with increased antibodies and C3. There are B lymphocytes around the vessels but not in the muscle fibers as in polymyositis. Histopathology reveals perifascicular inflammation. Treatment is with steroids and physical therapy. 15% are associated with cancer and 30% also have Raynaud syndrome. The active phase of the disease lasts around 2 years, most people improve, 20% recover, and there is a 15% mortality rate. EMG demonstrates fibrillations and positive sharp waves.

6. Inclusion body myositis — peak age is 60 years with a male predominance. It is slowly progressive, painless lower limb weakness, steroid resistant, normal CPK, and microscopy is similar to polymyositis, but with intranuclear inclusions. It may be caused by a virus or prion.

7. Drug-induced inflammatory myopathies — caused by penicillamine and tryptophan. The CK is normal and there are perivascular eosinophils.

F. Miscellaneous

1. Rhabdomyolysis — destruction of striated muscle usually from ischemia or trauma. Myoglobin (smaller than hemoglobin and not bound to haptoglobin) enters the kidneys and may cause renal failure. There is fever, leukocytosis, pain, and albumin loss in the urine.

2. Familial periodic paralysis — due to a genetic defect coding for Na^+, Cl^-, or Ca^{2+} channels in the muscle fiber membranes (most commonly related to Ca^{2+} channels). There is autosomal dominant inheritance with a male predominance. It is characterized by intermittent episodes of paralysis with onset in late childhood and episodes occurring every few weeks, although the frequency decreases with age. Attacks are associated with hyperkalemia and hypokalemia, hyperthyroidism, and cold weather. It is

diagnosed by a very low serum K$^+$ (1.8 mEq/dL) and weakness exacerbated by glucose, NaCl, and exercise that is relieved with KCl. The muscle sarcoplasm develops vacuoles. Treat with KCl, 5–10 g orally per day, imipramine, acetazolamide, and limiting carbohydrates and NaCl.

3. Muscle cramps — caused by sustained contraction after muscle stretching. It is associated with pregnancy, dehydration, hypothyroidism, and dialysis. It is improved by massage and stretching and can be treated with quinine or diphenhydramine.

4. Energy is obtained from glycogen during exercise and from fatty acids/triglycerides during rest.

5. K$^+$ <2.5 or > 9mEq/dL — flaccid paralysis and decreased deep tendon reflexes

6. Ca^{2+} <7 mEq/dL (or with decreased Pco$_2$) — The muscles may overfire and cause tetany.

7. Ca^{2+} >12 mEq/dL — muscle weakness

8. Hypermagnesemia — tetany

9. Hypomagnesemia — weakness

10. Muscle fibers increase or decrease in size with exercise, etc., but the number of cells does not change. Deinnervation occurs with aging and causes group atrophy.

11. Differential diagnosis of peripheral weakness syndromes
    a. Ocular palsy (spare pupil) — hyperthyroidism and myasthenia gravis
    b. Bilateral facial palsy — myasthenia gravis, fasciohumeroscapular muscular dystrophy, Guillain–Barré syndrome, and Lyme disease
    c. Bulbar palsy — myasthenia gravis and botulism
    d. Cervical weakness (inability to lift head) — idiopathic polymyositis
    e. Weakness of respiratory muscles and trunk — polymyositis, glycogen storage diseases, and motor system diseases
    f. Bilateral upper limb weakness — ALS
    g. Bilateral lower limb weakness — polyneuropathy
    h. Limb-girdle weakness — polymyositis, dermatomyositis, and MD; Duchenne MD (lower limbs), and facioscapulohumeral MD
    i. Generalized weakness — familial hypokalemia/hyperkalemia
    j. Weakness of one muscle — neuropathy, seldom myopathy (except familial periodic paralysis)

4 Neurology

Associate Editor, **Greg Hawryluk**

I. Introduction

A. The fundamental questions in neurology are

   1. Is it neurologic?

   2. What is the lesion?

   3. Where is the lesion?

B. In general, the time course tells you the "what."

   1. Vascular events tend to be spontaneous and rapid in onset.

   2. Infectious or metabolic causes tend to evolve over days.

   3. Neoplasia and degeneration tend to evolve over months to years.

C. Knowledge of functional neuroanatomy/imaging tells you the "where."

   1. Brain, basal ganglia, cerebellum, brainstem, spinal cord, peripheral nerve, neuromuscular junction, muscle

II. Neurologic Development and Aging

A. Developmental milestones (**Table 4.1**)

   1. One year: Single words

   2. Two years: Climb 2 steps, 2 word sentences

Table 4.1 Developmental Milestones

Time	Gross Motor	Fine Motor	Speech	Social
6 Weeks	Lifts chin			Social smile
6 Months	Weight on hands, sitting up	Ulnar grasp	Responds to name	Stranger anxiety
9 Months	Pulls to stand	Finger-thumb grasp	"Mama, Dada"	Separation anxiety
1 Year	Walks with support	Pincer grasp	2 Word vocabulary	Drinks with cup
18 Months	Climbs stairs with support	Scribbling	10 Words, own name	Uses spoon
2 Years	Runs, kick ball	Undresses	2 Word sentences	Parallel play
5 Years	Catches ball	Ties shoelaces	Future tense	

3. Three years: Tricycle, Repeats 3 digits

4. Four years: Copies a square (4 sides)

B. Primitive reflexes

1. Should not persist beyond 3–5 months of age

2. Moro reflex — sudden withdrawal of support results in upper limb (UL) abduction and extension with hand opening followed by UL flexion and adduction; should disappear by 3–4 months; asymmetry or absence suggests focal motor lesion (e.g., brachial plexus injury)

3. Galant reflex — when suspended ventrally, stroking one side of back results in lateral curvature of the trunk toward that side; should disappear at 2–3 months

4. Grasp reflex — should disappear by 2–3 months

5. Tonic neck reflex ("fencing posture") — disappears by 2–3 months

6. Placing and stepping reflex — disappears by 2–5 months

7. Rooting/sucking disappears by 3–4 months

C. Abnormal development

1. Neurocutaneous syndromes
   a. Neurofibromatosis 1 — café-au-lait spots, axillary freckles, Lisch nodules of the iris, neurofibromas, bony lesions; seizures, scoliosis, optic glioma
   b. Neurofibromatosis 2 — bilateral vestibular schwannomas
   c. Sturge–Weber — port-wine nevus syndrome in V1 distribution, associated vascular malformations of brain with leptomeningeal enhancement, seizures
   d. Tuberous sclerosis — adenoma sebaceum, ash leaf macules (hypopigmentation), cardiac rhabdomyomas, kidney angioleiomyomas, mental retardation, seizures

2. Motor delay — increased tone with upper motor neuron (UMN) lesion or decreased tone (Werdnig-Hoffman disease [infant spinal muscular atrophy]), Down syndrome, Prader–Willi syndrome (paternally imprinted defect of 15q; Angelman's if maternally imprinted), basal ganglia, or cerebellar disease

3. Speech delay — male predominance; stuttering affects 2% of children, fluency is increased with ethanol or singing. 90% of lisps and articulation disorders resolve prior to or during adolescence.

4. Cognitive impairment
   a. Intelligence — the ability to act, think, and deal rationally and effectively with the environment. It is inherited and is located in many parts of the brain.
   b. Mental retardation — occurs in 3% of births, defined as intelligence quotient (IQ) < 70
   c. Learning disability — distinct from mental retardation. Academic difficulties exist in the presence of a normal IQ; rule out mental retardation, dyslexia, seizures, attention deficit disorder, etc.
   d. Autism — adequate motor and memory skills with decreased social development and communication. Only one third talk; may exhibit stereotypical movements
   e. Asperger syndrome — autistic but highly functioning in some areas such as math
   f. Dyslexia — difficulty with written language: poor reading and spelling, but verbal skills are normal. Affects 6% of children, is familial, and is more common in left-handed people.

5. Attention deficit-hyperactivity disorder — 3–5% prevalence. Characterized by inattention, forgetfulness, poor impulse control, distractibility. Highly genetic, 50% of cases persist into adulthood. Treatment is

with behavioral modification and stimulants such as methylphenidate. Prone to high-risk behaviors and substance abuse (i.e., "self-medication").

D. Aging

1. Changes with aging — decreased pupillary reactions, accommodation, high-tone hearing, taste, smell, strength, reflexes, vibratory sense (with normal proprioception), posture, and gait

2. Dividing cells decrease their rate of division. Nondividing nerve and muscle cells gradually die off. The brain shrinks by 230 g because of neuronal loss.

3. Collagen loses elasticity and contractility. The skull thickens with age, may rarely develop hyperostosis frontalis interna (thickening of frontal bone typically in obese hirsute women), and becomes strongly adhesed to the dura making epidural hematomas much less common than subdural hematomas.

4. Neuritic plaques (first in the hippocampus) and neurofibrillary tangles increase in number. Lipofuscin and iron deposits are increased, as is hippocampal granulovacuolar degeneration.

5. Ataxia develops from cervical spondylosis (spinocerebellar tract damage), cerebellar degeneration, posterior column dysfunction, vestibular degeneration, normal pressure hydrocephalus (NPH), or drugs.

III. Confusional States

A. Memory — involves the dorsomedial thalamus, hippocampus, temporal cortex, ascending reticular activating system (ARAS), and neocortex. Pathways include hippocampus to precommissural fornix to septal gray to diagonal band of Broca to the amygdala. Lesions of the amygdala, fornices, or mamillary bodies do not impair memory. Lesions of the dorsomedial thalamus, hippocampus, or temporal cortex cause memory impairment because these structures are needed for memory. Old memories are stored elsewhere in the brain.

B. Acute confusional state — characterized by a decrease in the speed, clarity, and quality of thinking, decreased coherence, orientation, concentration, and recall. There may or may not be illusions, hallucinations, or paranoid delusions. Electroencephalogram (EEG) has high-voltage slow waves. Origin may be drug intoxication, metabolic, concussion, and seizure.

C. Delirium — acute, transient, reversible confusion with a disorder of perception, overalertness to stimuli, and increased emotion. Typically autonomic symptoms (unlike other confusional states) such as dilated pupils, tachycardia, hyperthermia, and increased sweating. EEG is normal or has B-waves. Cause must be sought; may result from withdrawal from ethanol, barbiturates, sedatives, herpes simplex virus (HSV), poisons (atropine), respiratory disease, anemia, surgery, trauma, stroke, infection, etc. Delirium tremens has a 10% mortality rate.

D. Mood — overall attitude versus affect—outward facial expression in response to a particular stimuli. Mood and affect can be opposite.

E. Transient global amnesia — striking loss of memory for recent events and an impaired ability to retain new information, but preservation of remote and working memory. It occurs in middle age or older and typically resolves within 24 hours. Etiology controversial: may be caused by ischemia (thalamus, medial temporal structures), migraine, and temporal lobe seizure; may be functional. Precipitants include physical exertion, overwhelming emotional stress, pain, cold-water exposure, sexual intercourse, and Valsalva maneuver. Psychologic comorbidity is frequent. It has a benign course and seldom recurs.

F. Dementia

1. Decline in memory and one other cognitive function from a level previously attained. Interferes with normal social and occupational activities. Distinct from delirium, which is an acute onset disorder primarily of attention; not a part of normal aging

2. Risk factors include advancing age, positive family history, brain injury, and presence of the apolipoprotein E-4 allele.

3. Important to rule out reversible causes for dementia (10%) including intoxication, infectious, metabolic/nutritional, structural, neoplastic, vascular, or mood disorders. "Pseudodementia" results from psychosis or depression. Also consider NPH when there is a triad of dementia, urinary incontinence, and gait disturbance.

4. Alzheimer disease — accounts for over half of dementias with 85% of cases being familial. At age 65, 2–3% prevalence, at age 85, 25–50% have symptoms; progresses to death in 7–10 years. Early short-term memory loss is most striking. Later develops aphasia, apraxia, and agnosia. Characteristic pathologic findings are
    a. Neuronal loss and atrophy associated with generalized cortical atrophy — more pronounced in temporal and parietal lobes
    b. Neurofibrillary tangles — paired helical filaments formed by hyperphosphorylation of microtubule-associated protein tau (also seen in Creutzfeldt–Jakob disease and supranuclear palsy)
    c. Senile plaques – amyloid β peptides, proteolytic product of amyloid precursor protein (APP), average 50 μm in size; when deposited in the walls of small cerebral vessels this causes amyloid (congophilic) angiopathy predisposing to lobar hemorrhage. APP is located on chromosome 21 explaining why those with Down syndrome have symptoms of this disease by age 40. ApoE4 mutation leads to excessive accumulation of amyloid.
    d. Hirano bodies (intracellular aggregates of actin and associated proteins in neurons also seen in Creutzfeldt–Jakob disease).
    e. Lowered neurotransmitters, especially acetylcholine (ACh); increased glutamate levels
    f. Three theories: cholinergic, tau, and amyloid-β hypotheses
    g. Single photon emission computed tomography (SPECT) is approaching the accuracy of clinical exam (85–90%), although autopsy is required for definitive diagnosis.
    h. Acetylcholinesterase inhibitors such as donepezil, galantamine, rivastigmine can slow progression, but do not halt or reverse progression. Blockade of N-methyl-d-aspartate receptor excitotoxicity with memantine is showing promise.

G. Vascular dementia — second most common dementia, typified by stepwise decline. May be seen concurrently with other forms of dementia. More common in men. Somewhat treatable by treating vascular risk factors. Binswanger disease/subcortical leukoencephalopathy are rare forms of vascular dementia involving deep white matter.

H. Pick disease — frontotemporal atrophy; occurs more frequently in young patients; aphasia rare unlike Alzheimer. Socially inappropriate behavior typifies the condition (i.e., inappropriate sexuality, stealing). Genetic causes identified but account for only 5–10% of Pick cases.

I. Lewy body disease — 10–15% of dementia; overlaps with Alzheimer and Parkinson, typified by α-synuclein cytoplasmic inclusions referred to as Lewy bodies. Loss of both ACh and dopamine-producing neurons. Recurrent visual hallucinations early in the disease along with features of Parkinsonism help establish the diagnosis.

J. Wernicke–Korsakoff syndrome — severe, acute deficiency of thiamine (vitamin B1), usually found in chronic alcoholics. Atrophy of mamillary bodies pronounced. Wernicke encephalopathy typically presents with ataxia and nystagmus; Korsakoff psychosis with anterograde and retrograde amnesia and confabulation.

IV. Brain Structure and Function

A. Cortical structure

1. 2–4 mm thick, forms vertical cortical columns (of Lorente de No), which are functional units

2. Developmentally, inner layers form first with subsequent superficial migration.

3. Three types of cortex: neocortex (90%), paleocortex (base of hemispheres, olfactory system), archicortex (hippocampal formation)

4. Alternate classification
   a. Allocortex (olfactory cortex and hippocampus) — by definition, variable number of layers
   b. Isocortex has six layers (refer back to **Fig. 1.22**):
       (1) Molecular layer
       (2) External granular layer
       (3) External pyramidal layer
       (4) Internal granular layer
       (5) Internal pyramidal layer
       (6) Multiform layer

5. Layer 4 is the chief input layer; layer 5 provides efferent output. Layer 6 is responsible for corticothalamic interconnection. Layers 1, 2, and 3 mediate connections with other parts of the cortex.

6. Pyramidal cells are chief cortical efferents; stellate or granule cells are the main interneurons and are much more numerous.

B. Brain zones

1. The central zone (hypothalamus and allocortex) — mediate internal functions

2. The peripheral zone (cortex of sensorimotor and association areas) — mediates perception and interaction with the outside world

3. The border zone (limbic system) — between the central and peripheral zones, adapts the organism to the environment (**Fig. 4.1**)

C. Brain lobes

1. In 1909, Brodmann mapped the cerebral cortex into regions based on cytoarchitecture; this was later found to correlate closely with function.

2. Frontal lobe
   a. Constitutes about ⅓ of the entire human cortex
   b. Function — executive functions: personality, motivation, abstract thinking, introspection, and planning
   c. Components

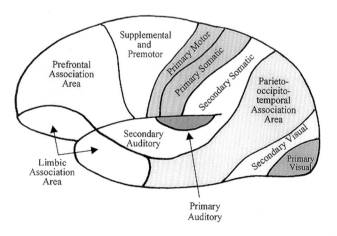

Fig. 4.1   Sensory, motor, and association cortical areas.

(1) Primary motor (area 4) — controls contralateral body with size of representation corresponding to finesse movement of associated body part. Lesion: contralateral loss of fine movements

(2) Premotor (area 6) — contains programming for movements; electrical stimulation produces contralateral movement. Lesion: inability to perform complex movements in the absence of paralysis (apraxia)

(3) Supplementary motor (extension of areas 6 and 8, medial frontal lobe) —contains programming for complex movements of several parts of the body. Stimulation results in aversive movements of head, eyes, and contralateral UL. Lesion: transient contralateral weakness, spasticity, and release of suck and grasp reflexes generated by the parietal lobe. Also results in decreased speech initiation that lasts around 3 weeks.

(4) Frontal eye field (area 8) — induces contralateral gaze (as in seizure). Lesion: impaired contralateral gaze

(5) Prefrontal cortex (areas 9, 10, 45, 46) — divided into the orbitofrontal region (visceral and emotional activities) and the dorsolateral area (intellectual abilities and executive functions). It has multiple connections with the visual, auditory, and somatosensory cortices. Stimulation does not elicit a motor response; however, stimulation of the orbitofrontal and cingulate gyri causes autonomic changes such as altered respiratory rate and blood pressure. Lesion: decreased motor activity, compulsive manipulation of objects, and release of some reflexes. Even large lesions here can be asymptomatic.

(6) Broca speech (area 44, 45) — pars opercularis, pars triangularis, and pars orbitalis — responsible for the motor component of speech. Lesion: impaired expressive speech distinct from dysarthria, comprehension intact; agraphia and facial apraxia

d. Additional frontal lobe symptoms

(1) Bilateral frontal lesions — impaired gait and incontinence (lack of warning), pseudobulbar palsy (degeneration of corticobulbar pathways to V, VII, X, XI, and XII cranial nerve nuclei with sparing of III, IV, and VI)

(2) Cognitive function — especially with dorsolateral lesions; impaired memory, attention, problem solving, and concentration

(3) Initiative — abulia (decrease in thought, movement, speech, will, or initiative) especially with bilateral and anteriorly located lesions. Akinetic mutism is more severe (following eye movements, but no speech or voluntary motor responses), lasts several weeks following lesion.

(4) Personality — especially with medial orbital lesions; decreased social consciousness, inappropriate behavior

e. Apraxia — the inability to perform a previously learned skill without significant motor, sensory, or ataxic deficits

(1) A planned action starts in the dominant parietal cortex and then goes to the premotor and supplemental motor cortices. The parietal area concerned may be near the supramarginal gyrus in the receptive speech center.

f. Apraxia types

(1) Ideational apraxia — inability to create a plan for a skilled movement. Damage is in the dominant parietal lobe. Test by having the patient act as if he or she is combing the hair without a comb.

(2) Ideomotor apraxia — inability to carry out a skilled command. Patient can conceive the movement, but not perform it. Damage is to connections between parietal and frontal lobes. Test by having the patient dress or eat with utensils. Most frequent apraxia.

(3) Limb apraxia

        (4) Limb-kinetic — deficits specifically involving fine limb movements

        (5) Nonverbal oral/buccofacial — difficulty demonstrating facial movements on command

        (6) Verbal — impairment of movements necessary for speech

        (7) Constructional — inability to draw or construct simple structures

        (8) Oculomotor — impaired eye movement

        (9) Dressing — impairment in ability to put on clothing

   g. Motor fibers

        (1) 30,000 Betz cells in the fifth layer of the motor cortex (area 4), but 1 million axons in each pyramid. The pyramid (in a monkey) contains fibers from the parietal lobe (40%; areas 1, 3, 5, and 7), motor cortex (31%; area 4), and premotor cortex (29%; area 6). Some input also occurs from the supplementary motor area.

        (2) The corticospinal pathway runs from the motor and sensory cortices diffusely to the intermediate and dorsal horns (nucleus proprius) to control sensory afferent projections and motor function, especially in the face and hands.

        (3) 80% of the fibers cross, and the uncrossed fibers travel mainly in the ventral corticospinal tract. Most corticospinal fibers synapse on internuncial neurons in the intermediate zone of the spinal gray, and 20% synapse directly on anterior horn cells.

        (4) Cortical fibers synapse directly on the CN V, VII, nucleus ambiguous, and XII, whereas there is no direct connection to CN III, IV, VI, and dorsal motor nucleus of X.

        (5) Patients with pseudobulbar palsy are unable to close their eyes or move their mouth or tongue, but are able to yawn, cry, cough, etc., which are reflexes of the pons and medulla.

        (6) The premotor cortex (area 6) can elicit motor activity with stimulation, but requires a higher amplitude than area 4.

        (7) Both the premotor and supplementary cortices send fibers directly to the spinal cord.

        (8) The supplementary motor cortex (anteromedial area 6) elicits gross bilateral movements with stimulation. It receives input from the premotor cortex for planned movements and from the posterior parietal cortex for activity initiated by visual, tactile, and auditory information. Output is to the motor cortex (area 4).

        (9) A lesion in area 4 produces hypotonia and weakness of the contralateral distal limb, but no spasticity.

      (10) A lesion in area 6 produces spasticity by increased stretch reflexes.

      (11) A lesion in the supplemental motor cortex produces involuntary grasping (it normally inhibits this reflexive activity).

      (12) The ventromedial pathway runs from the tectum, vestibular nuclei, and pontine and medullary reticular nuclei to the internuncial neurons in the ventromedial spinal cord to control axial movements and posture.

      (13) The lateral pathway runs from the red nucleus to the internuncial neurons in the dorsolateral spinal cord to control the limbs, especially the hands.

3. Parietal lobe

   a. Functions — body schema; integrating somatosensory, auditory, and visual information. Dominant lobe involved with mathematical calculations and language. Nondominant lobe involved with visuospatial relationships and geographic memory.

   b. Components

        (1) Primary somatosensory area (areas 3, 1, 2) — organized like primary motor cortex, size of representation based on sensitivity of a body part rather than size. Stimulation produces contralateral paresthesias. Lesion: loss of contralateral tactile sense and proprioception

(2) Secondary somatosensory area — Pain may be perceived here. Bilateral cortical representation with poor somatotopic organization

(3) Primary gustatory cortex (area 43) — anterior portion of parietal operculum. Lesion: contralateral ageusia

(4) Association area (areas 5, 7) — consists of superior and inferior parietal lobules; processes tactile and visual information; important for awareness of body and environment, performance of sequential tasks, especially if they involve the hands. Stimulation produces no sensation. Lesion: astereognosis, neglect

(5) Supramarginal gyrus (area 40) — caps the sylvian fissure

(6) Angular gyrus (area 39)—caps the superior temporal sulcus

(7) Wernicke area (areas 39, 40, 22) — supramarginal, angular, and posterior portion of the superior temporal gyri

   c. Additional parietal lobe deficits

(1) Vision — deep parietal lesion may interrupt superior geniculocalcarine fibers and produce contralateral inferior quadrantanopsia and also may abolish ipsilateral opticokinetic nystagmus and impair perception of spatial relationships.

(2) Cortical sensory functions — lesion may produce astereognosia, graphesthesia, and decreased two-point discrimination, with the deficits bilateral, but more pronounced on the contralateral side. There is decreased localization of touch and pain, but the perception of pain, temperature, touch, and pressure remains intact.

(3) Some apraxias can result from parietal lesions — dressing apraxia (mainly nondominant parietal lobe lesion) and constructional apraxia (mainly right side superior parietal lobule)

   d. Agnosias ("nonknowledge," or loss of knowledge) — inability to ascribe meaning to stimuli; loss of ability to recognize objects, persons, sounds, shapes, or smells in the absence of sensory deficit or memory loss. Three classifications: visual (occipital lobe), auditory (temporal lobe), tactile (cannot recognize objects placed in hand)

   e. Gerstmann syndrome — dominant parietal lobe lesion causes right/left dissociation, finger agnosia, acalculia, and agraphia

  4. Temporal lobe

   a. Function — integrates emotion, behavior, and sensation, which merge to create the idea of self. Also plays important roles in hearing, memory, and speech.

   b. All of the temporal lobe has six layers of cortex (isocortex) except the hippocampus and dentate gyrus, which have three layers (allocortex).

   c. Vascular supply — medial temporal lobe supplied by the posterior cerebral artery (PCA), superior and lateral temporal lobe supplied by the middle cerebral artery (MCA).

   d. Anterior and inferomedial temporal lobe have strong connections to the limbic system and are important for visceral activity, emotion, behavior, and memory. Posterior temporal lobe may store experiences; stimulation here produces illusions of past events.

   e. Left temporal lobe important for learning/memory of verbal information; right temporal lobe is more important for visual information.

   f. Seizure in the temporal lobe may produce auditory illusions, gustatory sensations, or hallucinations.

   g. Connections — anterior commissure and middle corpus callosum connect the two temporal lobes. Uncinate fasciculus connects the anterior temporal lobe to the orbitofrontal gyrus. Arcuate fasciculus connects Wernicke to Broca area.

   h. Components

(1) Superior temporal gyrus — involved with acoustic language with output to the limbic and prefrontal areas. Heschl gyrus (areas 41, 42) is the primary auditory cortex located in the

posterior superior temporal lobe deep in the sylvian fissure. Stimulation produces humming, buzzing, clicking, or ringing. Lesion: bilateral Heschl gyri injuries may cause deafness. A lesion on one side produces partial loss of hearing on the contralateral side.

(2) Areas 22, 21 comprise the auditory association area; stimulation produces sensation of bell or whistle. Lesion: auditory agnosia

(3) Middle and inferior temporal gyri — involved with visual discrimination with input from striate and peristriate cortices and output to contralateral visual association cortex, prefrontal, superior temporal, and limbic cortices

(4) Vestibular cortex lies just posterior to Heschl gyrus. Lesion: Unilateral lesion results in decreased opticokinetic nystagmus.

i. Additional temporal lobe deficits

(1) Kluver–Bucy syndrome — from bilateral amygdala damage; absence of emotional response, compulsion to explore all objects visually, tactilely, and orally; hypersexuality and visual agnosia

(2) Visual function — interruption of the inferior geniculocalcarine fibers (Meyer loop) produces "pie in the sky" contralateral superior quadrantanopsia. Bilateral lesions of middle and inferior temporal gyri may produce psychic blindness (one can see the object, but not understand what it is or what it is for). Temporal seizures may produce visual hallucinations.

(3) Time perception — may be altered by a lesion on either side, a seizure, or Korsakoff psychosis

(4) Smell and taste — Smell is affected by a lesion in the posterior orbitofrontal, subcallosal, anterior temporal, or insular cortex. Taste is affected by a lesion in the posterior insula. Olfaction plays a critical role in taste, as in a CN I deficit, commonly seen following brain injury.

j. Auditory agnosia — occurs with a lesion in association areas 22 and 21; sounds and tones are discriminated, but there is an inability to recognize words, music, and sounds. It can be separated into auditory agnosia (nonverbal auditory cues) and pure word deafness.

5. Occipital lobe

a. Represents one eighth of the cortex. The occipital lobes are connected by the posterior third of the corpus callosum.

b. Left side — more involved with naming, symbols, and color

Right side — more involved with spatial relationships, forms, faces, constructional praxis, and emotion

c. Hallucination — the perception of a stimulus that does not exist versus illusion —the distorted perception of an existing stimulus

d. Components

(1) Primary visual cortex (area 17) also known as the striate area and receives the optic radiations. Band of Gennari divides the fourth layer of the cortex into two granular layers with a thick myelin layer. Macular vision is represented in the posterior half of area 17.

(2) Parastriate cortex (area 18) and peristriate cortex (area 19) have no line of Gennari. These receive input from area 17 and perform complex visual processing (i.e., color, movement direction)

e. Deficits

(1) Cortical blindness — usually from bilateral PCA strokes and associated with the absence of α waves on electroencephalogram (EEG) (**Fig. 4.2**)

(2) Anton syndrome — an anosognosia; cortical blindness with an affected association area such that the patient denies that he or she is blind

(3) Impaired spatial localization — bilateral parietooccipital lesions

(4) Balint syndrome —psychic paralysis of gaze with normal extraocular function. Associated with inattention to the peripheral visual field and simultanagnosia; caused by a bilateral lesion in the parietooccipital cortices

f. Visual agnosia — inability to recognize objects, lesions of the left occipital and temporal lobes

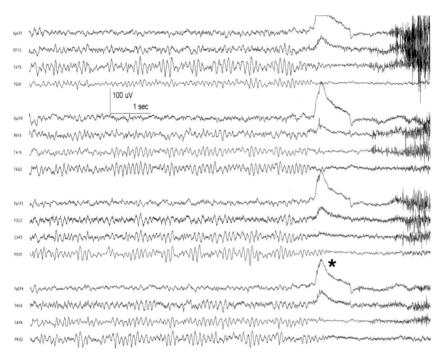

Fig. 4.2 Awake, resting electroencephalogram. Normal posterior α rhythm disappears with eye opening (*). High frequency activity at end of figure after eye opening is muscle artifact. Anteroposterior bipolar montage. (Courtesy of Dr. Richard Wennberg)

V. Speech and Language

A. 95% of people are right-hand dominant and have language dominance in the left hemisphere. Of left-handed people, 85% still have language dominance in the left hemisphere, 15% have bilateral dominance, and a very small number have right hemisphere dominance.

B. There are two receptive areas — (1) spoken language is received in Heschl's gyrus (areas 41 and 42) and the posterior superior temporal gyrus (areas 39, 40, 22, and part of Wernicke's area) and (2) written language is received in the angular gyrus in the inferior parietal lobule (area 39, part of Wernicke area). The supramarginal gyrus lies between these two centers.

C. There is one expressive area — the posterior inferior frontal gyrus (area 44, Broca area).

D. All speech areas border the sylvian fissure. The arcuate fasciculus connects these areas.

E. Aphasias (**Fig. 4.3**) — evaluate comprehension, reading, speech, writing, repetition, and naming

1. Expressive — lesion in Broca area. Speech output is decreased, with less fluency and impaired repetition (unable to write from dictation but can copy letters). Usually caused by upper branch MCA stroke

2. Receptive — lesion in Wernicke area. Decreased speech comprehension (both written and auditory), fluent paraphasic speech (using inappropriate, malformed words, or neologisms), impaired reading and repetition, inability to write or say what is wanted. Usually caused by lower branch MCA stroke

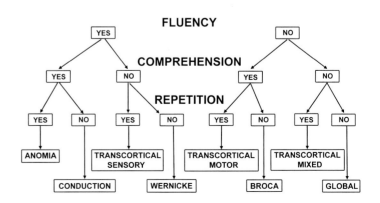

Fig. 4.3 Classification of aphasia.

3. Global — both Broca and Wernicke areas and is usually caused by large left MCA stroke

4. Conduction — lesion of the arcuate fasciculus. Fluent paraphasic speech, impaired repetition, writing, and reading aloud similar to Wernicke aphasia except with retained understanding of words read and heard. Awareness of the problem preserved. Usually caused by an embolic stroke in the posterior temporal branch of the MCA

5. Transcortical aphasias — lesions at the borderzone of the anterior cerebral artery (ACA), MCA, and PCA; associated with preserved repetition. Transcortical sensory aphasia often associated with hemianopsia and has a good prognosis.

6. Pure word deafness — impaired auditory comprehension and repetition with normal reading, writing, and speaking. Bilateral or unilateral middle third of the superior temporal gyrus between the primary auditory cortex and Wernicke area, often caused by a lower MCA embolic stroke

7. Pure word blindness — alexia without agraphia. Lesion of the left geniculocalcarine tract and corpus callosum

VI. Emotion

A. The amygdala plays an important role in emotion, especially fear; interconnected with olfactory system (afferent) and the hypothalamus (efferent).

B. Hunger and thirst are feelings centered more in the hypothalamus.

C. Pleasure is concentrated in the nucleus accumbens and septal nuclei.

D. Stimulation of the globus pallidus can produce an experience of joy.

E. Guilt, anxiety, and paranoia may be associated with the orbitofrontal cortex.

F. Anxiety, fear, and depression can be caused by stimulation of the temporal or cingulate gyrus.

G. Fear — involves both the sympathetic and parasympathetic systems. Fear is decreased with destruction of the amygdala.

H. Anxiety — mainly sympathetic and is associated with depression, hypoglycemia, pheochromocytoma, hyperthyroidism, and steroids

I. Depression — related to low levels of serotonin (5-HT) and norepinephrine (NE)

J. Emotional lability — increased control of emotional response with age; may result from cerebral disease

K. Pathologic laughing or crying — involuntary and uncontrollable, seen with injury to bilateral corticobulbar tracts from lacunar infarction, multiple sclerosis (MS), and amyotrophic lateral sclerosis (ALS)

L. Two paths control the pontomedullary facial movements involved with laughing and crying. The voluntary pathway involves the corticobulbar tract in the genu of the internal capsule. The involuntary pathway is anterior to the genu of the internal capsule. Damage to the anterior path causes unilateral decreased movement with emotion. Damage to the posterior path causes unilateral increased movement with emotion.

M. Aggression — may result from birth injury, trauma, encephalitis, or psychomotor seizures. Stimulation of the medial amygdala elicits anger. Bilateral amygdala ablation or section of the stria terminalis reduces anger.

N. Placidity or apathy — exploratory behavior is controlled by cortical and limbic dopaminergic pathways to the diencephalon and midbrain through forebrain bundles. Apathy is seen with frontal tumors, NPH, and Alzheimer disease. Abulia or akinetic mutism is caused by bilateral septal nuclei lesions.

O. Altered sexuality — disinhibition caused by orbitofrontal damage. Diminished drive is caused by superior frontal damage, depression, and drugs. Erections and orgasms can be produced by stimulation of the thalamic medial dorsal nucleus, medial forebrain bundle, and septal nuclei.

VII. Seizures

A. Epilepsy is a chronic condition of various etiologies characterized by a predisposition to recurrent seizures. It is an abnormal and excessive discharge of brain neurons with hypersynchrony and behavioral change.

B. 1% of the population. 8% of the population will have a seizure in their lifetime.

C. Epileptics have 2–4 times the mortality rate as compared with normal, highest in the first 10 years after diagnosis. A single seizure generally does not constitute epilepsy unless accompanied by a cortical lesion or epileptiform anomalies on EEG.

D. 70% are well controlled on anticonvulsants; many refractory patients (usually complex partial seizures) are surgical candidates. If a single first-line anticonvulsant fails, all other agents are likely to fail.

E. Kindling: Seizures beget seizures.

F. Classification

  1. Remote symptomatic — due to a known or identifiable brain lesion

  2. Cryptogenic — acquired brain lesion that is unknown or not identified

  3. Idiopathic — unknown etiology, presumed genetic

G. Epilepsy "zones"

  1. Irritative zone — area of cortex that generates interictal spikes

  2. Ictal onset zone — area of cortex where seizures are generated

  3. Epileptogenic lesion — structural abnormality of the brain that is the direct cause of epileptic seizures

  4. Symptomatogenic lesion — portion of the brain responsible for initial clinical symptomatology

  5. Functional deficit zone — cortical area of nonepileptic dysfunction

  6. Epileptogenic zone — area of brain necessary and sufficient for initiating seizures; removal or disconnection required for amelioration of seizures

H. Seizure pathophysiology

  1. May involve increased excitation (glutamate) or decreased inhibition (i.e., gamma-aminobutyric acid [GABA]), but this certainly oversimplifies the situation.

  2. Some have hypothesized "sick neuron" theory where a neuron becomes hyperexcitable or bursts when it usually would not.

  3. Many genetic anomalies are being identified; often involve Ca^{2+}, K^+, or Na^+ channels or neurotransmitter receptors.

  4. Neural synchrony may result from electrotonic interactions via neuronal/glial gap junctions, field effects (lamellar organization of cortex and limbic structures allows for the generation of large electric fields).

5. Findings in seizure foci — increased extracellular K$^+$ in glial scars, defect in voltage-gated Ca^{2+} channels; focus slower to bind and remove ACh, decreased GABA and taurine, increased glycine and increased or decreased glutamate. The surrounding neurons are hyperpolarized and have increased GABA.

6. Depolarization spreads until the surrounding neurons inhibit it. Seizures start in the cortex, spread to the deep nuclei, and then return to the cortex. The impulses go to the basal ganglia, thalamus, and reticular formation where they are amplified (tonic phase, decreased consciousness, autonomic changes, and polyspike pattern). As the diencephalon inhibits the impulse, the pattern changes to clonic with a spike and wave pattern. The depolarizations gradually slow and then stop by the exhaustion of neurons and increased blood–brain barrier breakdown.

7. Todd postictal paralysis may be caused by decreased glucose or increased lactate.

8. Seizure patients demonstrate the frequent loss of hippocampal CA1 neurons and Purkinje cells, possibly caused by hypoxia and ischemia.

9. Febrile seizures — 5% of the population has one; as long as they are not complex, do not increase risk of developing epilepsy. Epilepsy risk increases to 6–15% with 2 or more of the following:
   a. Seizure duration greater than 15 minutes
   b. Focal seizure
   c. Abnormal preexisting neurologic exam
   d. Seizure recurrence within 24 hours
   e. Family history of epilepsy

I. Partial seizures

1. Focal onset; must rule out a structural cause; this is the predominant seizure type after age 40, frequently secondary to stroke

2. Simple (no change of consciousness) or complex (altered consciousness)

3. Also classified as motor, somatosensory, autonomic, or psychic

J. Generalized seizures

1. May have bilateral onset or may evolve from a partial seizure

2. May be tonic, clonic, tonic-clonic, myoclonic, or atonic

3. Absence (petit mal) is also a generalized seizure; results from abnormal thalamocortical activity similar to what generates sleep spindles. Seen in 6–12% of epileptics, peak age 4–13 years, and there are frequent automatisms or other clonic activity. The EEG has a characteristic 3 Hz spike and wave appearance (**Fig. 4.4**).

K. Temporal lobe epilepsy (**Fig. 4.5**)

1. Semiology — may include foul smell (uncus, corticomedial nucleus of the amygdala), Déjà vu (hippocampus), fear and anxiety (central and basolateral nuclei), rising feeling in abdomen (autonomic nuclei)

2. Mesial temporal sclerosis — most frequent cause of intractable temporal lobe epilepsy; typically normal birth history, febrile seizures in 75%; pathology classically notes hippocampal atrophy with gliosis and neural loss in CA1, CA4, and dentate gyrus (**Fig. 4.6**).

L. Pediatric seizure syndromes

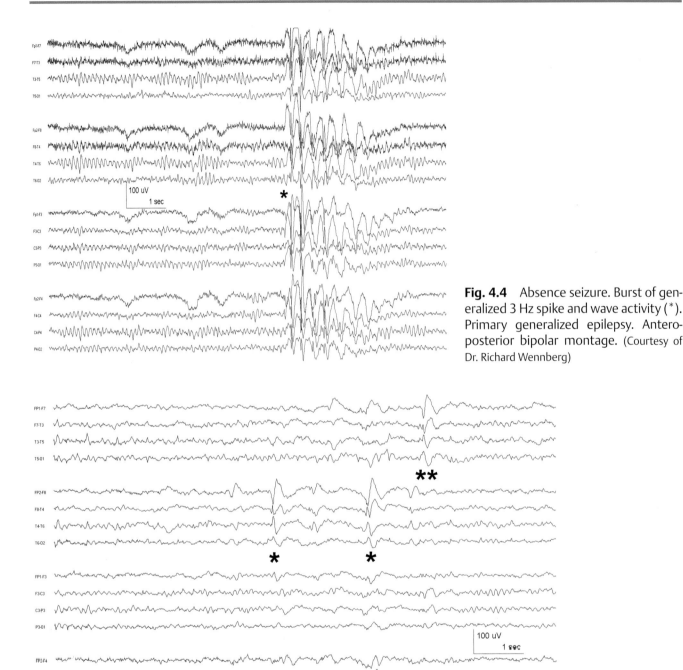

Fig. 4.4 Absence seizure. Burst of generalized 3 Hz spike and wave activity (*). Primary generalized epilepsy. Anteroposterior bipolar montage. (Courtesy of Dr. Richard Wennberg)

Fig. 4.5 Temporal lobe epilepsy. Bilateral temporal lobe interictal epileptiform activity. Independent sharp and slow wave complexes over right (*) and left (**) anterior-midtemporal regions. Anteroposterior bipolar montage. (Courtesy of Dr. Richard Wennberg)

1. Infantile spasms (West syndrome) — repeated flexion and extension of neck trunk and extremities lasting 10–30 seconds; onset typically 4–8 months and often associated with developmental delay; those with known cause typically more resistant to treatment. Hypsarrhythmia is typical on EEG. Treatment: adrenocorticotropic hormone (ACTH), vigabatrin, or ketogenic diet

2. Benign epilepsy of childhood with rolandic spikes — focal motor seizures typically involving the face during sleep–wake transition states; conscious but aphasic postictally. Remits spontaneously in adolescence

3. Juvenile myoclonic epilepsy — myoclonus in the morning. Onset is typically 12–16 years; autosomal dominant condition, variable penetrance; children have normal IQ; 5–10% of cases of epilepsy. Treat with valproic acid for life.

4. Lennox–Gastaut syndrome — multiple seizure types, frequent status epilepticus peak onset 2–6 years. Associated with encephalopathy and brain malformations: children have decreased IQ. Very difficult seizure to treat, frequently proceeded by infantile spasms

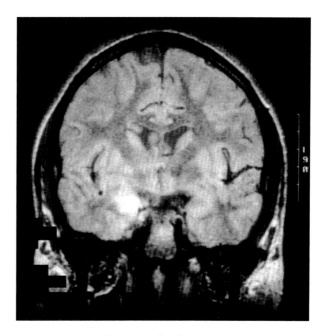

Fig. 4.6 Mesial temporal sclerosis. Coronal proton-density magnetic resonance image with increased signal intensity in the right medial temporal lobe. (From Albright AL, Pollack IF, Adelson PD, Eds. Principles and Practice of Pediatric Neurosurgery. New York, NY: Thieme; 1999. Reprinted by permission.)

M. Miscellaneous seizure phenomena

1. Jacksonian march — tonic activity spreading from the fingers, face, followed by lower limbs (LLs), followed by clonic activity

2. Epilepsia partialis continua — persistent focal motor seizures every few seconds. It responds poorly to medications.

3. Reflex epilepsy — induced by auditory, visual, or somatosensory stimuli, or words or eating

4. Neonatal seizures — usually focal. In the first few days, they are ominous and usually related to cerebral damage. In the first few weeks, they are usually due to metabolic disease with decreased glucose, Ca^{2+}, vitamin B6, etc.

5. Pseudoseizures — more frequent in those who have other neurologic conditions. History is key to diagnosis and used to decide who should instead undergo placement of invasive electrodes in the face of an unremarkable EEG.

N. Seizure treatment — Because of significant impact of seizures on quality of life, complete seizure freedom is the goal, not a reduction in frequency; may be medical or surgical

1. Anticonvulsants — can be teratogenic (4% birth defects versus 2% in general population, especially cleft lip or palate), but are less damaging than active seizures during pregnancy. Three modes of action, some drugs have multiple modes of action:
   a. Voltage-dependent Na+ channel blockade

(1) Phenytoin — hold channels longer in their inactive state; allows neurons to fire at moderate, but not very rapid rates. Effective against many seizure types. Half-life is 24 hours, and it is not removed by dialysis (**Fig. 4.7**). Side effects include allergy (fever, rash, polyarthritis), ataxia, diplopia, stupor, hirsutism, gingival hyperplasia, coarse facial features, cerebellar degeneration, peripheral neuropathy, and decreased vitamin K (supplement pregnant women before delivery). Can cause Stevens–Johnson syndrome. Avoid using with Coumadin (Bristol-Myers Squibb, New York, NY), sulfa, disulfiram, and chloramphenicol. Serum level is increased by cimetidine, chloramphenicol, valproic acid, and uremia.

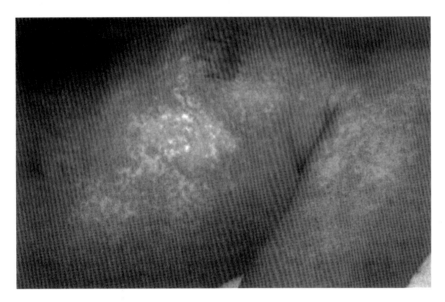

Fig. 4.7 Dilantin rash characterized by maculopapular trunk and proximal limb rash.

(2) Carbamazepine — similar mechanism to phenytoin. Half-life is 12 hours. Side effects include leukopenia, pancytopenia (monitor blood counts), diplopia, and hyponatremia from the syndrome of inappropriate antidiuretic hormone (SIADH). Serum levels increased with erythromycin.

b. Enhancement of GABA-A system

(1) GABA channels mediate inward Cl⁻ current, which hyperpolarizes neurons making them less excitable. Includes barbiturates (which can directly activate these channels) and benzodiazepines (increase channel activity, but cannot activate them). Valproic acid acts by increasing GABA activity. It is hepatotoxic if < 2 years; serum levels are increased with phenytoin (Dilantin, Pfizer Pharmaceuticals, New York, NY) and phenobarbital. Half-life is 8 hours.

c. Bind to L-type Ca^{2+} channels

(1) Some anticonvulsants are thought to bind to L-type voltage-gated Ca^{2+} channels, which are particularly important in the thalamus and thought to be important in absence seizures. Ethosuximide is such a drug (side effects: lethargy, hiccoughs, rare eosinophilia, leukopenia).

2. Other anticonvulsant agents

a. Acetazolamide — direct inhibition of carbonic anhydrase or due to resulting acidosis, may be useful in absence and nonfocal epilepsies. Side effects: teratogenic, risk of sulfonamide allergy

b. Gabapentin — does not interact with GABA receptors. May be used for generalized or partial seizures, but not absence seizures. Side effects: few side effects include somnolence, dizziness, ataxia, fatigue, nystagmus, increased appetite

      c. Lamotrigine — may inhibit presynaptic glutamate release, used as adjunctive therapy for partial seizures and Lennox–Gastaut syndrome; may have a role in generalized seizures. Side effects: somnolence, rash, dizziness, diplopia

      d. Felbamate — Used as an adjunct for partial seizures, Lennox–Gastaut syndrome. Side effects: aplastic anemia and hepatic failure; use with caution

      e. Topiramate — may have activity at Na^+ channels, GABA, and glutamate receptors. Adjunct to treating partial seizures. Side effects: cognitive impairment, weight loss, dizziness, ataxia

      f. Tiagabine — GABA uptake inhibitor

3. Treatment strategy — generalized seizures treated with valproic acid. Ethosuximide has a unique role in absence seizures. Dilantin and carbamazepine are generally used for partial seizures but may also have utility in generalized seizures. Phenobarbital is frequently used in children.

4. Status epilepticus — a medical emergency. Continuous seizure or recurrent seizures without normalization of consciousness for 30 minutes; however, many now consider 10 minutes sufficient for diagnosis. High mortality rate; often require intubation and intensive care management. Subclinical status should be considered in patients who have a depressed level of consciousness not otherwise explained. Typically treat with lorazepam 0.2 mg/kg up to 9 mg. Load with Dilantin — 20 mg/kg at maximum rate of 50 mg/min (or 150 mg/min for Fosphenytoin). If patient is already on Dilantin, administer 500 mg.

5. Seizure surgery — Considered for those with disabling, medically refractory seizures for > 1 year. Can perform resections or disconnections. Imaging, EEG, and seizure semiology should be concordant for highest chance of operative success.

      a. Complex partial seizures — Randomized, controlled trial showed 58% seizure-free in those treated surgically versus 8% in medical group. Extent of hippocampal, parahippocampal, and amygdala resection is a source of debate. Must assess laterality of memory preoperatively (Wada test) to ensure unilateral resection would not be debilitating. Unilateral resection may cure bilateral temporal lobe epilepsy.

      b. Corpus callosotomy — may be used for atonic seizures (drop attacks) and seizures with secondary generalization; involves division of anterior two thirds; does not stop seizures but prevents bilateral involvement allowing for preservation of consciousness; risks include disconnection syndrome; seizure recurrence can occur with time.

      c. Lesionectomy for lesional epilepsy — When a lesion seems responsible, removing it is often effective for seizure cure.

      d. Hemispherectomy — generally accepted that "functional hemispherectomy," which preserves basal ganglia, has lower risk than "anatomic." May have a role in intractable infantile seizures.

      e. Multiple subpial transections — Based on the notion of cortical columns. 5 mm linear incisions can be made for partial seizures emanating from eloquent cortex.

VIII. Multiple Sclerosis and Variants

A. Multiple sclerosis

1. Autoimmune demyelination affecting the white matter of the central nervous system (CNS) with a predilection for periventricular areas. Lesions in different locations, separated in time, are important for the diagnosis (i.e., a single case of optic neuritis or transverse myelitis may not progress to MS).

2. Prevalence ~50/100,000, more common in temperate zones, female predominance, onset usually in young adulthood.

3. Many lesions demonstrated on magnetic resonance imaging (MRI) are asymptomatic. MR lesions are high intensity on T2 and fluid attenuated inversion recovery (FLAIR).

4. Precise cause remains unclear; abnormal immune response clearly important in disease process, however. Associated with perivascular infiltration of monocytes and lymphocytes pathologically. Both environment and genetics seem important. Abnormal cytokine activity reported (interleukin-12); also associated with HLA-DR2.

5. Elevated immunoglobulin G (IgG) in cerebrospinal fluid (CSF) seen — oligoclonal band pattern

6. Uhthoff phenomenon — optic nerve dysfunction after heat exposure. Neuromyelitis optica (Devic disease)

7. Treatment
   a. Acute exacerbations treated with intravenous methylprednisolone (speeds recovery, but does not affect degree of recovery).
   b. Immunomodulatory drugs approved as first line therapies for MS (interferon β-1a, interferon β-1b). Decrease the rate of relapses by one third.
   c. Traditionally, cyclosporine, azathioprine, and methotrexate have been used to treat progressive disease/prevent relapses.

B. Other neuroinflammatory disorders

   1. Acute demyelinating encephalomyelitis — considered an isolated postinfectious or postvaccinial attack on the CNS

   2. Schilder disease — massive demyelination in children, adolescents with malignant course

   3. Baló concentric sclerosis — Disease pattern suggests alternating spared and damaged white matter progressing from the ventricles outward.

IX. Basal Ganglia

A. Physiology — Involved in the sequencing and modulation of motor activity by controlling the initiation, amplitude, and velocity of a movement. Also tonically inhibit unwanted movements. The caudate loop is involved with planning and selecting appropriate patterns of movement. When the basal ganglia are dysfunctional, hypokinesia occurs because fewer motor units are recruited and several cycles are needed to produce the intended action. Neurotransmitters are glutamate (from the cortex), ACh (from the caudate and putamen), dopamine (DA, from the substantia nigra pars compacta [SNpc]) and GABA (from the SN pars reticulata [SNpr]). The basal ganglia output is in a constant balance between ACh (positive) and DA (negative). Low levels of DA from the SN allow an increase in the effect of the ACh (positive) from the caudate and putamen on the globus pallidus (GP).

B. Symptoms of basal ganglia dysfunction

   1. Hypokinesia — reduced number of movements; no deterioration in strength. Examples are decreased blinking, difficulty swallowing saliva, mask facies, and monotone soft speech.

   2. Bradykinesia — slow movements

   3. Posture — normally controlled by the visual, proprioceptive, and labyrinthine input with motor responses. Basal ganglia disease associated with stooped posture, abnormal righting mechanism.

   4. Rigidity — bidirectional increased tension of all muscle groups, most prominent in flexors. No associated change in deep tendon reflexes (DTR). Cogwheel rigidity may be caused by the disinhibition of a tremor associated with basal ganglia disease.

5. Decreased SN input → increased striatal output → decreased medial globus pallidus (GPm) output → increased thalamic and pontine output and rigidity. Therefore, rigidity may be caused by decreased output of the SN or GPm. With this model, the rigidity and bradykinesia of Parkinson disease may be treated by a lesion of the GPm or ventrolateral thalamus (receives input from the GPm) (refer back to **Fig. 2.7**).

6. Athetosis or hemiballism may result if output from the subthalamus or striatum is decreased because this causes increased GPm output.

7. Dyskinesias — difficulty in or distortion of voluntary movements

8. Tremor — the most frequent dyskinesia. It is caused by alternating motion of agonist/antagonist muscles with regular frequency and amplitude. A resting tremor of 4–5 per second in the lips, head, and digits (pill rolling) is seen with Parkinson disease. Tics may be related to caudate disease.

9. Chorea — brisk, graceful, arrhythmic, involuntary movements. These are jerky actions (more complex than myoclonus) associated with Huntington disease (caudate and putamen lesions), haloperidol, hyperthyroidism, systemic lupus erythematosus (SLE), rheumatic heart disease (Sydenham chorea), and polycythemia vera. Associated with hypotonia, pendular reflexes (swings back and forth 4–5 times instead of 1–2 times), or hung-up reflexes (by a superimposed chorea movement).

10. Hemiballismus — unilateral violent flinging-type movement of the proximal upper or lower extremity seen with a contralateral subthalamic nucleus (of Luys) lesion and associated with hypotonia. Ballistic (phasic) movements have a triphasic pattern with an initial agonist burst, followed by an antagonist and then agonist. They are made with segmental spinal reflexes with proprioceptive guidance.

11. Athetosis — slow involuntary movements that flow into each other in a wormlike fashion. They occur contralateral to a lesion and are associated with spasticity. They may be seen with Huntington, Wilson, Hallervorden–Spatz (rare, progressive extrapyramidal dysfunction, and dementia), Leigh, Niemann–Pick (abnormal lipid metabolism) diseases, hepatitis, haloperidol, and 3,4-dihydroxy-L-phenylalanine (L-dopa).

12. Myoclonus — irregular, arrhythmic, shocklike contraction of muscle groups. May be seen with cerebellar, brainstem, and spinal cord disease. Includes polymyoclonus (widespread), segmental (spinal lesion), palatal (60–100 Hz, lesion of the central tegmental tract, removing inhibition of the nucleus ambiguous), essential (occurs in childhood, autosomal dominant inheritance, causes myoclonus multiplex, and is suppressed with ethanol), intention (posthypoxic and associated with cerebellar ataxia).

13. Dystonia — persistent posture at the flexion/extension ends of an athetotic movement, especially in the axial muscles. It is associated with Parkinson other conditions and especially medications (phenothiazines). Treat with botulinum toxin, benzodiazepines, baclofen, and anticonvulsants.

14. Tics — stereotyped and irresistible movements (i.e., blinking or sniffing). They most commonly occur at ages 5–10 years.

C. Evaluation

1. Boundaries between abnormal movements (chorea, athetosis, and ballism) blur. They are abolished by sleep and increased by stress.

2. Evaluation should include liver function tests (hepatolenticular degeneration), slit-lamp examination (Kayser–Fleischer rings), serum ceruloplasmin, and urine copper excretion to rule out Wilson disease.

D. Tourette syndrome — repetitive tics that may be simple (sniffing, snorting, involuntary vocalization) or complex (sexual or aggressive impulses, coprolalia); associated with obsessive–compulsive disorder. Transmission is autosomal dominant, and treatment is with haloperidol or benztropine. The mechanism may be impaired DA reuptake.

E. Parkinson disease

    1. Hallmarks are 4–7 Hz resting tremor, cogwheel rigidity, and bradykinesia.

    2. Affects 1% of aged population, slight male predominance. Genetics and environment appear causative. Gene mutations identified in 20% of cases, but present in about half of young cases. Age is the biggest risk factor.

    3. Differentiated from other causes of Parkinsonism because it is often asymmetrical and responds well to levodopa. Suspect secondary Parkinsonism when rapid progression, poor response to levodopa, early midline symptoms, early dementia, autonomic disturbance, or extraocular movement anomalies.

    4. Results from degeneration of DA neurons of SNpc; net result is decreased activity in supplemental motor cortex. Lewy bodies are seen pathologically.

    5. Treatment
        a. Levodopa — DA precursor that is actively transported across the blood–brain barrier. Typically combined with a peripheral aromatic acid decarboxylase inhibitor (benserazide or carbidopa). May extend duration of action with catechol-O-methyl transferase (COMT) inhibitors (entacapone, tolcapone) or monoamine oxidase B inhibitors (selegiline, rasagiline). Result of administration is synthesis of DA in a nonphysiologic fashion.
        b. Complications of levodopa — on–off effect, wearing off, and dystonia. Amantadine may help motor-induced dyskinesias.
        c. Other DA agonists (pramipexole, cabergoline, pergolide) induce fewer motor complications and are now usually prescribed before levodopa.

F. Secondary Parkinsonism

    1. Olivopontocerebellar degeneration — multiple system atrophy associated with ataxia; cerebellar degeneration starts in pons progressive anterograde to cerebellar cortex (pontocerebellar fibers) and retrograde to the inferior olives.

    2. Striatonigral degeneration — more aggressive course, a form of multiple system atrophy in which parkinsonian features predominate although autonomic and cerebellar symptoms can be seen.

    3. Shy–Drager syndrome — multiple system atrophy with autonomic dysfunction predominating; orthostatic hypotension is a key finding, poor response to levodopa.

    4. Progressive supranuclear palsy (Steel–Richardson–Olszewski syndrome) — triad of progressive supranuclear ophthalmoplegia (impaired voluntary vertical gaze, but preserved doll's eyes), pseudobulbar palsy, axial dystonia. Tend to have mask-like facies, dysarthria, dysphagia, emotional incontinence. Onset is typically around age 60 with slight male predominance.

    5. Drug/toxin induced — antipsychotics, phenothiazine antiemetics, metoclopramide, 1-methyl-4-phenyl-1,2,3,6-tetrahydropyridine (MPTP), carbon monoxide, manganese

G. Huntington disease

    1. A terminal illness first described in 1872 by George Huntington

2. Prevalence 8/100,000, more common in North Americans, less in Asians. Survival is typically 10–25 years from time of onset.

3. Polyglutamine disease associated with expansion of the Huntingtin gene. Defect at 4p16.3; 36 or fewer trinucleotide repeats is considered normal. Mutation is autosomal dominant with heterozygotes and homozygotes clinically indistinguishable. Forty or more repeats are the abnormal form of the gene. The disorder expresses an anticipation effect with subsequent generations having more repeats and thus earlier onset of symptoms.

4. Chorea, typically with onset in the 40s. Onset before age 20 is juvenile Huntington (Westphal variant). Cognitive and psychiatric problems eventually manifest.

5. Degeneration of neurons in the frontal lobes and caudate nucleus are typical leading to impairment in the basal ganglia's inhibitory functions. Brain imaging reveals dilatation of the frontal horns of the lateral ventricles due to caudate atrophy.

6. Treat symptomatically with benzodiazepines or DA depleting agents such as reserpine or tetrabenazine, neuroleptics.

X. Headaches

A. Head sensation — face (CN V1–3), supratentorial compartment (CN V1 and 2), mastoid air cells and posterior middle fossa (CN V3), and infratentorial compartment (CN IX, CN X, and C1–C3 posterior roots). CN VII, IX, and X supply a small area around the ear, and the sphenopalatine branches of CN VII supply some of the nasoorbital region. C2 supplies the back of the head.

B. Supratentorial pain is referred to the anterior head (V1). Infratentorial pain is referred to the neck and the back of the head. Inflammation of CN VII, IX, and X is referred to the nasal area, orbit, ear, and throat.

C. Head pain — usually from the dura, sinuses, and blood vessels (especially proximal). Intracranial and extracranial blood vessel dilation causes headache and may be induced by seizure, histamine, ethanol, monosodium glutamate, and nitrites. Sudden severe headache (like a bomb going off in the head) mandates ruling out aneurysmal rupture. Differential diagnosis includes thunderclap headache, benign orgasmic cephalgia exercise-induced headache.

D. Tension headache — bilateral, dull, aching, band-like pain, either predominantly occipital, temporal, or frontal. More common in women, may persist for days. One third of patients have depression. Treatment includes massage, relaxation, amitriptyline, diazepam, and codeine.

E. Cluster headache — severe, unilateral orbitofrontal headache that lasts 45 minutes. It is more common in young adults, has a male predominance, and tends to occur at the same time daily for 6–12 weeks before remitting for an average of 12 months (**Table 4.2**). Associated with rhinorrhea, lacrimation, and conjunctival injection. Mechanism may be parasympathetic discharge, swelling in the wall of the internal carotid artery (ICA) with sympathetic dysfunction (it is associated with Horner syndrome) or histamine release. Attacks may be triggered by ethanol. Prophylaxis includes β-blockers, lithium, naproxen, ergotamines, or methysergide. Acute treatment is 100% O_2 by facemask, ergotamine, sumatriptan, or steroids. If refractory, sphenopalatine ganglion lesioning may be considered.

F. Migraine headache — familial, periodic, usually unilateral, pulsatile, with onset in childhood or early adulthood, female predominance, less frequent with age (**Table 4.2**).

Table 4.2   Cluster versus Migraine Headache

Cluster Headache	Migraine Headache
Ipsilateral flushing	Ipsilateral pallor
Increased intraocular pressure	Normal intraocular pressure
Increased local skin temperature	Decreased local skin temperature
Male predominance	Female predominance
Older patients	Younger patients

1. Migraine aura — may be due to spreading oligemia with cortical impairment at a rate of 2–3 mm/minute. The aura may cause depolarization of autonomic and pain trigeminal fibers around blood vessels that lead to pain, increased permeability, etc.

2. Common migraine — characteristic migraine headache, but has no aura or neurologic deficit

3. Classic migraine — aura is usually visual (scintillating scotomas, fortification spectra, spark photopsia, etc.), but can involve numbness, weakness, dysphasia, etc. Symptoms progress over 5 to 15 minutes. About 1 hour after aura onset, the headache begins, which is typically unilateral and throbbing. It slowly increases in intensity to a peak in 1 hour and may last from a few hours to 2 days. May be associated with neurologic deficit (which resolves within 24 hours), which has a slow, march-like progression. Associated with nausea, vomiting, photophobia, and sonophobia. May be triggered by the ingestion of chocolate, cheese, foods containing tyramine, and red wine; decreases in frequency during pregnancy.

4. Migraine equivalent — typically pediatric, developing into typical migraine with age; headache may be absent, and it increases in frequency with age. Various types include hemiplegic migraine (may persist after headache resolves), basilar artery migraine (symptoms referable to vertebrobasilar system such as vertigo, ataxia, visual symptoms), cyclic vomiting, abdominal migraine, benign paroxysmal vertigo of childhood, ophthalmoplegic migraine (in children, periorbital pain and diplopia occurring several days after), ocular migraine (visual disturbance), acute confusional migraine, complicated migraine (prolonged deficit resolving by 30 days), migrainous infarction.

5. Migraine treatment
    a. Aura or early-stage headache — acetylsalicylic acid, nonsteroidal antiinflammatory drugs, or ergotamine (70% success); use promethazine or metoclopramide for nausea and vomiting
    b. Late stage — codeine, meperidine, and subcutaneous sumatriptan (a 5-HT agonist)

6. Migraine prevention — propranolol (75% success), methysergide (5-HT antagonist), Ca^{2+} channel blockers, monoamine oxidase inhibitors (phenelzine), and phenytoin (Dilantin)

G. Tolosa–Hunt syndrome — painful ophthalmoplegia caused by nonspecific inflammation of the cavernous sinus, superior orbital fissure; characterized by ocular and retroorbital pain, ocular motor paralysis (pupil may be involved), and possibly sensory loss over the forehead. May be mild proptosis, optic disk edema. Treatment is with steroids.

H. Trigeminal neuralgia — characterized by paroxysmal, stabbing, intense pain in the face, with sudden onset, lasts for a few seconds, and episodes may occur frequently over several weeks. It is incited by touch or other stimuli to trigger zones on the face. Typically, CN V is compressed by something such as the superior cerebellar artery or brainstem veins.

1. Most commonly, it affects the CN V2 and V3 distributions, and it is associated with minimal or no neurologic deficit.

2. It is more commonly bilateral with MS (which must always be ruled out). Brainstem or cranial nerve tumor must also be ruled out with imaging.

3. Medical treatment is with carbamazepine, phenytoin (Dilantin), gabapentin, pregabalin, and baclofen. Opiates offer little relief. Excellent response to carbamazepine (at least initially) is diagnostic; if no relief occurs, the diagnosis should be questioned.

4. If medications provide inadequate relief or are not well tolerated, surgical options include balloon gangliolysis, radiofrequency or glycerol rhizotomies, microvascular decompression, stereotactic radiosurgery, and peripheral neurectomy.

I. Other head pains

1. Raeder paratrigeminal syndrome — pain of trigeminal neuralgia in V1 and V2 with oculosympathetic paralysis (ptosis, miosis, but normal hidrosis). Associated with decreased facial sensation and masseter weakness.

2. Sluder sphenopalatine neuralgia (lower-half headache) — pain behind the eye, nose, or jaw with a blocked nostril or lacrimation

3. Temporal arteritis — temporal headache or jaw claudication resulting from granulomatous inflammation with giant cells involving branches of the external carotid artery. Onset typically after 60 years, thick and tender scalp arteries, with or without fever, erythrocyte sedimentation rate (ESR) typically > 50; 50% have polymyalgia rheumatica. Might lead to blindness because of thrombosis of the ophthalmic arteries or posterior ciliary arteries and is associated with amaurosis fugax and ophthalmoplegia. Diagnosed by temporal artery biopsy. Treatment is with prednisone to prevent blindness.

4. Glossopharyngeal neuralgia — paroxysmal pain in the tonsillar fossa or ear elicited by swallowing. May be due to neurovascular compression. Associated with syncope and bradycardia and treated with carbamazepine, phenytoin (Dilantin); surgical options include decompression or division of CN IX and the upper rootlets of CN X.

5. Postherpetic neuralgia — severe, constant, burning pain that occurs after zoster infection. It affects older ages. Treated with carbamazepine (Tegretol, Novartis Pharmaceuticals, East Hanover, NJ), gabapentin, phenytoin (Dilantin), amitriptyline, pregabalin, and local capsaicin. Results are poor.

6. Ramsay Hunt syndrome — geniculate ganglion (CN VII) herpes with ear pain and vesicles (in the external auditory meatus), facial weakness, possible hearing deterioration, vertigo, and tinnitus

7. Otalgia — diverse causes such as referred pain from CN V, VII, IX, and X

8. Occipital neuralgia — may be from the greater or lesser occipital nerve, C2 nerve. Treatment is with nonsteroidal antiinflammatories, steroids, or local injections.

9. Other facial pain syndromes include temporomandibular joint disease, atypical facial pain, sinusitis, headache with flushing due to pheochromocytoma or carcinoid, malignant hypertension, and facial reflex sympathetic dystrophy.

XI. Cerebellum

A. 3s are key — lobes, nuclei, cortical layers. Contains more neurons than the rest of the brain. Ipsilateral representation of body parts; does not contribute directly to consciousness. Consistent cytoarchitecture, from superficial to deep: molecular layer (few neurons), Purkinje layer (single layer of huge neurons unique to the cerebellum), granular layer (numerous, densely packed granule cells which is the only excitatory cerebellar cortical neuron).

B. Input is climbing and mossy fibers. Climbing fibers arise from olivocerebellar afferents from the inferior olivary nucleus; virtually no branches; enter via the inferior cerebellar peduncle. Mossy fibers arise from all other afferents, branch repeatedly in cerebellar white matter; enter via the middle cerebellar peduncle.

C. Purkinje neurons are the sole output of the cerebellar cortex, and are inhibitory neurons that inhibit the deep cerebellar nuclei.

D. Horizontal segments

   1. Flocculonodular lobe (archicerebellum, vestibulocerebellum) — input is from the vestibular apparatus and nuclei; important role in equilibrium. Lesion: positional nystagmus and impaired equilibrium

   2. Anterior lobe (paleocerebellum) — input is from the spinocerebellar tracts, which carry information from muscle tendons; arises from dorsal nucleus of Clarke (nucleus thoracicus), which forms a column of neurons in the medial part of lamina VII from C8–L2; functions in posture and muscle tone. Lesion: slight hyperreflexia

   3. Posterior lobe (neocerebellum) — input is from corticopontine fibers via the brachium pontis, functions in coordination. Lesion: causes decreased tone, clumsiness, and intention tremor (if the dentate nucleus is involved)

E. Longitudinal segments

   1. Vermis (output via fastigial nucleus) — responsible for medial motor pathways and trunk control

   2. Intermediate zone (output via interposed nuclei – globose and emboliform) — involved in lateral motor pathways and limb control. Input is from area 4 and the spinocerebellar tract. Lesion causes intention tremor.

   3. Lateral zone (output via dentate nucleus) — input is from the cortex. Involved in voluntary motor planning. Dentate input is from the premotor and supplemental motor cortices by way of the pons. It sends fibers to the ventrolateral thalamus and motor cortex (area 4).

F. Lesions

   1. Lesion of the flocculonodular lobe (lateral vestibular nucleus) — nystagmus, truncal ataxia

   2. Ethanol and malnutrition damage the anterior lobe — Lower limb/gait ataxia results.

   3. Posterior lobe syndrome — ataxia, decreased muscle tone, intention tremor

   4. Lesion of the vermis (fastigial nucleus) — truncal ataxia, scanning speech, or cerebellar mutism, and hypotonia

   5. Lesion of the intermediate hemisphere (interposed nuclei) — appendicular ataxia and hypotonia

   6. Lesion of the lateral hemisphere — terminal tremor, delay in initiating movements, and mild ipsilateral weakness. Symptoms are worse if the dentate nucleus or superior cerebellar peduncle is damaged.

G. Cerebellar symptoms

   1. Hypotonia — caused by decreased input to the α and γ motor neurons and improves with time following a lesion.

2. Dyscoordination — involves abnormal rate, range, and force. Slowness in responding to and initiating a movement may be present. Movements are decomposed into parts.

3. Titubation — 3 Hz anterior-posterior head bob (thalamic head bob is slower)

4. Dysarthria — scanning speech with variable intonation (increased or decreased force) and is explosive with individual syllable pronunciation. Slurred speech is caused by corticobulbar tract interruption.

5. Myoclonus, dysequilibrium, and poor eye saccades may also be caused by cerebellar lesions.

6. Tremor — rhythmic, regular, oscillating action of alternating agonists/antagonists. It is biphasic unlike clonus.
   a. Physiologic tremor — occurs while awake and asleep at 8–13 Hz, exacerbated by fear, hyperthyroidism, hypoglycemia, ethanol withdrawal, caffeine, steroids, and pheochromocytoma
   b. Pathologic tremor — only occurs while awake (except palatal and ocular myoclonus) at 4–7 Hz
   c. Parkinsonian (resting) tremor — occurs at rest, involves 3–5 Hz hand movements, is decreased with activity, has a pill-rolling quality, is persistent when walking (unlike essential tremor), increased amplitude with stress, and is treated with anticholinergics or contralateral ventrolateral thalamic lesion.
   d. Intention tremor — occurs at 2–3 Hz, at the end of a movement, is absent at rest; rubral tremor more severe (red nucleus or brachium conjunctivum lesion) and is associated with titubation (rhythmic oscillation of the head on the trunk). Treatment is with contralateral ventrolateral thalamic lesion.
   e. Essential tremor — 4–8 Hz, may be familial, autosomal dominant inheritance, onset is in early adulthood and it persists throughout life. Senile tremor if it has very late onset. The rate decreases and the amplitude increases with aging. It mainly involves ULs, also head and voice, but rarely legs. Suppress the tremor with β-blockers, primidone, or ventrolateral thalamic lesion.

H. Friedreich ataxia — autosomal recessive condition resulting from mutation on chromosome 9. Results from degeneration of neurons in spinal cord and spinal roots. See demyelination of posterior columns and corticospinal, ventral, and lateral spinocerebellar tracts; unmyelinated nerves are characteristically spared. Associated with chronic interstitial myocarditis/hypertrophic cardiomyopathy and kyphoscoliosis from spinal muscular imbalance. Gait ataxia predominates.

XII. Vision and Eye Movements

A. Moving objects are seen better than stationary objects. Red and green are seen better than white. Bilateral visual extinction occurs with right parietal lesions. The most frequent visual disorder in children is nearsightedness (myopia). In adults, it is farsightedness (hyperopia). In the elderly, cataracts, glaucoma, retinal hemorrhages and detachment, macular degeneration, and tumors are relatively common.

B. Pupils

1. Anisocoria — Up to 1 mm difference in pupil diameter is normal.

2. Fixed and dilated pupil — results from compression of CN III in uncal herniation. Down and out eye deviation from a complete CN III palsy occurs late: parasympathetic fibers mediating pupillary constriction are at the periphery of CN III and are affected first by compressive lesions. More reliable than hemiparesis in predicting sidedness of a lesion; however, it indicates the correct side in only 83% of cases. Fixed and dilated pupils are very rare without appreciable decline in consciousness, but consciousness may be maintained on rare instances early in the course.

3. Traumatic mydriasis (look for hyphema) is an important cause of pupillary dilation in trauma.

4. Pontine lesion — pinpoint pupils due to unblocked parasympathetic input from loss of sympathetic input from the hypothalamus to the superior cervical ganglion

5. Argyll Robertson pupil — reacts to accommodation but not light, seen with syphilis (**Fig. 4.8**). The pupil is small, irregular, and does not dilate with mydriatics.

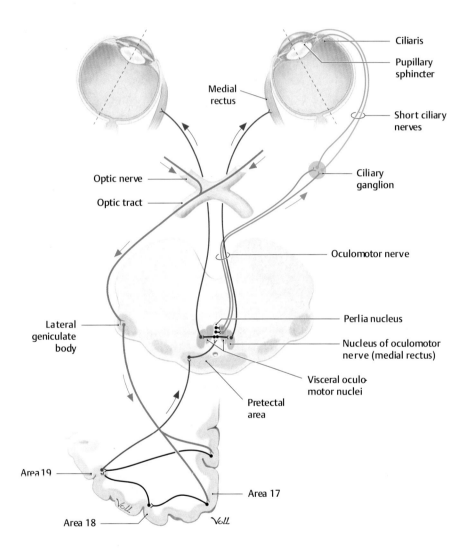

Fig. 4.8 Pathways for convergence and accommodation. For near vision, the eyes converge and the lens accommodates, which may be conscious or unconscious. Axons in the optic nerve (third neuron in the optic pathway) travel to the lateral geniculate body, synapse, and the fourth neuron goes to the visual cortex. Axons from area 19 (secondary visual area) reach the pretectal area through synapses and interneurons and then relay to the Perlia nucleus located between the two Edinger Westphal nuclei. Perlia nucleus contains neurons for accommodation that innervate the medial rectus for convergence and neurons for pupil constriction and accommodation (parasympathetic neurons). After synapsing here, preganglionic parasympathetic neurons travel to the ciliary ganglion and synapse and postganglionic neurons go to the ciliary body and papillary sphincter. Because Argyll Robertson pupil shows loss of pupil reaction with preserved accommodation and convergence, the connections to the ciliary and papillary sphincter muscles may be different, although the basis for this is unclear. (From THIEME Atlas of Anatomy, Head and Neuroanatomy, © Thieme 2007, Illustration by Markus Voll.)

6. Adie tonic pupil — mydriasis and blurry vision that occurs at 20–40 years with female predominance from degeneration of the ciliary ganglion (parasympathetics). Eyes respond to accommodation, but not light. Denervation supersensitivity to pilocarpine causes constriction. Benign condition associated with mild polyneuropathy with decreased DTRs in the lower extremities. No treatment indicated.

7. Ptosis — if associated with ipsilateral pupillary dilation, consider CN III palsy; if associated with ipsilateral pupillary constriction, consider Horner syndrome.

8. Horner syndrome — impairment of sympathetic supply to the eye. Sympathetic fibers from the long ciliary nerves travel with CN V1 to supply the Müller muscle of the eyelid explaining the ptosis classically seen in this condition. Reaction to amphetamine is seen with preganglionic, but not postganglionic lesions.

9. Pilocarpine — should constrict any pupil unless dilated by atropine

10. Near-light dissociation — lesion presumed to be near the nucleus of Edinger–Westphal, fibers mediating accommodation come from the occipital lobe via the internal capsule, follow a deeper course and are spared. Seen with pineal region lesions, MS, alcoholism, diabetes, Argyll Robertson pupil, Adie syndrome

C. Retina

1. Macula — region responsible for high visual acuity, located 4 mm lateral to the optic disk. Region in the center is the fovea centralis. The fovea has only cones, whereas the macula has both rods and cones.

2. Axons in the retina are unmyelinated before entering the optic nerve.

3. Subarachnoid hemorrhage (SAH) — associated with intraocular hemorrhages, often between the internal limiting membrane and the vitreous (subhyaloid or preretinal hemorrhages). Terson syndrome is classically vitreous hemorrhage associated with intracranial hemorrhage, though many consider retinal hemorrhage to be included in this syndrome as well.

4. Roth spot — a pale spot in the retina from the accumulation of white blood cells and fibrin, associated with subacute bacterial endocarditis or embolic plaques

5. Amaurosis fugax — transient monocular blindness usually from a fibrin embolus. 16% have a stroke with hemianopsia and/or unilateral blindness within 4 years. 25% will also involve the opposite eye.

6. Causes of sudden painless visual loss — central retinal artery or vein occlusion, ischemic optic neuropathy, retinal detachment, macular or vitreous hemorrhage, and acute glaucoma

7. Diabetic retinopathy — forms as fibrous tissue contracts and pulls the retina away from the choroid causing retinal detachment

D. Optic nerve

1. Papilledema — causes an enlarged visual blind spot and constricted visual field without visual acuity change. It develops as increased CSF pressure in the optic sheath, compresses nerve fibers, resulting in axonal swelling and leaking (see **Fig. 3.101**).

2. Optic neuritis — causes rapid partial or total loss of vision in one eye. It usually occurs in young adults and may be associated with retrobulbar neuritis or papillitis (edema of the optic nerve head). Usually local tenderness or pain is present with eye movements. It is bilateral in 10% of cases, and 75% develop MS. It is the first symptom in 15% of MS cases. Vision returns to normal within a few weeks, although color blindness frequently lingers (dyschromatopsia). Steroids speed recovery. In children, it is more frequently bilateral and viral (Fig. 3.100).

3. Ischemic optic neuropathy — the most common cause of painless monocular blindness in patients older than 50 years. Abrupt onset and is caused by occlusion of the central retinal artery. It produces an altitudinal field deficit, flame hemorrhage, and edema with disk atrophy. Occasionally bilateral, especially with diabetes or hypertension

4. Toxic and nutritional optic neuropathies — cause bilateral, symmetric central, or centrocecal scotomas (unlike demyelinating disease) with normal peripheral fields. Seen with B vitamin deficiencies, ethanol, or methanol

5. Episodic visual loss in early adulthood is usually caused by migraines and in late adulthood by transient ischemic attacks (TIAs).

E. Nonneurologic causes of visual loss

1. Cornea — scar, deposits (copper with Wilson disease), infection, and trauma

2. Anterior chamber — hemorrhage, infection, open-angle glaucoma (90% of glaucoma cases, drainage pathway is partially open, there is gradual visual loss, and the eye looks normal), and closed-angle glaucoma (red and painful eye). The visual loss with glaucoma is an arcuate defect in the upper and lower nasal fields.

3. Lens defects — associated with cataracts, diabetes (sorbitol accumulation), Wilson disease, Down syndrome, and spinocerebellar ataxia

4. Vitreous humor — hemorrhage from retinal or ciliary vessels by trauma, aneurysm, and arteriovenous malformation (AVM). Floaters are opacities in the vitreous humor. A sudden increase in floaters with a flash of light occurs with retinal detachment.

5. Uveitis — Inflammation of the iris, ciliary body, and adjacent structures accounts for 10% of blindness in the United States and is caused by toxoplasma, MS, cytomegalovirus, autoimmune disease (i.e., Behçet disease).

6. Leber hereditary optic atrophy — Onset is at 18–25 years, with male predominance, and inheritance by maternal mitochondrial DNA. Causes optic atrophy with deterioration of central, then peripheral, vision with stabilization.

7. Retinitis pigmentosa — affects children and adolescents, with male predominance and autosomal recessive or dominant inheritance (chromosome 3). It causes bilateral degeneration of all layers of the retina with foveal sparing. Symptoms include decreased night vision progressing to blindness. Associated with multiple diseases (Refsum disease, Leber disease, etc.)

8. Stargardt disease — Onset is at 6–20 years; it causes slow macular degeneration, especially of the central cones (opposite of retinitis pigmentosa).

F. Visual fields

1. Hemianopia — blindness in half of the visual field

2. Homonymous — The same field is involved in each eye.

3. Concentric visual field constriction (tunnel vision) — may be psychogenic or caused by glaucoma, papilledema, and retinitis pigmentosa. If psychogenic, the field does not change with distance.

4. Prechiasmatic lesion deficits
   a. Monocular blindness
   b. Visual loss extends to the periphery
   c. Scotoma — island of decreased vision surrounded by normal vision

5. Chiasmatic lesion deficits
   a. Junctional scotoma — caused by a lesion at the optic nerve/chiasm junction where the fibers from the ipsilateral eye and the fibers of von Willebrand knee from the contralateral eye are com-

pressed, resulting in ipsilateral monocular blindness and contralateral superotemporal quadrantopia "pie in the sky."

b. Bitemporal hemianopia — due to pituitary tumors, sarcoid, aneurysms, and Hand–Schüller–Christian disease (abnormal lipid accumulation particularly involving the skull). Patients typically bump into things they walk past.

6. Retrochiasmatic lesion deficits
   a. Homonymous hemianopia
   b. Congruous — identical field defect in each eye. Lesions closer to the cortex create more congruous deficits.
   c. Meyer loop — fibers of the inferior temporal lobe representing the contralateral superior visual field; a lesion involving them causes a "pie in the sky" deficit in the contralateral visual field
   d. Macular sparing — Macular representation in the primary visual cortex is in the most posterior aspect; caused by a PCA stroke with the occipital pole being supplied by MCA collaterals.
   e. Bilateral central scotomas — caused by occipital pole strokes
   f. Homonymous altitudinal hemianopsias — caused by bilateral occipital strokes. Monocular altitudinal deficits are usually caused by ischemic optic neuropathies.

G. Ocular movements

1. Saccadic movements — rapid voluntary movements to search a visual field. They are controlled by area 8 of the middle frontal gyrus to initiate contralateral eye deviation. Saccadic movements may also be elicited by sound or movement reflexes.

2. Pursuit movements — slow, involuntary movements keeping the eyes fixated on a moving target. They are controlled by the ipsilateral parietooccipital cortex with flocculonodular input. If a cortical injury is present, saccades are needed to keep an object in a field, and the opticokinetic reflex (pursuit of objects with stationary head such as telephone poles while in a car) is impaired on that side.

3. Vertical eye movements — controlled by fibers from the cortex through the anterior limb of the internal capsule and through the thalamus to the pretectum, superior colliculi, interstitial nucleus of Cajal, ipsilateral rostral interstitial nucleus of the medial longitudinal fasciculus (MLF), and the CN III nucleus.

4. Horizontal eye movements — controlled by fibers from the cortex through the posterior limb of the internal capsule to the prepontine reticular formation (PPRF) to ipsilateral CN VI and contralateral CN III nuclei.

5. Horizontal gaze center — PPRF and CN VI nuclei. Fibers from the CN VI nucleus cross to the contralateral CN III nucleus to innervate the medial rectus for conjugate lateral gaze. If these fibers are disrupted, the contralateral eye does not adduct, causing unilateral internuclear ophthalmoplegia (INO) (**Fig. 4.8**). A lesion of one CN VI nucleus impairs both eyes from moving to the side of the lesion.

6. Vertical gaze center — rostral interstitial MLF at the junction of the midbrain and thalamus, and also the interstitial nucleus of Cajal.

7. Stimulation of the
   a. Rostral PPRF — vertical eye movements
   b. Caudal PPRF — ipsilateral horizontal conjugate eye movements
   c. Superior colliculus — contralateral horizontal conjugate eye movements
   d. Middle frontal gyrus — contralateral horizontal conjugate eye movements

8. Cerebellar control — the flocculonodular lobe and vermis project to the vestibular nuclei and to CN III, IV, and VI. Disruption of this pathway impairs smooth pursuit and causes gaze-paretic nystagmus. If Purkinje cell inhibitory input is removed, the medial vestibular nucleus causes eye deviation away from the lesion.

9. Parinaud syndrome — impaired upgaze, impaired convergence, mydriasis, convergence nystagmus, and lid retraction (Collier sign). Dissociated near-light response is also present. Results from damage to the dorsal midbrain and tectum from tumor, MS, or stroke

10. Cortical lesion — causes eye deviation toward the lesion

11. Midbrain lesion — causes eye deviation toward the lesion (the descending fibers have not yet crossed in the midbrain/pontine junction)

12. Pontine lesion — causes eye deviation away from the lesion

13. Skew deviation — where one eye is more vertical than the other; seen with INO, brainstem, or cerebellar pathology

14. Downward eye deviation — caused by thalamic hemorrhage

15. Decreased upgaze — aging, increased intracranial pressure (ICP), Parinaud syndrome, and Niemann–Pick disease

16. Decreased downgaze — progressive supranuclear palsy

17. INO (**Fig. 4.9**) — caused by ipsilateral MLF lesion rostral to the abducens nucleus. The ipsilateral eye does not adduct completely when looking to the contralateral side; the contralateral eye exhibits nystagmus as it abducts. MS is the most common cause in the young. Bilateral INO causes bilateral adduction weakness. Anterior INO caused by a lesion in the high midbrain. There is decreased convergence with bilateral adduction weakness. Posterior INO caused by a pontine lesion. There is normal convergence with bilateral adduction weakness. Convergence occurs by means of paths to the CN III nuclei that are not in the MLF.

18. One-and-a-half syndrome — INO on one side and horizontal gaze palsy on the other. One eye is fixed at midline for horizontal movements and one eye can only abduct. It is seen with bilateral MLF (PPRF) and unilateral CN VI palsy and is caused by vascular or demyelinating disease.

19. Nystagmus — involuntary rhythmic eye movements. Convention uses the direction of the fast component when referring to its direction. Divided into jerk (has the traditional slow/fast components, may be caused by drug intoxication, ethanol, phenytoin [Dilantin] and barbiturates) and pendular, which has the same speed in both directions (seen where vision is lost early in life). Downbeat nystagmus caused by cervicomedullary junction lesion. Convergence nystagmus (nystagmus retractorius) is slow abduction of the eyes followed by rapid adduction caused by a midbrain lesion, typically part of Parinaud syndrome.

20. Ocular bobbing — abrupt, fast downward movement of the eyes with slow return to midposition; classically seen with pontine lesion, but it may not be specific for such a lesion

XIII. Smell and Taste

A. Olfactory receptor cells undergo constant turnover with new cells made from the basal cells. Other neurons that grow in adult humans are in the subventricular zone and dentate gyrus.

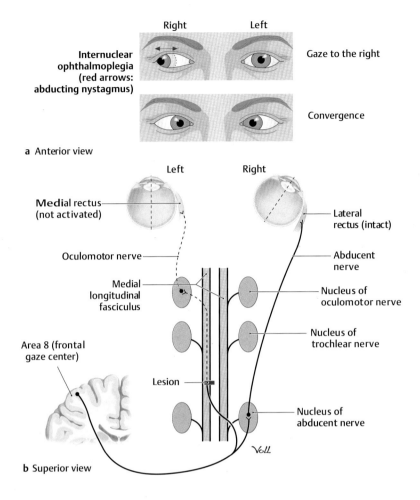

Right Left

Internuclear
ophthalmoplegia
(red arrows:
abducting nystagmus)

Gaze to the right

Convergence

a Anterior view

Left   Right

Medial rectus
(not activated)

Lateral
rectus (intact)

Oculomotor nerve

Abducent
nerve

Medial
longitudinal
fasciculus

Nucleus of
oculomotor nerve

Area 8 (frontal
gaze center)

Nucleus of
trochlear nerve

Lesion

Nucleus of
abducent nerve

b Superior view

Fig. 4.9 Ocular findings with left internuclear ophthalmoplegia. The left medial rectus muscle is no longer activated during gaze to the right so the eye does not adduct. The right eye shows abducting nystagmus. (From THIEME Atlas of Anatomy, Head and Neuroanatomy, © Thieme 2007, Illustration by Markus Voll.)

B. Anosmia is caused by trauma, radiation, infection, esthesioneuroblastoma, inflamed nasal mucosa, and tobacco. Kallmann syndrome (hypothalamic hypogonadism) is characterized by congenital anosmia from failure of the olfactory bulbs to form.

C. Decreased olfactory discrimination in Korsakoff psychosis (caused by dorsomedial thalamic lesion) and medial temporal lobe lesions

D. Olfactory hallucinations are caused by temporal seizures (uncinate fits), schizophrenia, and depression.

E. Decreased taste sensation caused by tobacco and inadequate saliva production (cystic fibrosis or Sjögren syndrome). Taste sensation is decreased in half of the tongue in Bell palsy.

XIV. Hearing

A. Auditory nerve contains 50,000 fibers (5% of those seen in the optic nerve).

B. Hearing loss

1. Conductive — decrease in low-pitch sounds and is caused by otosclerosis, otitis, and cholesteatoma

2. Sensorineural — decrease in high-pitched sounds and is caused by cochlear or nerve disease

3. Central — rare, caused by a lesion from the cochlear nuclei to the cortex, and must involve both temporal lobes

C. Testing

1. Weber test — place the tuning fork on the forehead. The sound is better in the normal ear if there is sensorineural hearing loss; the sound localizes to the worse ear in conductive hearing loss.

2. Rinne test — compares air and bone conduction by placing tuning fork on mastoid and then outside ear. If air conduction is not better, the problem is conductive.

D. Symptoms and signs

1. Tinnitus — nontonal can result from contraction of muscles (i.e., stapedius, tensor tympani) or bruit from an arteriovenous fistula or malformation (AVM); tonal is from middle or inner ear pathology. Physiologic tinnitus is present in 90% of people; it is usually masked by surrounding noise and may be due to vascular compression with ephaptic transmission.

2. Auditory hallucinations/illusions — described with dorsal pontine lesions

E. Hair cells — may be damaged by trauma, loud noise, drugs (aminoglycosides), and hypoxia

F. Nerve damage — occurs with age

G. Middle ear deafness — caused by trauma, otitis media, and otosclerosis (20–30 years, dominant inheritance, and treated with hearing aids or stapedectomy)

H. Sensorineural deafness — caused by infection (the CSF contacts the perilymph), vascular disease, demyelination, and tumors. High-frequency loss occurs with age and exposure to loud noises.

I. Vestibular schwannoma — causes high-tone hearing loss

XV. Vertigo

A. Vertigo — from Latin "vertere" meaning "to turn"; distinct from dizziness, it is the sensation of spinning or pulling to one side. It is associated with nausea, vomiting, sweating, and difficulty ambulating. Different positions may affect severity of symptoms. It is usually due to labyrinth, CN VIII, or vestibular nucleus dysfunction. When caused by a CN VIII lesion, symptoms are less severe than with labyrinthine disease. Brainstem disease may produce nystagmus without vertigo and does not cause hearing loss.

B. Meniere disease — recurrent vertigo with fluctuating unilateral tinnitus and low-tone hearing loss (these are more likely later in the disease course). Onset is around age 40 years with no sex predominance. Onset is abrupt, and it may last minutes to hours. The horizontal nystagmus is contralateral to the affected side and falling is ipsilateral. The abnormality is distention of the endolymphatic duct with rupture into the perilymph. This dumps K^+ that causes dysfunction of the apparatus; nerve degeneration is eventually seen. Treatment is with bed rest, dimenhydrinate, and diuretics. If severe, one labyrinth can be sacrificed after hearing has been lost. Other options include sectioning the vestibular portion of CN VIII, microvascular decompression, or endolymph-subarachnoid shunt. Most cases resolve spontaneously in a few years.

C. Benign positional vertigo — paroxysmal vertigo and nystagmus only elicited with certain head positions. It is more common and may be due to dislocation of posterior semicircular canal otoliths. Diagnosed with the Dix–Hallpike maneuver, it may be treated with the Epley maneuver.

D. Vestibular neuronitis — a single attack of vertigo without tinnitus or deafness. Onset is in young to middle-aged adults, and there is no sex predominance. There is frequently a history of previous upper respiratory infection. The patient falls to the ipsilateral side. It normally resolves in days and can be treated with antihistamines.

E. Labyrinthitis — similar to vestibular neuronitis but can include tinnitus and deafness

XVI. Syncope

A. Syncope — abrupt, brief loss of consciousness and tone because of decreased cerebral blood flow (CBF). There is slower loss of consciousness than with seizures. Seizures lack pallor and presyncopal dizziness and typically have a prolonged postictal phase. When the CBF drops to < 30 mL/100 g/min, the patient loses consciousness.

B. Differential diagnosis

    1. Circulatory failure

        a. Impaired vasoconstriction — vasovagal, postural hypotension, primary autonomic insufficiency, sympathectomy, and carotid sinus hypersensitivity

        b. Hypovolemia — blood loss and Addison disease

        c. Decreased venous return — Valsalva maneuver, coughing, and straining

        d. Decreased cardiac output — dysrhythmia (Adams–Stokes syndrome) or obstructive

    2. Altered delivery — decreased O_2, erythrocytes, and glucose

    3. Emotional

C. Vasodepressor (vasovagal) syncope

    1. Most common cause of syncope. Female more than male, younger people, associated with emotional situations, hunger, and hot crowded environments

    2. On standing, patient experiences a prodrome with gray pallor, coldness, sweatiness, nausea, vomiting, and salivation.

    3. Followed by loss of consciousness and falling, but usually enough time exists to protect oneself during the fall. Sphincter control is maintained. There is papillary dilation, systolic blood pressure < 60 mm Hg, bradycardia, and decreased respiratory rate.

    4. Symptoms reverse quickly upon positioning the patient supine, which increases CBF.

    5. It is caused by the sudden dilation of intramuscular arterioles with decreased peripheral vascular resistance and hypotension. Vagal stimulation causes bradycardia, hypotension, sweating, increased peristalsis, and salivation. The drop in peripheral vascular resistance is more important than the drop in heart rate. The skin vessels become constricted causing pallor.

    6. Anticholinergics (e.g., propantheline 15 mg 3 times a day) are a treatment option.

D. Postural (orthostatic) hypotension — occurs on rising. The patient faints without exhibiting all of the vasovagal-type symptoms. Associated conditions include peripheral nerve disease, autonomic insufficiency, L-dopa, antihypertensive medications, sedatives, hypovolemia, and spinal cord injury above T6. It is due to poor reflex contraction of the arteries and muscles.

E. Primary autonomic insufficiency — It has adult onset and is caused by sympathetic ganglion or intermediolateral spinal cord degeneration. Associated diseases are Shy–Drager syndrome and olivopontocerebellar degeneration.

F. Other causes

    1. Micturition syncope — occurs after urinating by reflex vasodilation elicited by bladder emptying

    2. Tussive syncope — occurs in men who are heavy smokers, where a coughing episode decreases venous return

3. Vagoglossopharyngeal neuralgia — Pain causes bradycardia and then syncope.

4. Cardiac syncope — Stokes–Adams syndrome (complete atrioventricular block with pulse < 40), sick sinus syndrome, myocardial infarction (MI), aortic stenosis, etc.

5. Carotid sinus hypersensitivity, atherosclerosis of the vertebrobasilar system, and subclavian steal

XVII. Coma

A. Consciousness — awareness of self and environment. Consciousness is impaired if the ARAS is damaged or a significant portion of the cortex and thalamus (typically bilateral) is dysfunctional and prevents the feedback required to stimulate the ARAS.

B. Common causes of coma — trauma, ethanol, drugs, and stroke. Consider intoxications, metabolic, infectious, shock, seizures, hypertensive encephalopathy, hyperthermia or hypothermia, SAH, other intracranial hemorrhage (ICH), and tumor.

C. Cherry-red skin — caused by carbon monoxide poisoning

D. Other conditions — Obtundation or stupor is when the patient rouses only with strong and repeated stimuli. In coma, the patient cannot be roused and there are no purposeful responses to stimulation. Sleep is a rousable resting state with decreased tone, blinking, swallowing, and DTRs. In persistent vegetative state, the eyes open and sleep/wake cycles return, but no real interactions with the environment are present.

E. Locked-in syndrome — the inability to respond because of a lesion involving the corticospinal and corticobulbar pathways with sparing of the ARAS. The lesion is usually near the basis pontis and only eye movements (such as the ability to look upward) may be spared.

F. Normal wakefulness with a desynchronized EEG requires the ARAS of the upper pons and midbrain to connect to the intralaminar/centromedian thalamic nuclei. EEG may show no activity in hypothermia, drugs, electrolyte disorders, etc.

G. Breathing in coma

1. Kussmaul respirations — rapid deep breathing associated with acidosis

2. Cheyne–Stokes breathing — slow irregular breathing with periodic bursts of a rapid rate. Results from impaired ability of the respiratory center to respond to alterations in serum O_2 or CO_2 levels. Multiple causes including increased ICP, congestive heart failure, altitude sickness, toxic-metabolic encephalopathy.

3. Central neurogenic hyperventilation — caused by a lesion at the midbrain/pons junction that removes the inhibition of the respiratory center and results in alkalosis. May need to sedate, paralyze, and ventilate to control respirations

4. Apneustic breathing — caused by a lesion in the low pons. Inspiration is followed by a 3-second pause.

5. Irregular (Biot) breathing — caused by a dorsomedial lesion in the medulla. Distinct from Cheyne–Stokes in that all breaths are of equal volume.

6. As a patient dies from cerebral herniation, first there is Cheyne–Stokes respiration, followed by neurogenic hyperventilation, and then Biot breathing as the lesion progresses from the upper to lower brainstem.

K. Pupillary reaction with coma

1. Midbrain lesion — dilated pupils

2. Pons lesion — pinpoint pupils

3. Opiates — pinpoint pupils

4. Anesthesia — midsized fixed pupils

5. Atropine toxicity — dilated pupils

L. Barbiturate and phenytoin (Dilantin) toxicity — may abolish ocular movements with maintenance of normal papillary reactions

M. Decerebrate rigidity — described by Sherrington with intercollicular lesions in cats and monkeys. Decerebrate posturing is caused by sectioning between the red nucleus and the vestibular nuclei.

N. Decorticate rigidity — caused by a lesion at a higher level (white matter or thalamus) and manifests as UL flexion and adduction with LL extension

XVIII. Cerebrospinal Fluid Diseases

A. Lundberg pressure waves — A, B, and C, and are independent of respiratory or cardiovascular waveforms. A-waves are plateau waves that can occur every 15–30 minutes; these are sustained, reach levels around 50 mm Hg, and may cause death.

B. Normal pressure hydrocephalus — urinary incontinence, memory deterioration, and gait disturbance ("magnetic gait" with unsteady, short steps and poor balance): remember wet, wacky, and wobbly. May be a sequela of trauma, SAH, infection; no preceding cause in 30%. Computed tomographic (CT) scan reveals enlarged ventricles without appropriate atrophy. Test by removing CSF by lumbar puncture to evaluate for possible improvement with ventriculoperitoneal shunting. Guidelines for management recently published.

C. Pseudotumor cerebri — idiopathic increase in ICP with papilledema. Usually affects overweight women. It may be related to vitamin A toxicity, retinoic acid treatment for acne, or steroid withdrawal; it causes headaches and visual loss. Patients should be followed by Goldman perimetry fields to monitor for peripheral visual loss. An enlarged blind spot is also characteristic. May be treated with weight loss (decreased intraabdominal pressure reduces venous pressure, increasing CSF reabsorption), acetazolamide, serial lumbar punctures, or shunting (lumboperitoneal or ventriculoperitoneal). Visual deterioration may be treated with optic nerve sheath fenestration (unilateral procedure causes bilateral improvement in 66% of cases). Subtemporal decompression may be performed by some neurosurgeons.

XIX. Cerebrovascular Disease

A. Stroke — sudden nonconvulsive focal deficit caused by a decrease in blood flow or O_2 delivery. Embolic strokes tend to reach a peak deficit quickly, whereas thrombotic and hemorrhagic strokes peak more slowly.

B. Stroke risk factors — hypertension, diabetes, tobacco (decreases high-density lipoprotein [HDL] levels and CBF), hypercholesterolemia, family history, age, and heart disease (atherosclerosis, CHF, or dysrhythmia).

C. Stroke etiologies — embolism (30–60%), thrombosis (30%), and hemorrhage (10%; hypertensive or SAH)

D. Stroke mortality — at 1 month: 19%, 1 year: 23%, 3 years: 46%, and 7 years: 60%. 65% remain functionally independent.

E. Atherothrombotic stroke

1. Atherosclerosis causes vessel stiffening and compounds the effects of hypertension, aggravating arterial damage. It forms mainly at branch points or bends of vessels such as the ICA bifurcation and cavernous portion, MCA bifurcation, ACA curve over the corpus callosum, and PCA where it winds around the midbrain. Plaques seldom form distal to the first branch point intracranially.

2. The normal ICA lumen is 7 mm, and symptoms will likely occur when it is < 1.2 mm.

3. 65% of thrombotic strokes are preceded by minor signs and frequently have progressive symptoms (rare with embolic [except when TIA occurs] or hemorrhagic strokes).

4. Evaluation with an angiogram carries the risk of stroke, 1–3% in the general population, but up to 5% in patients with atherosclerotic disease.

5. Thrombotic stroke mortality is 3–6% if small and up to 40% if basilar.

6. Most patients improve, although if no improvement is seen in 2 weeks, the prognosis is poor. Most motor and language deficits that persist for 6 months do not improve.

7. Seizures are a sequela of 20% of cortical embolic strokes. Stroke is the most common reason for new onset seizures in the elderly.

F. Transient ischemia attacks (TIAs)

1. Definition — transient loss of neurologic function from vascular insufficiency lasting < 24 hours (most last < 15 minutes). They occur mainly with thrombotic atherosclerotic lesions and are associated with hypertension, male sex, and occasionally with migraines.

2. TIAs are thought to be due to emboli, spasm, or decreased flow. TIAs with recurrent, similar symptoms are likely due to decreased flow (thrombus), whereas TIAs with different symptoms are more likely to be embolic.

3. The risk of a stroke developing after a TIA is 26% over 2 years (front-loaded risk with 20% occurring in 1 month). The risk of MI is 21% over 5 years.

4. A carotid circulation TIA may produce ipsilateral monocular visual loss (amaurosis fugax or transient monocular blindness) or contralateral hemispheric symptoms such as sensorimotor loss (usually hand).

5. A vertebrobasilar TIA may produce dizziness, diplopia, dysarthria, homonymous visual field deficit, etc.

G. Treatment of TIA or thrombotic stroke

1. Acute phase
    a. Maximize CBF by keeping the patient supine and allowing the blood pressure to remain elevated (up to around 180 mm Hg).
    b. If < 3 hours, consider thrombolysis with tissue plasminogen activator (tPA, if no contraindications), surgical clot removal, or vascular bypass. Endovascular tPA administration or clot retrieval may be performed up to 6 hours after onset of deficit.
    c. Anticoagulation may help to decrease thrombus progression in some cases but is of no proven short-term benefit for completed stroke.
    d. Other medical options such as hypothermia, Ca^{2+} channel blockers, and barbiturates have not proven helpful.
    e. Surgery — decompressive hemicraniectomy has been shown in randomized, clinical trials to improve survival and produce reasonable functional outcomes in patients under 60 years of age with MCA territory infarct > 145 cm3, surgery within ~48 hours of onset who are at high risk of herniation and death.

H. Embolic stroke

1. It is most frequently from a cardiac source (i.e., atrial fibrillation with a mural thrombus). It usually involves the upper division of the MCA and there is no right/left predominance; may progress to hemorrhage

2. Symptoms are of sudden onset and usually without warning. Unlike thrombotic strokes, there is less time for collaterals to develop.

3. Noncardiac sources include a fragment of plaque from the aorta, cervical carotid, or intracranial vessels.

4. Evaluation should include electrocardiogram (20% of MIs are silent), echocardiogram (to search for an embolic source), carotid Doppler ultrasonography, and CT (30% become hemorrhagic).

5. 20% have a second embolus within 10 days and 80% have a subsequent stroke develop.

6. Treat with tPA if deficit onset < 3 hours.

7. Treat rheumatic heart disease with valvuloplasty or lesion removal.

I. Lacunar stroke — small, deep, and usually multiple strokes of the putamen, caudate, thalamus, pons, internal capsule, and white matter caused by occlusion of small perforating vessels; associated with hypertension, atherosclerosis, and diabetes. Pathologic findings demonstrate lipohyalin degeneration of small vessels and Charcot–Bouchard aneurysms.

J. Ischemic penumbra

1. With CBF of 8–23 mL/100 g/min there is an isoelectric EEG associated with loss of synaptic function, but neurons are still viable. At a CBF of 18 mL/100 g/min, ischemia can have a long duration without cell death. This region is the penumbra.

2. As the duration of ischemia increases, there is increased intracellular Ca^{2+} (which triggers several damaging intracellular cascades); decreased adenosine triphosphate (ATP) and creatine phosphate; decreased NE, 5-HT, and substance P; increased free fatty acids and glycerol from membrane breakdown; increased prostaglandins, leukotrienes, and free radicals; increased protein denaturation; and cellular swelling.

3. The accumulation of excitatory neurotransmitters glutamate and aspartate also leads to increased intracellular Ca^{2+} and cellular damage/death.

4. A decrease in temperature 2–3°C decreases the metabolic requirements of neurons and increases the tolerance to hypoxia 30%. Elevated serum glucose leads to astrocytic anaerobic glycolysis and lactic acid accumulation with increased neuronal death.

K. Anticoagulation

1. Effective treatment for cardiogenic stroke (secondary to MI, atrial fibrillation, or valve prosthesis), decreasing embolic rate from 5.5% to 2% per year. Be cautious with anticoagulation in the face of larger strokes or poorly controlled hypertension. Do not anticoagulate a patient with subacute bacterial endocarditis.

2. 10% of TIAs develop stroke at 6 months with or without anticoagulation.

3. The risk of anticoagulation is early hemorrhage (20%), death (1%), and long-term hemorrhage (5%).

4. The risk of hemorrhage from Coumadin is increased with phenobarbital, carbamazepine, cephalosporins, sulfas, penicillin, and ethanol.

5. Antiplatelet agents are typically prescribed following stroke: aspirin, aspirin plus dipyridamole, ticlopidine, or clopidogrel.

L. Surgery — Carotid endarterectomy has been proven as better medical management in decreasing stroke in (1) symptomatic patients with > 70% stenosis. Reduces stroke from 26% to 9% over 2 years (North American Symptomatic Carotid Endarterectomy study [NASCET]) and (2) asymptomatic patients with > 60% stenosis. Reduces stroke from 11% to 5% over 5 years (ACAS).

M. Hemorrhagic stroke

   1. Intracerebral hemorrhage is associated with poorer outcomes than cerebral infarction or SAH.

   2. Early signs of ICP elevation (decreased level of consciousness, nausea) may help clinically distinguish these from ischemic stroke. CT scan is still required to rule out hemorrhagic stroke before tPA therapy.

   3. Hematoma volume can be measured with the ABC/2 method.

   4. Prognostic factors for outcome include increased age, larger hematoma volume, intraventricular extension, level of consciousness. Hematoma volume > 80 cm3 is rarely survivable.

N. Neurovascular syndromes

   1. Carotid occlusion — thrombotic. 25% have amaurosis episode before stroke.

   2. Middle cerebral artery
      a. Usually embolic
      b. Supplies — putamen, part of the head and body of the caudate, outer GP, and posterior limb of the internal capsule. The superior division supplies Rolandic and pre-Rolandic areas (may result in hemiparesis or hemianesthesia) and Broca area (aphasia). The inferior division supplies the inferior parietal and lateral temporal lobes (may result in Wernicke aphasia or homonymous hemianopsia).

   3. Anterior cerebral artery
      a. Supplies — anterior ¾ of the medial hemispheres and anterior ⅕ of the corpus callosum, anterior limb of the internal capsulae, inferior head of the caudate, and anterior GP
      b. Bilateral occlusion — paraplegia (mainly lower limb), incontinence, abulia, and personality changes
      c. Unilateral occlusion — contralateral hemiparesis (mainly of the lower limb) and mild sensory changes. A left-sided occlusion affecting the artery of Huebner may cause transcortical motor aphasia.

   4. Anterior choroidal artery
      a. Supplies — the internal GP, posterior limb of the internal capsule, and temporal horn choroid plexus
      b. Occlusion causes hemiplegia, hemianesthesia, and homonymous hemianopsia.

   5. Posterior cerebral artery
      a. Interpeduncular branches — supply red nucleus, substantia nigra, medial cerebral peduncles, CN III and IV, reticular formation, superior cerebellar peduncle, MLF, and medial lemniscus. Occlusion causes Weber syndrome (CN III nerve palsy with contralateral hemiplegia), impaired vertical gaze, and coma.
      b. Thalamoperforator branches — supply the anterior, inferior, and medial thalamus. Occlusion causes hemiballismus, choreoathetosis, and Korsakoff syndrome (medial dorsal thalamus).
      c. Thalamogeniculate branches (medial and lateral) — supply the geniculate bodies, central and posterior thalamus. Occlusion causes contralateral hemianesthesia and transient hemiparesis with delayed hyperpathia from thalamic sensory relay nuclei ischemia (Dejerine–Roussy syndrome, typically refractory to treatment).

     d.   PCA perforators — supply lateral cerebral peduncle and pineal gland

     e.   Posterior choroidal branches — supply the posterosuperior thalamus, choroid plexus, and hippocampus

     f.   PCA trunks supply — inferomedial temporal lobe and medial occipital lobe. Occlusion causes cortical symptoms with visual loss (sparing the macula), alexia, anomias (especially color), and impaired memory. Bilateral occlusion causes cortical blindness, central scotomas (from bilateral poles), Balint syndrome, and prosoprognosia.

    6.   Basilar artery

     a.   Paramedian branches — 7–10 branches that supply the medial pons

     b.   Short circumferential branches — 5–7 branches that supply the lateral ⅔ of the pons and the superior and middle cerebellar peduncles

     c.   Long circumferential branches — branches of the basilar, anterior inferior cerebellar, and superior cerebellar arteries that supply the cerebellar hemispheres

     d.   Interpeduncular branches — supply the subthalamus and midbrain

     e.   Complete basilar syndrome — impaired ARAS, upper CN deficits (diplopia), motor and sensory deficits (quadriparesis), and occasionally locked-in syndrome

     f.   Superior cerebellar artery occlusion — ipsilateral cerebellar ataxia, nausea, vomiting, ataxic speech, and decreased contralateral pain and temperature sensation in the body

     g.   Anterior inferior cerebellar artery occlusion — vertigo, nystagmus, nausea, vomiting, tinnitus, Horner syndrome, and decreased contralateral pain, and temperature sensation in the body

    7.   Vertebral artery

     a.   Supplies the medulla, inferior cerebellar peduncle, and posteroinferior cerebellar hemispheres (by way of the posterior inferior cerebellar artery [PICA])

     b.   In general, with the stroke syndromes of the brainstem, medial lesions affect the corticospinal tracts or hypoglossal nuclei and lateral lesions affect the spinothalamic tract or the cerebellum.

     c.   Medial medullary syndrome — involves the pyramid, medial lemniscus, and CN XII, causing contralateral upper and lower limb paralysis, contralateral impaired posterior column function, and ipsilateral tongue weakness

     d.   Lateral medullary syndrome (Wallenberg syndrome) — involves CNs V, VIII, IX, and X, sympathetic fibers, spinothalamic tract, and cerebellum. Causes decreased contralateral pain and temperature of the body, ipsilateral Horner syndrome, ipsilateral decreased facial pain and temperature (descending fibers and spinal nucleus of V), nystagmus, nausea, and vertigo (vestibular nuclei), decreased gag, hoarseness, dysphagia, and cord paralysis (IX and X), decreased taste (solitary tract), ipsilateral falling, and ataxia (restiform body). Hiccoughs are also common.

   8.   Lacunar stroke — Syndromes include pure motor (involving the internal capsule and pons), pure sensory (involving the internal capsule), pure dysarthria, hemisensory (thalamus), hemiparesis-ataxia, and dysarthria-clumsy hand (pons). Multiple lacunes are the most common cause of pseudobulbar palsy.

XX. Back Pain

A.   The sinuvertebral nerves branch from the posterior divisions of the spinal nerves just distal to the dorsal root ganglion and reenter the intervertebral foramina to innervate the ligaments, periosteum, outer anulus, and facet capsules. Branches of the L5 and S1 roots innervate the lumbosacral and sacroiliac joints.

B.   After 20 years of age, the glycosaminoglycans in the nucleus pulposus are replaced by collagen and elastin, and the water content of the disk decreases from 90% to 65%. The end plates become less vascular. By 50 years of age, 70% of people have MRI abnormalities. The shrinking disks alter the alignment of the facets and lead to degenerative changes. Back pain may be local, referred, or radicular.

C. Referred pain — upper lumbar disease may cause pain in the flank, groin, or anterior thigh by irritation of the superior cluneal nerves from L1–L3 that innervate the buttocks. Lower lumbar disease may be referred to the lower buttocks or posterior thigh, but never below the knee. The pain is usually diffuse and aching.

D. Radicular pain — sharp, "shock-like," intense, and elicited by the straight-leg raises (Lasègue sign) for lower lumbar disk disease. The reverse straight-leg raise and femoral stretch signs are positive for upper lumbar disease. L3 and L4 radicular pain is to the groin and anterior thigh. L5 and S1 radicular pain is to the leg and foot.

E. Disk disease is exacerbated by flexion (from the increased disk protrusion), whereas spondylosis and lumbar stenosis are exacerbated by extension (from the buckling of the ligamentum flavum).

F. Assess hip pathology by rotating the thigh (Patrick test). Consider vascular claudication in those complaining of leg pain.

G. Assess sacroiliac joint pathology by directly pressing on the sacroiliac joint or abducting the lower limb in the side position.

H. Disk disease peaks in middle age, then declines in incidence. L5–S1 is more common than L4–L5. C5–C6 (20%) and C6–C7 (70%) are the most common sites in the cervical spine. Thoracic disks account for 0.5% of herniated disks and occur mainly at T8–T12. The first reported case of a herniated disk was by Mixter and Barr.

I. Ankylosing spondylitis — a chronic, progressive seronegative arthritis that typically occurs in young men. It is an enthesopathy, which has a predilection for the axial skeleton. It is associated with HLA-B27 and causes back pain, decreased range of motion, and kyphotic deformity of the spine (poker spine). It destroys the sacroiliac joints and forms a bony bridge between the vertebral bodies (bamboo spine). It is associated with Reiter syndrome, psoriasis, iritis, and inflammation of the intestine.

J. Spine metastases — most commonly from **b**reast, **l**ung, **t**hyroid, **p**rostate, **k**idney, and multiple **m**yeloma (**Mnemonic: BLT with PKM**: bacon, lettuce, and tomato with pickles, ketchup, and mustard).

XXI. Peripheral Nerve

A. Consists of cranial and spinal nerves

B. Peripheral neuropathy/polyneuropathy — diffuse lesion of peripheral nerves producing motor, sensory, or reflex changes in combination or isolation

   1. Pure sensory involvement is rare and raises suspicion of a paraneoplastic disorder.

   2. Diabetes, ethanol, and Guillain–Barré syndrome account for the great majority of cases of polyneuropathy.

   3. Differential diagnosis of neuropathy (DANG THE RAPIST, see Chapter 3 section XXXI A):

C. Mononeuropathy — anomaly of a single nerve frequently from compression or trauma

D. Mononeuropathy multiplex — impairment of two or more nerves typically from a systemic process such as vasculitis, diabetes.

E. Ephaptic transmission — transmission of an impulse from one nerve to another as a result of nonsynaptic physical contact

F. Workup — hemoglobin A1c test, thyroid function tests, ESR, vitamin B12, EMG/nerve conduction velocities (NCV).

G. Charcot–Marie–Tooth syndrome — (peroneal muscular atrophy), the most common inherited neurologic disorder. Distal muscle weakness and wasting starting in the legs. Results from a mutation of peripheral myelin protein 22 leading to unstable myelin that breaks down spontaneously. Pain and temperature are spared because these nerves are not myelinated anyway. Onion-bulb appearance is seen as a result of repeated cycles of demyelination and remyelination.

H. Guillain–Barré syndrome — 1–3/100,000 incidence, several forms, classically an acute inflammatory demyelinating polyneuropathy with ascending weakness, paralysis, and hyporeflexia ± sensory or autonomic involvement. Thought to be an autoimmune response; recovery is dependent upon remyelination. 40% of patients are seropositive for Campylobacter jejuni. The Miller–Fisher variant is the triad of ataxia, areflexia, and ophthalmoplegia and is associated with anti-GQ1b antibodies. Recovery is usually in 1–3 months. Can see enhancement of nerves on MRI, delay in F wave on NCV suggesting demyelination

I. Chronic inflammatory demyelinating polyneuropathy — a chronic form of Guillain–Barré; > 8 week duration is required for diagnosis. Autoimmune condition with perivascular endoneurial infiltration of lymphocytes and macrophages that affects 1–2/100,000; most common in fifth and sixth decades. Motor symptoms are typically more prominent than sensory. Treatment: plasmapheresis, intravenous IgG, immunosuppression

J. Amyotrophic lateral sclerosis (Lou Gehrig disease) — degeneration of anterior horn motor neurons resulting in a mixed upper and lower motor neuron disease. Affects voluntary muscles with ocular and bladder sparing. Onset is after age 40. Etiology not certain; incidence 1/100,000, prevalence 5/100,000. About 10% of cases demonstrate autosomal dominant, or less commonly, autosomal recessive inheritance. Tongue atrophy and fasciculations are classic. Cognition affected in only 1–2%. Must be distinguished from cervical spondylotic myelopathy. Median survival is 3 years from diagnosis.

K. Martin–Gruber anastomosis — median to ulnar nerve crossover in the forearm; important to identify to prevent confusion with NCV

L. Thoracic outlet syndrome (TOS; superior thoracic aperture syndrome)

   1. Anatomy — the anterior and medial scalene muscles insert onto the first rib, and the subclavian artery and brachial plexus pass between them. The subclavian vein passes between the anterior scalene and the clavicle.

   2. Can be vascular (arterial or venous) or neurogenic from brachial plexus compression. Compression of any of these structures can cause UL and shoulder pain. Numerous causes including an incomplete cervical rib with a fascial band to the first rib, a long transverse process from C7 to the first rib, or rarely by a complete cervical rib articulating with a T1 rib.

   3. Compression of the vein may cause UL swelling.

   4. Compression of the artery causes a unilateral Raynaud-type phenomenon. The Adson test is where the patient sits with the ULs dependent, holds his or her breath, tilts the head back, and turns it to the affected side to determine whether the radial pulse is obliterated.

   5. Neurogenic TOS is typically unilateral and most frequent in middle-aged women. Asthenic, long neck, and droopy shoulders are associated. Neurogenic TOS causes wasting of the muscles supplied by the lower trunk of the brachial plexus and ulnar nerve (hypothenar eminence, etc.). Pain and paresthesias are rare. May be a dull ache in medial forearm, sensory loss in digits 4 and 5. Can see positive Tinel sign over supraclavicular plexus. It may be mistaken for ulnar neuropathy or cervical disk disease.

   6. An x-ray can reveal a cervical rib or elongated transverse process. EMG/NCV can be very helpful. Median nerve compound muscle action potential typically affected (with preservation of median nerve sensory potential), may see reduced ulnar sensory potential. Abductor pollicis brevis is typically affected.

7. If patients fail conservative management (i.e., physical therapy to strengthen the shoulders), surgery may be performed via the following approaches: anterior supraclavicular, transaxillary, or posterior subscapular. Goal is to decompress, removing the offending structure such as a cervical rib, or compressing band.

M. Peripheral nerve testing (**Figs. 4.6–4.13**)

1. Evoked potentials — helpful in diagnosing acoustic neuroma, MS, brainstem lesions

a. Visual evoked potentials (VEP) — monitor the visual pathway and are positive in 33% of patients with MS without obvious optic neuritis. P100 peak is monitored. Flash VEP can be performed through closed eyelids; pattern reversal VEP requires patient cooperation.

b. Brainstem auditory evoked responses — monitor the auditory pathway. Changes are usually ipsilateral even though most fibers cross to the contralateral side. Abnormal in 50% of MS cases (**Fig. 4.14**).

c. Somatosensory evoked potentials (SSEPs) — monitor the posterior column pathway of the sensory system. Painless electric stimuli (5 Hz) are placed over the median, peroneal, and tibial nerves. Recordings for the upper limb are made over Erb point (above the clavicle), over the C2 spine, and over the contralateral parietal cortex. Recordings for the lower limb are made over the lumbar and cervical spines and the contralateral parietal cortex. Normal peaks are Erb point (N9), cervical cord (N11), lower medulla (N13), and thalamocortical area (N19/P22). For intraoperative monitoring > 50% decrease in N20–P25 amplitude is significant.

2. Motor stimulation — tests of the motor cortex, facial nerve, and other peripheral nerves may be accomplished intraoperatively to elicit motor responses to locate eloquent areas. Thresholds for intraoperative monitoring > 80% decrease in amplitude (baseline motor evoked potential [MEP] must be > 100 µV), total loss of

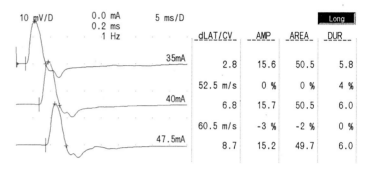

	dLAT/CV	AMP	AREA	DUR
35mA	2.8	15.6	50.5	5.8
	52.5 m/s	0 %	0 %	4 %
40mA	6.8	15.7	50.5	6.0
	60.5 m/s	-3 %	-2 %	0 %
47.5mA	8.7	15.2	49.7	6.0

Fig. 4.10 Median motor nerve responses in a normal subject. Recording site: abductor pollicus brevis, amplitude measures from baseline to peak. (Courtesy of Drs. Vera Bril and Mylan Ngo)

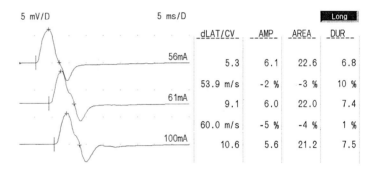

	dLAT/CV	AMP	AREA	DUR
56mA	5.3	6.1	22.6	6.8
	53.9 m/s	-2 %	-3 %	10 %
61mA	9.1	6.0	22.0	7.4
	60.0 m/s	-5 %	-4 %	1 %
100mA	10.6	5.6	21.2	7.5

Fig. 4.11 Median motor nerve responses in a patient with carpal tunnel syndrome showing prolonged median distal latency at wrist. Recording site is abductor pollicus brevis. (Courtesy of Drs. Vera Bril and Mylan Ngo)

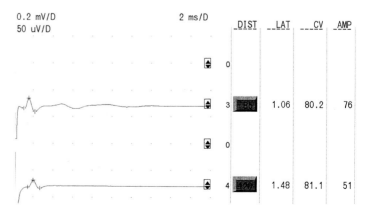

	DIST	LAT	CV	AMP
0				
3		1.06	80.2	76
0				
4		1.48	81.1	51

Fig. 4.12 Median sensory nerve responses in a normal patient. Recording at wrist stimulating at palm and digit 2. (Courtesy of Drs. Vera Bril and Mylan Ngo)

MEP, or > 100 V stimulus increase in MEP threshold. Risks include tongue lacerations and seizures.

3. Nerve conduction velocity
   a. Axonal disease — decreases wave amplitude
   b. Myelin disease — increases latency and decreases velocity
   c. Repetitive nerve stimulation — increases amplitude (incremental response) with Eaton–Lambert syndrome and decreases amplitude (decremental response) with myasthenia gravis
   d. H reflex — elicited by submaximal stimulation of an S1 sensory fiber that sends the impulse to the spinal cord where a monosynaptic reflex elicits a plantar flexion motor impulse. It is the electrical equivalent of the Achilles reflex and is caused by submaximal stimulation of a mixed motor-sensory nerve that is not strong enough to obtain a direct motor response.
   e. M wave — a direct motor response caused by stimulation of a motor nerve
   f. F response — elicited by supramaximal stimulation of a mixed motor-sensory nerve, which causes antidromic impulse transmission back to the anterior horn. If appropriately timed, it can depolarize the cell body leading to an orthodromic impulse to the muscle eliciting contraction. This avoids sensory pathways and is useful if few sensory fibers are available to test.

0.1 mV/D   2 ms/D
20 uV/D

DIST	LAT	CV	AMP
5 75	2.3	32.6	55
0			
0			
5 100	3.1	32.3	22

Fig. 4.13 Median sensory nerve responses in a patient with carpal tunnel syndrome showing slow conduction velocity and prolonged latency. Recording at wrist stimulating at palm and second digit. (Courtesy of Drs. Vera Bril and Mylan Ngo)

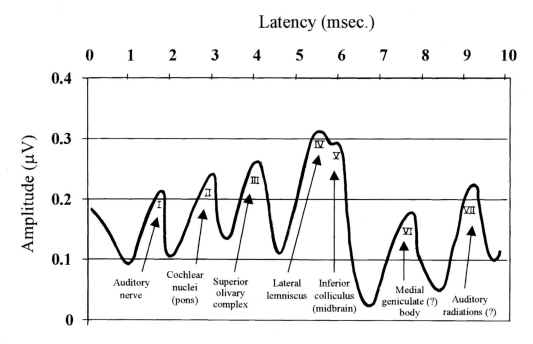

Fig. 4.14 Brainstem auditory evoked responses. Wave 1 is auditory nerve or organ of Corti, wave 2 is cochlear nuclei (pons), wave 3 is superior olivary complex, wave 4 is lateral lemniscus or nucleus, wave 5 is inferior colliculus, wave 6 is medial geniculate body possibly, but of questionable origin, and wave 7 is possibly auditory radiation.

g. Sensory nerve action potential (SNAP) — pure sensory nerves are stimulated and the signal is detected over the proximal skin. Signal is 1000 times weaker than the M-wave. Useful with injury proximal to the nerve cell body (i.e., brachial plexus avulsion).

XXII. Muscle

A. Electromyelogram

1. Each motor unit (one lower motor neuron) supplies a few to 200 muscle fibers. The motor unit potential is triphasic.

2. Resting muscle is either silent or with brief (1 millisecond) monophasic negative potentials (from miniature endplate potentials caused by the spontaneous release of 1 quantum of ACh).

3. Normal insertional activity is caused by damage from the needle and the stimulation of fibers. Increased insertional activity is caused by denervation or primary muscle disease. Decreased insertional activity is caused by advanced myopathy with replacement by fibrous tissue.

4. A few days after a motor nerve is cut, denervation hypersensitivity may be present as the muscle contracts from circulating ACh. Fibrillations may be detected on EMG.

5. Muscle contraction causes an interference pattern.

6. Fibrillation potential — a triphasic potential lasting 1–5 milliseconds caused by the activity of one fiber. It is not able to be seen through the skin. It is caused by denervation, starts around 3 weeks from the injury, and may be associated with positive sharp waves (diphasic potential of greater amplitude and duration than fibrillation potentials because of the nerve injury by electrode insertion). Fibrillation potentials are seen with poliomyelitis, ALS, and peripheral nerve injuries.

7. Fasciculation potential — has 3–5 phases lasting 5–15 milliseconds and is caused by activity of a group of fibers (motor unit). It can be seen through the skin and is associated with nerve fiber irritability (not destruction) from hypocalcemia, hypothermia, nerve entrapments, ALS, poliomyelitis, and shivering.

B. Diseases

1. Polymyalgia rheumatica — onset in middle age with diffuse aching pain and stiffness of the proximal limbs. Lasts 6 months–2 years and is associated with an increased ESR and temporal arteritis. Treatment is with steroids.

2. Myokymia — spontaneous firing of a motor unit. There is constant muscle "rippling" as a result of a peripheral nerve branch lesion.

3. Denervation — decreased amplitude of the motor unit potential, increased duration

4. Reinnervation — exhibits decreased amplitude and increased duration and a polyphasic potential due to nerves growing back with varying degrees of myelination. A "giant unit" may form.

5. Myopathy or neuromuscular junction disease — exhibits decreased amplitude, decreased duration, and may be polyphasic from reinnervation.

XXIII. Motility

A. Movement disorders may be caused by problems with UMNs, parietal area (apraxia), lower motor neurons (LMNs), basal ganglia (posture, involuntary movement), cerebellum (ataxia), peripheral nerves, and muscles.

B. UMN injury causes slight disuse atrophy, spasticity, increased DTRs, but no fasciculations.

C. LMN injury causes severe atrophy, flaccidity, decreased tone, fasciculations, and EMG with fibrillations; individual muscles are affected.

D. Flaccidity causes absence of resistance to passive movement or hypotonia. Muscle normally has a slight resistance to movement (muscle tone).

E. Spasticity

1. Spasticity is a unidirectional velocity-dependent increase in muscle resistance caused by an increase in tonic stretch reflexes. It is associated with hyperreflexia (**Table 4.3**) and is most prominent in antigravity muscles (lower limb extensors and upper limb flexors).

Table 4.3   Differences between Spasticity and Rigidity

Spasticity	Rigidity
Resistance to passive movement is	
Unidirectional	Bidirectional
Velocity dependent	Velocity independent
Increased DTRs	Normal DTRs
Clasp knife	Lead pipe
Clonus	No clonus

Abbreviations: DTR, deep tendon reflex

2. Due to UMN paralysis, but not pure pyramidal tract disease. The associated injury produces an absence or reduction in inhibitory influences on α motor neurons but not from the corticospinal neurons. With isolated motor cortex lesions, only loss of fine movements is produced. Lesions confined to the pyramid produce flaccid paralysis that recovers well.

3. UMN syndrome (spasticity, spontaneous spasms, weakness, loss of discrete movements, abolished abdominal reflexes and extensor plantar responses) is caused by injuries that involve the cortex and underlying white matter with other tracts involved (corticobulbar, reticulospinal, and rubrospinal tracts).

4. Clasp knife phenomenon occurs when little resistance is present initially, followed by significant velocity-dependent resistance, and finally a drop in resistance. It is elicited by slowly imposing a passive movement on an involved limb and is associated with reticulospinal lesions.

5. Medications to treat spasticity include diazepam (activates GABA-a receptors and increases presynaptic inhibition of α motor neurons), baclofen (GABA-b receptor agonist, mechanism of action uncertain), and dantrolene (reduces depolarization-induced Ca^{2+} influx into skeletal muscle.

6. Surgery to treat spasticity includes
   a. Nonablative — botulinum toxin, intrathecal baclofen, or morphine pump implantation
   b. Ablative surgery with preservation of function — nerve blocks, selective neurectomies, percutaneous radiofrequency rhizotomies, myelotomies, and selective dorsal rhizotomies (with intraoperative monitoring to cut only selected dorsal roots)
   c. Ablative surgery with sacrifice of ambulatory function — intrathecal phenol, anterior rhizotomy, neurectomies and tenotomies, and cordotomy

F. Clonus is rhythmic involuntary, brief muscle contractions at 5–7 Hz that occur with spasticity; uniphasic (muscles contract then relax) versus tremors, which are biphasic (agonist then antagonist contraction). Classically elicited by the continued stretching of the gastrocnemius muscle and is due to sustained hyperexcitability of the α and γ motor neurons with synchronization of the contraction and relaxation phases of the muscle spindles.

G. Spasms — arrhythmic, brief or prolonged, spontaneous muscle contractions

    1. Spasmodic torticollis — spasms of the face and neck with female predominance. Onset is in mid-adulthood with slow progression. The neck is rotated, partially extended, and painful. Symptoms improve when lying down or the muscles are touched. The sternocleidomastoid, trapezius, and posterior cervical muscles are involved. Treatment is with botulinum toxin injections or sectioning of the ipsilateral CN XI and bilateral cervical roots C1–C3.

    2. Blepharospasm — eyelid spasms in which the eyelids may completely close shut. Onset is in late adulthood. Treatment is with botulinum toxin injections or possibly partial muscle section.

    3. Lingual, facial, oromandibular spasms — spasms consisting of jaw opening and tongue protrusion or jaw closing. Onset is in late adulthood. There is a female predominance. Treatment is with botulinum toxin injections.

XXIV. Sensory Syndromes

A. Cortical sensory loss — decreased two-point discrimination, graphesthesia, and astereognosia. Tactile agnosias are caused by dominant parietal lesions and involve both hands. Decreased two-point discrimination and extinction are more common with right parietal lesions but may also occur with left-sided lesions.

B. Medullary lesions — decreased pain and temperature in the contralateral body and ipsilateral face (caused by disruption of the spinal trigeminal tract before it decussates as the trigeminothalamic tract in the upper medulla).

C. Alloesthesia (Bamberger sign) — characterized by a painful stimulus on one side of the body that is thought to be on the other side. It is caused by a right putamenal lesion or a cervical spine lesion affecting the uncrossed spinothalamic tract.

D. Tabes dorsalis — involves the posterior columns and roots, classically a rare sequela of tertiary syphilis; more loosely defined, causes can include diabetes and trauma. It is characterized by lower-extremity numbness, pain, decreased vibration, proprioception, reflexes and tone, abnormal gait, atonic bladder, and normal strength.

E. Syringomyelia — dissociated, "suspended" sensory loss of pain and temperature with sparing of touch and proprioception; important cause of delayed deterioration following spinal cord injury

F. Polyneuropathy — usually affects distal nerves in a stocking-glove fashion

XXV. Stance and Gait

A. Ambulation requires four components:

    1. Antigravity reflexes — from the brainstem

    2. Stepping — from the subthalamus and midbrain to the ventral spinal cord with cortical control

    3. Equilibrium — by proprioception from peripheral stretch reflexes, central vestibulocerebellar input, and visual input

    4. Propulsion — a motor function of the legs

B. Abnormal gait — may be impaired by damage to motor, visual, labyrinthine, proprioceptive, or cerebellar systems

1. Cerebellar — wide-based, unsteady, veering to the side of the lesion, irregular steps and pendular reflexes (poor damping of reflexes because of poor agonist/antagonist coordination). It is seen with MS, tumors, and cerebellar degeneration.

2. Sensory ataxia — impaired joint position sense, irregular steps, and wide-based gait. The lower limbs fling out as the patient watches them to see where they are and the feet slap the ground. Positive Romberg sign is seen as the patient falls when visual input is removed. Associated with MS, tabes dorsalis, Friedreich ataxia, and subacute combined degeneration (B12 deficiency)

3. Spastic — circumduction or scissoring gait (with the stiff, straight legs swinging out to compensate for lack of flexion). It is seen with postanoxic injury, cerebral palsy, and MS.

4. Festinating — characterized by short jerky steps, rigidity, shuffling, bending forward, and speeding up to chase the center of gravity. It is seen with Parkinson disease.

5. Steppage — high-stepping gait associated with footdrop, Charcot–Marie–Tooth disease (peroneal muscular atrophy), peroneal nerve compression, poliomyelitis, and disk disease.

6. Waddling — weak gluteal muscles (especially the medius), which cause the pelvis to drop to the side of the raised leg. It is seen with proximal myopathy (e.g., muscular dystrophy).

7. Apraxic — slow, short, shuffling "magnetic" steps, with a wide base; seen with NPH and frontal lobe injuries

8. Senile — slow and stooping, may have some Parkinsonian features

9. Hysterical — characterized by inconsistent and exaggerated movements

XVI. Sleep

A. Circadian rhythms — regulated by the suprachiasmatic nuclei. The newborn sleeps 16–20 hours, a child 10–12 hours, and an adult 6.5 hours per day.

B. Sleep stages (**Fig. 4.10** and **Fig. 4.15**)

1. Awake — α waves (10 Hz)

2. Stage 1 — decreased voltage, loss of α waves

3. Stage 2 — sleep spindles (0.5–2-second bursts of 13 Hz) and K complexes (sharp slow waves of high amplitude) (**Fig. 4.10** and **Fig. 4.15**)

4. Stage 3 — slow-wave sleep, high-amplitude δ waves (1–2 Hz)

5. Stage 4 — δ waves

6. Rapid eye movements (REM) — decreased muscle tone (α and γ motor neuron inhibition, decreased H response, and decreased reflexes), rapid eye movements, pupillary dilation and constriction, increased blood pressure, pulse, respiratory rate and CBF, penile erections, visual dreaming (dreaming also occurs in stage 4 sleep), decreased responsiveness, and desynchronized EEG with increased frequency and decreased amplitude.

C. The first REM cycle is at 1.5 hours, and then it repeats every 4–6 hours. Later cycles have decreased stage 4 and increased REM components (mainly stage 2 and REM). Newborns have 50% REM and 60-minute cycles.

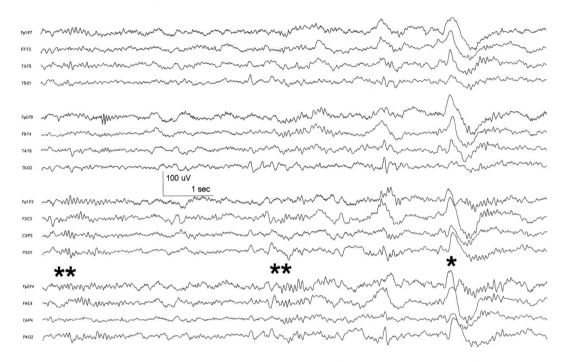

Fp1-F7
F7-T3
T3-T5
T5-O1

Fp2-F8
F8-T4
T4-T6
T6-O2

100 uV
1 sec

Fp1-F3
F3-C3
C3-P3
P3-O1

**   **   *

Fp2-F4
F4-C4
C4-P4
P4-O2

Fig. 4.15 Stage II sleep. K-complex (*); sleep spindles (**). Anteroposterior bipolar montage. (Courtesy of Dr. Richard Wennberg)

Young adults have 25% REM, 5% stage 1, 50% stage 2, and 20% stages 3 and 4. Older people have decreased stages 3 and 4 sleep (5%).

D. Non-REM sleep (stages 1–4) is associated with decreased temperature, blood pressure, respiratory rate, CBF, and cerebral metabolism. Decreased stage 4 and REM sleep are associated with hypothyroidism, Down syndrome, dementia, and phenylketonuria.

E. Cycling (~90 minutes) of gastric motility, hunger, and alertness during the day is likely a persistence of circadian rhythms.

F. The REM and non-REM cycles are controlled by 5-HT, NE, and ACh in the pons. The awake stage has increased 5-HT, NE, and decreased ACh, and the REM stage has increased ACh and decreased 5-HT, NE. The pedunculopontine nucleus contains ACh and NE.

G. Cortisol and thyroid stimulating hormone (TSH) decrease with sleep onset. Cortisol increases with awakening. Luteinizing hormone and prolactin levels increase with sleep, and growth hormone levels surge in the first 2 hours of sleep. Melatonin is only made at night.

H. Sleep deprivation — widespread effects on metabolism, hormone secretion, and brain function. In rats, causes death in a few weeks. When sleep eventually ensues, the time in stage 4 increases. Monoamine oxidase inhibitors increase NE and suppress REM sleep.

I. Insomnia — Benzodiazepines and ethanol are helpful for sleep onset, but prevent a good sleep at later stages. Barbiturates decrease stage 4 and REM sleep, certain benzodiazepines decrease stage 4 sleep.

J. Restless leg syndrome — 10–15% of the population with no gender predominance. There is a common genetic variant that increases risk for the condition. Can develop secondary to iron deficiency, peripheral neuropathy. Treated pharmacologically with DA agonists, benzodiazepines, opioids, anticonvulsants, or clonidine

K. Night terrors — mainly in childhood, occurs in stage 3 or 4 sleep, onset is 30 minutes after falling asleep; typically no memory of precipitating event and may be treated with benzodiazepines to decrease stage 4 sleep. More common in boys, it remits with adolescence.

L. Nightmares — occur in children and adults during REM sleep

M. Parasomnias — undesirable motor, verbal, or experiential events during sleep

N. Somnambulism (sleepwalking) — usually at 4–6 years, occurs during stage 4 sleep in the first third of the night; associated with enuresis and night terrors. 15% of children have one episode and 20% have a family history. May be a disorder of slow-wave sleep. No gender predominance. Treat with lorazepam or tricyclic antidepressants.

O. REM sleep behavior disorder — paralysis normally seen with REM sleep is diminished or absent; patients "act out" their dreams. Most common in older men; may precede Parkinson disease

P. Nocturnal epilepsy — occurs mainly during stage 4 and REM

Q. Hypersomnia — associated with trypanosomiasis, hypercarbia, myxedema, and lesions in the midbrain or thalamus.

R. Sleep apnea

    1. Central sleep apnea is caused by lower brainstem lesions.

    2. Obstructive sleep apnea is caused by soft tissues surrounding the airway such as the tongue, tonsillar hypertrophy. Typically seen in obese middle-aged men, especially those with acromegaly, and is associated with noisy snoring and daytime somnolence. Treat with a continuous positive airway pressure, sleeping in the lateral position, and avoidance of ethanol. Surgical resection of soft tissue can also be employed.

S. Narcolepsy — classic tetrad of excessive daytime sleepiness (may fall asleep while eating, talking), cataplexy (sudden loss of muscle tone with no loss of consciousness elicited by emotion), hypnagogic hallucinations, and sleep paralysis (paralysis on awakening, sparing eyes and breathing function).

    1. Results from abnormal regulation of REM sleep, peak age 15–35 years, no sex predominance, strongly associated with HLA-DR2.

    2. 70% develop cataplexy. All patients with cataplexy have narcolepsy.

    3. Treatment is with scheduled naps, methylphenidate, and amitriptyline (for cataplexy).

T. Enuresis — male predominance, peak age 4–14 years, family history is common, can be secondary to numerous causes (diabetes, cystitis, structural anomalies), which must be ruled out. Can be treated pharmacologically with desmopressin acetate (DDAVP), anticholinergics, or imipramine

XXVII. Autonomic Diseases

A. The anterior hypothalamus is involved with parasympathetic control, whereas the posterolateral hypothalamus is involved with sympathetic control.

B. There are 3 cervical, 11 thoracic, and 4–6 lumbar sympathetic ganglia.

C. The head — supplied by the superior cervical ganglion (C8–T2)

D. Stellate ganglion — the fused inferior cervical and upper thoracic ganglia. It innervates the upper limbs.

E. The abdomen — innervated by the celiac, superior, and inferior mesenteric (splanchnic) ganglia

F. The lower limbs — innervated by ganglia from L3–S1

G. The sympathetic system acts diffusely, whereas the parasympathetic system has more precise effects. The entire body has sympathetic innervation; only parts have parasympathetic innervation.

H. Postganglionic fibers are unmyelinated and travel with vessels.

I. Atropine — only blocks muscarinic receptors; thus only the parasympathetic postganglionic synapses are affected. The autonomic ganglia and muscles are spared.

J. Curare — blocks the nicotinic receptors, affecting the autonomic ganglia and neuromuscular junction

K. Adrenergic receptors

   1. α — increases blood pressure, relaxes gastrointestinal tract, and dilates the pupils. α1-adrenergic receptors are postsynaptic and α2-adrenergic receptors are presynaptic (decreases neurotransmitter release).

   2. β — increases heart rate and contractility, vasodilates and relaxes bronchi. β1-adrenergic receptors are in the heart and β2-adrenergic receptors are in the bronchioles and smooth muscles.

L. In denervation hypersensitivity, an end organ becomes hypersensitive to neurotransmitters 2–3 weeks after denervation by upregulation of receptors.

M. Select pathology

   1. Botulism — exotoxin from Clostridia botulinum. There is decreased release of presynaptic ACh causing minimal autonomic effects. The very diluted toxin is used for innumerable medical and nonmedical indications.

   2. Orthostatic hypotension
        a. Normally, 600 mL of blood collects in the capacitance veins in the legs with standing. This drops the venous return and thus the cardiac output 10%. The effect is a transient decrease in systolic blood pressure that is corrected as the baroreceptors signal via CNs IX and X, stimulating the medulla to increase sympathetic tone.
        b. Idiopathic orthostatic hypotension — occurs in mid- to late adulthood from postganglionic sympathetic degeneration
        c. Shy–Drager syndrome — Chapter 3 section XVIII
        d. Olivopontocerebellar degeneration and striatonigral degeneration are other variants of MSA. Both may have degeneration of lateral horn cells but lack Lewy bodies.
        e. Peripheral neuropathy with secondary orthostatic hypotension — Guillain–Barré syndrome, diabetes, ethanol, etc.

   3. Horner syndrome — ipsilateral ptosis, miosis, and anhidrosis from deficient sympathetic supply to the eye. It may be central or peripheral. The ganglion involved is usually the superior cervical ganglion, but the fibers pass through the stellate ganglion, and a lesion there (i.e., Pancoast tumor) may cause Horner syndrome with upper limb findings (warm and dry). A CN III deficit includes decreased near vision from ciliary muscle paralysis.

   4. If the CN VII parasympathetic fibers are injured, they may undergo aberrant regeneration with connections of the fibers of the chorda tympani reaching the sphenopalatine ganglion, producing crocodile tears (lacrimation from gustatory stimuli).

5. Spinal shock— see Chapter 2 Section XI

6. Hyperhidrosis — treated by ablating the T2 and T3 ganglia (sympathectomy), but leaving T1 to prevent Horner syndrome

7. Raynaud syndrome — episodic digital arterial spasms with female predominance and elicited by cold or stress. 50% have an associated collagen vascular disease. Constriction is mediated by sympathetic input and vasodilation is mediated by mast cells and histamine release locally. The main problem with Raynaud syndrome is the mast cell dysfunction; thus sympathectomy has not proven helpful. Avoid β blockers; consider prostaglandin injection.

N. Bladder

1. Pertinent musculature is the detrusor, which empties the bladder, the involuntary internal sphincter, and the voluntary external sphincter.

2. Sympathetic input — from T12–L2 the inferior mesenteric ganglion to the hypogastric nerve to the pelvic plexus, bladder dome detrusor (β), and internal sphincter (α). Alpha-adrenergic stimulation closes the bladder neck.

3. Parasympathetic input — causes detrusor to contract and internal sphincter to relax. Originate in intermediolateral gray of spinal cord at S2–S4 level, travel via pelvic splanchnic nerves, terminating in ganglia in bladder.

4. External sphincters of the bladder and anus — voluntary control mediated by striated muscles innervated by the pyramidal tract. Following a synapse, these signals travel via the pudendal nerve from S2–S4 (from the nucleus of Onuf).

5. Bladder afferents travel in the pudendal nerves followed by the spinothalamic tract.

6. Micturition center — locus ceruleus of the pons; pontine reflex coordinates sphincter relaxation with detrusor contraction. Output is through the reticulospinal tract to the caudal spinal cord. Input is from the cortex (diffusely), limbic system, thalamus, and cerebellum.

7. The corticospinal tract (anteromedial frontal lobes, genu of corpus callosum) and midbrain inhibit micturition and the pons and posterior hypothalamus facilitate micturition.

8. LMN lesions — atonic bladder; treat with bethanechol

9. UMN lesions — spastic bladder (by loss of corticospinal inhibition); treat with propantheline (muscarinic receptor blocker) or oxybutynin (Ditropan, Ortho-McNeil Pharmaceutical Inc., Raritan, NJ).

O. Bowel — Hirschsprung disease is characterized by congenital megacolon resulting from absence of ganglionic cells in the myenteric plexus (especially the internal anal sphincter and rectosigmoid colon). The aganglionic segment is constricted (unable to relax) with proximal dilation. It occurs in children, has male predominance, and is treated surgically.

XXVIII. Endocrine Diseases

A. Sympathetic input — stimulates increased melatonin (pineal), increased glucagon and insulin (pancreas), increased renin (kidney juxtaglomerular apparatus), and increased catecholamines (adrenal medulla).

B. Diabetes insipidus — polyuria from insufficient vasopressin (central) or impaired response to it (nephrogenic). Central can be caused by tumors (hypothalamic hamartoma, craniopharyngioma, and glioma), trauma, surgery, histiocytosis X, and sarcoid. After surgery, there is a triphasic response: (1) low ADH secondary to posterior pituitary damage, (2) transient increase in ADH by hormone released from dying cells, and (3) low ADH because of loss of cells.

C. Syndrome of inappropriate antidiuretic hormone (secretion) — may be caused by stroke, tumor (CNS or pulmonary oat cell), hemorrhage, infection, hypothalamic lesions, and drugs (carbamazepine, thiazides, chlorpromazine, and vincristine). Symptoms include seizures and decreased consciousness as the serum Na$^+$ drops to < 120 mEq/L. Rapid correction of chronic hyponatremia can cause central pontine myelinolysis, especially in the face of malnutrition.

D. Cushing syndrome — caused by increased serum cortisol. Findings include truncal obesity, abdominal striae, fragile skin, increased facial hair, baldness, osteoporosis, weakness, hypertension, and psychologic changes. 85% are caused by a pituitary tumor (Cushing disease), which has survival rates equivalent to breast cancer if untreated. Microadenomas are 3 times more common than macroadenomas. Pituitary tumors have a positive high-dose dexamethasone suppression test. Cushing syndrome may also be caused by an adrenal tumor or ectopic ACTH secretion (pulmonary oat cell or squamous carcinoma, negative dexamethasone suppression tests), or it may be iatrogenic (most common).

E. Addison syndrome — insufficient aldosterone with increased skin pigmentation (melanocyte stimulating hormone is high along with ACTH). Symptoms include hypotension, oliguria, hyperthermia, hyperkalemia, hyponatremia, and hypoglycemia. Causes include tuberculosis, adrenoleukodystrophy, and autoimmune disease (Hashimoto thyroiditis, diabetes). Treat with both mineralocorticoids and glucocorticoids.

F. Precocious puberty — in males can be caused by teratoma (pineal or mediastinal) and adrenal or testicular tumors. In females, it is caused by estrogen-secreting or hypothalamic tumors/hamartomas (neurofibromatosis type 1 and polyostotic fibrous dysplasia).

G. Obesity — ventromedial hypothalamic lesions result in increased food intake; lesions of the ventrolateral hypothalamus result in decreased food and water intake. Prader–Willi classically associated with hyperphagia along with underdeveloped gonads, decreased tone, mental retardation, short stature, and decreased growth hormone-releasing hormone.

H. Hyperthermia — due to anterior hypothalamic lesion, malignant hyperthermia (treat with dantrolene), and neuroleptic malignant syndrome

I. Hypothermia — due to posterior hypothalamic lesion, hypothyroidism, hypoglycemia, uremia, ethanol, and barbiturates

XXIX. Effects of Neoplasia on the Nervous System

A. Paraneoplastic disorders — polyneuropathy, polymyositis, and myasthenic-myopathic syndrome (Eaton–Lambert syndrome). Theory holds that malignant cells have epitopes leading to antibodies that cross-react with normal tissues. Investigations required to rule out occult malignancy.

B. Anti-Yo antibodies (anti-Purkinje cell) — associated with breast and ovarian carcinomas and thus have female predominance; cause cerebellar degeneration

C. Anti-Hu antibodies (antineuronal nucleoprotein) — seen in pulmonary oat cell carcinomas and lymphoma; cause sensory neuropathy

D. Anti-Ri antibodies — associated with breast carcinoma; cause opsoclonus

E. Antibodies to presynaptic terminals — Eaton-Lambert syndrome, associated with oat cell pulmonary carcinoma

F. Cerebellar degeneration — associated with lung (44%) and ovarian (17%) carcinomas and lymphoma (14%). 50% have anti-Yo. Associated with brainstem atrophy, perivascular inflammation, vertigo, impaired ocular motility, and cognitive changes

G. Stiff-man syndrome — minor stimuli (i.e., sounds) can trigger severe spasms of trunk, limbs, which can be incapacitating. Associated with tumors, and elevated glutamic acid decarboxylase level is diagnostic. Responds to intravenous IgG, benzodiazepines, anticonvulsants.

H. Encephalomyelitis — associated with oat cell tumors. It may be related to antibodies and affects the limbic system (limbic encephalitis), medulla, cerebellum, and spinal gray matter. Limbic encephalitis causes anxiety, depression, confusion, hallucinations, memory impairment, and dementia.

I. Necrotizing myelopathy — associated with pulmonary carcinoma

J. Motor neuropathy — associated with Hodgkin disease; loss of anterior horn cells

5 Neurosurgery

Associate Editor, Scellig Stone

Cranial Procedures

I. Vascular Disease

A. Aneurysms

    1. Epidemiology
        a. Adult prevalence 2%
        b. Annual incidence of aneurysmal subarachnoid hemorrhage (SAH) ~ 6–8/100,000, peak age 50s
        c. Modifiable risk factors for SAH — hypertension, smoking, excessive alcohol

    2. Presentation / Natural history
        a. Saccular aneurysms
            (1) 10–15% of SAH fatal before reaching hospital, ~50% by 1 month
            (2) Overall, ~⅓ die, ⅓ have severe permanent disability, and ⅓ return to baseline.
            (3) Major morbidities include rebleeding, hydrocephalus (~15–20%), cardiac (up to 50%), vasospasm, hyponatremia, and seizures.
            (4) See **Tables 5.1–5.4** for risk of rupture data and grading scales.
        b. Fusiform aneurysms
            (1) Treatment options are medical (antiplatelet therapy or anticoagulation for emboli) and surgical (trapping with or without bypass or resection with vessel reconstruction).

Table 5.1 Risk of Rupture over 5 Years (%) According to International Study of Unruptured Intracranial Aneurysms (Prospective)

Type of Aneurysm	< 7 mm and No Prior SAH	< 7 mm and Prior SAH	7–12 mm	13–24 mm	>24 mm
Carotid cavernous	0	0	0	3.0	6.4
Anterior circulation	0	1.5	2.6	14.5	40.0
Posterior circulation	2.5	3.4	14.5	18.4	50.0

Abbreviation: SAH, subarachnoid hemorrhage.

Table 5.2 Hunt and Hess Clinical Grading Scale

Grade	Description	Clinical Vasospasm (%)	Good Outcome (%)
I	Asymptomatic or minimal headache and slight nuchal rigidity	20–30	~70
II	Moderate-to-severe headache, nuchal rigidity, ± cranial nerve palsy only		
III	Drowsy, confusion, or mild focal deficit	50	~15
IV	Stupor, moderate-to-severe hemiparesis, possibly early decerebrate rigidity		
V	Deep coma, decerebrate rigidity, moribund appearance	75	~0

Table 5.3   World Federation of Neurosurgical Societies Clinical Grading Scale

Grade	GCS	Motor Deficit
I	15	No
II	13–14	No
III	13–14	Yes
IV	7–12	Yes or no
V	3–6	Yes or no

Abbreviations: GCS, Glasgow coma score.

Table 5.4   Fisher Grading for Appearance of SAH on Computed Tomography (CT)

Grade	CT Findings	Incidence of Clinical Vasospasm (%)
I	No hemorrhage evident	0
II	Diffuse SAH with vertical layers < 1 mm thick	0
III	Localized clots and/or vertical layers of SAH > 1 mm thick	95
IV	Diffuse or no SAH, but with intracerebral or intraventricular hemorrhage	0

Abbreviation: SAH, subarachnoid hemorrhage.

  c. Dissecting aneurysms
   (1) Antiplatelet or anticoagulants if extracranial and associated with ischemia, surgical or endo-vascular obliteration if intracranial and associated with hemorrhage
  d. Traumatic aneurysms
   (1) Pseudoaneurysms from arterial rupture and containment of hematoma by surrounding tis-sue, associated with penetrating (more common) or blunt head injury, can lead to carotid cavernous fistulas (CCFs)
   (2) Often present with delayed hemorrhage (but variable), treated surgically or endovascularly
  e. Infectious (mycotic) aneurysms
   (1) Rare, usually distal, occur in 5–15% with bacterial endocarditis
   (2) Most fusiform and friable, may cause stroke or hemorrhage
   (3) Usually resolve within 6 weeks with antibiotics. If associated with hemorrhage, is enlarging, or not resolved on follow-up angiogram after antibiotic treatment, treatment is needed.

 3. Treatment
  a. Endovascular coiling or neurosurgical clipping — Goal is exclusion of aneurysm from circulation; second line options include trapping or parent vessel sacrifice.
  b. Randomized controlled trial (RCT) of surgery versus coiling for ruptured intracranial aneurysms (International Subarachnoid Aneurysm Trial [ISAT]) found 31% surgical and 24% endovascular patients dead or dependent at 1 year so coiling is a good option for some cases, but durability of coiling and generalizability of results remain uncertain.
  c. For unruptured aneurysms, natural history must be weighed against mortality (1–2% for sur-gery/coiling) and morbidity (4% coiling and 8% surgery, but these are variable).
  d. Most consider endovascular for posterior circulation, surgery for middle cerebral artery (MCA), variable for anterior cerebral artery (ACA) and other sites.

e. Surgical approaches are pterional for most anterior circulation aneurysms; anterior interhemispheric can be used for anterior communicating artery and must be for more distal ACA aneurysms (**Fig. 5.1**). Posterior circulation aneurysms at basilar apex can be approached by pterional, subtemporal, or combined approach.

B. Arteriovenous malformations (AVMs)

1. Epidemiology
   a. Prevalence 15–18/100,000, incidence 1/100,000, typically present before age 40
   b. Account for 1–2% of all strokes (3–4% in young adults)

2. Presentation / Natural history
   a. Presentations include hemorrhage (50%), seizures (25%), headache, and incidental, focal deficits (due to arterial steal or venous hypertension)
   b. Hemorrhage rate 2–4% per year, rehemorrhage rate may be higher. Future hemorrhage is associated with hemorrhagic presentation, large size, deep venous drainage, associated aneurysms.
   c. Hemorrhage mortality 10–30%, morbidity 10–30%
   d. See **Tables 5.5** and **5.6** for Spetzler–Martin grading system and associated outcomes.

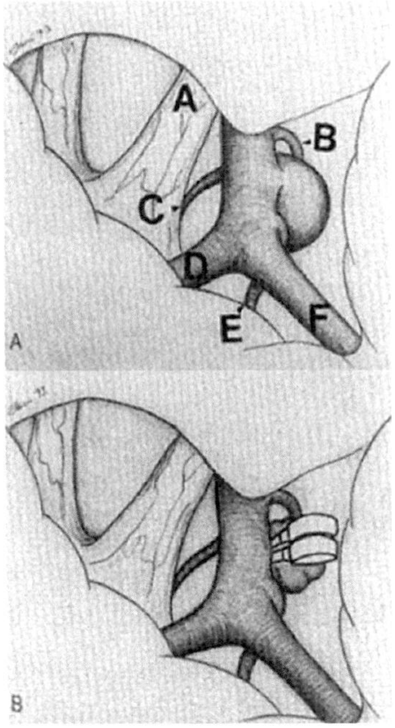

Fig. 5.1 (**A**) Right posterior communicating artery aneurysm exposed through a pterional approach. (A) optic nerve, (B) posterior communicating artery, (C) superior hypophyseal artery, (D) anterior cerebral artery, (E) anterior choroidal artery, (F) middle cerebral artery. (**B**) Same view after clipping of the aneurysm. (From Alleyne Jr. CH. Neurosurgery Board Review. New York, NY: Thieme; 1997. Reprinted by permission.)

Table 5.5   Spetzler–Martin Grading System

Feature	Points
Nidus size (cm)	
Small (< 3)	1
Medium (3–6)	2
Large (> 6)	3
Eloquence of adjacent brain	
Noneloquent	0
Eloquent (sensorimotor, language, visual, thalamus, hypothalamus, internal capsule, brainstem, cerebellar peduncles, deep cerebellar nuclei)	1
Pattern of venous drainage	
Superficial only	0
Deep	1

Table 5.6   Outcomes Based on Spetzler–Martin Grade

Grade	Surgery % Morbidity (Major Deficit)	Radiosurgery % Morbidity	% Obliteration
I	0	0	90
II	5 (0)	11	70
III	16 (4)	12	60
IV	27 (7)	21	45
V	31 (12)	–	–

3. Treatment

    a. Medical management (antiepileptics, etc.), embolization (cure rate generally low, but > 80% if pure fistula or single feeding artery), radiosurgery (hemorrhage risk still present during the ~2–3 years until obliteration, generally considered for < 3 cm nidus with deep and/or eloquent location), surgical excision, or combination of modalities

C. Dural arteriovenous fistulas (DAVFs)

   1. Epidemiology

    a. 10–15% of intracranial vascular malformations, incidence 0.2/100,000, slight female preponderance, typically present in midlife

   2. Presentation / Natural history

    a. Clinical presentations include incidental, tinnitus, headache, visual impairment, hemorrhage. Borden I generally benign (conversion rate to higher grade ~ 2%), but occasionally symptoms warrant treatment. Borden II and III have 15% annual event rate (8% hemorrhage) with 10% annual mortality rate and generally require treatment.
See **Table 5.7** for classification of DAVF III:

   3. Treatment

    a. Goal is to eliminate cortical venous reflux (CVR). Treatment options include endovascular (transarterial embolization – rarely cures, versus transvenous coiling – generally preferred), surgical disconnection of CVR, and radiosurgery (~⅔ cure rate, generally third choice modality).

Table 5.7   Dural Arteriovenous Fistula Classification Schemes

Borden		Cognard	
I	Dural venous drainage, no CVR	I	Dural venous drainage (anterograde), no CVR
		IIa	Dural venous drainage (retrograde), no CVR
II	Dural venous drainage and CVR	IIb	Dural venous drainage (anterograde) and CVR
		IIa+b	Dural venous drainage (retrograde) and CVR
III	CVR only	III	CVR only
		IV	CVR only with venous ectasias

Abbreviation: CVR, cortical venous reflux.

D. Moyamoya disease

   1. Epidemiology

    a. Incidence — rare (< 1/100,000), though higher in Japan

    b. Two peaks at mean ages 3 and 20s–30s

    c. Often linked to inflammatory conditions, also associated with atherosclerosis

   2. Presentation / Natural history

    a. Typical presentations are ischemic (80% in pediatric cases), hemorrhage (60% in adult cases), seizures, progressive cognitive decline. 73% major deficit or death within 2 years of diagnosis in children. Treatments address ischemia with less effect on hemorrhage risk; good prognosis in ~ 60%.

   3. Treatment

    a. Surgical revascularization including direct bypass, indirect revascularization (encephalomyosynangiosis, encephaloduromyosynangiosis), omental transposition, multiple burr holes

E. Cavernous malformations

1. Epidemiology
   a. Prevalence 0.5%, incidence 0.5/100,000/year, three autosomal dominant familial forms known (CCM1–3, particularly prevalent in Hispanic population)

2. Presentation / Natural history
   a. Presenting symptom seizures (50%, incidence 1–2%/year), focal deficit (25%, ~ 40% fully resolve), incidental, headaches. Risk of symptomatic hemorrhage 0.5–2%/year, may be higher in patients with previous hemorrhages (~ 5%/year), deep lesions (~10%/year), posterior fossa lesions, familial inheritance, and women (~ 4%/year).

3. Treatment
   a. Observation/medical for control of seizures, surgical excision has good–excellent outcome in ~ 90%, lower with deep lesions; radiosurgery does not alter radiographic appearance and has not been shown to alter the natural history

F. Intracerebral hemorrhage (ICH) — no structural lesion

1. Epidemiology
   a. Incidence ~12–15/100,000/year, 15–30% of all strokes
   b. Risk factors include age > 60, male sex, heavy ethanol use, drugs (cocaine, etc.), coagulopathy, hypertension (most common cause), amyloid angiopathy (most common cause in elderly)

2. Presentation / Natural history
   a. Poor prognosis with age > 60, increasing hematoma volume (particularly > 30 cc, **Table 5.8**), lower initial Glasgow Coma Scale (GCS), basal ganglia or brainstem (deep) location, presence of intraventricular hemorrhage (IVH)

Table 5.8   Natural History of Deep Basal Ganglia Hemorrhages

Volume (0.5 ABC) (cc)	30-Day Mortality (%)	Functional Independence (%)
< 30	23	18.0
30–60	64	1.4 (all cases > 30 cc)
> 60	93	

Abbreviation: 0.5ABC = method for measuring volume of hematoma as half the length times width times height on CT scan.

3. Treatment
   a. Medical management (target systolic blood pressure < 180 mm Hg, correct coagulation, control increased intracranial pressure [ICP]) or surgical evacuation. Surgery for supratentorial ICH not proven to benefit, decreases mortality without changing morbidity in putamen/thalamic hemorrhages, and evacuation of superficial hemorrhages may be life saving but may not alter recovery of deficits. Surgery may benefit patients < age 60 with lobar ICH, < 1 cm from surface and with initial GCS > 8. Cerebellar hemorrhage > 3 cm, neurologically deteriorating, brainstem compression, or obstructive hydrocephalus should have urgent evacuation.

G. Infarction (see Chapter 3 section XXI and Chapter 4 section XIX)

1. Natural history for surgical stroke
   a. Cerebellar infarct — Postinfarct edema can lead to brainstem compression and obstructive hydrocephalus (risk mainly 12–96 hours postictus, mortality up to 80%).

b. MCA territory infarct — "malignant" cerebral edema in up to 10%, mortality up to 80%

2. Treatment
   a. Cerebellar infarct — Early symptoms warrant emergent craniectomy / removal infarcted tissue, can be life saving with good outcome if brainstem not involved.
   b. MCA territory infarct — Early hemicraniectomy can reduce mortality to ~30–40%, but morbidity generally severe. Better outcomes (option) in young patients with nondominant hemispheric involvement.

H. Carotid stenosis

1. Epidemiology
   a. Prevalence (any degree): 2.5% < age 65, 35% > age 75
   b. Prevalence (> 50% stenosis): < 5% in general adult population, 10% of age > 60 with ≥ 1 cardio-vascular (CV) risk factor (↑ with ↑ age and number of CV risk factors)

2. Presentation / Natural history (**Table 5.9**)
   a. Presentations include transient ischemic attack (TIA), stroke, and amaurosis fugax.
   b. Recurrent or post TIA/stroke risk is front loaded: 20% are in first month.

Table 5.9   Natural History of Carotid Stenosis Managed Medically and Surgically

Degree of Stenosis	Best Medical Treatment	Carotid Endarterectomy	Absolute Risk Reduction
Asymptomatic: > 60% (ACST, ACAS) ≥ 50% (VAS)	11–12% at 5 years 5–9% at 4 years	5–6% at 5 years 5–9% at 4 years	6% at 5 years* –
Symptomatic (NASCET): ≥ 70% 50–69% < 50%	26% at 2 years 22% at 5 years 15–19% at 5 years	9% at 2 years 16% at 5 years 15–19% at 5 years	17% at 2 years 6% at 5 years –†

Abbreviations: ACAS, Asymptomatic Carotid Atherosclerosis Study; ACST, Asymptomatic Carotid Surgery Trial; NASCET, North American Symptomatic Carotid Endarterectomy Trial; VAS, Veterans Administration Study.

*Assumes perioperative morbidity and mortality rate of 3%.

†Similar results in European Carotid Stenosis Trial (ECST).

3. Treatment — medical management (Chapter 4 section XIX)
   a. Carotid endarterectomy generally appropriate for symptomatic patients with 70–99% stenosis, a consideration for symptomatic patients with 50–69% stenosis or asymptomatic patients with 60–99% stenosis (careful patient selection and low perioperative morbidity and mortality). Timing of surgery is preferable within a few weeks (↓ upfront stroke risk).
   b. Endovascular angioplasty ± stenting is under investigation; generally considered an option in high-risk patients where early benefit appears similar to surgery.

I. Arterial dissections

1. Epidemiology
   a. Associated with fibromuscular dysplasia, connective tissue diseases
   b. Intracranial
      (1) Traumatic/iatrogenic: less common than spontaneous
      (2) Spontaneous — ~70% vertebrobasilar, account for < 10% spontaneous SAH (mainly age > 30), rare cause of stroke (mainly age < 30)

    c. Extracranial

      (1) Traumatic/iatrogenic: more common than spontaneous

      (2) Spontaneous — more common in young women

  2. Presentation / Natural history

    a. Typical presentations include headache/neck pain, Horner syndrome (for internal carotid artery [ICA]), TIA/stroke

    b. Traumatic generally present < 24 hours

    c. Intracranial vertebrobasilar dissections — if presenting with hemorrhage, rebleed rate up to 30–70% with 70% occurring in first 24 hours, 80% in first week, 90% in first month; can also cause symptomatic embolization/stenosis; overall mortality ~30%.

  3. Treatment

    a. Extracranial — anticoagulate for 6–12 weeks, antiplatelet agents, or if emboli persist, repair of vessel with interposition vein graft, bypass, or endovascular angioplasty with or without stenting

    b. Intracranial — similar except if SAH presentation; requires preventative treatment for future hemorrhage. Surgical options include proximal clipping if collateral flow adequate, trapping, resection with or without bypass. Endovascular stenting or occlusion of dissection is also a viable option.

J. Carotid cavernous fistula (CCF)

  1. Epidemiology

    a. Traumatic — prevalence in head trauma 0.2%

    b. Spontaneous — includes direct high-flow (typically ruptured cavernous ICA aneurysms), low-flow dural shunts from meningeal branches of ICA, external carotid artery (ECA), or both

  2. Presentation / Natural history

    a. Orbital/retroorbital pain, chemosis, pulsatile proptosis, ocular/cranial bruit, visual deterioration, diplopia, and ophthalmoplegia

    b. 50% of low-flow CCFs spontaneously thrombose.

  3. Treatment

    a. Low-flow CCFs can be watched until they spontaneously thrombose if visual acuity stable and intraocular pressure < 25 mm Hg

      (1) Endovascular embolization transarterially through ICA or ECA (placing balloon in fistula or trapping with two balloons ± bypass) or transvenous coiling via petrosal sinus (from the jugular vein) or superior ophthalmic vein (enter supraoptic vein as it enters orbit to become superior ophthalmic vein, **Fig. 5.2**).

      (2) Rarely open surgery

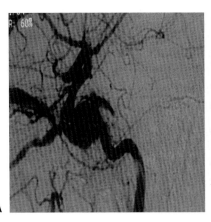
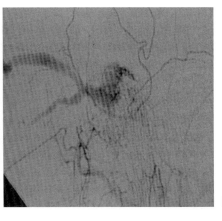

A   B

Fig. 5.2 Carotid cavernous fistula (CCF) seen on lateral angiography of internal carotid artery injection. (**A**) Early filling of the cavernous sinus in the arterial phase with dilated superior and inferior ophthalmic veins and (**B**) filling from the external carotid artery.

II. Infectious Disease

A. Cerebral abscess

1. Epidemiology
   a. Prevalence — ~ 2500 cases/year in U.S.; male:female (M:F) ratio is 2:1
   b. Contiguous spread (most common, 40%) — sinusitis, otitis media, dental abscess
   c. Hematogenous spread — lung infections, pulmonary AVF, congenital cyanotic heart disease, bacterial endocarditis, immunodeficiency, dental abscess, gastrointestinal infections
   d. Penetrating source — penetrating head trauma, neurosurgery, cerebrospinal fluid (CSF) leak
   e. Pathogens include *Streptococcus* (most common), *Streptococcus milleri* and *anginosis* (sinusitis), *Bacteroides, Proteus, Staphylococcus aureus* (trauma), *Staphylococcus epidermidis* (iatrogenic), *Actinomyces* (dental), fungal (immunocompromised)

2. Presentation / Natural history (**Table 5.10**)
   a. Symptoms nonspecific for brain lesion, history typically acute
   b. Mortality 10–20%, neurologic disability 45%

Table 5.10   Cerebral Abscess Stages

Stage (age)	Histology Highlights	CT and MRI	Resistance to Aspiration
I – Early cerebritis (up to 5 days)	Poorly demarcated inflammation	CT: Thick ring enhancement T1: hypo, T2 hyper	Slight
II – Late cerebritis (5 days–2 weeks)	Developing necrotic center		None
III – Early capsule (2–3 weeks)	Neovascular reticular network surrounds	CT: Thin ring enhancement T1: hypo edema/center, hyper capsule T2: hyper edema, capsule and center Restricted diffusion	None
IV – Late capsule (> 3 weeks)	Collagen capsule with surrounding gliosis		Firm capsule

Abbreviations: CT, computed tomography; hypo, hypointense; hyper, hyperintense; MRI, magnetic resonance imaging.

3. Treatment
   a. Antibiotics — can be sole treatment for cerebritis stage (< 2 weeks of symptoms), < 3 cm diameter, known organism; typically at least 6 weeks intravenous (IV) therapy
   b. Surgical indications — significant mass effect / elevated ICP, no improvement after 4 weeks of antibiotics, proximity to ventricle (increased likelihood of ventricular rupture), uncertain diagnosis of pathogen, trapped foreign material, and poor condition of patient
   c. Surgical options — stereotactic or computed tomographically (CT) guided aspiration; craniotomy and excision if encapsulated or foreign material

B. Subdural empyema / Epidural abscess

1. Epidemiology
   a. 5 times less common than cerebral abscess, subdural empyema more common than epidural abscess, M:F ratio 3:1
   b. Generally from contiguous spread or penetrating source (rarely hematogenous), can be secondary to meningitis
   c. Associated cerebral abscess in 25% cases

d. Common organisms — *Streptococci, Haemophilus influenza, Staphylococcus aureus* or *epidermidis*, anaerobes

2. Presentation / Natural history

   a. Presents as nonspecific brain lesion, meningismus common, more commonly febrile than with cerebral abscess alone
   b. Subdural empyema often leads to cortical venous infarct, secondary cerebritis/abscess
   c. Mortality 10–20%, morbidity ~50%, worse prognosis if age > 60 and poor presentation

3. Treatment

   a. Rarely antibiotic therapy alone (if patient well, collection is small, early response), multiple burr holes for drainage (if early), or craniotomy/debridement

C. Shunt infection

1. Epidemiology

   a. ~5% risk of early infection
   b. < 5% risk of late infection (> 6 months), typically seeding from septicemia
   c. Risk factors — length of procedure, younger age
   d. Pathogens — *Staphylococcus epidermidis* (60–75%), *Staphylococcus aureus*, gram-negatives

2. Presentation / Natural history

   a. Presents as systemic infection, abdominal pain, obstruction, tenderness along tubing
   b. Mortality 10–15%. Shunt nephritis (immune complex deposition in renal glomeruli), usually with ventriculoatrial shunts, rarely occurs.

3. Treatment

   a. Antibiotics alone — poor success, considered only in high surgical risk, terminally ill patients. Slit ventricles are difficult to catheterize in a highly shunt-dependent patient.
   b. Typically requires complete hardware removal, external drainage, IV antibiotics (typically vanco-mycin first line if gram-positive); await ≥ 3 days of sterile CSF, then place new shunt

D. Osteomyelitis/Infected bone flap

1. Epidemiology

   a. Very rare in absence of surgery (producing initially avascular bone flap), can result from contigu-ous spread or penetrating trauma (hematogenous rare)
   b. *Staphylococcus aureus* most common, followed by *Staphylococcus epidermidis*

2. Presentation / Natural history

   a. Variable, progressive/erosive
   b. Gradenigo syndrome (Chapter 3 section X)

3. Treatment

   a. Antibiotics alone rarely curative, generally requires surgical debridement/removal bone flap, 6–24 weeks antibiotics, cranioplasty at > 6 months

III. Neoplastic Disease

A. Approaches

1. Inferior frontal lobe and parasellar region — bicoronal incision with unilateral or bilateral subfrontal approach or pterional approach

2. Sellar region — transsphenoidal approach open or endoscopic, bicoronal incision with unilateral or bilateral subfrontal approach, or pterional approach

3. Frontal lobe — linear, curved, or horseshoe incision with frontal craniotomy

4. Anterior temporal lobe — linear incision with temporal craniotomy

5. Posterior temporal lobe — linear, reverse question mark, or Isle of Mann incision with temporal craniotomy

6. Parietal lobe — linear or horseshoe incision with parietal craniotomy

7. Occipital lobe — linear or horseshoe incision with occipital craniotomy

8. Trigone of the lateral ventricle — linear or horseshoe incision with appropriate craniotomy for superior parietal, middle temporal gyrus, lateral temporooccipital, or transoccipital approach

9. Anterior third ventricle — linear or horseshoe incision with frontal parasagittal craniotomy and interhemispheric/transcallosal or transcortical approach. The third ventricle can then be approached through the interforniceal or transchoroidal (displace the choroid plexus laterally, divide the tela choroidea, and enter the foramen of Monro between the choroid and fornix) approaches (**Fig. 5.3**).

10. Posterior third ventricle/pineal region — linear or horseshoe incision with (1) suboccipital transtentorial approach, (2) supracerebellar infratentorial approach, (3) interhemispheric transcallosal (splenium) approach, and (4) transcortical parietal approach (seldom used).

11. Midline posterior fossa/fourth ventricle — linear incision with suboccipital craniotomy

12. Lateral posterior fossa/CPA — linear incision with retrosigmoid craniotomy

13. Upper clivus — linear or horseshoe incision with subtemporal approach and anterior petrosectomy

14. Middle and lower clivus — curvilinear incision with combined retrosigmoid posterior temporal craniotomy and posterior petrosectomy

B. Localization

1. Nasion — located at the midline frontonasal suture

2. Glabella — the most forward point on the midline supraorbital ridge

3. Pterion — located at the junction of the frontal, parietal, temporal, and greater wing of sphenoid bones. It is located two fingerbreadths above the zygomatic arch and a thumb's breadth behind the frontal process of the zygomatic bone.

4. Asterion — located at the junction of the lambdoid, occipitomastoid, and parietomastoid sutures. It lies on top of the lower half of the transverse/sigmoid sinus junction.

5. Lambda — located at the junction of the lambdoid and sagittal sutures

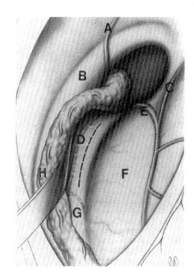

Fig. 5.3 Anatomy of the right foramen of Monro. (**A**) Septal vein, (**B**) column of fornix, (**C**) anterior caudate vein, (**D**) tela choroidea, (**E**) thalamostriate vein, (**F**) thalamus, (**G**) internal cerebral vein, (**H**) choroid plexus. (From Alleyne Jr. CH. Neurosurgery Board Review. New York, NY: Thieme; 1997. Reprinted by permission.)

6. Bregma — located at the junction of coronal and sagittal sutures

7. Inion — located at the indentation under the external occipital protuberance that overlies the torcula

8. Opisthion — located at the posterior margin of the foramen magnum in the midline

9. Sylvian fissure — located by (1) marking the 75% point on a line over the superior sagittal sinus from the nasion to the inion; (2) marking the frontozygomatic point, which is 2.5 cm up along the orbital rim past the zygomatic portion; and (3) the sylvian fissure extends along the line connecting the 75% point and the frontozygomatic point. The pterion is located 3 cm behind the frontozygomatic point along the sylvian line.

10. Rolandic fissure — located by (1) the upper rolandic point, with is 2 cm posterior to the 50% point of the midline nasion/inion line; and (2) the lower rolandic point is at the junction of the line from the upper rolandic point to the midzygomatic arch and the sylvian fissure line as previously defined. The rolandic fissure lies between these two points. The lower rolandic point is also 2.5 cm behind the pterion along the sylvian line. The motor strip is usually 4 to 5.4 cm behind the coronal suture.

11. Angular gyrus (part of Wernicke area) — usually just above the pinna, although it is quite variable

C. Neuroepithelial tumors

1. Astrocytic tumors
   a. Diffusely infiltrating astrocytomas
      (1) Epidemiology and natural history (**Table 5.11**)
         (a) Dedifferentiation from low grade to high grade occurs sooner with age > 45.
         (b) 1–20% present as multiple gliomas.
         (c) Gliomatosis cerebri — rare, involving ≥ 2 lobes, poor prognosis

Table 5.11 Epidemiology/Natural History of Diffusely Infiltrating Astrocytomas

	GBM (IV)	Anaplastic (III)	Low Grade (II)
Relative frequency as % of Astrocytomas	50%	30%	20%
Peak age of incidence	50s	40s	30s
Median survival	1 year	2–3 years	5–10 years

Abbreviation: GBM; glioblastoma multiforme, most common primary brain tumor of adulthood.

      (2) Treatment
         (a) Diagnostic surgical biopsy or partial resection recommended in almost all cases. Gross total resection is the best option if tumor location and patient condition permit.
         (b) Treatment options for low-grade lesions include serial follow-up, radiation and/or chemotherapy, surgery (no clearly superior strategy). Aggressive treatment may be appropriate for more aggressive tumors (young patients, large tumors that enhance, or patients with short clinical history or progression on imaging).
         (c) Standard treatment for high-grade lesions is gross total resection followed by external beam radiation and temozolomide chemotherapy. Poor prognosis with older patients (> 60), glioblastoma multiforme (GBM) histology, poor preoperative (preop) performance status
   b. Pilocytic astrocytoma
      (1) Epidemiology and natural history (**Table 5.12**)

Table 5.12 Epidemiology/Natural History

Type/Location	Affected	Common Presentation	Natural History
Cerebellar	Children > young adults	Posterior fossa mass	All generally indolent / slow growth, but variable
Optic glioma	Associated with neurofibromatosis type I	Proptosis, vision	
Hypothalamic*	Children	Diencephalic syndrome	
Hemisphere	Young adults > children	Like low-grade glioma	

*Some are pilomyxoid astrocytoma variants – more aggressive; grade II lesion.

        (a) All can cause obstructive hydrocephalus.
     (2) Treatment
        (a) Cerebellar/hemispheric — treatment of choice is surgical excision. Cyst wall need not be completely removed if nodule is resected.
        (b) Hypothalamic/optic — surgical excision if involving single nerve and sparing chiasm, otherwise biopsy + chemotherapy/radiation

2. Oligodendroglioma
    a. Epidemiology
       (1) ~ 25% of glial tumors, M:F ratio 3:2, mean age 40
    b. Presentation / Natural history
       (1) Often present with seizures and/or hemorrhage, nonspecific mass effect
       (2) 5-year survival rate 40–70% (grade dependent), overall median 3 years postoperation
       (3) Oligoastrocytoma variant behaves similarly to oligodendroglioma; both have more aggressive anaplastic forms.
    c. Treatment
       (1) Surgical resection followed by chemotherapy (favorable response rate associated with allelic losses of chromosomes 1p and 19q)
       (2) Radiation for anaplastic transformation

3. Ependymoma
    a. Epidemiology
       (1) 5% of intracranial gliomas, 70% pediatric (peak age is 10–15 years), commonly fourth ventricle floor
       (2) Subependymoma is rare form, generally incidental in older patients, rarely surgical
    b. Presentation / Natural history
       (1) Generally presents as slow-growing posterior fossa mass, anaplastic form more aggressive
       (2) Up to 80% 5-year survival in treated young patients, 40% in those < age 4 or elderly
    c. Treatment
       (1) Maximal possible resection (extent affects survival) followed by fractionated radiation
       (2) Spinal magnetic resonance imaging (MRI) + lumbar puncture for cytology to rule out subarachnoid metastases; spinal radiation if positive

4. Choroid plexus papilloma and carcinoma
    a. Epidemiology
       (1) 1% of intracranial tumors, 70% occur at age < 2. Majority are benign papillomas.
    b. Presentation / Natural history
       (1) Typically present with hydrocephalus

(2) 5-year survival rate 85% with benign lesions, 40% with carcinoma (atypical papilloma has intermediate prognosis)
c. Treatment
(1) Benign lesions require total surgical excision and adjuvant chemotherapy; use radiation only for carcinoma.

5. Pediatric brainstem gliomas
a. Epidemiology
(1) 10–20% pediatric brain tumors, mean age 7
b. Presentation / Natural history
(1) Tectal glioma — typically present with hydrocephalus, otherwise very benign, 80% 5-year progression-free survival rate
(2) Focal tegmental mesencephalic — often present with hemiparesis, slowly progress
(3) Diffuse pontine glioma — present with multiple cranial nerve palsies, ataxia, increased ICP, median survival < 1 year
c. Treatment
(1) Tectal gliomas require vigilant follow-up and often CSF diversion. Focal tegmental mesencephalic tumors are resected with adjuvant chemotherapy and radiation if they recur. Radiation +/− experimental chemotherapy and/or palliative are used for diffuse pontine glioma.

6. Other low-grade glial tumors
a. Angiocentric glioma
(1) Rare, slow growth, typically present with seizures in children/young adults. Resection is generally curative.
b. Chordoid glioma of the third ventricle
(1) Rare, typically in adults causing hydrocephalus/chiasm compression/hypothalamic dysfunction, resection generally curative
c. Astroblastoma
(1) Rare, mainly in children/young adults, surgically resected, adjuvant radiation/chemotherapy if rare high-grade form

7. Neuronal and mixed neuronal-glial tumors
a. Lhermitte–Duclos disease (dysplastic cerebellar gangliocytoma)
(1) Epidemiology
(a) Rare, affects young adults (mean age 34), associated with Cowden syndrome (multiple hamartomas)
(2) Presentation / Natural history
(a) Typically present with increased ICP/hydrocephalus, cerebellar signs, occasionally mental retardation
(b) May progress slowly
(3) Treatment
(a) Surgical resection
b. Desmoplastic infantile ganglioglioma (DIG)
(1) Epidemiology
(a) Virtually all < age 2 (peak 3–6 months), M:F ratio 2:1
(2) Presentation / Natural history
(a) Commonly present with increased head size, bulging fontanelles, paresis, seizures
(b) Median survival > 75% at 15 years, anaplasia very rare

(3) Treatment

    (a) Complete surgical resection curative for most, chemotherapy for anaplasia

c. Dysembryoplastic neuroepithelial tumor (DNET)

  (1) Epidemiology

    (a) < 1% primary brain tumors, affects children and young adults (< age 20)

  (2) Presentation / Natural history

    (a) Typically presents with epilepsy, benign with no or very slow growth

  (3) Treatment

    (a) Surgical resection of lesion ± neighboring epileptogenic foci

d. Ganglioglioma / gangliocytoma

  (1) Epidemiology

    (a) < 12% intracranial tumors, generally present < age 30 (peak 11)

  (2) Presentation / Natural history

    (a) Typically presents with epilepsy, benign, slow growth

    (b) 5–10 year survival, 80–90% with treatment

  (3) Treatment

    (a) Complete surgical excision, radiation considered for rare anaplastic ganglioglioma

e. Central neurocytoma

  (1) Epidemiology

    (a) Rare, ~10% intraventricular neoplasms (rarely extraventricular), 75% in ages 20–40

  (2) Presentation / Natural history

    (a) Typically present with increased ICP/hydrocephalus, seizures

    (b) Benign, slow growing, rarely hemorrhage, 5-year survival rate > 80%

  (3) Treatment

    (a) Resection usually cures, stereotactic radiosurgery/chemotherapy options if rare recurrence

f. Cerebellar liponeurocytoma

  (1) Epidemiology

    (a) Rare adult tumor of posterior fossa

  (2) Presentation / Natural history

    (a) Presents as posterior fossa mass, behaves as World Health Organization (WHO) grade II lesion

  (3) Treatment

    (a) Complete surgical excision, radiation may prevent recurrence

g. Papillary glioneuronal tumor

  (1) Epidemiology

    (a) Rare adult tumor

  (2) Presentation / Natural history

    (a) Typically presents with seizures, benign with slow growth

  (3) Treatment

    (a) Complete surgical excision generally curative

h. Rosette-forming glioneuronal tumor of fourth ventricle

  (1) Epidemiology

    (a) Rare tumor in young adults

  (2) Presentation / Natural history

    (a) Typically presents with hydrocephalus and ataxia, indolent behavior, recurrence rare

  (3) Treatment

    (a) Surgical excision generally curative

    i. Paraganglioma

      (1) Epidemiology

         (a) Rare, **Table 5.13** lists specific names associated with location.

Table 5.13 Names of Paragangliomas

Site	Designation
Carotid bifurcation	Carotid body tumor
Superior vagal ganglion	Glomus jugulare tumor
Auricular branch of vagus	Glomus tympanicum
Inferior vagal ganglion	Glomus intravagale
Adrenal medulla and sympathetic chain	Pheochromocytoma

      (2) Presentation / Natural history

         (a) Presents as slow growing mass, systemic features of catecholamine release, carcinoid-like syndrome with cranial nerve palsies related to location

         (b) Slow growth, benign, 5-year survival rate ~ 90%, rarely hemorrhage

      (3) Treatment

         (a) Medical therapy includes α/beta blockers to prevent blood pressure lability and arrhythmias.

         (b) Radiation therapy is used generally if surgery is not possible.

         (c) Embolization prior to surgery can reduce intraop blood loss.

         (d) Surgical resection is preferred.

8. Pineal region tumors

    a. Pineocytoma

      (1) Epidemiology

         (a) < 1% primary brain tumors, mainly children and young adults (peak incidence age 10–20)

      (2) Presentation / Natural history

         (a) Typically present with increased ICP/hydrocephalus, Parinaud syndrome

         (b) Stable or slow growth, 5-year survival rate ~ 90%, rarely hemorrhage

      (3) Treatment

         (a) Surgical resection, stereotactic biopsy high risk

    b. Pineoblastoma

      (1) Epidemiology

         (a) < 1% primary brain tumors, along with pineocytomas and intermediate tumors (features of both) account for 15% pineal region tumors, most in children (peak age 3), M:F ratio 1:2

      (2) Presentation / Natural history

         (a) Typically present with increased ICP/hydrocephalus, Parinaud syndrome

         (b) Primitive neuroectodermal tumor (PNET) with CSF seeding in ~ 50%, median survival 2 years

      (3) Treatment

         (a) Surgical resection + cranial/spinal radiation if age > 3 + chemotherapy

    c. Papillary tumor of the pineal region

      (1) Epidemiology

         (a) Rare tumor in children and young adults

      (2) Presentation / Natural history

         (a) Typically presents with hydrocephalus and WHO grade II–III behavior; can recur

(3) Treatment

    (a) Surgical resection followed by focal radiation

9. Embryonal / Primitive neuroectodermal tumors (PNETs)

    (1) All tend to disseminate via CSF (often into the spinal subarachnoid space), 20–50% at diagnosis

  a. Medulloblastoma

    (1) Epidemiology

        (a) 15–20% of total and ~⅓ of posterior fossa pediatric brain tumors, rare in adults, most diagnosed by age 5, M:F ratio 3:1

    (2) Presentation / Natural history

        (a) Rapid presentation with increased ICP/hydrocephalus, cerebellar signs

        (b) Standard risk – no metastases, no gross residual postresection = 5-year survival approaches 100% if ERBB-2 tumor protein negative, 54% if ERBB-2 positive

        (c) High risk – metastases, residual postresection, 5-year survival ~ 20%

    (3) Treatment

        (a) Surgical excision, adjuvant chemotherapy, craniospinal radiation if age > 3

  b. CNS PNET / Supratentorial PNET

    (1) Epidemiology

        (a) 1% pediatric brain tumors, median age 3, M:F ratio 2:1

        (b) Variants include CNS neuroblastoma (including esthesioneuroblastoma), ganglioneuroblastoma, medulloepithelioma, pineoblastoma, and ependymoblastoma.

    (2) Presentation / Natural history

        (a) Presentation varies with site of origin (e.g., seizures if hemispheric, vision/endocrine if suprasellar, hydrocephalus/Parinaud syndrome if pineal).

        (b) 30% 5-year survival; survival associated with complete resection, no metastases, age > 2, heavily calcified lesion

    (3) Treatment

        (a) Aggressive surgical excision, adjuvant chemotherapy, craniospinal radiation if age > 3

  c. Atypical teratoid-rhabdoid tumor

    (1) Epidemiology

        (a) Almost always age < 3

    (2) Presentation / Natural history

        (a) Presents as raised ICP, developmental regression, seizure, torticollis

        (b) Median survival is 6 months.

    (3) Treatment

        (a) Gross total resection, radiation usually not option as age < 3, experimental chemotherapy

D. Tumors of cranial and paraspinal nerves

  1. Schwannoma

    a. Presentation / Natural history

      (1) 8% of intracranial tumors

      (2) Parenchymal typically present with epilepsy or focal deficit before age 30, vestibular schwannoma with sensorineural hearing loss/tinnitus/dizziness after age 30

      (3) Slow growth, < 10% recurrence postresection

      (4) Can be complicated by hydrocephalus requiring shunt

    b. Treatment

      (1) Audiology assessment helps treatment decisions/gives baseline.

      (2) Can follow symptoms/radiology/audiology every 6 months for < 3 cm lesions

(3) Stereotactic radiosurgery option for growing tumors < 3 cm; ~ 90% tumor control possible with rare facial palsy and 50–90% hearing preservation

(4) Surgical resection of lesions < 3 cm adds benefit of tumor removal, generally for all > 3 cm, 80% normal/near-normal cranial nerve (CN) VII and up to 40% hearing preservation overall with small vestibular schwannoma (generally total loss with large lesions)

(5) Surgical approaches include translabyrinthine (sacrifices hearing if still present, but may better preserve CN VII), suboccipital (may best preserve hearing), retromastoid, subtemporal

2. Neurofibroma (including plexiform)
   a. Epidemiology
      (1) Rarely intracranial, plexiform neurofibromas often in orbit (CN V1), scalp, parotid (CN VII)
      (2) Associated with neurofibromatosis (especially plexiform in neurofibromatosis type I [NF1])
   b. Presentation / Natural history
      (1) Typically present as painless mass, slow growth, benign, 2–12% degenerate into malignant peripheral nerve sheath tumor, recurrence rate high
   c. Treatment
      (1) Surgical resection (complete usually impossible) usually for symptomatic spinal cord or neural compression

3. Other
   a. Perineurioma
      (1) Rare lesion, rarely intracranial affecting cranial nerves, plexiform variant described
      (2) Presents as benign mass, treated with surgical resection
   b. Malignant peripheral nerve sheath tumor
      (1) Rarely intracranial affecting cranial nerves, can arise from neurofibromas or radiation exposure, malignant/aggressive, treated with surgical resection ± chemotherapy/radiation

E. Tumors of the meninges

1. Meningiomas
   a. Epidemiology
      (1) Autopsy prevalence 3% in > age 60, 15–20% of primary intracranial tumors (second to GBM)
      (2) Multiple in up to 8%, females twice as commonly affected as males, higher in NF, rare in childhood unless NF1
   b. Presentation / Natural history
      (1) Incidental presentation in up to 50% cases, typically grow slowly, ~1% malignant
      (2) Overall 5-year survival > 90%, 20-year recurrence rate 20–50%
      (3) Most important risk factors for recurrence are atypical histology and extent of resection **(Table 5.14)**

Table 5.14 Simpson Grading System for Meningioma Resection

Grade	Extent of Resection	Recurrence Rate* (%)
I	Complete including dural attachment and abnormal bone	10
II	Complete with cauterization of dural attachment	15
III	Complete without dural attachment	30
IV	Incomplete resection	Up to 85
V	Biopsy	100

*Length of follow-up varies around 5 years; numbers may increase with longer follow-up.

c. Treatment
   (1) Surgical resection is treatment of choice

2. Benign mesenchymal tumors and tumor-like lesions
   a. Epidemiology
      (1) Rare lesions affecting meninges and/or adjacent skull/scalp
      (2) WHO classification subtypes include rhabdomyoma, angiolipoma, chondroma, leiomyoma, osteochondroma, benign fibrous histiocytoma, osteoma, solitary fibrous tumor, lipoma, and hemangioma.
   b. Presentation / Natural history
      (1) Typically incidental or cosmetic concern, typically stable or very slow change
      (2) Lipoma can expand with systemic steroids.
   c. Treatment
      (1) Rarely require treatment by excision

3. Malignant mesenchymal tumors (primary CNS sarcomas)
   a. Epidemiology
      (1) 0.1–3% of intracranial tumors in children and adults
      (2) Fibrosarcoma is most common overall; hemangiopericytoma is 40 times less common than meningioma.
      (3) Others include rhabdomyosarcoma, leiomyosarcoma, chondrosarcoma, Ewing sarcoma (PNET), osteosarcoma, Kaposi sarcoma, liposarcoma, epithelioid hemangioendothelioma, angiosarcoma, and malignant fibrous histiocytoma.
      (4) Radiation-induced sarcomas have been reported.
   b. Presentation / Natural history
      (1) Aggressive course, can metastasize, median survival variable with subtype, but generally 6–24 months (exceptions include hemangiopericytoma with ~80% 5-year survival rate)
      (2) Long-term survival possible with radical resection of well-circumscribed lesions
      (3) Meningeal sarcomatosis can occur (diffuse spread with no known primary)
   c. Treatment
      (1) Radical surgical excision is primary goal; adjuvant chemotherapy/radiation may help.

4. Hemangioblastoma
   a. Epidemiology
      (1) 1–2% primary intracranial tumors, 25–40% associated with von Hippel–Lindau
      (2) Sporadic peak age 50, von Hippel–Lindau-associated occur in young adults, slight male predominance, 10% of posterior fossa tumors
   b. Presentation / Natural history
      (1) Present with mass effect due to cyst expansion; new lesions develop with von Hippel–Lindau
      (2) Typically benign/slow growth. 85% 10-year survival postresection rate, 15% recur
   c. Treatment
      (1) Complete surgical resection ± preop embolization

5. Primary melanocytic lesions
   a. Melanocytoma
      (1) Rare benign lesions; clinical features and treatment similar to meningiomas
   b. Malignant melanoma
      (1) Rare, aggressive like systemic form; treated with resection + chemotherapy/radiation, prognosis poor

    c. Meningeal melanomatosis / Diffuse melanosis
      (1) Diffuse form of malignant melanoma, often found postmortem, can develop hydrocephalus requiring shunt; treated with chemotherapy ± radiation, prognosis poor

F. Lymphomas and hematopoietic tumors

  1. Primary CNS lymphoma
    a. Epidemiology
      (1) Incidence increasing, up to 10% primary intracranial tumors, 2–6% acquired immunodeficiency syndrome (AIDS) patients
      (2) Mean age 60 in immunocompetent, 35 in acquired and 10 in inherited immunodeficiencies, slight male predominance
    b. Presentation / Natural history
      (1) Can present as mass lesion, often neuropsychiatric changes
      (2) Median survival 1–4 months without treatment, 1–4 years treated (2–6 months in AIDS)
    c. Treatment
      (1) Resection typically not required due to radiation/chemosensitivity
      (2) Stereotactic biopsy followed by radiation/chemotherapy
      (3) Intrathecal methotrexate for young patients
      (4) Dramatic but short-lived response to steroids

  2. Plasmacytoma
    a. Epidemiology
      (1) Rarely intracranial not involving skull
    b. Presentation / Natural history
      (1) Often mimics meningioma
      (2) High risk to develop multiple myeloma within 10 years (though parenchymal lesion may have lower risk)
    c. Treatment
      (1) Rule out systemic multiple myeloma with urinalysis for protein, serum protein electrophoresis
      (2) Complete surgical excision followed by radiation

  3. Granulocytic sarcoma
    a. Epidemiology
      (1) Mainly pediatric, often precedes development of or occurs with systemic acute myelogenous leukemia
    b. Presentation / Natural history
      (1) Typically presents as extraaxial mass with short history, median survival 2–20 months
    c. Treatment
      (1) Surgical biopsy followed by chemotherapy and radiation generally first line, surgical resection typically reserved for emergent mass effect

G. Germ cell tumors

  1. Germinoma
    a. Epidemiology
      (1) 1–2% CNS tumors, 50% pineal region tumors; more common in Japan
      (2) Peak age 10, 90% < age 20; M:F ratio 10:1 for pineal region, whereas suprasellar germinomas more common in females

b. Presentation / Natural history
 (1) Pineal region — Parinaud syndrome, hydrocephalus
 (2) Suprasellar — diabetes insipidus, visual decline, hypothalamic–pituitary dysfunction
 (3) Tumor markers (Chapter 3 section IX)
 (4) Favorable prognosis, especially with low human chorionic gonadotrophin secretion
 (5) 5-year survival rate > 90% (very radiation/chemotherapy responsive)
c. Treatment
 (1) Biopsy, radiation + chemotherapy first line
 (2) Ventriculoperitoneal shunt or third ventriculostomy (may allow biopsy)

2. Nongerminomatous germ cell tumors
 a. Epidemiology
  (1) Predominate over germinomas in ages 0–3
 b. Presentation / Natural history
  (1) Generally worse prognosis than germinoma (< 50% 5-year survival rate)
  (2) Tumor markers (Chapter 3 section IX)
 c. Treatment
  (1) Mature teratomas curable with resection, treatment algorithm unclear for other subtypes (attempted resection + chemotherapy/radiation versus primary chemotherapy/radiation has no survival difference)
 d. Types
  (1) Embryonal carcinoma (malignant germ cell tumor) — < 1% CNS tumors, affects prepubertal children (rare < age 4), associated with Klinefelter syndrome, malignant and invasive
  (2) Yolk sac tumor (endodermal sinus tumor) — Typically in infants or adolescents, malignant/aggressive
  (3) Choriocarcinoma — Malignant, highly hemorrhagic
  (4) Teratoma
  (5) Mixed germ cell tumor

H. Tumors of the sellar region

1. Pituitary adenoma
 a. Epidemiology
  (1) 10% of intracranial tumors, M=F, peak incidence 30s–40s, associated with multiple endocrine neoplasia syndromes
  (2) 50% present as microadenomas (< 1 cm diameter), 50% as macroadenomas
 b. Presentation / Natural history
  (1) Present due to mass effect or endocrine disturbance, rarely apoplexy
  (2) Functional/secreting typically present earlier than nonfunctioning
  (3) Treatment outcomes generally very good with exception of thyroid stimulating hormone-secreting and nonfunctional lesions (cure in ~ 40%)
 c. Treatment
  (1) Endocrinologic, ophthalmologic, visual field workup
  (2) Prolactin (ng/mL) < 25 normal, 25–150 "stalk effect," > 150 ~ diagnostic of prolactinoma
  (3) Rapid corticosteroids ± emergent surgical decompression for apoplexy

(4) Surgical options include transsphenoidal (± endoscopic), open, or combined (latter two typically for large/suprasellar lesions)

(5) Radiation (focal or stereotactic) reserved for refractory cases

(6) Endocrinologic follow-up important

(7) See **Table 5.15** for classic presentations and associated treatments.

Table 5.15 Pituitary Adenoma Presentation and Treatment

Tumor	Classic Presentation	Treatment
Prolactinoma	Amenorrhea/galactorrhea (females), impotence (males), infertility (both)	Dopamine agonists (e.g., bromocriptine) generally provide complete control.
Adrenocorticotrophin	Cushing disease, hyperpigmentation	Surgery first line, ketoconazole
Growth hormone	Acromegaly in adults, gigantism in prepubertal children	Surgery first line, octreotide, some respond to dopamine agonists
Thyroid-stimulating hormone	Thyrotoxicosis	Surgery first line
Gonadotropin-secreting	As for nonfunctional	Surgery first line
Nonfunctional	Mass effect, stalk compression, bitemporal hemianopsia, cranial nerve deficits	Surgery first line

2. Craniopharyngioma
   a. Epidemiology
      (1) 2–5% intracranial tumors, 50% in children, peak incidence age 5–10
   b. Presentation / Natural history
      (1) Presents as sellar mass, benign but relentless behavior
      (2) 5-year survival rate 55–85%, recurrences typically occur < 1 year
      (3) Postoperative (postop) complications include diabetes insipidus, hypothalamic injury, 5–10% mortality
   c. Treatment
      (1) Medical optimization prior to surgery important (often adrenal cortical insufficiency needing hydrocortisone coverage perioperatively)
      (2) Attempt gross total surgical removal if risk appropriate
      (3) Postop radiation for subtotal resection may benefit but adds morbidity

3. Other
   a. Pituicytoma (granule cell tumor)
      (1) Rare, peak 50s (never < age 20), presents like nonfunctional adenoma, benign / slow growing but can recur, treated via surgical resection
   b. Spindle cell oncocytoma of the adenohypophysis
      (1) Rare adult tumor, presents like nonfunctional adenoma, benign, treated via resection

I. Metastatic tumors

1. Epidemiology / Natural history
   a. Most common brain tumor (> 50% of total), though account for 6% in pediatric cases, multiple in 50–70%, most common posterior fossa tumor in adults
   b. **Table 5.16** summarizes epidemiology of brain metastases.

Table 5.16 Epidemiology of Brain Metastases

Primary	% of Cerebral Metastases	% with Cerebral Metastases	Median Survival with Treatment (Months)
Lung	44	20	6–12
Breast	10	10	12–18
Renal cell	7	20	6–9
Gastrointestinal	6	5	6–12
Melanoma	3	40	3–4
Other (e.g., testicular)	20	(40 for testicular)	6–12
Unknown	10	—	

    2. Treatment
        a. Steroids (typically dexamethasone) reduce vasogenic edema, anticonvulsants generally only if have a seizure
        b. Unknown primary or unconfirmed diagnosis: stereotactic biopsy or excision
        c. Widespread systemic involvement, short life expectancy, and/or poor preop status: consider biopsy and/or whole brain radiotherapy, palliation
        d. Solitary metastasis goal is total surgical excision + whole brain radiotherapy; stereotactic radiosurgery generally if surgery is not feasible
        e. Multiple metastases consider excision of symptomatic lesion or multiple lesions (controversial) + whole brain radiotherapy, or radiotherapy alone (stereotactic radiosurgery generally if surgery is not feasible)

J. Cysts and tumor-like lesions

    1. Rathke cleft cyst
        a. In up to ⅓ autopsies, typically incidental, but can cause sellar mass and pituitary dysfunction symptoms, generally stable but aspiration/partial excision if symptomatic

    2. Epidermoid and dermoid cysts
        a. ~1% of primary brain tumors, linear slow growth, typically present as mass lesion, may cause bouts of meningitis (epidermoid: aseptic Mollaret recurrent meningitis, dermoid: septic), treated by surgical excision. Perioperative steroids may reduce chemical meningitis

    3. Colloid cyst
        a. < 1% intracranial tumors, usually age 20–50, benign, slow growing, can cause hydrocephalus with sudden death, treated by surgical excision, generally ventriculoscopic or open (typically transcallosal or transcortical approach), stereotactic aspiration described

    4. Arachnoid cyst
        a. 1% intracranial masses, 3–5 times more common in males, typically incidental, but rarely cause symptomatic mass effect; rarely treated by excision, fenestration, or shunting of cyst

    5. Neurenteric cyst
        a. Rare, stable or slow growth, can get cervicomedullary compression, curable by excision

    6. Hypothalamic hamartoma (tuber cinereum hamartoma)

a. Heterotopic gray matter, common cause of precocious puberty due to luteinizing hormone releasing hormone (LHRH) release and/or gelastic seizures, treated with LHRH agonist ± antiepileptic, surgical resection if refractory (high morbidity) or stereotactic radiosurgery

K. Local extension of regional tumor

1. Chordoma (cranial)
    a. Epidemiology
        (1) Rare (< 1% CNS tumors), 35% clival (50% sacral), peak incidence age 50–60, no sex predilection
    b. Presentation / Natural history
        (1) Typically present with CN palsies (III, VI)
        (2) Malignant/osteolytic, slow growth, often mimics chondrosarcoma
        (3) Metastatic rate 5–20% (occur late), recurrence rate 85% following surgery
    c. Treatment
        (1) Wide en bloc resection with postop radiation (proton beam may be most effective)

IV. Functional

A. Neurovascular compression syndromes

1. Trigeminal neuralgia
    a. Epidemiology
        (1) Annual incidence 4/100,000, higher in multiple sclerosis (MS), typically > age 50, more common in men
    b. Presentation / Natural history: Chapter 4 section X
    c. Treatment
        (1) Medical — Chapter 4 section X
        (2) Surgery — when drugs lose effect or unacceptable side effects occur
        (3) Peripheral nerve block procedures (phenol/alcohol injection, neurectomy), causes sensory loss, transient benefit due to nerve regeneration in 1–2 years
        (4) Percutaneous trigeminal rhizotomy via radiofrequency thermocoagulation (highest risk of facial numbness), glycerol injection, microcompression via balloon catheter — all have initial success rates ~90–95% with 20% recurrence in 6 years, 80% at 12 years; can be repeated. Severe complications: anesthesia dolorosa, neuroparalytic keratitis
        (5) Subtemporal extradural or intradural retrogasserian rhizotomy and transection of descending trigeminal tract in medulla (rarely used)
        (6) Microvascular decompression (typically by superior cerebellar artery), initial success rate ~85–95%, 20% recurrence in 6 years, 30% at 10 years, no sensory impairment
        (7) Stereotactic radiosurgery of root entry zone, initial success ~80–95% after median latency 3 months, recurrence rate ~ 25% at 3 years

2. Hemifacial spasm
    a. Epidemiology
        (1) Annual incidence 1/100,000, more common in females, typically young adult or older
    b. Presentation / Natural history
        (1) Intermittent painless unilateral spasmodic facial contractions, often starting with orbicularis oculi and progressing to hemiface
    c. Treatment
        (1) Local botulinum toxin injection is typically highly effective but temporary.

(2) Microvascular decompression (typically by anterior-inferior cerebellar artery), main risk is hearing loss (up to 10%), results better with shorter duration of symptoms and younger patients (> 80% complete resolution with ~10% recurrence that generally occurs within 2 years)

B. Movement disorders (Chapter 4 section IX)

   1. Parkinson's disease

     a. Medical first line (levodopa)

     b. Surgery considered in patients with acceptable operative risk with levodopa responsiveness, but unacceptable frequency of "off" periods and dyskinesias (can reduce "off" period, allowing levodopa dose reduction resulting in less dyskinesias)

     c. Pallidotomy and deep brain stimulation (DBS) of the globus pallidus interna (GPi) offers ~ 40% improvement in motor scores and ~ 65% improvement in dyskinesias with < 1% mortality and 5% significant morbidity.

     d. Subthalamic nucleus DBS offers ~10% better motor and dyskinesia improvement over GPi, generally preferred, but pallidotomy is an option if close patient follow-up is not possible.

   2. Essential tremor

     a. Medical first line; surgery for refractory/debilitating cases only

     b. Unilateral ventrointermedius (Vim) thalamotomy improves or abolishes contralateral tremor in 80–90%, temporary contralateral weakness/dysarthria/numbness common but rarely permanent

     c. Unilateral Vim DBS achieves similar results with titratability (can adjust settings to lessen unwanted sensory side effects) generally outweighing extra need for follow-up and hardware complications, likely that ability to change settings prevents late recurrence

     d. Stereotactic radiosurgery thalamotomy offers similar early success rates, avoids low morbidity of surgery (benefits mainly higher surgical risk patients); however, long-term follow-up is uncertain.

   3. Dystonia

     a. Medical first line, surgery for refractory cases only (predominantly primary generalized and cervical dystonias that tend to respond better than secondary forms)

     b. Pallidotomy and GPi DBS offer ~40% improvements in motor function and quality of life; DBS adds titratability benefit and is generally preferred.

     c. Stereotactic radiosurgery pallidotomy has been shown to be effective in case reports.

     d. Intrathecal baclofen pumps provide some relief in certain refractory cases (see below).

   4. Spasticity

     a. Medical/physical therapy first line, then orthopedic (tendon release etc.) / neurosurgery

     b. Multitude of procedures described with limited efficacy, common practice includes

       (1) Intrathecal baclofen pump (~ 30% catheter complication rate, including potentially life-threatening withdrawal)

       (2) Selective dorsal rhizotomy (interrupts afferent reflex arc)

C. Epilepsy — Chapter 4 section VII

   1. 20–30% patients refractory to medical therapy (several drugs over several years)

   2. Overall outcomes for properly selected epilepsy surgeries (lesional and nonlesional) are ~60% good or seizure free, further 20% some improvement

   3. Workup includes structural imaging, electroencephalography (EEG), functional imaging/testing, and neuropsychological testing if eloquent brain is at risk.

4. Precise localization of epileptogenic focus using depth electrodes and subdural strips/grids is often necessary in staged procedure.

5. Potentially surgical conditions include
   a. Focal onset temporal lobe seizures
      (1) Includes idiopathic, mesial temporal sclerosis, and lesional
      (2) Unless lesional, typically involves standard anterior temporal lobectomy with amygdalohippocampectomy (4.5 cm from temporal tip on dominant side to preserve speech, 6 cm on nondominant side to preserve vision)
   b. Focal onset extratemporal seizures
      (1) Includes idiopathic and lesional
      (2) Typically involves resection of epileptogenic focus or lesion
      (3) Radiosurgery option for hypothalamic hamartoma causing gelastic seizures
   c. Catastrophic epilepsies
      (1) Includes lesional, hemimegalencephaly, diffuse cortical dysplasias, Rasmussen encephalitis, Sturge–Weber, porencephalic cysts
      (2) Commonly require anatomic (resective) or functional (disconnection) hemispherectomy of the involved side; latter less morbid
   d. Generalized epilepsy
      (1) Drop attacks (atonic) improve by ~ 70% with corpus callosotomy (generally anterior ⅔ divided to reduce risk of disconnection syndrome).
      (2) Refractory generalized tonic-clonic seizures can improve to a lesser extent with corpus callosotomy and vagal nerve stimulators (~ 50% of patients improve by ~ 50%).

D. Pain
   a. Pain procedures are last resort for medically intractable pain.

   1. Ablative procedures
      a. Cordotomy
         (1) Unilateral percutaneous C1–C2 lesion of spinothalamic tract, complete or significant relief of contralateral pain in ~ 85% for up to 1 year, ideal for unilateral pain below C5 in terminally ill patient; small risk of Ondine curse (respiratory arrest and death during sleep)
      b. Dorsal root entry zone (DREZ) procedure
         (1) Microincisions of root entry zone, typically indicated for refractory cervical root avulsion pain or pain at transition zone in spinal cord injury, ~ 65% benefit at 10 years
      c. Sympathectomy
         (1) For refractory complex regional pain syndrome, see Sympathectomy for Hyperhidrosis section below

   2. Neuromodulatory procedures
      a. Spinal cord stimulation and peripheral nerve stimulation
         (1) Provides ~50% reduction in neuropathic pain (often for failed back surgery syndrome)
      b. Motor cortex stimulation and DBS in periaqueductal/periventricular gray matter
         (1) ~50% receive benefit in neuropathic pain, most often attempted for intractable facial pain
      c. Intrathecal drug infusion
         (1) Primarily used for cancer pain, ~ 90% good pain relief, equipment complications common

E. Sympathectomy for hyperhidrosis
   a. Also rarely for sympathetic-mediated pain, Raynaud disease, intractable angina

1. Epidemiology
    a. Incidence ~1%

2. Presentation / Natural history
    a. Manifests mainly with hyperhidroses of palms

3. Treatment
    a. Medical therapy (topical agents, anticholinergics, etc.) first line
    b. T2–T3 sympathectomy for refractory cases, ~100% success rate
    c. Conventionally performed via posterior paravertebral approach, thorascopic procedure associated with less morbidity
    d. Horner syndrome can occur if stellate ganglion is divided.

V. CSF Diseases

A. Hydrocephalus

1. Epidemiology
    a. Congenital (Chiari malformations, aqueductal stenosis, Dandy–Walker)
    b. Acquired (infectious, posthemorrhagic, neoplasia)

2. Presentation / Natural history
    a. Presents with raised ICP, CN VI palsy, Parinaud syndrome, macrocrania if chronic, and neonatal/infantile onset

3. Treatment
    a. Serial spinal taps for communicating hydrocephalus option if posthemorrhagic (can be temporary)
    b. Third ventriculostomy for obstructive hydrocephalus when third ventricle is wide enough, basilar artery not compressed against the clivus, success rate 60–90%; extremely rare acute closure and deterioration reported
    c. Shunts (ventriculoperitoneal [VP] / atrial / pleural, lumboperitoneal – for communicating hydrocephalus), valves include low-med-high pressure, flow-regulated, programmable
    d. Shunt complications — incidence of failure 25–40% in first year (most in first few months) then 5%/year, 50% fail at 5 years. Complications include mechanical failure (proximal and distal occlusions and disconnections), migration, overdrainage or underdrainage, infection, ventricular loculation, skin erosion, craniosynostosis in infants, abdominal hernia, peritoneal pseudocyst, shunt nephritis, and subdural hematoma (SDH).

B. Normal pressure hydrocephalus

1. Epidemiology
    a. Age usually > 60, males > females, accounts for ~1% of dementias

2. Presentation / Natural history
    a. Normal CSF pressure with classic triad: dementia, "magnetic gait," urinary incontinence
    b. Slow continual decline without treatment

3. Treatment
    a. Best results if secondary to identifiable cause like prior SAH, trauma, or infection
    b. VP shunt treatment of choice in carefully selected patients
    c. Incontinence and gait respond best, dementia less likely to improve unless short history
    d. Overall ~ ⅓ improve, ⅓ halt decline, ⅓ no response

C. Idiopathic intracranial hypertension (pseudotumor cerebri)

1. Epidemiology
   a. Peak age 15–40 years, M:F ratio 1:4–8, associated with obesity and dural sinus thrombosis

2. Presentation / Natural history
   a. Typically presents with headache and papilledema without hydrocephalus
   b. Usually self-limited but recurrences are common; severe visual deficits in ~10% if untreated

3. Treatment
   a. Workup including opening pressure measurement, CSF analysis, ophthalmologic evaluation with visual fields (enlarged blind spot in most)
   b. Medical management includes weight loss (of 6% usually causes full resolution), dietary salt restriction, acetazolamide (reduces CSF production), and short-term steroids if severe.
   c. Surgical treatment highly successful; options include serial lumbar punctures, shunt (typically lumboperitoneal), optic nerve sheath fenestration (relieves optic nerve pressure only), subtemporal decompression.

VI. Congenital Disease

A. Craniosynostosis

1. Presentation / Natural history
   a. Typically presents as cosmetic concern, ~10% develop raised ICP
   b. Treatment generally is indicated for cosmesis only.

2. Treatment
   a. Surgical strip craniectomies/cranial remodeling, typically in conjunction with craniofacial surgery, most significant complication risk is blood loss requiring transfusion(s)
   b. Positional plagiocephaly responds satisfactorily to repositioning ± helmet therapy.

B. Encephaloceles

1. Epidemiology
   a. 1–4/10,000 live births, more common in males
   b. 80% cranial (usually occipital), 15% frontoethmoidal (sincipital), others mainly basal
   c. Associated with spina bifida, split cord, Chiari II and III, Klippel–Feil, Dandy–Walker

2. Presentation / Natural history
   a. Generally identified prenatally, anterior can present later with facial/ocular manifestations or CSF leak

3. Treatment
   a. Excision of sac and contents with watertight dural closure (generally combined intracranial and transnasal approach for basal), treatment of hydrocephalus if needed

C. Chiari malformations (Chapter 3 section V)

1. Epidemiology
   a. Chiari I typically presents in young adults (0.01% of population), Chiari II in infants (1/3000 live births).
   b. ~25% Chiari I is associated with other skeletal abnormalities (basilar invagination, Klippel–Feil, atlantooccipital fusion, cervical spina bifida), not brain abnormalities.

   c. Chiari II associated with many CNS abnormalities (myelomeningocele in 100%, migrational abnormalities, hindbrain abnormalities, aqueductal stenosis), lacunar skull, incomplete C1 arch, low-lying torcula
   d. ~50% both types associated with syringomyelia (generally improves with treatment)

  2. Presentation / Natural history
   a. Chiari I — cervical pain, suboccipital headache, Lhermitte sign, central cord syndrome
   b. Hydrocephalus in 25% Chiari I, in 90% Chiari II
   c. Natural history variable, surgery considered if symptomatic

  3. Treatment
   a. Principle to treat from above down — hydrocephalus first if present, then posterior fossa decompression, and finally the syringomyelia
   b. Posterior fossa decompression with duraplasty (~80% improve); syrinx often then resolves

D. Dandy–Walker malformation

  1. Epidemiology
   a. 1–4/100,000 live births, ⅔ associated with other developmental anomalies, 80% hydrocephalus

  2. Presentation / Natural history
   a. Macrocephaly, cognitive impairment, incidental in mild form (mega cisterna magna)
   b. Virtually 100% survival with treatment, but 50% normal intelligence; ataxia, spasticity, fine motor impairment common

  3. Treatment
   a. Standard treatment is shunting of cyst.

VII. Trauma

A. ICP Monitoring

  1. Indications
   a. GCS ≤ 8 with abnormal CT (edema, contusion, hemorrhage) or two of the following with a normal-appearing CT: age > 40, decerebrate or decorticate posturing, and/or episode of systolic blood pressure < 90 mm Hg
   b. Elevated ICP develops in 3% of mild head injuries (GCS 13–15), 10–12% of moderate head injury (GCS 9–12), and 50% of severe head injury (GCS ≤ 8).

  2. Techniques
   a. External ventricular drain
    (1) Gold standard, permits CSF drainage, typically right frontal (inserted perpendicular to Kocher point of 1–2 cm anterior to coronal suture, 2–3 cm lateral to midline)
   b. Intraparenchymal monitor
    (1) Simpler insertion, accuracy tends to drift after few days
   c. Other
    (1) Subarachnoid screw/bolt, etc., rarely used as less reliable

B. ICP Management (escalating steps)

  1. Action required if ICP > 20 for > 5 minutes or cerebral perfusion pressure (CPP) < 60 for 5 minutes

  2. **Table 5.17** describes management of increased ICP.

Table 5.17 Management of Increased Intracranial Pressure (ICP)

Action	Notes
Elevate head of bed 30–45 degrees	Balances venous outflow and arterial inflow
Relieve any jugular compression	Straighten neck, loosen bandages, etc.
Adequate analgesia	Avoid excess initially as can alter neurologic status
Avoid hypoxia and hypercarbia	Airway intubation for GCS ≤ 8; target normocarbia, brief hyperventilation in emergencies, avoid PEEP, hyperventilation vasoconstricts as long as there is no vasomotor paralysis, decreases ICP but may cause ischemia by decreasing CBF, use as a brief temporizing measure in general
Maintain mean blood pressure > 90 mm Hg	Can maintain CPP > 60 mm Hg if ICP monitored
Correct hyponatremia, fever, hyperglycemia	Reduces ICP / cerebral metabolic demand
CSF drainage if ventricular drain present	
Mannitol, hypertonic saline	Typically are bridge to further treatment, must keep serum osmolarity < 320 mOsm/L to avoid renal injury, expands plasma volume, reduces hematocrit, increases erythrocyte deformability, osmotic diuresis decreases brain volume, hypertonic saline similar, but avoid if there is hyponatremia
Surgical evacuation of mass lesion, CSF drainage, decompressive craniectomy	Early decompressive craniectomy favored by some
Barbiturate coma/paralysis	To burst suppression on EEG

Abbreviations: CBF, cerebral blood flow; CPP, cerebral perfusion pressure; CSF, cerebrospinal fluid; EEG, electroencephalogram; GCS, Glasgow Coma Scale; PEEP, positive end-expiratory pressure.

C. Prophylactic anticonvulsants

    1. Early posttraumatic seizure (< 7 days) in 4–25% and late in 9–42%. Administer anticonvulsants in acute setting to avoid seizures increasing ICP and metabolic demand. Discontinue after 1 week. Risk factors for early seizures are GCS < 10, cortical contusion, extra- or intraaxial hemorrhage, penetrating head wound, depressed skull fracture, and seizure < 24 hours from trauma.

D. Skull fractures

    1. Depressed

        a. Epidemiology

           (1) Complicate up to 6% head injuries, ≥ 5 mm depression highly associated with dural tear

        b. Presentation / Natural history

           (1) No evidence that elevating reduces risk of subsequent posttraumatic seizures

           (2) Early surgery may reduce risk of infection in compound fractures (up to 10% risk)

           (3) Overall 15% develop posttraumatic seizures, 10% neurologic morbidity, 2–20% mortality

        c. Treatment

           (1) Surgical debridement / elevation (± dural repair and cranialization of frontal sinus) generally indicated for fracture causing significant mass effect, in cosmetically sensitive area (forehead), compound (open) fractures with evidence of dural tear (depression >1 cm, CSF leak clinically or radiographically), displaced posterior table of sinus fracture, significant underlying hematoma requiring surgery

           (2) Conservative approach generally for other scenarios or if over major dural venous sinus

2. Traumatic CSF fistula
   a. Epidemiology
      (1) 3% of all head injury patients (10% of penetrating), 10-fold ↑ overall infection rate
      (2) 60% manifest within days, 95% within 3 months.
   b. Presentation / Natural history
      (1) 70–85% cease spontaneously by 2 weeks, most by 6 months.
      (2) Meningitis incidence is 5–10% (highest after 7 days).
   c. Treatment
      (1) General measures — expectant, bed rest only if low pressure symptoms, avoid Valsalva
      (2) Acetazolamide / fluid restriction to reduce CSF production, rarely used
      (3) Persistent leak (generally > 5–7 days) — lumbar drain; surgery if drain fails (attempt to clinically / radiographically localize fistula, close bone / dural defects, and provide barrier / patch)
      (4) Prophylactic antibiotics may select resistant organisms; evidence for use controversial

E. Penetrating trauma

1. Epidemiology
   a. Less common than blunt trauma, the majority are gunshot wounds (mortality ~ 90%).

2. Presentation / Natural history
   a. High impact velocity (rifle bullet) causes tissue cavitation exceeding bullet diameter (Chapter 3 section XXII).

3. Treatment
   a. Stabilize protruding object, remove only in operating room
   b. Preop angiography if large named artery or dural sinus at risk and hemorrhage controlled
   c. Empiric antibiotics for low velocity objects (knife, etc.), optional for bullets (controversial)
   d. Surgical debridement of missile tract / extraction bone fragments only if mass effect

F. Cerebral contusion

1. Epidemiology
   a. 10% of head injuries with GCS ≤ 8, typically evident within 72 hours of injury

2. Presentation / Natural history
   a. Common in sudden deceleration / angular acceleration injuries (coup and contrecoup impact on bony prominences at temporal, occipital, frontal poles)
   b. Often enlarge / coalesce (especially in first 48–72 hours), mortality ~ 50% overall

3. Treatment
   a. ICP management as above including consideration of early surgical evacuation

G. Epidural hematoma

1. Epidemiology
   a. 1% of head trauma admissions, rare < age 2 or > age 60
   b. 85% arterial source (most commonly middle meningeal artery)
   c. 20% have underlying acute subdural hematoma, 85% associated with skull fracture

2. Presentation / Natural history
   a. Classically brief traumatic loss of consciousness, lucid interval, then deterioration / contralateral weakness / ipsilateral blown pupil

b. Ipsilateral weakness seen in Kernohan phenomenon (opposite cerebral peduncle compressed on tentorial notch) – false localizing sign

c. Overall mortality is ~ 20%, 10% if treated within first few hours.

3. Treatment
a. Emergent correction of coagulopathy, nonsurgical option if ≤ 1 cm thick with minimal signs
b. Emergent surgical evacuation for all other cases

H. Subdural hematoma

1. Epidemiology
a. Acute — 2% of head trauma admissions, generally more underlying brain injury than epidural hematoma, source typically cortical laceration or bridging vein tear, anticoagulation therapy increases risk 10–30-fold
b. Chronic — Mean age is 65; risk factors: trauma, ethanol abuse, seizures, coagulopathy

2. Presentation / Natural history
a. Acute — typically lacks lucid interval due to greater underlying brain injury, overall mortality > 50% (> 80% if > age 65, > 90% if anticoagulated or GCS III), functional survival in ~⅓ of survivors, mortality/morbidity ~ halved if operated on within 4 hours in a classic study, the results of which are controversial
b. Chronic — can present with minor headache, cognitive and higher cortical functional changes, or as focal mass effect

3. Treatment
a. Emergent correction of coagulopathy, observation with follow-up imaging if ≤ 1 cm thick with minimal signs
b. Emergent surgical evacuation via craniotomy for acute subdural
c. Chronic subdural typically treated initially with burr hole drainage ± temporary subdural drain placement (~ 85% success rate), craniotomy generally for loculated / refractory cases

Spinal Procedures

I. Vascular Disease

A. Spinal arteriovenous malformation

1. Epidemiology
a. 4% primary intraspinal masses, generally present in adults
b. Dural AVM — most common, dural artery to spinal vein in intervertebral foramen
c. Other types — Intradural-extramedullary, intramedullary, perimedullary AVF

2. Presentation / Natural history
a. 80% present as progressive myelopathy/back pain, 20% acute (typically hemorrhage)
b. Foix–Alajouanine syndrome – Chapter 3 section XXVI

3. Treatment
a. Localization with angiography (gadolinium-enhanced magnetic resonance angiography [MRA] or CT angiography [CTA] can permit focused catheter angiography)
b. Surgical disconnection of venous outflow / resection required, occasionally can embolize

B. Spinal epidural/subdural hematoma

    1. Epidemiology

        a. Rare, can be traumatic (including after lumbar puncture, especially in patients with recognized or unrecognized coagulation disorders) or spontaneous (spinal AVM, etc., ~⅓ associated with anticoagulation), low cervical and thoracolumbar most common

    2. Presentation / Natural history

        a. Acute back pain, followed by acutely progressive myelopathy

        b. Better neurologic recovery associated with, time to decompression (especially < 48 hours)

    3. Treatment

        a. Normalization of coagulation

        b. Conservative/close observation option if pain only, otherwise urgent decompressive laminectomy / evacuation

C. Cavernous malformation

    1. Spinal:cranial ratio is ~1:20, treated as for cranial counterparts (see Cranial Procedures section)

II. Infections

A. Epidural abscess

    1. Epidemiology

        a. 1/10,000 hospital admissions, mean age 50–60

        b. 50% thoracic, 30% lumbar, 20% cervical

        c. > 50% *Staphylococcus aureus*, followed by *Streptococcus*, coliforms, others

        d. Risk factors include diabetes, IV drug use, chronic renal failure, ethanol abuse

    2. Presentation / Natural history

        a. Classically, back pain, fever, and local tenderness; can develop myelopathy rapidly

        b. Often associated with osteomyelitis

        c. Poor neurologic recovery with delayed surgery

    3. Treatment

        a. Early surgical evacuation followed by antibiotics (~ 6 weeks IV, then ~ 6 weeks orally)

B. Diskitis

    1. Epidemiology

        a. *Staphylococcus aureus* > *Staphylococcus epidermidis* (most common if postop) > gram-negative (*Pseudomonas* in IV drug users)

        b. Spontaneous usually in IV drug users, diabetics, other immunocompromised patients

        c. Postoperative (< 0.5% from lumbar diskectomy or anterior cervical diskectomy) typically weeks after surgery

    2. Presentation / Natural history

        a. Primary symptom localized pain/tenderness, > 50% radicular symptoms, < 50% febrile

        b. Elevated erythrocyte sedimentation rate/C-reactive protein highly sensitive in immunocompetent

        c. Outcomes generally good with appropriate treatment

3. Treatment
    a. Radiographically guided percutaneous needle aspiration (~ 60% positive)
    b. ~75% managed with antibiotics (IV for 6 weeks, orally for 6 weeks) and immobilization
    c. Surgery required for diagnosis or if neural decompression needed or instability persists despite treatment

C. Vertebral osteomyelitis

    1. Epidemiology
        a. Incidence 1:250,000, lumbar > thoracic > cervical/sacral
        b. *Staphylococcus aureus* > *E. coli*, others including *Pseudomonas* in IV drug users
        c. Pott disease — tuberculosis
        d. Risk factors include IV drug abuse, diabetes, dialysis, immunocompromised, endocarditis, post-operative
        e. Infection sources — genitourinary tract (most common), respiratory, soft tissue/dental infections

    2. Presentation / Natural history
        a. Primary symptom localized pain/tenderness, > 50% radicular symptoms, < 50% febrile
        b. Elevated erythrocyte sedimentation rate/C-reactive protein highly sensitive in immunocompetent

    3. Treatment
        a. Blood cultures positive in ~ 50%
        b. Radiographically guided percutaneous needle aspirate (~ 60% positive)
        c. ~ 90% managed with antibiotics (IV for 6 weeks, orally for 6 weeks) and immobilization

III. Spine Neoplasia

A. Intramedullary

    1. Ependymoma — 45%
        a. Epidemiology
            (1) Peak in young adults, common in neurofibromatosis type 2 (NF2)
            (2) Most commonly cervical and filum (typically myxopapillary ependymoma)
        b. Presentation / Natural history
            (1) Months to years of pain (nocturnal) initially, then sensory/motor loss, sphincter disturbance; can also get central cord symptoms due to syrinx formation
            (2) Prognosis good and recurrence low if complete resection achieved
        c. Treatment
            (1) Complete surgical resection (usually a distinct plane); while minimizing deficit, most use intraoperative neuromonitoring
            (2) Most important predictor of postop function is preop status.
            (3) Adjuvant radiation is generally reserved for high grade or multiple recurrent lesions

    2. Astrocytoma — 35% in adults, 90% in age < 10
        a. Epidemiology
            (1) Peak in young adults, most commonly thoracic and cervical
        b. Presentation / Natural history
            (1) Indistinguishable from ependymoma
            (2) ~25% malignant in adults, less in pediatric population
            (3) 50% 5-year survival for low-grade (recurrences common), poor prognosis for high grade

  c. Treatment
   (1) Surgical resection while minimizing deficit (plane of dissection can be indistinct), most use intraoperative neuromonitoring
   (2) Most important predictor of postop function is preop status.
   (3) Adjuvant radiation is generally reserved for multiple recurrent lesions.

 3. Hemangioblastoma — 5%
  a. Epidemiology
   (1) ⅓ associated with von Hippel–Lindau, mean age 30–40, most thoracic or cervical
  b. Presentation / Natural history
   (1) Classically present over years with sensory deficit (often proprioceptive due to tendency for a location in the dorsal columns near the sensory root entry) early, pain, then sensory/motor loss, sphincter disturbance
   (2) Prognosis good and recurrence low if complete resection achieved
  c. Treatment
   (1) Complete surgical resection while minimizing deficit, most use intraoperative neuromonitoring

 4. Other
  a. Lipoma
   (1) Rare without associated dysraphism, peak in young adults, motor > sensory symptoms, typically indolent, but can acutely progress, typically require subtotal removal as adherent
  b. Ganglioglioma
   (1) Rare, typically pediatric/young adult, slow progression, treated like ependymomas

B. Intradural extramedullary

 1. Meningioma — 40%
  a. Epidemiology
   (1) M:F ratio 1:4, peak onset age 50, 75% thoracic, often multiple in NF2
  b. Presentation / Natural history
   (1) Most present with localized back pain or slow-onset myelopathy.
   (2) Recurrence rate 5%, 15% with subtotal resection (better than cranial prognosis)
  c. Treatment
   (1) Total surgical excision
   (2) Radiotherapy for recurrences that cannot be completely excised, rare malignant forms

 2. Schwannoma — 30%
  a. Epidemiology
   (1) No sex predilection, peak onset age 30, associated with NF2
  b. Presentation / Natural history
   (1) 80% present with radicular pain.
   (2) Recurrence rate 5–10%, 40% with NF2
  c. Treatment
   (1) Total surgical excision (can often preserve uninvolved rootlets)

 3. Neurofibroma — 10%
  a. Epidemiology
   (1) No sex predilection, peak onset age 20, highly associated with NF (60% with NF1)
  b. Presentation / Natural history
   (1) 80% present with radicular pain.

(2) Recurrence rate 10–15%, malignant degeneration rare unless in NF1 (5–10%)
  c. Treatment
    (1) Aim for total excision but typically only possible with significant neurologic consequence. Goal is to decompress the spinal cord; pain relief is good even if partial excision (85%)

4. Other
  a. Myxopapillary ependymoma
    (1) Present in filum, mean age 30, generally benign, treated with complete excision with radiotherapy if recurrent (10–20%)
  b. Spinal paraganglioma
    (1) Incidence 0.07/100,000, benign, typical near cauda equina, treated with complete excision with radiotherapy for recurrence (5–10%)

C. Extradural

1. Primary malignant tumors
  a. Universally rare and highly recurrent
  b. Typically present with subacute persistent/nocturnal pain, acute neurologic deterioration
  c. Treated generally by wide en bloc resection with margins and chemotherapy/radiation
  d. Extradural primary malignant spine tumors see **Table 5.18**

2. Primary benign tumors
  a. Generally rare, typically present incidentally or like malignant lesions but generally with less acute symptom onset
  b. Extradural primary benign tumors see **Table 5.19**

3. Plasmacytoma and multiple myeloma
  a. Epidemiology
    (1) Spectrum of disseminated (multiple myeloma, common) to focal (plasmacytoma, rare)
    (2) Plasmacytoma — more common in males, mean age > 50, spinal in 25–50%
    (3) Multiple myeloma — no sex predilection, mean age > 60, annual incidence 0.002%, spine common location for symptomatic lesions
  b. Presentation / Natural history
    (1) Spinal involvement typically with pain or compression (root or cord)
    (2) ~ 50% of plasmacytoma progress to multiple myeloma within 5 years
    (3) Multiple myeloma median survival rate is 2.5 years.
  c. Treatment
    (1) Rule out additional lesions with skeletal survey.
    (2) Urine/serum protein electrophoresis (oligoclonal bands and Bence–Jones proteins in myeloma), 24-hour creatinine clearance, serum calcium (hypercalcemia common), complete

Table 5.18 Extradural Primary Malignant Spine Tumors

Tumor	Key Features	Median Treated Survival
Osteosarcoma	1–3% of osteosarcomas, peak age 20–30	6–10 months
Chondrosarcoma	5% of chondrosarcomas, typically elderly men	1–3 years
Chordoma	See Cranial section 3, subsection K	6 years
Ewing sarcoma	3–4% of Ewing, mainly sacral, typically 5–15 years	2–3 years

Table 5.19 Extradural Primary Benign Spine Tumors

Tumor	Key Features
Eosinophilic granuloma	Emobilization (rarely low-dose radiation) and analgesia sufficient unless spinal cord compression then surgery
Osteochondroma	5% in spine, often asymptomatic but otherwise typically pain, generally conservative treatment unless suspect chondrosarcoma (1–5% degenerate) – do needle or open biopsy if neurologic compromise surgery generally curative
Osteoid osteoma	Chapter 3 section XXV, surgical resection curative
Osteoblastoma	Chapter 3 section XXV, requires en bloc resection to prevent recurrence
Aneurysmal bone cyst	Preop endovascular embolization and surgical curettage generally cure
Hemangioma	Up to 11% prevalence in autopsies, often incidental, rarely compressive (often thoracic), female > male, preop embolization with surgical resection generally cures
Giant cell tumor	Rare, generally sacral, female > male, peak age 20s, most present with pain, can be aggressive, preop embolization and complete resection required (high recurrence)

Abbreviation: preop, preoperative.

blood count (marrow suppression in myeloma), coagulation parameters (coagulopathy due to paraproteinemia common)

(3) Radiotherapy first if no rapid neurologic deterioration (control rates > 90%) or instability, otherwise complete resection / instrumented fusion, add chemotherapy for myeloma

4. Metastatic
   a. Epidemiology
      (1) Most common extradural tumor, M:F ratio 1.5:1, 25% have multiple lesions
      (2) Overall symptomatic spinal metastases occur in 10% cancer patients, 40% by autopsy
      (3) 95% extradural, 4.5% intradural, 0.5% intramedullary
      (4) In order of frequency, breast (20%), lung (20%), prostate (10%); others including renal, gastrointestinal, unknown
   b. Presentation / Natural history
      (1) Classically, initially pain (90%), progresses to motor/sensory loss/sphincter dysfunction
      (2) Can also be constitutional symptoms, hypercalcemia, pathologic fracture/instability
   c. Treatment
      (1) Seek primary clinically and diagnostically
      (2) Medical — steroids (typically 10 mg dexamethasone followed by 16 mg/day)
      (3) Radiation — used for all, generally primary modality for lymphoma and myeloma (highly radiosensitive) or for patients without spinal cord compression, life expectancy < 3–4 months, diffuse involvement, high surgical risk, complete deficit for > 48 hours, breast and prostate intermediate
      (4) Surgery — complete/aggressive resection with stabilization for spinal cord compression followed by radiation is primary treatment for single level disease, failure of radiotherapy, instability or bony compression, or unknown diagnosis
      (5) A comparison of radiation versus surgery for treatment of single level spinal cord compression is given in **Table 5.20**.

Table 5.20 Surgery versus Radiation for Single-Level Spinal Cord Compression

Group	Mean Days Survival	% Ambulatory at 3 Months	Mean Days Ambulatory	% Regained Ambulation	Mean Days Continent
Radiation	100*	57	13	19	17
Surgery + radiation	126*	84	122	62	156

*Not significant.

IV. Degenerative Spinal Disease

A. Cervical disk disease

1. Epidemiology
   a. Byproduct of aging, spondylosis present in 80% of people > age 55, disk space narrowing in ⅔ people > age 65, 70% C6–C7, 25% C5–C6
   b. Typically caused by soft disk in younger patients, osteophytic spurs in older

2. Presentation / Natural history
   a. Presentation includes neck pain, radiculopathy, and myelopathy.
   b. Soft disk — The majority improves spontaneously over a few months.
   c. Osteophytic — can be intermittent, often progressive, and rarely spontaneously recovers

3. Treatment
   a. Conservative therapy first line — short course of immobilization, nonsteroidal antiinflammatories (NSAIDs), opiates, epidural cortisone injections, physical therapy, and home cervical traction. 95% recover from acute cervical radiculopathy with these measures.
   b. Surgical management — anterior cervical diskectomy ± fusion, posterior keyhole laminotomy (far lateral disks), or posterior decompressive laminectomy (multiple levels with spondylosis). The long-term success of single-level diskectomy is very similar with no operative fusion (no bone graft placed), fusion with autologous or allograft bone graft, or fusion with bone graft and anterior cervical plating. All groups had 73–83% long-term symptomatic success and nearly 100% fusion at 4 years, but kyphosis developed in 63% of patients without bone grafts and in only 42% of patients in the other groups. Poor fusion rates were found for three or more levels done anteriorly.
   c. Postop sequelae include C5 radiculopathy in up to 3% (cause unknown), adjacent level degeneration can occur

B. Thoracic disk disease

1. Epidemiology
   a. Cause of back pain in 1–2/1000 patients
   b. Autopsy incidence 7–15%, 75% between T8–T12

2. Presentation / Natural history
   a. Presentation variable, diagnosis often late
   b. Can have back or radicular pain (60%), sensory changes (25%), and myelopathy (20%)

3. Treatment
   a. Posterior — laminectomy, transpedicular, or far lateral costotransversectomy if a trajectory can be achieved that will reach the herniation without having to retract the spinal cord (never retract the spinal cord); easier for soft disks, more difficult if the disk is calcified

b. Anterior — generally preferred as any cord manipulation is avoided; includes thoracoscopic procedures, right-sided thoracotomy to avoid the heart in the upper thoracic spine, left-sided thoracotomy lower down because the aorta is easier to mobilize and the liver hinders exposure on the right

c. Outcomes of surgical procedures for thoracic disk disease are given in **Table 5.21**.

Table 5.21 Surgical Outcome for Thoracic Disk Disease

Procedure	Normal (%)	Improved (%)	Unchanged (%)	Worse (%)
Laminectomy	15	42	11	32
Transpedicular	37	45	11	7
Costotransversectomy	35	53	12	0
Transthoracic	67	33	0	0

C. Lumbar disk disease (Chapter 3 section XXIX)

1. 75% with acute lumbar radiculopathy will improve by 1 month, > 85% in total

2. Conservative therapy first line (unless cauda equina syndrome – surgical emergency, or progressive deficit) — bed rest, NSAIDs, analgesia, physiotherapy after acute phase

3. Surgical management — generally consider if no improvement in 6–12 weeks, 90–95% effective. Options include intradiskal therapy (only 50–75% success rate), laminectomy, microdiskectomy, and microendoscopic diskectomy. Complications include infection (0.5–2%), increased motor deficit (1–8%), dural tear (1–5%), and reherniation (5%).

4. Surgical outcome better than conservative at 1 year, little difference at 4 years (thus surgery effective for prompt pain relief)

D. Cervical spondylosis/stenosis

1. Epidemiology
   a. Cervical spondylotic myelopathy is the most common myelopathy in patients > age 55.

2. Presentation / Natural history
   a. Presents with myelopathy or radiculopathy, neck pain (controversial); amyotrophic lateral sclerosis can mimic
   b. ~ 50% improve with surgery if symptoms < 1 year, 16% if > 1 year, > 50% halt progression, better for relief of radicular pain

3. Treatment
   a. Medical treatment with bracing only temporizes
   b. Surgical decompression, typically anterior cervical diskectomy and fusion for anterior compression at one to two levels, laminectomy ± fusion for posterior compression at three or more levels (see Cervical Disk Disease section)

E. Lumbar spondylosis/stenosis

1. Epidemiology
   a. Associated with achondroplasia, congenital narrow canal, spondylolisthesis / spondylolysis (typically L5-S1), acromegaly, Paget's disease, ankylosing spondylitis, posttraumatic

b. L4–L5 > L3–L4 > L2–L3 > L5–S1

2. Presentation / Natural history
    a. Presents with neurogenic claudication, less commonly radicular symptoms (lateral recess syndrome)
    b. Treatment typically relieves lower limb pain and halts neurologic progression, less commonly improves neurologic function or relieves back pain
    c. Good or excellent surgical outcome in 70% at 5 years

3. Treatment
    a. Medical with NSAIDs, physical therapy first line if mild symptoms (typically at least 3-month trial)
    b. Surgery involves posterolateral decompression ± foraminotomies for all, posterolateral fusion if evidence of instability and/or spondylolisthesis; adjunct pedicle screw instrumented fusion an option for significant instability (but adds morbidity)
    c. Early ambulation is important to minimize risk of venous thromboembolism, see Lumbar Disk Disease section for risks.

V. Rheumatologic Disease

A. Rheumatoid spine disease

1. Epidemiology
    a. > 85% have radiographic C-spine involvement, including subaxial subluxations and upper involvement (atlantoaxial subluxation, pannus formation, basilar invagination)

2. Presentation / Natural history
    a. Mean onset of atlantoaxial subluxation from diagnosis of rheumatoid arthritis = 15 years, progressive
    b. **Table 5.22** presents the Ranawat scale for neurologic symptoms from rheumatoid arthritis.

Table 5.22 Ranawat Scale for Neurologic Symptoms from Rheumatoid Arthritis

Class	Deficit
I	None
II	Subjective weakness, hyperreflexia, dysesthesia
IIIa	Objective weakness, long tract signs, ambulatory
IIIb	Objective weakness, long tract signs, nonambulatory

3. Treatment
    a. Atlantoaxial subluxation treated via C1–C2 fusion if symptomatic, asymptomatic if atlas-dens interval ≥ 8 mm (range used includes 6–9 mm)
    b. Reduction and extension of surgery to occiput if basilar invagination present
    c. C1–C2 fusions typically done via C1 lateral mass/C2 pars screw fixation, C1–C2 transarticular screws or C2 laminar screws
    d. Transoral odontoidectomy if compression due to pannus or nonreducible basilar invagination; surgical morbidity 5–15%

B. Ankylosing spondylitis

1. Epidemiology
    a. Male preponderance, onset typically in young adult, 90% positive for human leukocyte antigen (HLA) B27

2. Presentation / Natural history
    a. Presenting symptoms include back pain and stiffness with progressive limitation in motion, sacroiliac joint pain, and uveitis
    b. Benign for most patients; progression typically slow
    c. Spinal fractures common in late stages, 75% cervical, can lead to pseudarthroses
    d. Can also develop spinal stenosis from ossification of the posterior longitudinal ligament (OPLL)

3. Treatment
    a. Surgical treatment rarely to correct functionally debilitating fixed flexion deformities (via osteotomies) and repair fractures (external orthoses favored in most cases)

C. OPLL

1. Epidemiology
    a. Prevalence ~2% in asymptomatic adults, incidence ~ 0.5%, increases with age
    b. Higher prevalence in men and Japanese (over 10% Japanese men > age 60)
    c. Average clinical onset age 50, 75% cervical

2. Presentation / Natural history
    a. Typically presents as mild/subjective complaint, can present as progressive myelopathy, radiculopathy, dysesthesia, neck pain
    b. Acute symptomatic onset after minor trauma can occur

3. Treatment
    a. Surgery indicated for myelopathy, refractory radicular pain
    b. Anterior cervical decompression and fusion generally favored for segmental and localized cervical involvement of fewer than three levels, posterior for continuous involvement (laminectomy and expansive laminoplasty options)
    c. Poor recovery in patients > age 65, severe disability, myelopathy > 2 years

D. Diffuse idiopathic skeletal hyperostosis (DISH)

1. Most common in male Caucasians, typically present at 60–70 years

2. 97% involve thoracic spine, 90% lumbar, 78% cervical, all three in 70%

3. Important to neurosurgery as flowing osteophytic fusion creates torque leading to high fracture risk

4. Surgery rarely to remove anterior osteophytes causing dysphagia

VI. Syringomyelia/Hydromyelia

A. Epidemiology

1. Often associated with Chiari malformation, myelomeningocele, tumor, infection, trauma

B. Presentation / Natural history

1. Classically as central cord syndrome

C. Treatment

    1. Craniocervical decompression (for Chiari malformation), syringoperitoneal, syringopleural, and syringosubarachnoid shunts and lysis of subarachnoid adhesions. Patients with multiple adhesions tend to do poorly. Overall results are that 33% improve, 33% remain stable, and 33% continue to deteriorate.

VII. Congenital/Developmental

A. Dysraphism

    1. Epidemiology
        a. Occulta occurs in 20–30% of North Americans.
        b. Myelomeningocele > meningocele, occur in 1/1000 live births, but increases to 2–3% risk with previously affected child, 6–8% with two previous affected children
        c. Most myelomeningoceles have Chiari II malformation and many developmental abnormalities.

    2. Presentation / Natural history
        a. Occulta typically incidental (but can have split cord malformation, tethered cord, etc.)
        b. Hydrocephalus in 75% of myelomeningocele
        c. 80% mortality without treatment, 15% with treatment (80% normal intelligence, 50% some degree of ambulation, 10% continent of urine)

    3. Treatment
        a. Limit examinations of defect until repaired, prophylactic antibiotics if ruptured, keep moist to prevent desiccation, keep pressure off lesion, surgical repair within 36 hours ideal (earlier closure reduces infection rate, no effect on neurologic recovery), often need VP shunt

B. Tethered cord

    1. Epidemiology
        a. Typically pediatric, adult cases reported
        b. Associated with thickened filum or lipoma, most common in myelomeningocele

    2. Presentation / Natural history
        a. Classically presents with lower limb weakness and pain, bladder dysfunction, local cutaneous changes (tuft hair, nevus flammeus, dimple, etc.), cavovarus feet

    3. Treatment
        a. Laminectomy and surgical detethering ± lipoma resection, often recurs as children grow

C. Split cord malformations

    1. Epidemiology
        a. Type I (diastematomyelia) — two hemicords in separate dural tubes separated by osteocartilaginous septum
        b. Type II (diplomyelia) — two hemicords in same dural tube separated by fibrous septum

    2. Presentation / Natural history
        a. Type I often exhibits cutaneous changes, foot deformities like tethered cord, present like tethered cord but can be older age at onset, most in lumbar spine

    3. Treatment
        a. Resection septum, dura reconstituted as single tube if separate, detethering
        b. Watertight closure — CSF leaks common

D. Dermal sinus tracts

    1. Epidemiology

        a. Rare, spine (most lumbar) > occipital, 50% end in dermoids or epidermoids

    2. Presentation / Natural history

        a. Associated with skin dimples, hyperpigmentation, hairy nevi, capillary malformation

        b. Typically present as either cosmetic concern or infection (can lead to meningitis)

    3. Treatment

        a. Resection down to spinal canal with closure of the dura

VIII. Trauma

A. Spinal cord injury (SCI) treatment

    1. Epidemiology

        a. ~14,000/year in North America, cervical most common, peak in young adult men

    2. Presentation / Natural history

        a. The ASIA Impairment Scale is given in **Table 5.23**, and spinal cord injury patterns are outlined in **Table 5.24**.

    3. Treatment

        a. Transport with rigid collar on spine board

        b. If alert, not intoxicated, without neck pain or tenderness, no other major injuries, no underlying condition predisposing to fractures, normal exam including range of motion, then can clear clinically (all others require CT ± MRI)

Table 5.23 ASIA Impairment Scale

Class	Description	Ambulatory at Follow-Up (%)
A	Complete	<3
B	Incomplete (some sensory only, can include perianal)	50
C	Incomplete, > 50% muscles below level of injury have < grade 3 power	75
D	Incomplete, > 50% muscles below level of injury have ≥ grade 3 power	95
E	Normal	100

Note. Level of injury typically described as lowest level with grade 3 or better power.

Table 5.24 Spinal Cord Injury Patterns

Type	Key Findings / Notes
Complete	Entire cross-sectional area of cord affected
Brown–Séquard (hemi) syndrome	Lost contralateral pain/temp, ipsilateral motor/proprioception
Anterior cord syndrome	Lost bilateral motor/pain/temp, preserved proprioception
Posterior cord syndrome	Lost proprioception only
Central cord syndrome	Weakness upper > lower limbs, associated with hyperextension of narrow canal

Abbreviation: temp, temperature.

     c. Early closed reduction with traction recommended for awake / examinable patients who have bony displacement with spinal cord compression

     d. Maintain mean blood pressure at 85–90 mm Hg for up to 7 days to reduce secondary injury

     e. Steroid therapy associated with slight neurologic benefit but significant additional morbidity, thus considered option if can start within 8 hours of SCI (methylprednisolone 30 mg/kg over 1 hour then 5.4 mg/kg/h for 23 hours)

     f. Venous thromboembolism prophylaxis (low-molecular-weight heparin, heparin, pneumatic compression stockings, or vena caval filter)

     g. Surgical decompression/stabilization (indications and timing controversial)

     h. Penetrating injuries — prophylactic broad-spectrum antibiotics, surgery for CSF fistula or neurologic deterioration with retained foreign body

B. Upper cervical spine fractures

   1. Epidemiology

     a. 5–10% of patients with significant head injury have cervical spine injury.

     b. 20% with one injury have another at another level.

   2. Types / Treatment

     a. Occipital condyle fractures

       (1) Typically due to axial load

       (2) Type I — stable comminuted fracture, treated with collar

       (3) Type II — stable basal skull fracture involving condyle, treated with collar

       (4) Type III — alar ligament avulsion of medial condyle fragment, unstable, treated with halo vest for 6–12 weeks

     b. Atlantoaxial dislocation

       (1) Typically due to violent mechanism of injury, frequently fatal or associated with severe neurologic compromise (cervicomedullary syndrome), typically treated with immediate external immobilization prior to surgical reduction/instrumented fusion from occiput to C2

     c. Atlantoaxial rotatory subluxation

       (1) Occur spontaneously (usually children), after trauma, with an upper respiratory infection or in rheumatoid arthritis

       (2) Treat with reduction by traction (7–15 lb in children and 15–20 lb in adults), consider C1–C2 fusion if unable to reduce or subluxation recurs

     d. Jefferson fracture

       (1) Fractures through anterior and posterior arches of C1 caused by axial loading

       (2) Unstable, though usually no neurologic deficit because fractures push bones outward

       (3) Rule of Spence — on open-mouth view, total overhang of both C1 lateral masses > 7 mm = probable transverse ligament disruption and rigid immobilization is required

       (4) Treated with immobilization for 12 weeks if transverse ligament intact (typically with halo vest), surgical C1–C2 fusion if transverse ligament disrupted

     e. Odontoid fracture

       (1) Usually due to flexion injury, classified by Anderson and D'Alonzo

         (a) Type I — through tip of odontoid, rare, usually stable

         (b) Type II — at base of odontoid, least likely to heal with immobilization, 30% nonunion overall with 10% nonunion if < 6 mm displacement, but up to 70% nonunion if ≥ 6 mm displacement. Children < 7 years old usually heal with immobilization. Surgery indicated if age ≥ 50, displacement ≥ 6 mm, instability in halo vest, and nonunion (usually presents with posterior high cervical pain)

(c) Type III — through body of C2. 90% heal with immobilization (halo vest preferred).
(2) Surgical options include odontoid screw (mainly for type II) or posterior C1–C2 fusion.
f. Hangman fracture
(1) Traumatic spondylolisthesis of axis caused by hyperextension and axial loading (classic diving accidents), fracture through pedicle or isthmus (between the superior and inferior articulating processes) of C2, classified by Effendi into three types
(2) Type I — fracture through isthmus with < 3 mm displacement, stable injury, neurologic injury rare, treatment is collar
(3) Type II — fracture through isthmus with disruption of C2–C3 disk and posterior longitudinal ligament (PLL) with increased displacement, slight angulation, and anterolisthesis C2 on C3; may be unstable, neurologic deficit is rare, treated with reduction and halo vest for 12 weeks
(4) Type IIa — fracture has less displacement but more angulation than type II, unstable, treated with reduction and halo vest for 12 weeks
(5) Type III — fracture in which C2–C3 facet capsules disrupted followed by isthmus fracture and possibly anterior longitudinal ligament disruption and C2–C3 locked facets, unstable and most associated with neurologic deficit, treatment typically open surgical reduction of facet dislocation and posterior C1–C2 or C1–C3 instrumented fusion with lateral mass plates/wires

C. Lower cervical spine fractures
a. Treatment depends if stable (generally conservative) or unstable
b. The White and Panjabi Score for lower cervical spine instability is given in **Table 5.25**.

1. Facet dislocation / fracture
a. Occur with flexion ± distraction injuries
b. Unilateral facet dislocation — generally present with radiculopathy, treated with attempted closed reduction with traction. If facet fractures present, injury is likely to heal with 12 weeks of external immobilization (e.g., halo vest). If primarily ligamentous injury or dislocation cannot be reduced, consider open reduction and surgical stabilization with posterior wiring, lateral mass plates, or anterior cervical diskectomy and fusion (particularly if disk herniation present – consider MRI before traction to ensure that no disk material will be pushed into the cord)

Table 5.25 White and Panjabi Score for Lower Cervical Spine Instability*

Element	Point
Anterior elements damaged	2
Posterior elements damaged	2
Sagittal plane translation > 3.5 mm	2
Sagittal plane angulation > 11 degrees	2
Positive stretch test (rarely done)	2
Spinal cord injury	2
Radiculopathy	1
Disk narrowing	1
Dangerous loading anticipated	1

*≥5 = Unstable.

    c. Bilateral facet dislocation — generally presents with spinal cord injury, has anterior displacement that is at least 50% of the vertebral body. Management similar to unilateral locked facets with greater urgency for closed traction-reduction (small risk of reduction-induced disk herniation generally outweighed by urgency to decompress cord)

2. Clay shoveler fracture
    a. Spinous process avulsion, usually C7, caused by hyperflexion or direct trauma, stable if in isolation

3. Simple wedge fracture
    a. Flexion-compression, involves anteroinferior edge of vertebral body, usually stable, treated with collar for 6–12 weeks if flexion–extension x-rays normal, halo fixation if unstable

4. Burst fracture
    a. Compression injury, can cause retropulsed bone into spinal canal, treated with traction to restore height (may pull retropulsed fragments back through ligamentotaxis) followed by external fixation (halo if reduction satisfactory) or anterior fusion (corpectomy if significant retropulsion)

5. Teardrop fracture
    a. Hyperflexion causing injury to disk, facet joints, and all ligaments (highly unstable), associated with small bone chip off anteroinferior vertebral body edge (often mistaken as stable minor avulsion) and posterior displacement of fractured vertebral body into spinal canal. Typically present with severe SCI or anterior cord syndrome. Surgical stabilization required and typically combines anterior decompression and posterior fusion

6. Distraction-extension fracture
    a. Appears similar to teardrop except disk space widens with anterior longitudinal ligament (ALL) disruption (can have anteroinferior vertebral body bone chip avulsion and retrolisthesis of vertebral body), typically treated with closed reduction followed by anterior cervical diskectomy and fusion

D. Thoracolumbar fractures

1. Epidemiology
    a. Most common type = burst fracture
    b. Can be classified using three-column model of Denis:
       (1) Anterior column — anterior half of disk space and vertebral body with anterior anulus and ALL
       (2) Middle column — posterior half of disk space and vertebral body with posterior anulus and PLL
       (3) Posterior column — posterior arch with facets, supraspinous and interspinous ligaments, and ligamentum flavum; injury to this column alone does not cause instability

2. Types / treatment
    a. Compression fracture
       (1) Isolated fracture of anterior column (stable), wedging of vertebral body anteriorly with no loss of posterior height or subluxation, no neurologic deficit is present, treated with early mobilization (orthosis for pain control) with radiographic follow-up
    b. Burst fracture
       (1) Three column compression injury, suggested by > 50% loss of vertebral body height and/or > 20 degrees segmental kyphosis and/or < 50% retained anteroposterior canal diameter due to retropulsed bone (50:20:50 rule). 50% of patients will have neurologic deficits. Generally treated by surgical decompression with instrumented fusion (approaches include posterior relying on ligamentotaxis, transpedicular posterolateral, and anterior – typically retroperitoneal)

  c. Flexion-distraction fracture
   (1) Anterior and middle column compression and posterior column distraction (tensile); unstable, surgery required.
  d. Chance fracture
   (1) Classically described as "seat-belt fracture," flexion injury with anterior column acting as a fulcrum (spinal segment fails in tension), usually no neurologic deficit, abdominal organ injury in ~50%, typically treated by posterior instrumented fusion
  e. Fracture-dislocation
   (1) Failure of all three columns with translation/rotation of spine, most cases have neurologic deficits, treated with reduction and instrumented fusion

Peripheral Nerve Procedures

I. Neoplasia

A. Benign neural sheath tumors

 1. Schwannoma
  a. Epidemiology
   (1) Most common peripheral nerve tumor in adults; associations: NF2 and schwannomatosis
  b. Presentation / Natural history
   (1) Slow growing, benign
   (2) Palpable mass in an extremity, typically on flexor surfaces, often radicular pain or paresthesias (exacerbated by manipulation), typically relatively mobile
  c. Treatment
   (1) Complete surgical resection without complication in ~ 90% cases, pain relief in ~ 90%
   (2) Steps — expose proximal and distal nerve + related structures, separate from uninvolved structures, open capsule longitudinally (in safe area based on intraoperative stimulation, avoid paralytic agents), interfascicular dissection to define mass, stimulation of entering and exiting fascicle (generally nonfunctional), if safe divide fascicle and remove tumor

 2. Neurofibroma
  a. Epidemiology
   (1) Associated with NF1
  b. Presentation / Natural history
   (1) Benign but ~10% transform into malignant peripheral nerve sheath tumor, clinically like schwannoma
  c. Treatment
   (1) Intrafascicular growth — complete resection less achievable than schwannoma without clinical nerve injury (similar technique used)
   (2) Dermal and subcutaneous lesions rarely require surgery

B. Common benign nonneural sheath tumors

 1. Desmoids, myositis ossificans, and osteochondromas
  a. All can encase/adhere to/invade adjacent nerves, treated with careful dissection and resection (radiation for desmoids because highly recurrent)

2. Ganglion cyst
   a. Can be intra- or extraneural, arise near joints, resected like neural sheath tumors

3. Lipoma
   a. Typically compresses nerve (e.g., in carpal tunnel), surgically resected

C. Malignant peripheral nerve sheath tumors

1. Epidemiology
   a. Annual incidence ~1/100,000, 5–10% of soft tissue sarcomas
   b. Generally present in adults, no gender predilection, 50% associated with plexiform neurofibromas in NF1

2. Presentation / Natural history
   a. Typically present as like a benign lesion but more painful, less mobile, some rapid growth
   b. Worse prognosis if > 5 cm size, high grade histology, NF1, lack of tumor-free margin
   c. 5-year survival rate 30–50%, can metastasize

3. Treatment
   a. Surgical goal — en bloc resection with tumor-free margins
   b. Typically add adjuvant radiation / chemotherapy (though benefit minimal)
   c. Metastatic disease typically treated with palliative debulking + chemotherapy / radiation

II. Entrapment Neuropathies

A. Median nerve entrapments

1. Carpal tunnel syndrome
   a. Epidemiology
      (1) Occurs at wrist by transverse carpal ligament, affects distal supply to LOAF muscles (lumbricals 1 and 2, opponens pollicis, and abductor and flexor pollicis brevis)
      (2) Associations include acromegaly, diabetes, pregnancy, hypothyroidism, and rheumatoid arthritis (should rule these out/treat underlying condition first)
   b. Presentation / Natural history
      (1) Dysesthesias (nocturnal), weakness of LOAF muscles, possible thenar atrophy, and hypesthesia (palmar side of hand and fingers lateral to middle of fourth digit)
      (2) Phalen test reproduces symptoms, 60% positive Tinel sign over carpal tunnel syndrome
      (3) Electromyography and nerve conduction studies usually abnormal (normal in 15–25%, Chapter 4 section XXII)
   c. Treatment
      (1) Rest, splinting, NSAIDs ± local steroid injections resolve ~50% cases, ⅓ relapse
      (2) Refractory cases treated with open or endoscopic division of transverse carpal ligament, rare complications include direct injury to nerve or recurrent motor branch

2. Pronator teres syndrome
   a. Entrapment in forearm between two heads of pronator teres, aching/fatiguing with grip weakness and index finger and thumb paresthesias
   b. Absence of nocturnal exacerbation and presence of palm numbness unlike carpal tunnel syndrome
   c. Treated with rest (typically due to repetitive pronation and hand gripping), rarely surgical decompression

3. Compression at Struthers ligament
    a. Ligament connecting medial epicondyle and supracondylar process (present in 2% of population), covers brachial artery and median nerve, requires decompression if symptomatic

4. Anterior interosseous neuropathy
    a. Motor branch of median nerve innervating flexor digitorum profundus 1 and 2, flexor pollicis longus, and pronator quadratus, manifests with "pinch sign" (poor flexion of distal phalanges of thumb and index finger) with no sensory loss
    b. Most resolve expectantly in 8–12 weeks; explore nerve origin and decompress if refractory

B. Ulnar nerve entrapment

1. Findings
    a. Wartenberg sign — abducted fifth digit caused by weak third palmar interosseous
    b. Froment prehensile thumb sign — proximal thumb phalanx extends while distal phalanx flexes when grasping (flexor pollicis longus compensates for adductor pollicis)
    c. Interossei wasting — most evident in thumb web space
    d. Claw hand deformity — fourth, fifth, ± third digits hyperextended at metacarpophalangeal (MCP) joints (extensor digitorum overrides ulnar lumbricals 3 and 4 and interossei) and flexed at interphalangeal joints (pull of long flexors)
    e. Ulnar distribution sensory loss

2. Entrapment locations
    a. Upper arm entrapment — under arcade of Struthers (thin flat aponeurotic band anterior to medial head of triceps), rare but can occur posttransposition
    b. Elbow entrapment — most vulnerable point (nerve superficial, flexed, crossing joint)
        (1) Treated initially conservatively by padding (avoid trauma)
        (2) Treated surgically by dividing medial intermuscular septum and arcade of Struthers proximal to elbow, and aponeurosis connecting two heads of flexor carpi ulnaris distal to elbow (cubital tunnel). Treatment options include decompression, transposition (subcutaneous, intramuscular, and submuscular), or medial epicondylectomy (overall outcomes 60% excellent, 25% fair, 15% poor or no change)
    c. Forearm entrapment — in cubital tunnel distal to elbow between two heads of flexor carpi ulnaris (covered by a facial band)
    d. Guyon canal — roof is palmar fascia and palmaris brevis, floor is flexor retinaculum of palm (above the transverse carpal ligament), treated similar to carpal tunnel syndrome (rare)

C. Radial nerve entrapments

1. Axillary entrapment
    a. Seen with crutch misuse, rare, weakness of triceps (unlike distal sites)

2. Mid–upper arm entrapment
    a. Occurs in spiral groove or at intermuscular septum
    b. Caused by improper positioning during sleep, "Saturday night palsy," or while under general anesthesia
    c. Clinically see wrist-drop without triceps involvement (mimicked by lead poisoning)

3. Forearm entrapment
    a. Posterior interosseous syndrome — finger extension weakness without wrist drop or sensory loss, may be due to constriction at arcade of Frohse, exploration indicated after 8 weeks

    b. Radial tunnel syndrome — tunnel extends from just above elbow to just distal, pain in elbow occurs with little muscle weakness, responds to decompression

D. Suprascapular nerve entrapment

  1. Occurs in suprascapular notch by transverse scapular ligament, causes deep shoulder pain and supraspinatus and infraspinatus muscle atrophy, can be treated by decompression if conservative management fails

E. Meralgia paresthetica (lateral femoral cutaneous nerve entrapment)

  1. Occurs as nerve emerges ~1 cm medial to anterior superior iliac spine (enters thigh between inguinal ligament and anterior superior iliac spine)

  2. Presents with burning dysesthesia in lateral / upper thigh (purely sensory branch – L2, L3)

  3. Risk increases with obesity, diabetes, pregnancy, and prone positioning during surgery

  4. Treatment usually conservative (success 91%) with weight loss, physical therapy, NSAIDs, and steroid injections

  5. Surgical decompression ± transposition if refractory

F. Peroneal nerve entrapment

  1. Involves common peroneal nerve as it passes behind fibular head (superficial and fixed making it vulnerable to trauma or pressure)

  2. Symptoms are weakness (usually extensor hallucis longus, tibialis anterior, toe extensors, and rarely peroneal muscles with weak foot eversion) and sensory changes (less common, involve lateral aspect of lower half of leg)

  3. Surgical decompression for failed conservative management

G. Tarsal tunnel syndrome

  1. Entrapment of posterior tibial nerve posterior and inferior to medial malleolus

  2. Symptoms are pain and paresthesias of toes and sole of foot, intrinsic weakness of foot

  3. Surgery indicated if conservative measures fail (ankle support, etc.)

H. Neurologic thoracic outlet syndrome

  1. Rare, typically unilateral, females more than males, etiologies include constricting band from first rib to cervical rib or C7 transverse process, constriction from pectoralis minor tendon

  2. Usually involves C8/T1 roots, lower trunk of brachial plexus, or medial cord

  3. Symptoms include medial forearm sensory changes, clumsy hand, often positional

  4. Treated with stretching/physical therapy, surgical decompression if refractory (first rib resection, see Chapter 4 section XXI)

III. Traumatic Neuropathies

A. General aspects

  1. Epidemiology

      a. Blunt > penetrating

      b. > 70% have nerve still in gross continuity

2. Natural history

      a. Classification (Chapter 3 section XXXI)

      b. Absence of Tinel sign over nerve suggests no ongoing regeneration

      c. Electromyography and nerve conduction velocities ≥ 3 weeks postinjury can differentiate neuropraxia from denervation (falsely normal if done earlier)

      d. Recovery proceeds as autonomic > sensory > motor function

      e. Target muscle loses ability to accept regenerating fiber after ~18–24 months.

3. Treatment

      a. Clean sharp injuries should be directly repaired (end–end) within days

      b. Contaminated/blunt lacerations should be acutely debrided, tag nerve ends/suture to surrounding tissue to preserve length, repair ~3 weeks later when healthy nerve ends declared/demarcated (often need graft)

      c. For closed injuries, early intervention only for vascular compression (hematoma, pseudoaneurysm, etc.); otherwise establish baseline exam, follow for 3 months to rule out neurapraxic injury; electromyography and nerve conduction studies useful > 3 weeks postinjury; repair in ~ 3 months if no recovery (involves gross evaluation of nerve, neurolysis, electrical studies – if no nerve action potential across injury then resect until fascicular pattern seen and graft (typically sural nerve used) tension-free

B. Brachial plexus injuries (classic)

1. Epidemiology

      a. Typically associated with multiple injuries (violent trauma), often associated with broken clavicle, scapula, humerus

      b. Perinatal brachial plexus injury occurs in ~1/1000 live births, most upper plexus injuries, 90% spontaneous recovery rate (much better than for injuries described below, recovery far better than in adults)

2. Presentation / Natural history

      a. Erb palsy — upper plexus injury (mainly C5–C6), associated with stretch from downward force on shoulder, arm hangs internally rotated with elbow extended, hand strength normal (30% recover spontaneously with evidence by 3–4 months)

      b. Klumpke palsy — lower plexus injury (mainly C8–T1), associated with upward traction of abducted arm, claw deformity (weak hand) ± Horner syndrome (T1), poor recovery

      c. Complete plexus injury — flail limb, most common overall, most severe/least recovery

      d. Determine if root(s) avulsed — this precludes direct surgical repair (suggested by Horner syndrome – interruption of rami communicantes, serratus anterior / rhomboid / phrenic weakness, normal sensory nerve action potentials in anesthetic region, normal motor action potentials – dorsal root ganglion cell / axon intact, pseudomeningoceles on MRI or myelogram)

3. Treatment

      a. As for general nerve injuries

      b. If plexo-plexal repair not possible or root avulsion, can reconstruct with nerve transfer (donors include CNs 11 / 12, cervical plexus, intercostals, phrenic, medial pectoral, sural, etc.), primary goal proximal (shoulder/elbow) stability/function, musculocutaneous nerve best recipient

      c. Good results in > 60% with surgical repair of upper plexus injuries

      d. Poor recovery and poor response to surgery with lower plexus injuries

6 Critical Care

Associate Editor, **Carlo Santaguida**

I. Trauma

A. Basics

1. Monro–Kellie doctrine — There is a fixed volume within the skull and any increase in volume of one intracranial component will require a decrease in another component to maintain normal pressure.

2. Cerebral perfusion pressure CPP = mean arterial pressure (MAP) – intracranial pressure (ICP) = (⅔ diastolic blood pressure [BP] + ⅓ pulse pressure [PP]) – ICP.

3. No clear optimal level for CPP, but should be > 50–70 mm Hg

4. Autoregulation
   a. Cerebral blood flow (CBF) pressure autoregulation is maintained at a constant level despite fluctuation of systolic BP from 50–160 mm Hg.
   b. Viscosity — alteration of vessel diameter in response to changes in blood viscosity
   c. Metabolic — CBF responds to brain metabolic demand.
   d. Blood gas — Hypoxia leads to vasodilatation and P_aCO_2 regulates cerebrovascular tone.

B. Prevention of secondary injury

1. Cerebral edema — peaks several days following injury, generally due to cytotoxic edema. May increase ICP and decrease CPP. Steroids are of no benefit and are detrimental in traumatic brain injury.

2. Hypotension — results in compensatory vasodilatation and increased ICP. Avoided to maintain CPP. Systolic blood pressure (SBP) < 90 mm Hg is associated with a twofold increase in mortality.

3. Hypoxemia — detrimental from the resultant vasodilatation and ICP increase and lack of O_2 to neurons

4. Pyrexia — metabolism increased, resulting in larger energy requirement of brain. 10% increase in metabolism per increased degree centigrade

C. Brain oxygen monitoring — may be measured by jugular venous saturation or brain tissue oxygen tension. Jugular venous saturation < 50% or oxygen tension < 15% is threshold to treat

D. Brain death

1. Considered in presence of catastrophic central nervous system (CNS) event, no medical conditions and no drug intoxication or poisoning that may confound assessment, temperature > 34°C.

2. Clinical exam — Glasgow Coma Score (GCS) 3, absent pupillary light, corneal, oculocephalic, oculovestibular and gag reflexes, absent cough while suctioning, absent sucking or rooting reflexes and fulfill criteria of apnea test.

3. Apnea test — core body temperature > 36.5°C, SBP > 90 and euvolemia. Absence of respiratory response with P_aCO_2 > 60 or increase of 20 mm Hg from baseline

4. May supplement with electroencephalogram, somatosensory or brainstem evoked potentials.

5. No CBF may be documented by cerebral angiography, transcranial Doppler or computed tomographic angiography (CTA) and may be necessary when cannot document other features above.

II. Cardiac

A. Narrow complex/supraventricular tachycardia (SVT) (**Table 6.1** and **Table 6.2**)

Table 6.1 Dysrhythmias

P Wave Type	Dysrhythmia
Uniform	Sinus tachycardia
Multiple forms	Multifocal atrial tachycardia
Inverted	Junctional tachycardia
Sawtooth	Atrial flutter
None	Paroxysmal atrial tachycardia, atrial fibrillation

Table 6.2 Tachydysrhythmias

QRS < 0.12 Seconds (Narrow Complex) Irregular Rhythm	Regular Rhythm	QRS > 0.12 Seconds (Wide Complex) Supraventricular Tachycardia
Atrial fibrillation	Sinus tachycardia	SVT with aberrant conduction
Multifocal atrial tachycardia	Atrial tachycardia	Ventricular tachycardia
Atrial flutter	Atrial flutter	Torsades de pointes
	Junctional tachycardia	

Abbreviation: SVT, supraventricular tachycardia.

1. SVT includes a rate >100 with QRS complex < 0.12 seconds wide (< small 3 squares), and it implies a supraventricular rhythm (originating at or above the atrioventricular [AV] node) because the His-Purkinje system is utilized to allow for fast conduction.

2. Irregular SVT is generally multifocal atrial tachycardia if P waves are present or atrial fibrillation if P waves are not present. Multifocal atrial tachycardia is seen with chronic obstructive pulmonary disease (COPD) and is associated with theophylline. Atrial fibrillation is caused by cardiac disease or hyperthyroidism.

3. Regular SVT has a wider differential, and characterization of P waves may help determine rhythm.

4. If the P wave is normal in rate and morphology then it is likely a sinus tachycardia.

5. If the P waves have a sawtooth pattern with a rate ~250 then it is likely an atrial flutter.

6. If there is no P wave the SVT is likely a junctional tachycardia or a reentrant form.

7. If it is difficult to assess rhythm or there are no visible P waves then you can slow down the rate with vagal maneuvers (i.e., Valsalva or carotid sinus massage) or administer adenosine. If these maneuvers reverse the tachycardia, the underlying condition is likely a reentrant tachycardia.

8. AV reentrant tachycardia has an accessory pathway outside of the AV node, most commonly the bundle of Kent. When there is anterograde conduction through the bundle of Kent, δ waves are present, which is a major characteristic of Wolff–Parkinson–White syndrome.

9. If SVT is in an unstable patient then cardioversion is indicated.

10. If stable then attempt to establish the diagnosis and treat with β-blocker (metoprolol) or Ca^{2+} channel blocker (verapamil).

B. Wide complex tachycardia

1. Wide complex tachycardia (> 0.12 seconds or 3 small squares QRS duration) is often a ventricular rhythm but may also be an SVT with aberrancy (bundle branch block), a pacemaker, or relating to AV reentrant tachycardia.

2. Ventricular tachycardia (VT) may often be caused by QT prolongation from hypomagnesia, hypokalemia, or iatrogenic (quinidine, digoxin).

3. Polymorphic VT is generally found in an unstable patient following myocardial ischemia but may be seen in Torsades de pointes when a prolonged QT interval is present. May resolve with K^+ or Mg^{2+} replacement.

4. In the stable patient, elective synchronized cardioversion is appropriate treatment for VT. If the patient is unstable, then conscious synchronized cardioversion is recommended; defibrillation if patient is unconscious.

C. Bradycardia

1. Bradycardia — heart rate < 60. If associated P wave with every beat then it is a sinus bradycardia. Sign of increased ICP. Common in athletes or iatrogenic relating to drugs, it may be due to sick sinus syndrome in patients with heart disease.

2. If intermingled with SVT known as tachycardia–bradycardia syndrome.

3. If PR interval longer than 0.2 seconds then it is first degree AV block.

4. Second degree AV block is divided into Wenckebach and Mobitz.

5. Wenckebach is a cyclic progressive blocking of conduction at an AV node, which results in a dropped QRS, characterized by progressive lengthening of the PR interval.

6. Mobitz refers to a series of P waves that cannot conduct through an AV node.

7. Third AV degree block is a complete dissociation of P and QRS waves generally resulting in an escape junctional rhythm.

8. If the patient is symptomatic may treat with atropine, transcutaneous pacer, dopamine, or epinephrine drip. If the patient is not symptomatic but has a Mobitz or third degree AV block may need transvenous pacer.

D. Other electrocardiogram (ECG) findings

1. Digoxin — gradual downward curve of ST segment; causes multiple dysrhythmias and AV blocks

2. Hypocalcemia — increased QT interval

3. Hypokalemia — U-wave

4. Hyperkalemia — peaked T-wave

5. Hypothermia — J-point elevation

6. Hyperthyroidism — atrial fibrillation

7. Quinidine toxicity — prolonged QT interval, notched P wave, wide QRS, ST depression

8. Subendocardial ischemia — ST depression

9. Transmural ischemia — ST elevation

10. Pericarditis — flat or concave ST segment elevation often in all leads

11. Brugada syndrome — right bundle branch block with ST elevation in V1–V3 predisposes to sudden cardiac death

12. Long Q-T syndrome — QT interval is > 50% of cardiac cycle, predisposes to arrhythmias

13. Wellens syndrome — T wave inversion in V2–V3 due to anterior descending coronary artery stenosis

14. Subarachnoid hemorrhage (SAH) — shows peaked T wave and ST depression

15. Pulmonary embolism — Most frequent ECG changes are nonspecific ST and T changes (66%), tachycardia (63%), and rarely the classic "S1Q3T3."

E. Cardiac medications

1. Antiarrhythmics — class 1 (Na^+-channel blockers), class 1A (quinidine and procainamide; may lead to reversible K+-channel blockade resulting in prolonged QT), class 2 (β-blocker), class 3 (K^+-channel blocker such as amiodarone, sotalol), class 4 (Ca^{2+}-channel blockers)

2. Adrenergic receptors – $α_1$-receptor stimulation leads to vasoconstriction. $β_1$ receptors increase cardiac rate (chronotropy) and strength of contraction (inotropy). $β_2$ receptors vasodilate.

3. Dopamine receptor — leads to vasodilatation in cerebral, renal, coronary, and mesenteric vasculature

4. Dobutamine — $β_1$ agonist, mild β + $α_2$ agonist, inotropic, causes peripheral vasodilation (reduces afterload), increases cardiac output (CO) with a reflex decrease in systemic vascular resistance (SVR), no change in BP. Side effects include tachycardia if hypovolemic. Contraindications include hypertrophic cardiomyopathy. Dose is 5–15 µg/kg/min up to 40.

5. Dopamine — causes renal, splanchnic, and cerebral vasodilation, increased renal Na^+ excretion independent of blood flow and vasoconstriction with higher doses. Useful with cardiogenic or septic shock. Doses are 1–2 µg/kg/min for renal effect and selective vasodilatation. Doses of 5–10 µg/kg/min have more $β_1$ effect leading to higher stroke volume; 10–20 µg/kg/min for $α_1$ and $β_1$ effects. Side effects include tachydysrhythmias.

6. Epinephrine — Strong $β_1$, moderate $β_2$ + $α_1$, drug of choice for anaphylaxis. $α_1$ effects predominate over $β_2$ at higher doses. Dose is 3–5 mL of 1:1000 or 2–4 µg/min. Side effects include myocardial ischemia, dysrhythmia, and acute renal failure.

7. Phenylephrine — Mostly a_1 effects with minimal effects on inotropy and chronotropy.

8. Norepinephrine — Agonist for $α_1$ and $β_1$ receptors, may lead to reflex bradycardia following increase in MAP. Drug of choice in septic shock. Dose is 8–70 µg/min. Use with dopamine 1 µg/kg/min for renal protection. Contraindications include renal failure.

9. Vasopressin — noradrenergic pressor, appropriate for late vasodilatory shock

10. Digitalis — When therapeutic it slows AV conduction and sinoatrial node. If serum levels are excessive then may cause AV block, sinus block, and premature atrial beats. Hypokalemia enhances digoxin toxicity. Digitalis toxicity may cause ventricular tachycardia and fibrillation. Treatment is with K^+, Mg^{2+}, lidocaine, digoxin antibody, and charcoal.

11. Furosemide — a diuretic that increases SVR and decreases CO. Diuresis occurs in 20 minutes–2 hours. Nonsteroidal antiinflammatories (NSAIDs) may block the response. Use for early oliguric renal failure. Dose is 1 mg/kg. Side effects include ototoxicity, hypokalemia, hypomagnesemia, hypochloremia, and metabolic alkalosis. Contraindications include sulfa allergy, hepatorenal syndrome, and edema from nephrotic syndrome.

12. Glucagon — increases heart rate and contractility independent of its β effect. It reverses a β-blocker overdose to help as an inotrope, but not a chronotrope. Consider use with electromechanical dissociation. Dose is 1–5 μg up to 1–20 μg/h mixed with 10 mL saline intravenously (IV). Side effects include hypokalemia and hyperglycemia.

13. Labetalol — blocks α and β receptors to lower BP and does not increase heart rate or change CO. Dose is 2 mg/min or 20–80 mg every 10 minutes up to 300 mg IV.

14. Nitroglycerine — relaxes arteries (> 200 μg/min) and veins (< 50 μg/min) and increases coronary blood flow. Use with myocardial ischemia/infarction (if normotensive), pulmonary hypertension, and heart failure. Dose is 10–200 μg/min. There is decreased tolerance with intermittent infusion (12 hours on/12 hours off) or N-acetylcysteine that replenishes sulfhydryl groups in vessel walls. Side effects include methemoglobinemia that causes cyanosis with a normal blood gas when it is >10% (70% is usually fatal). Treat with methylene blue, 2 mg/kg IV over 10 minutes. Contraindications include increased ICP and closed-angle glaucoma.

15. Sodium nitroprusside — dilates arteries and veins, increases stroke volume, and does not change heart rate. Drug of choice for hypertensive emergencies. Dose is 2–3 μg/kg/min for < 72 hours. Side effects include cyanide toxicity, especially in smokers with decreased thiosulfate. Cyanide is converted to thiocyanate in the liver and is excreted from the kidneys. Symptoms include headache, nausea, vomiting, weakness, hypotension, lactic acidosis, and tolerance to nitroprusside. Keep the cyanide < 5 μg/mL. Prevent toxicity by mixing with 1% thiosulfate solution. Also try to keep the B_{12} level normal. Thiocyanate toxicity causes acute renal failure, mental status changes and occurs with levels >10 mg/dL. Contraindications include B_{12} deficiency and renal failure.

F. Cardiopulmonary resuscitation (CPR) — 30% survive and 10% recover to baseline. Postresuscitation injury is caused by poor reflow from vasoconstriction (treatment is with Ca^{2+}-channel blockers or Mg^{2+}) and reperfusion injury by free radicals. Consider giving $MgSO_4$ 2 g IV over 20 minutes to prevent "no reflow" from vasoconstriction. Consider Ca^{2+}- channel blockers when not hypotensive. Steroids and barbiturates have not been shown to be of value. Prognosis is related to the ischemic time before and during CPR. 30% of patients in postresuscitation coma regain consciousness. After 48 hours, only 2–7% of patients still in a coma recover; after 7 days, none recover.

G. Air embolism — associated with dyspnea, substernal chest pain, millwheel murmur, focal neurologic deficits, and cardiorespiratory failure. May be diagnosed with echocardiography (presence of air, ventricular dilatation, pulmonary artery hypertension), end tidal CO_2 (fall in end-tidal CO_2), computed tomography (CT) scan, and pulmonary angiography. The most sensitive monitor is the precordial Doppler. Treated with left lateral decubitus position, nitrogen washout (high flow O_2), hyperbaric O_2, or aspiration of air from venous circulation. Mortality rate is 15%.

III. Respiratory

A. Oxygenation

1. O_2 content = 1.34[Hb g/dL] × O_2 saturation + (0.003 × PaO_2) = O_2 mL/100 mL

2. O_2 delivery = O_2 content × CO. Normal 520–570 mL/min/m^2

3. O_2 uptake = CO × (arterial O_2 content – venous O_2 content). Normal 110–160 mL/min/m^2

4. O_2 extraction ratio = Uptake/Delivery × 100 (22–32%)

5. If the O_2 extraction ratio exceeds 60%, uptake becomes dependent on delivery.

6. All tissues increase O_2 extraction in the face of decreased blood flow except the coronary circulation, which is always at its maximal extraction rate (flow dependent).

7. Mixed venous O_2 is measured in the pulmonary artery, and normal is 68–77%. It is lower with hypoxemia, increased metabolic rate, decreased CO, and anemia.

8. Lactate increases if the O_2 delivery is less than the metabolic demand and the cells are forced to use anaerobic glycolysis. Normal blood level is < 2 mmol/L, and > 4 mmol/L is abnormal.

9. Lactate may be elevated without hypoxemia, but with hepatic insufficiency (decreased clearance), thiamine deficiency (interferes with glucose metabolism), infection (endotoxin release affects glucose metabolism), and respiratory alkalosis.

10. The plateau of the oxygen–hemoglobin dissociation curve begins at PO_2 60 mm Hg, and O_2 saturation 90%. Below this point, the O_2 saturation drops much more quickly with decreases in O_2 pressure.

11. Bohr effect
    a. Right shift — occurs in tissues and there is decreased O_2 affinity. A right shift occurs with increases in H^+, CO_2, temperature, and 2,3-diphosphoglycerate (DPG).
    b. Left shift — occurs in the lung and there is increased O_2 affinity. A left shift occurs with decreases in H^+, CO_2, temperature, and DPG, as well as with banked blood (due to decreased DPG). Hemoglobin has less affinity for O_2 in the tissues where there are higher H^+ and CO_2 levels.

12. Oximetry detects red oxyhemoglobin and infrared deoxyhemoglobin in a photodetector. Pulse oximetry samples only pulsatile vessels (arteries) because it detects volume fluctuations. It is not affected by most skin tissue thickness, pigments, or nail polish. Oximetry becomes less accurate when the O_2 saturation is below 70%.

13. Nasal cannula providing 100% O_2 at 1–6 L/min produces a FiO_2 of 0.21–0.46.

14. The maximum FiO_2 that can be achieved with a nasal cannula is 46%. This is with 6 L/min minute ventilation, and it is even less with tachypnea.

15. Standard mask providing 5–10 L/min of 100% O_2 can produce a FiO_2 of 40–60%. This level is lowered with increased respiratory rates caused by inhalation of ambient air.

16. Partial rebreather mask (no ambient air allowed, rebreathing done into mask) at 5–7 L/min provides a FiO_2 of 75%.

17. Nonrebreather mask (no ambient air allowed, exhaled breath is not reinhaled) at 4–10 L/min provides a FiO_2 of 100%.

B. Ventilation

1. Anatomic dead space (= 150 mL) includes the trachea, bronchi, and distal parts of the respiratory tree that are not used for gas exchange.

2. Physiologic dead space includes the alveoli where gas is not equilibrating with the capillary blood.

3. Total dead space normally makes up 20–30% of minute ventilation. In the normal alveoli, the arterial and expired PCO_2 are equal because no dead space is present.

4. Increased dead space is caused by overdistended alveoli (COPD and positive end-expiratory pressure [PEEP]), destroyed alveolar–capillary interface (emphysema), or decreased blood flow (congestive heart failure, pulmonary embolus).

5. The O_2 pressure in the alveolus — $(P_AO_2) = FiO_2 (Pb - P_{water}) - (P_aCO_2/RQ) = 0.21 (713 \text{ mm Hg}) - P_aCO_2/0.8$, where Pb is atmospheric pressure and RQ is the respiratory quotient.

6. The A-a gradient is the alveolar to arterial O_2 gradient $(P_AO_2 - P_aO_2)$. The $P_AO_2 = FiO_2 (Pb - P_{water}) - (P_aCO_2/RQ)$ and is normally 100 mm Hg at FiO_2 of 0.21 producing an A-a gradient of 10–20 mm Hg. The normal A-a gradient increases 6 mm Hg for each 10% increase in FiO_2 and is 60–70 mm Hg at a FiO_2 of 1.0. Increased FiO_2 causes an increased A-a gradient because there is less hypoxic vasoconstriction in the poorly ventilated areas.

7. In hypoxemia if the A-a gradient is normal, there is likely no primary cardiopulmonary problem so consider neuromuscular or central nervous system (CNS) causes. If there is an increased A-a gradient and the venous PO_2 is > 40 mm Hg, the problem is caused by increased dead space or shunting. If the venous PO_2 is < 40, the problem is caused by decreased blood flow or a high metabolic rate.

8. Hypercapnia can be caused by increased production of CO_2 from sepsis, trauma, burns, increased carbohydrate intake, and acidosis.

9. $RQ = VCO_2/VO_2$ and is the ratio of molecules of CO_2 created for each O_2 used. Normal is 0.8; carbohydrates are 1, proteins are 0.8, and lipids are 0.7. Therefore, an increased carbohydrate load creates more CO_2 molecules to expel.

10. Hypercapnia can also be caused by hypoventilation with a normal A-a gradient as with sleep apnea, myasthenic syndrome, Guillain–Barré syndrome, phrenic nerve injury, peripheral neuropathy, muscle weakness (from decreased phosphate or Mg^{2+}, sepsis, and shock), opiates, and lidocaine.

C. Pulmonary disorders

1. Acute lung injury (ALI) — defined as lung inflammation resulting in increased pulmonary capillary permeability. Characterized by bilateral chest infiltrates with pulmonary capillary wedge pressure (PCWP) < 18 mm Hg (or no suspected heart failure) and PaO_2/FiO_2 between 201 and 300 mm Hg

2. Acute respiratory distress syndrome (ARDS) — more severe ALI with worsening hypoxia (PaO_2/FiO_2 < 200 mm Hg). There is diffuse alveolar damage. Protein leaves vascular space losing colloid osmotic pressure gradient, which prevents fluid reabsorption from alveoli. The alveoli fill with inflammatory fluid. Acute onset and may persist for weeks. Causes include sepsis, aspiration, infectious pneumonia, trauma, burns, and pancreatitis. Mortality rate is over 30%.

3. Differentiating ARDS from cardiogenic pulmonary edema — pleural effusions more common in heart failure and PCWP >18 mm Hg. ARDS has high protein levels from bronchioalveolar lavage (**Table 6.3**).

Table 6.3 Acute Respiratory Distress Syndrome (Capillary Leakage) versus Hydrostatic Edema

ARDS	Hydrostatic Edema
Early hypoxemia	Late
Diffuse infiltrate	Patchy
Peripheral vascular prominence	Perihilar vascular prominence
No Kerley B lines	Kerley B lines
Clear lung bases	Obscured bases
More protein in fluid	Less protein in fluid
Associated with sepsis, trauma, and multisystem organ failure	Associated with hypertension, myocardial infarction, and acute renal failure

Abbreviation: ARDS, acute respiratory distress syndrome.

4. Diuretics are of no benefit in ARDS because the fluid leaking into the alveoli is the result of acute inflammation.

5. CO can be increased (with dobutamine) to increase the O_2 delivery.

6. Vasodilators are not indicated because they may increase the pulmonary shunt fraction.

7. Steroids have not been proven to be of benefit.

8. Cheyne–Stokes breathing — gradually increasing and decreasing tidal volume mixed with periods of apnea. Often an ominous sign, the respiratory center does not respond properly to PCO_2 or PO_2.

D. Respiratory medications

1. β_2-agonists — work best when inhaled with a nebulizer such as albuterol 5 mg (0.1 mL of 5%) every 4 hours. Also consider terbutaline, metaproterenol, and isoetharine. At high doses they may stimulate β_1-receptors and cause tachycardia, hypokalemia, or tremors. If this happens, decrease the dose. They work best with asthma, but occasionally help with COPD.

2. Theophylline — questionable benefit for asthma. Works by increasing the cyclic adenosine monophosphate (cAMP) level. Side effects include seizures, dysrhythmias, hypokalemia, and hypotension. These are much more likely with a level > 20. Treat overdose with oral charcoal 20 g orally every 2 hours for 6 doses, even if it is already removed from the blood.

3. Anticholinergics — atropine 0.025–0.075 mg/kg inhaled every 3 hours. Ipratropium, 0.02–0.03 mg/kg inhaled every 3 hours (less systemic side effects). They work by decreasing the parasympathetic input that constricts small airways.

4. Steroids — synergistic with β-agonists in the treatment of asthma but not with COPD, ARDS, sepsis, or anaphylaxis. Hydrocortisone 2 mg/kg IV or 0.5 mg/kg hourly; methylprednisolone 40–125 mg IV every 6 hours.

5. Doxapram — stimulates both peripheral chemoreceptors and brainstem respiratory centers. Side effects include hypertension, tachycardia, and seizures. The dose is 1–3 mg/min IV up to 600 mg.

6. *N*-acetylcysteine inhaler — The dose is 2.5 mL of 10% and 2.5 mL normal saline via nebulizer. It may cause bronchospasm with reactive airway disease or asthma. Overuse for more than 2 days increases airway irritation. It helps with mucous plugs and thick secretions. Humidification alone helps to break up sputum to a lesser extent.

7. Heliox — a combination of helium and O_2 that results in a reduction of turbulent air flow. Greatest benefit in acute upper airway obstruction

E. Paralytics, sedatives, muscle relaxants

   1. Side effects — decreased ability to clear pulmonary secretions even with suctioning (increased risk of pneumonia and mucous plug) and increased risk of venous thromboemboli

   2. Halothane — causes central depression and bronchodilation

   3. Vecuronium — a nondepolarizing blocker, has the least histamine release, dose is 0.1 mg/kg, duration is 30 minutes

   4. Pancuronium — a nondepolarizing blocker, dose is 0.01 to 0.05 mg/kg every hour, duration is 1 hour, side effects include tachycardia

   5. Succinylcholine — a depolarizing blocker, short acting, increases the K^+ level; contraindicated with hyperkalemia, hemiplegia, or other neurologic disorders associated with weakness

   6. Reversal agents — used to counteract muscle paralysis of competitive acetylcholine receptor blockade. The local acetylcholine levels are increased by acetylcholinesterase inhibitors such as neostigmine 2.5–5 mg/70 kg. Pretreat with atropine (0.6–1.5 mg/70 kg) to prevent bradycardia from the increased parasympathetic stimulation by the increase in acetylcholine levels. Onset may be delayed 15–30 minutes.

   7. Haloperidol — does not cause respiratory depression or hypotension (unless used with propranolol). Dose is 3–5 mg IV up to 10 mg, wait 20 minutes and double the dose. If this is ineffective, change agents or add benzodiazepines. There are less extrapyramidal side effects with the IV route. This condition is associated with neuroleptic malignant syndrome characterized by hyperthermia, muscle rigidity autonomic dysfunction, and confusion. This condition may occasionally be fatal and should be treated with dantrolene. Haloperidol also lowers seizure threshold.

   8. Diazepam — 1–10 mg IV

   9. Lorazepam — 0.04–0.05 mg/kg, good amnestic

   10. Midazolam — 1 mg IV every 3 hours up to 0.15 mg/kg or 0.4 µg/min, good amnestic

   11. Morphine — increases histamine release and worsens asthma

K. Mechanical ventilation

   1. Four modes — volume-, pressure-, time-, or flow-cycled

   2. Volume-cycled — Ventilation is entirely dependent on preset tidal volume, respiratory rate, and inspiratory flow.

      a. Controlled mechanical ventilation — Ventilation is only dependent on rate and tidal volume settings, which is appropriate if the patient is not making respiratory efforts.

    b. Assist-control — A preset tidal volume is delivered when patient attempts to make inspiratory effort.

    c. Intermittent mandatory ventilation — Preset tidal volume and rate is delivered at a regular interval and patient may breathe spontaneously as well.

3. Flow-cycled — pressure support once the patient triggers a breath, a preset pressure is delivered until flow tapers

4. Tidal volume — normally at 5–6 cc/kg in humans

5. Rate — Start at 12 for adults.

6. Sigh — a breath 1.5 × tidal volume, not shown to be of benefit

7. Monitoring lung mechanics — assess without mechanical ventilation. Test lung volume for elastic recoil and expiratory flow rate for resistance.

8. Proximal airway pressure — The peak end-inspiratory pressure is proportional to the inflation volume, the resistance of the airways, and the lung and chest wall compliance. It is proportional to $R + 1/C$, where R is airway resistance and C is lung and chest wall compliance.

    a. At a constant volume, an increased inflation pressure is due to either increased resistance or decreased compliance.

    b. The plateau pressure is proportional to $1/C$.

    c. Increased plateau pressure is due to decreased compliance. Increased peak pressure with no change in plateau pressure is due to increased airway resistance.

    d. Increased peak and increased plateau pressures are due to decreased lung/chest wall compliance. Compliance = Volume change/Pressure change = tidal volume/plateau pressure cm H_2O. Normal is 0.05–0.07 L/cm H_2O.

9. Acute respiratory failure — usually caused by pneumonia, edema, and COPD. These do not respond to steroids or bronchodilators. If the patient is not on a ventilator, check for airway obstruction at the bedside with a peak expiratory flow rate (positive if >15% increase noted). If the patient is on a ventilator, assess the peak inspiratory pressure.

10. If there is a sudden respiratory deterioration:

    a. Peak pressure increased with normal plateau pressure — likely increased airway resistance. Treat with suction or bronchodilation.

    b. Peak and plateau pressure increased — likely decreased compliance or auto PEEP (with obstructive lung disease). Likely due to pneumothorax, atelectasis, edema, or abdominal distension

    c. Peak pressure decreased — assess for air leak

11. PEEP should help increase compliance and decrease plateau pressure. In determining efficacy, be sure to subtract the PEEP setting from the measured plateau pressure to obtain the correct value.

12. Increased PEEP causes decreased preload and decreased contractility (by decreasing coronary blood flow). Determine the O_2 delivery and assess if there is decreased plateau pressure (from increased compliance) to find best PEEP setting. The O_2 saturation value may be misleading because it may be associated with decreased O_2 delivery. The relationship between O_2 saturation and O_2 delivery depends on the cardiac output (**Table 6.4**).

Table 6.4 Relationship between O$_2$ Saturation and O$_2$ Delivery

O$_2$ Saturation	Cardiac Output	O$_2$ Delivery
Increased	No change	Increased
Increased	Decreased	No change
Increased	More decreased	Decreased

13. PEEP is not very effective for localized disease. It works mainly on the normal areas of the lung, over-distending the alveoli and redirecting the blood to areas with poor ventilation. Complications include barotrauma, fluid retention (by atrial compression that increases atrial natriuretic factor secretion), decreased CO, and increased ICP.

14. After extubation, the most frequent respiratory problem is laryngeal edema. When severe, treatment is with reintubation or emergent tracheotomy. Epinephrine and steroids are not proven to be helpful.

15. Tracheotomy
    a. benefits — clearing of secretions, decreased laryngeal injury and better patient comfort
    b. Complications — 5% of cases, include pneumothorax, laryngeal injury, nerve injury, hemorrhage, decannulation, and tracheal stenosis

16. Barotrauma — occurs in 43% of patients if the peak inspiratory pressure is > 70 cm H$_2$O, and in 0% if it is < 40 cm H$_2$O. Assess for subcutaneous emphysema, interstitial emphysema, pneumothorax, and pneumoperitoneum.

17. Weaning from the ventilator — Typical parameters are PO$_2$ > 60 mm Hg with FiO$_2$ < 0.6 without PEEP, tidal volume > 5 mL/kg, vital capacity >10 mL/kg, minute ventilation < 10 L/min, and negative inspiratory force > 25 mm H$_2$O. 30% that fulfill these parameters still fail, and 30% who do not fulfill them tolerate extubation. Consider a continuous positive airway pressure (CPAP) trial and check arterial blood gases in 30 minutes as opposed to intermittent mandatory ventilation or pressure support weaning.

IV. Renal

A. Creatinine clearance = (140 – age) × weight (kg)/ 72 × serum creatinine (mg/dL)

B. Fractional excretion = (urine Na$^+$/plasma Na$^+$)/(urine creatinine/plasma creatinine) × 100

C. Oliguria — urine production < 400 mL/24 hours

D. Anuria — defined as urine output < 100 mL/24 hours

E. Prerenal causes of renal failure — decreased renal blood flow from hypovolemia, vasodilation, and heart failure, or iatrogenic with drugs that lower glomerular filtration pressure (angiotensin converting enzyme inhibitors). Urine Na$^+$ is < 20 meq/L and the fractional excretion of Na$^+$ is < 1%.

F. Renal causes of renal failure — acute tubular necrosis (ATN; caused by sepsis, toxins, drugs, and myoglobin), acute interstitial nephritis (caused by an immunogenic reaction to penicillins, NSAIDs, furosemide, and cimetidine; associated with fever, rash, eosinophilia, and arthralgia) and acute glomerulonephritis. The urine Na$^+$ is > 40 meq/L and the fractional excretion of Na$^+$ is > 2%.

G. Postrenal conditions — obstruction of urine outflow; acutely may appear like a prerenal condition and chronically like a renal condition

H. When there is decreased renal blood flow, Na+ resorption increases and urine Na+ decreases. In renal failure, there is decreased Na+ resorption and increased urine Na+ (but this is also seen with diuretics).

I. Urine microscopic examination is helpful in determining the condition (**Table 6.5**).

Table 6.5 Urine Microscopic Examination

Condition	Cast Type
Prerenal	Hyaline and finely granular casts
Renal	
ATN	Epithelial and coarse granular casts
Acute interstitial nephritis	White cell casts
Acute glomerulonephritis	Red cell casts
Postrenal	No casts

Abbreviation: ATN, acute tubular necrosis.

J. Approach to acute renal failure

1. Rule out hypovolemia by raising the PCWP to >15 mm Hg and the central venous pressure (CVP) to >10 mm Hg. If the CO is decreased in the face of euvolemia, evaluate for myocardial infarction and cardiac tamponade. If CO is impaired, then treat with dobutamine if normotensive or dopamine if hypotensive.

2. Assess the urine electrolytes and microscopic examination.

3. Furosemide increases renal tubular flow and decreases the back pressure in the glomeruli. Consider giving volume with colloid or mannitol. Furosemide at high doses may decrease the CO and may increase vasoconstriction, so avoid its use in the presence of hypovolemia.

4. Discontinue nephrotoxic drugs — Change aminoglycosides to aztreonam, discontinue amphotericin B for 24 hours and then restart it at half dose and alternate pentamidine and sulfamethoxazole.

5. Consider dialysis in acute renal failure in the following conditions: K^+ > 6.5 meq/L, metabolic acidosis (pH < 7.1), refractory hypervolemia azotemia (blood urea nitrogen [BUN] > 80 mg/dL), Na^+ < 120 meq/L or >155 meq/L, and overdose of dialyzable drug.

K. Drug adjustments in acute renal failure — Discontinue Mg^{2+} antacids and use AlOH or sucralfate, decrease the digoxin dose to 25% or change to verapamil, change sodium nitroprusside to trimethaphan camsylate and lower the procainamide dose to 50%; closely follow the *N*-acetylprocainamide (NAPA) levels.

L. Rhabdomyolysis — consider if creatinine increases >1 mg/dL, BUN increases > 30 mg/100 mL, and K^+ increases > 0.5 mEq/L – all in 24 hours. There is elevated creatine phosphokinase and aldolase (only found in skeletal muscle). Treatment is with aggressive hydration. May lead to ATN-like illness

M. Renal tubular acidosis (RTA)

1. Type 1 (distal) — nonanion gap metabolic acidosis, hypokalemia, increased nephrocalcinosis, and urine pH > 5.5

2. Type 2 (proximal) — nonanion gap metabolic acidosis, hypokalemia, and a defect in reabsorption of HCO_3^-

3. Type 3 — combined proximal and distal, known as juvenile RTA

4. Type 4 (hypoaldosteronism) — nonanion gap metabolic acidosis, hyperkalemia

N. Loop diuretics — Compete with chloride on the Na-K-2Cl pump interfering with Na⁺ absorption at thick ascending limb of the Loop of Henle. Furosemide is the most commonly used loop diuretic and it may lead to excretion of 20% of filtered Na⁺.

O. Thiazide diuretics — Inhibit Na^+-Cl^- cotransporter leading to excretion of 5% of filtered Na⁺. These diuretics are significantly less potent then loop diuretics; contraindicated in anuria, renal insufficiency, gout, hypercholesterolemia, hypokalemia, and systemic lupus erythematosus (may exacerbate symptoms).

P. K⁺-sparing diuretics – Amiloride or spironolactone interfere with the function of Na⁺ channels in the cortical collecting tubule. Spironolactone disrupts the Na⁺ channels through competitively inhibiting the mineralocorticoid receptors.

Q. Osmotic diuretics — Mannitol is nonreabsorbable and interferes with the water gradient in the proximal tubule and the loop of Henle leading to the excretion of water in excess of Na⁺.

R. Urodynamic testing — Uroflowmetry measures rate of urine flow, cystometrogram measures bladder filling pressure, pressure-flow study determines if reduced flow is due to obstruction or detrusor weakness.

S. Treat urinary retention due to neurogenic or atonic bladder with bethanechol.

V. Gastrointestinal

A. Stress ulcers

1. Caused by mucosal ischemia that decreases mucus formation and leads to superficial erosions.

2. The hemorrhage rate of stress ulcers is 20% and the massive hemorrhage rate is 5%. The hemorrhage rate can be lowered to 5% with H2 blockers or antacids, both are equally effective. Antacids have been shown to be more effective in decreasing occult blood. Both have the same efficacy for preventing frank blood. Enteral feedings are as helpful as H2 blockers and antacids.

3. Cytoprotective therapy (sucralfate) causes an increase in mucosal blood flow that may be prostaglandin mediated. It is very effective if the problem is caused by barrier breakdown and not by increased acid secretion. Benefits include normal pH, lowest cost, and no known side effects. In a low flow state, the splanchnic bed is affected first.

4. Gastric emptying is considered adequate if one can aspirate < 50% of the infused volume (50–100 mL) after 30 minutes.

B. Pseudomembranous colitis

1. Caused by *Clostridium difficile*

2. Characterized by fever, leukocytosis, watery diarrhea, and abdominal pain. It may progress to toxic megacolon and require surgery. Evaluate by sending the *C. difficile* toxin for culture or doing colonoscopy.

3. Treatment is with isolation, discontinuation of antibiotics (except aminoglycosides) and start oral vancomycin, 500 mg every 6 hours or oral or IV metronidazole 500 mg every 6 hours for 7–14 days. Cholestyramine binds the toxin but also binds the antibiotics, so only use it between doses.

VI. Shock States and Body Fluids

A. Shock (**Table 6.6**)

1. Shock occurs when inadequate tissue perfusion results in decreased tissue oxygen delivery to tissues. Mortality rate from shock is 35–40%

Table 6.6 Cardiovascular Findings with Different Types of Shock

Shock Type	HR	SVR	CO	CVP
Cardiac	↓	↑	↓	↑
Hypovolemic	↑	↑	↔/↓	↓
Septic	↑	↓	↑	↔/↓

Abbreviations: HR, heart rate; SVR, systemic vascular resistance; CO, cardiac output; CVP, central venous pressure.

2. Hypovolemic shock is characterized by decreased PCWP, decreased CO, and increased SVR. Causes include hemorrhage, fluid loss, and third spacing.

3. Cardiogenic shock has increased PCWP, decreased CO, and increased SVR. It is caused by myopathic (severe myocardial infarction), arrhythmic, mechanical (severe valve regurgitation), obstructive (pulmonary embolus, tension pneumothorax, cardiac tamponade) conditions.

4. Distributive (vasodilatory) shock has decreased PCWP, increased CO, and severely decreased SVR. Causes include septic shock, anaphylaxis, and neurogenic causes, following spinal cord injury.

5. Assess by determining PCWP, CO, SVR, oxygen delivery and uptake, and lactate level.

6. O_2 extraction is normally 22–32%.

7. Serum lactate level is normally 0–4 mEq/L.

8. Mixed venous PO_2 is normally 33–53 mm Hg and mixed venous O_2 saturation is 68–77%.

9. The treatment is goal-directed to achieve central venous pressure >8 + central venous oxygen saturation >70%.

10. If there is decreased CO with an increased SVR, use dobutamine (a pure β-agonist that increases CO, decreases BP, and decreases SVR).

11. If the SVR is normal, use dopamine (the α contribution increases SVR).

12. If the SVR is decreased, use dopamine or norepinephrine (NE) because both have α and β effects.

B. Anaphylaxis — Treat with airway maintenance, epinephrine (IV, endotracheal, subcutaneous, 3–5 mL of 1:10,000, 2–4 mg/min), albumin 5% 250 mL, dexamethasone, and diphenhydramine.

C. Body fluids

1. 60% of body weight is water. 20% of the body weight is extracellular fluid (**Table 6.7**).

2. 5 L of increased free water is needed for edema to become noticeable.

Table 6.7 Distribution of H_2O in the Body

Compartment	Volume (L)	Total Body Water (%)
Intracellular	23	55
Interstitial	8.4	20
Bone	6.3	15
Plasma	3.2	7.5
Body cavities	1.1	2.5
Total body water	42	100

3. Plasma osmolarity = $2 \times (Na^+ + K^+)$ + glucose/18 + urea/2.8. Normal is 290 mOsm/kg H_2O. During shock, replace the volume and Na^+ deficit quickly. Otherwise, replace free H_2O slowly to prevent edema. The free H_2O deficit = $0.6 \times kg \times ((serum\ Na^+/140) - 1)$.

4. Blood volume is 70 mL/kg (60 mL/kg for females).

5. Average adult male blood volume is 5.7 L.

6. Acute blood loss > 35% may be fatal (**Table 6.8**).

Table 6.8 Hemorrhage Classification (American College of Surgeons)

Class	Blood Loss (%)	Findings
1	15	Tachycardia and orthostatic tachycardia > 20 beats/minute
2	20–25	Orthostatic hypotension (decrease 15 mm Hg systolic)
3	30–40	Supine hypotension, oliguria (<400 mL/24 h)
4	> 40	Coma, cardiovascular collapse

7. Blood loss of 15% does not require IV replacement. The body initially recovers fluid from the interstitial space (this leaves a 1 L deficit) and the renin system absorbs Na^+, which fills interstitial space to replace deficit. There is also an increase in red blood cell (RBC) production.

8. Replace blood and fluid with short thick catheters to minimize the resistance to flow. Flow = (pressure difference $\times \pi \times r^4$)/($8 \times$ viscosity $\times$ length). Use either a large peripheral vein or infusion into a central vein, but with a short large-bore catheter.
    a. Viscosity is the resistance to concentric layers of fluid sliding over each other. The scale is relative to water, with water equaling 1.
    b. Raising the lower limbs does not help to increase the circulating blood volume. Colloid helps to increase CO more than blood because it has less viscosity, but it has less O_2 carrying capacity.
    c. Initial treatment should be to use colloid to raise the CO, and then monitor the VO_2 to determine whether blood is needed.
    d. Three times the amount of crystalloid is needed to achieve the same volume increase as a similar volume of colloid.

9. 80% of the crystalloid enters the extravascular space and only 20% stays intravascular. Its main component is Na⁺. Isotonic saline has 9 g/L NaCl or 0.9%.

10. Colloid is composed of large molecular weight products that do not pass through the capillary walls.
    a. 500 mL of 5% albumin increases the intravascular volume > 500 mL. 50 mL of 25% albumin increases the vascular volume 250 mL and the effect lasts 24–36 hours. 50% of the albumin resides outside of the vascular space.
    b. Rarely albumin may elicit an allergic response, cause a coagulopathy, or transmit viral hepatitis.
    c. Hetastarch is a colloid that contains no protein. It does not cause a coagulopathy and is removed from the bloodstream over several days.
    d. Dextrans are polysaccharide colloids that are 50% cleared from the blood in 6 hours. They are associated with increased bleeding by inhibition of platelets, decrease in the factor VIII level, and increase in fibrinolysis. They are also associated with renal failure and anaphylaxis.

11. Crystalloid versus colloid — crystalloid is less expensive. Colloid provides a more rapid increase in intravascular volume (2–4 times more than the same volume of crystalloid) and 50% less resuscitation time. It improves CO and oxygen transport. Both may leak from capillaries and cause pulmonary edema. There is no proven difference in survival from shock. Use crystalloid to fill the interstitium and colloid to fill the vascular space quickly.

VII. Blood Products and Coagulation

A. Whole blood — One unit contains 450 mL of blood and 50 mL of anticoagulant citrate (binds Ca²⁺), dextrose (feeds erythrocytes), and phosphate (maintains a normal pH, decreases the breakdown of DPG). Store at 1–6°C. Shelf life is 21 days, but the platelets lose function after 2 days. The K⁺ slowly leaks from the RBCs for 21 days and much more dramatically after that.

B. Packed red blood cells — Infusion volume includes 300 mL (200 mL of cells and 100 mL of plasma because ⅔ of the plasma has been removed) and normal saline to lower viscosity. The main indication is anemia. It is not a good source of volume because it is very viscous.

C. Fresh frozen plasma — One unit contains 200–250 mL of plasma. Store at –18°C for up to 1 year and use 6 hours after thawing. Transfuse to provide coagulation factors with a coagulopathy from liver disease or Coumadin (Bristol-Myers Squibb, New York, NY). Do not use as a volume expander. The risk of non A-non B hepatitis (hepatitis C) can be as high as 1%.

D. Cryoprecipitate — obtained by centrifuging fresh frozen plasma to create concentrated factors. It is rich in fibrinogen, factor VIII, von Willebrand factor (vWF), fibronectin, and antithrombin III. Store at –18°C. Use 6–10 units at a time for hemophilia, volume overload, uremia, or cardiac bypass (vWF reverses platelet abnormalities). There is a relatively high risk of hepatitis (each unit has the same hepatitis risk as one unit of whole blood) and it is expensive.

E. Fibronectin — a blood product found in cryoprecipitate. It is an opsonin that increases the phagocytosis of encapsulated gram-positive bacteria by neutrophils. There is no proven benefit if given to infected patients.

F. Infusion strategies
    1. Flow (Q) = P × π × r⁴/8 × viscosity × L; for nonpulsatile laminar flow of Newtonian fluids in rigid tubes
    2. Flow is increased by increasing pressure or radius and decreasing length and viscosity.

3. The viscosity is decreased by infusing blood products with normal saline (avoid Ca^{2+}-containing products that will cause clotting) and warming the blood (decreases viscosity 2.5 times and decreases hypothermia). The blood should be delivered at $> 35°C$. Dysrhythmias may occur when it is $< 28°C$.

4. The pressure is increased by using pressure bags up to 200 mm Hg that increases flow 2–3 times over gravity alone.

5. The length is decreased by using a 2-inch catheter. This is 50% faster than an 8-inch catheter.

6. The radius is increased by using a 14-gauge catheter. This is 75% faster than a 16-gauge catheter. The fastest is a Cordis catheter (Cordis Endovascular, Warren, NJ).

7. Filters help to trap decomposed platelets and white blood cells with fibrin. They should be replaced every 4 units.

8. Massive transfusions are when the entire blood volume is replaced in 24 hours (10 units of whole blood). There are frequent coagulation abnormalities, but no correlation with volume has been proven. Adding platelets and fresh frozen plasma has not been shown to diminish the coagulopathy. Dilutional thrombocytopenia does not occur until 1.5 times the blood volume has been replaced. The increased citrate load may decrease the serum Ca^{2+} level (of unclear significance) and be broken down to bicarbonate causing metabolic alkalosis. Rarely, there is hyperkalemia, but occasionally hypokalemia with a metabolic alkalosis.

G. Transfusion reactions — occur in 10% of all transfusions

1. Febrile nonhemolytic reaction — occurs with 1–4% of transfusions and is caused by accumulated cytokines (interleukin-1, interleukin-6, tumor necrosis factor α) in donor blood product and an interaction of donor leukocytes with recipient. The fever onset is in 1–6 hours. Stop infusion and determine if there is underlying hemolysis. Treat with acetaminophen. Only 15% of patients develop recurrent febrile nonhemolytic reactions, less common in leukoreduced packed erythrocytes.

2. Allergic transfusion reaction — occurs with 1–3% of transfusions and is caused by antibodies to plasma proteins. They are usually seen with a history of prior transfusions or with IgA deficiency without prior exposure. Findings include mild urticaria, pruritus with or without fever, and rarely anaphylaxis (with hypotension and wheezing). There is no need to stop the transfusion if there is only urticaria. Treat with diphenhydramine. Treat anaphylaxis with epinephrine 1:10,000 0.1 mL IV or 0.5 mL subcutaneously. Use washed erythrocytes in the future.

3. Transfusion-related acute lung injury — occurs with 1 in 2000 transfusions and is caused by a pulmonary agglutinin reaction. This causes a toxic response and is clinically similar to ARDS. Unlike ARDS, however, it resolves in 4 days. The respiratory symptoms begin in 1–2 hours and are associated with fever. Treatment is by stopping the transfusion and instituting supportive care.

4. Acute hemolytic reaction — occurs with 1 in 6000 transfusions, is caused by ABO antibodies to erythrocytes and is fatal in 1 in 100,000 cases. Lysis of one unit occurs in < 1 hour, and within a few minutes of the transfusion there may be fever, dyspnea, chest pain, lower back pain, hypotension, disseminated intravascular coagulation, multisystem organ failure, and death. The mortality is increased with a larger volume transfused. If there is an early fever, stop the transfusion and check the blood pressure. If it is low, give colloid and dopamine to increase the renal blood flow. Obtain a blood sample, check the plasma and urine for hemoglobin (gives it a pink color) and the blood with a direct Coombs' test. This test is positive during active lysis, but may be negative if all of the cells are already lysed.

5. Delayed hemolytic reaction — occurs between 2–10 days after transfusion. Caused by an antibody response to foreign red cell antigen. Hemolysis is less dramatic than acute hemolytic reaction. Future blood products transfused to the patient should be screened for offending antigen.

6. If using uncrossmatched blood, check the donor cells with recipient plasma (takes only 45 minutes). If there is no time, use O negative blood (the universal donor), but the serum still has antibodies to the A, B, and Rh antigens that may cause a minor reaction. Type-specific blood (type ABO and Rh) can be determined in 5 minutes.

H. Platelets

1. Transfusions
   a. Transfusion is indicated if there are < 50,000/mm^3 and there is active bleeding or an elevated bleeding time.
   b. A blood volume transfusion decreases the platelet count from 250,000 to 80,000. The platelets only last 1 day in whole blood.
   c. Consider transfusing platelets if a large blood transfusion is >1.5 times the blood volume or more than 15 units of whole blood are used.
   d. A platelet count of < 10,000 is associated with spontaneous hemorrhage. A platelet count of 80,000 is adequate for surgery if the bleeding time is normal.
   e. One unit contains 5.5 billion platelets from 10 donors in 50–70 mL of plasma. It can be stored for 7 days, but is more effective if used in less than 3 days. One-unit transfusion increases the platelet count from 5,000 to 10,000 and lasts for 8 days.
   f. If there is a transfusion reaction, consider using a single HLA-matched donor. Platelets have ABO antigens, but there are rarely serious reactions.

2. Thrombocytopenia (quantitative dysfunction)
   a. Heparin-induced thrombocytopenia (HIT) — Thrombocytopenia is noted in up to 10% of cases where heparin is used. There are two types, one of which is antibody mediated caused by heparin-induced antiplatelet antibodies that results in thrombosis, not hemorrhage. Thrombocytopenia is seen within 4–10 days. Treat by discontinuing the heparin and continue anticoagulation with lepirudin, argatroban, or danaparoid.
   b. Sepsis — associated with increased platelet consumption
   c. Thrombotic thrombocytopenic purpura —Treatment is with plasmapheresis or exchange transfusions, antiplatelet agents, and rarely splenectomy. Do not treat with platelets. (see Chapter 3 section XXI)
   d. Idiopathic thrombocytopenic purpura — immune mediated, not related to an exogenous cause, and occurs in children or adults. The marrow has increased megakaryocytes. Treatment is with steroids and splenectomy (the spleen normally sequesters 30% of platelets, but may hold 90% with splenomegaly).
   e. Drugs — various antibiotics, H$_2$-blockers, and diuretics
   f. Marrow dysfunction with decreased production
   g. Disseminated intravascular coagulation — widespread microvascular thrombosis resulting in depletion of platelets and coagulation proteins

3. Impaired platelet adhesion (qualitative dysfunction)
   a. Renal failure/uremia — Treat with dialysis.

b. von Willebrand disease — congenital or acquired. vWF may be absent or have qualitative abnormalities.

c. Cardiac bypass — caused by interaction with surface components of bypass machine

d. Drugs — acetylsalicylic acid (effect lasts the 10-day life of a platelet), dipyridamole, NSAIDs, ticlopidine, clopidogrel

e. Liver disease

f. Dysproteinemia — Multiple myeloma and Waldenstrom macroglobulinemia can lead to platelet dysfunction from presence of abnormal paraprotein.

g. Treat platelet dysfunction with desmopressin acetate (DDAVP; especially with vWF). It releases vWF into the blood to increase platelet adhesion. Dose is 0.3 µg/kg IV over 30 minutes and it works for 4 hours. There is no vasoconstriction (unlike vasopressin). Cryoprecipitate may also help.

I. Coagulation disorders (**Table 6.9**)

Table 6.9 Coagulation Cascade

Intrinsic Pathway (Affects PTT)	Extrinsic Pathway (Affects PT)
XII	Tissue thromboplastin
T	T
XI	VII
T	
IX (With VIII)	
	X (With V)
	T
	II (Prothrombin)
	T
	Thrombin
	T
	I (Fibrinogen)
	T
	Fibrin (With XIII)
	T
	Stabilized fibrin

Abbreviations: PTT, partial thromboplastin time; PT, prothrombin time.

1. Disseminated intravascular coagulation increases prothrombin time (PT), activated partial thromboplastin time (PTT), and bleeding time; it decreases platelets and fibrinogen. The decrease in fibrinogen most closely correlates with the increased bleeding. It is associated with sepsis, hemolytic transfusion reaction, and malignancy. Treatment is by removing the causative agent and using heparin, cryoprecipitate (with fibrinogen), platelets, and whole blood.

2. Bleeding time is increased by thrombocytopenia, decreased vWF, NSAIDs, and uremia.

3. PTT is increased by heparin and deficiencies of factors XII, XI, IX, and VIII, as well as X, II, and so on.

4. PT is increased by Coumadin and deficiencies of factors VII, X, V, and II.

5. PT and PTT are increased by deficiencies of factors X, V, II, and I.

6. Vitamin K-dependent factors — shortest to longest half-life proteins C and S, factors VII, IX, X, II.

7. Factor XIII deficiency — normal bleeding parameters, delayed bleeding problems.

8. Factor XII deficiency — increased PTT, normal bleeding

9. Factor IX deficiency (hemophilia B, Christmas disease, X-linked recessive) — increased PTT, normal PT, and bleeding time. Treat with fresh frozen plasma.

10. Factor VIII deficiency (hemophilia A — classic, the most common hereditary coagulopathy, X-linked recessive, absence of procoagulant portion with normal antigenic portion) — increased PT and PPT, and bleeding time (however, there is abnormal bleeding with severe deep hematomas and hemarthrosis). Treat with cryoprecipitate.

11. vWF disease (autosomal dominant, absence of the complete factor VIII) — normal PT, increased PTT, and bleeding time. Treat with cryoprecipitate.

12. Factor VII deficiency — shortest half-life, associated with malnutrition, increased PT, normal PTT, and bleeding time

13. Fibrinogen (factor I) deficiency and disseminated intravascular coagulation — increased PT, PTT, and bleeding time

14. Antithrombin III, protein C, and protein S deficiencies — hypercoagulability with mostly venous thrombotic complications

15. Heparin — works by binding to and increasing the action of antithrombin III, as well as other factors. It prevents the generation of thrombin and antagonizes its actions. It increases the PTT and has a half-life of 90 minutes. Heparin therapy is less effective in patients with antithrombin III deficiency. Heparin reversed with protamine sulfate.

16. Coumadin — prevents the synthesis of active coagulation factors that are vitamin K dependent (factors II, VII, IX, and X). It therefore has a slow onset of anticoagulation that requires a few days to be effective. It also prevents the formation of proteins C and S, which have a shorter half-life than the coagulation factors. This causes a hypercoagulable state for the first few days of therapy. Therefore, Coumadin should be started after the patient is anticoagulated with heparin. It increases the PT and lasts 48 hours. Vitamin K normalizes the PT in 12–36 hours. Fresh frozen plasma or factor isolates can normalize the PT immediately for 4–6 hours and are indicated to reverse Coumadin when there is intracranial hemorrhage.

17. Coumadin is metabolized by the cytochrome P450 system. Effectiveness is increased with sulfamethoxazole, phenytoin (Dilantin [Pfizer Pharmaceuticals, New York, NY], acutely), cimetidine, and ciprofloxacin. It is decreased with phenytoin (Dilantin, chronically), carbamazepine, phenobarbital, cyclosporine, nafcillin, rifampin, and cholestyramine.

18. Thrombolytic agents such as streptokinase, urokinase, and tissue plasminogen activator accelerate fibrinolysis within minutes. The antidote is fresh frozen plasma.

19. Patients with a cardiac valve should be anticoagulated to an international normalized ratio (INR) of 3–3.5 if they have a mechanical valve. If they have a xenograft valve, no anticoagulation is needed if it is aortic and only 6 weeks of treatment is needed if it is mitral.

J. Recombinant factor VII — binds directly to the surface of activated platelets resulting in thrombin burst. Appears to reduce clot size of intracerebral hemorrhage and may improve mortality. Theoretically, increases risk of thromboembolic phenomenon.

VIII. Acid–Base Disorders

A. pH

1. $pH = 6.10 + \log (HCO_3^- / (0.03\ PCO_2))$

2. The respiratory system compensates for acid/base abnormalities rapidly. The renal system compensates in 6 hours–3 days mainly by proximal tubule HCO_3^- resorption.

3. Normal pH is 7.35–7.44.

4. Normal pCO_2 is 36–44 mm Hg.

5. Normal HCO_3^- is 22–26 mEq/L.

6. The expected degree of compensation:
   a. Metabolic acidosis — change of $PCO_2 = 1.5\ HCO_3^- + 8$
   b. Metabolic alkalosis — change of $PCO_2 = 0.7\ HCO_3^- + 20$
   c. Acute respiratory acidosis — change of $pH = 0.008 \times (PCO_2 - 40)$
   d. Chronic respiratory acidosis — change of $pH = 0.003 \times (PCO_2 - 40)$
   e. Acute respiratory alkalosis — change of $pH = 0.008 \times (40 - PCO_2)$
   f. Chronic respiratory acidosis — change of $pH = 0.017 \times (40 - PCO_2)$

B. Metabolic acidosis

1. Metabolic acidosis — increased acid generation (lactic or ketoacidosis), decreased renal acid excretion (RTA type 1), loss of bicarbonate (RTA type 2, diarrhea)

2. Compensation — 1.2 mm Hg drop in PCO_2 for every drop in 1 meq/L of bicarbonate

3. Anion gap (AG) = $Na^+ - (Cl^- + HCO_3^-)$. Normal is 7–12 mEq/L. The accumulation of fixed acids provides H+ ions to decrease the HCO_3^- level and thus the AG increases. A decreased anion gap is caused by decreased albumin (an unmeasured anion). A 50% decrease in albumin lowers the AG by 6 mEq. The AG is also decreased by hyponatremia. Unmeasured anions include protein, phosphoric acid, sulfuric acid, and organic acids. Unmeasured cations include K^+, Ca^{2+}, and Mg^{2+}.

4. Normal anion gap acidosis — caused by a decreased HCO_3^- level, whereas the serum Cl^- increases to replace it. This is seen with diarrhea, mild renal insufficiency, increased Cl^- volume, and RTA type 2.

5. High anion gap acidosis — caused by increased fixed acids with lactic acidosis, ketoacidosis, renal failure, acetylsalicylic acid toxicity, methanol, and ethylene glycol.

6. The treatment of metabolic acidosis is to treat underlying cause, but consider treatment with HCO_3^- if the pH is < 7.20. HCO_3^- may cause hypotension. The HCO_3^- deficit is calculated as $0.5 \times kg \times$ (desired – serum HCO_3^-). Give a 50% bolus and then replace the remaining 50% over 6 hours.

7. The urine AG = (urine N^+ + urine K^+) – urine Cl^-. It is useful in differentiating the bicarbonate loss from diarrhea versus RTA. If the urine AG is negative with a pH < 5.5, it is normal. If it is negative with a pH > 5.5, it is due to diarrhea. If it is positive with a pH > 5.5, it is due to RTA.

8. Lactic acidosis — Lactic acid is the end product of glucose metabolism. The body normally produces < 2 mEq/L or up to 4 mEq/L with exercise. The liver clears it by using it for gluconeogenesis in energy production. Causes of lactic acidosis include sepsis, cardiogenic shock, multisystem organ failure, O_2 debt, epinephrine, sodium nitroprusside, bowel infarction, seizure, thiamin deficiency, and alkalosis.

Shock is associated with an increase in lactic acid from decreased blood flow and decreased CO, not from decreased O_2, hepatic dysfunction, or anemia. The AG may be as high as 30.

9. Ketoacidosis — Ketones form when there is decreased glucose use and the liver breaks down fatty acids for fuel. The AG is usually 15–20, lower than with lactic acidosis. Diabetic ketoacidosis results from insulin deficiency and a body reaction similar to starvation. There is hyperglycemia, anion gap acidosis, and urine and blood ketones. Rarely, the pH may be > 7.4, the AG may be normal, and the glucose may be < 350. The ketones are excreted in the urine, so the serum levels increase with dehydration. 50% have a concurrent illness. Treatment is with volume (colloids), K^+ 10–40 mEq/hour, insulin 10 units IV, and then 0.1 units/kg/hour IV. If the phosphorus is < 1, give 0.25 mmol/L over 6 hours. Do not give HCO_3^-. Alcoholic ketoacidosis is caused by starvation, dehydration (decreased clearance of ketones), and metabolism of ethanol. It is associated with a more normal glucose. Treat with volume using normal saline with 5% dextrose.

C. Metabolic alkalosis

1. Caused by decreased H^+ ions (from gastric acid loss through emesis or nasogastric suctioning), diuretics with depletion of Cl^- and retention of HCO_3^- from the kidneys, hydrogen shifting intracellularly, or volume contraction

2. Gastrointestinal loss — Loss of gastric acid secretions does not stimulate the excretion of pancreatic fluid, which is high in bicarbonate.

3. Renal loss — Hyperaldosteronism, loop, or thiazide diuretic leads to excretion of H^+.

4. Intracellular shift — Hypokalemia leads to H^+ shift into the cell to maintain electroneutrality.

5. Volume contraction — loss of bicarbonate-free fluid

6. Alkalosis — decreases CO, shifts the oxygen-hemoglobin dissociation curve to the left (decreases O_2 delivery), and increases O_2 consumption by increasing glycolysis. When severe, with HCO_3^- < 50 and pH > 7.6, it may be associated with seizures, dysrhythmias, and hypoventilation. These may be due to hypocalcemia. The expected $PCO_2 = 0.7 \times HCO_3^- + 20$.

7. Therapy — aimed at repleting the electrolyte losses to allow the kidney to excrete HCO_3^-. Cl^- deficit = $0.27 \times kg \times (100 - Cl^-)$. Give NaCl to correct the deficit at X liters = Cl^- deficit/154. The 154 is the Cl^- mEq in 1 L of 0.9% Na Cl solution. KCl is needed to normalize the K^+. Acetazolamide (500 mg) inhibits bicarbonate resorption, but decreases volume and K^+ levels, so it does not help to increase the Cl^-. Therapy for Cl^--resistant alkalosis (where the extracellular fluid volume is elevated) consists of repleting the K^+ and using the mineralocorticoid antagonist aldactone.

D. Respiratory acidosis — caused by hypoventilation

E. Respiratory alkalosis — caused by hyperventilation

IX. Electrolytes

A. Na^+

1. Hypernatremia (Na^+ >145 meq/L)
   a. Hypovolemic — due to insensible, diuretic, or gastrointestinal loss of hypotonic fluid. Hyperglycemic nonketotic syndrome is caused by a glucose > 900 mg/dL and severe volume depletion. It is more frequent with noninsulin-dependent diabetes mellitus. It is most commonly seen with mild

diabetes, where there is enough endogenous insulin to prevent ketosis. There is less accumulation of fatty acids. Predisposing factors include infection, total parenteral nutrition, β-blockers, diuretics, and steroids. Findings include altered mental status or coma. Elevated level of glucose may draw intracellular fluid to the extracellular space leading to dilution of Na^+ but in severe cases the glucose acts as an osmotic diuretic, which leads to excretion of water in excess of Na^+ resulting in hypernatremia. Treatment is with insulin 2–5 units IV hourly and volume restoration.

b. Euvolemic diabetes insipidus (DI) — due to impaired H_2O resorption in the distal tubules and loss of free water. Central DI caused by inhibition of antidiuretic hormone (ADH) release from posterior stalk of the pituitary from meningitis, trauma, or anoxia. Urine osmolarity is < 200 mOsm/L. Nephrogenic DI is due to ineffective responsiveness of the distal tubule to ADH from the use of aminoglycosides, lithium, amphotericin B, or ATN. Urine osmolarity is generally between 200–500 mOsm/L. Treatment is with fluids and if needed, aqueous vasopressin 5–10 units subcutaneously every 4–6 hours.

c. Hypervolemic hypernatremia — rare, caused by excessive hypertonic saline or $NaHCO_3$. Treat with diuretics and 5% dextrose in water.

d. Na^+ correction should be over in 48–72 hours to prevent cerebral edema and central pontine myelinolysis.

2. Hyponatremia (Na^+ < 135)

a. Pseudohyponatremia — The Na^+ is falsely lowered by increased triglycerides or plasma proteins.

b. Hyponatremia types

(1) Hypervolemic — urine Na^+ > 20 meq/L consistent with renal failure, urine Na^+ < 20 meq/L more consistent with hepatic failure or cirrhosis

(2) Euvolemic — urine osmolarity >100 (syndrome of inappropriate antidiuretic hormone [SIADH]), urine osmolarity < 100 (psychogenic polydipsia)

(3) Hypovolemic — urine Na > 20 (diuresis, adrenal insufficiency, hypovolemic hyponatremia, cerebral salt wasting [CSW]), Na < 20 (extrarenal losses, diarrhea)

c. SIADH — associated with tumors (oat cell pulmonary tumors), CNS abnormalities (seizures, tumors, stroke, trauma, and infection), pulmonary disease, medications (phenytoin [Dilantin], carbamazepine, and thiazides), chronic illness, and old age. Diagnosis is made by urine osmolarity > serum osmolarity, serum Na^+ < 135 mEq/L, serum osmolarity < 280 mOsm/L, and urine Na^+ > 20 mmol/24 hours with normal renal function, adrenal function, thyroid function, and euvolemia. Treatment is with fluid restriction, demeclocycline (induces nephrogenic DI), and furosemide with 3% NaCl solution if needed.

d. CSW — excessive renal excretion of Na^+, which also results in a hypovolemic state. Often associated with SAH, but may be associated with any intracranial process (hyponatremia in SAH patients is most commonly salt wasting not SIADH). Etiology is disruption of sympathetic input to the proximal tubule involved with salt reabsorption or brain and atrial natriuretic peptide is released after brain injury.

e. Severe hyponatremia — Na^+ < 120 mEq/L; may cause encephalopathy or ARDS. Avoid increasing Na^+ faster than 0.5 mEq/L/hour. Be especially careful with alcoholics or malnourished people because they have an increased risk of central pontine myelinolysis. Na+ deficit = total body water × (130 – Na^+). Correct with 3% NaCl 1 mL for each mEq of Na^+ deficit.

B. K^+

1. Normal body store of K^+ is 3500 mEq (50 mEq/kg); only 70 mEq (62%) is extracellular.

2. Hypokalemia < 3.5 mEq/L
    a. There is a transcellular shift of K^+ into the cells with epinephrine, dobutamine, albuterol, insulin, and alkalosis (hyperventilation).
    b. K^+ depletion occurs with diuretics (urine K^+ > 30), nasogastric suctioning, diarrhea, emesis, steroids, Mg^{2+} depletion, and cirrhosis.
    c. Findings include weakness, mental status changes, and ECG abnormalities (increased U wave and decreased T wave).
    d. Hypokalemia does not cause dysrhythmias, but it does increase digoxin toxicity.
    e. Treatment (**Table 6.10** and **Table 6.11**) — Use KCl if there is metabolic alkalosis and $KHCO_3$ if there is RTA. Replace carefully if there is an acidic pH. The dose is 0.7 mEq/kg IV over 1 hour (or 80–100 mEq/hour) if the K^+ is < 2 and there are dysrhythmias. The K^+ replacement must include Cl- if there is metabolic alkalosis or the K^+ is lost in urine. K^+ infusion > 40 mEq/hour causes sclerosis of veins.

3. Hyperkalemia
    a. K^+ > 5.5. If there is increased urine K^+, consider transcellular shift (myonecrosis, decreased insulin, and acidosis). If there is decreased urine K^+, consider a renal cause (angiotensin converting enzyme inhibitors, NSAIDs, and spironolactone).
    b. Findings — weakness, dysrhythmias, and ECG changes (peaked T waves, decreased P waves, and increased QRS duration).
    c. Treatment — if the serum K^+ is > 6 and there are ECG changes: (1) stabilize the membrane: Ca^{2+} gluconate 20 mL 10% IV over 3 minutes, repeat every 5 minutes (lasts 30 minutes); (2) increase intracellular shift: use insulin 10 units IV with 500 mL 20% dextrose over 1 hour (lowers the K^+ 1 mEq over 1 hour) and use $NaHCO_3$ 1–2 ampules over 5–10 minutes; and (3) increase clearance: use furosemide 40 mg IV, Na^+ polystyrene sulfonate resin oral 30 g in 50 mL 20% sorbitol or rectal enema 50 g in 200 mL 20% sorbitol and retain 45 minutes. If there is an AV block without

Table 6.10 Treatment of Hypokalemia

Serum K^+ (mEq)	Replacement (mEq)
3.5	200
3.0	350
2.5	470
2.0	700

Table 6.11 Evaluation of Urine K^+

Urine K^+ < 30	Urine K^+ > 30		
Diarrhea	Serum HCO_3^- < 24	Serum HCO_3^- > 24	
	RTA	Urine Cl^- < 10	Urine Cl^- > 10
		Emesis	Diuretics
		Nasogastric suctioning	Steroids
		Hyperventilation	Decreased Mg^{2+}

Abbreviation: RTA, renal tubular acidosis.

a response to Ca^{2+}, consider a pacemaker. If there is concomitant digoxin toxicity, treat with 2 g $MgSO_4$ and avoid Ca^{2+}.

C. Magnesium

1. The second most abundant intracellular cation (after K^+). It is a cofactor for all enzymes with adenosine triphosphate (ATP) and affects electrical stability of muscles and nerves. It is difficult to measure total body stores and the serum level is unreliable. 50% is in the bones and only 0.3% is in the serum. The daily intake should be 6–10 mg/kg/day.

2. Hypomagnesemia
   a. Causes — IV fluids without Mg^{2+} and diuretics that blunt the urine conservation attempts. This must be diagnosed by documenting decreased intracellular levels in erythrocytes or lymphocytes. Mg^{2+} is resorbed in the loop of Henle and is lost with loop diuretics, aminoglycosides, alcohol, and diarrhea.
   b. Findings — myocardial ischemia, dysrhythmias, digoxin toxicity, seizures, psychologic disorders, increased QT interval, and neuromuscular excitability
   c. It is associated with hypokalemia in 40% of cases (it is needed for the membrane pump that keeps K^+ intracellular), decreased PO_4^- (30%), decreased Na^+ (27%) and decreased Ca^{2+} (22%). Parathyroid hormone is decreased if the Mg^{2+} level is low.
   d. Replacement (if renal function is normal) — give $MgSO_4$ 1 mEq/kg in 24 hours and then 0.5 mEq/kg/d for 5 days. 1 g of $MgSO_4$ contains 8 mEq Mg^{2+}, so use $MgSO_4$ 3 g every 8 hours. Use MgCl if there is decreased Cl^-.
   e. If there are severe arrhythmias or seizures, give 2 g $MgSO_4$ IV in 1 minute, 5 g in 6 hours, and then 5 g every 12 hours for 5 days. If there is moderate depletion, give 6 g over 3 hours, 5 g over 6 hours and then 5 g every 12 hours × 5 days. Use caution with renal failure. Serum levels do not represent total body stores.

3. Hypermagnesemia
   a. Causes — renal failure, diabetic ketoacidosis, pheochromocytomas and Mg^{2+} ingestion (antacids, Mg^{2+} citrate and milk of magnesia). Use aluminum antacids to bind PO_4 and clear it. Aluminum causes constipation whereas Mg^{2+} causes diarrhea.
   b. Findings — hypotension (Mg^{2+} > 3), heart block (Mg^{2+} > 7.5), respiratory depression (Mg^{2+} >10), and coma
   c. Treatment — with Ca^{2+} gluconate 2 10 mL ampules, furosemide, and dialysis if needed

D. Ca^{2+}

1. In the blood 50% is bound to proteins (80% of these are albumin), 10% is complexed with anions (HCO_3^-) and 40% is free or ionized. Total serum Ca^{2+} is 8.5–10.5 mg/dL. Ionized Ca^{2+} is 4.8–7.2 mg/dL. The actual total serum level is increased over the measured level 0.8 mg/dL for each 1 mg/dL decrease in albumin below 4.

2. Hypocalcemia
   a. Causes — sepsis, hypomagnesemia (decreases parathyroid hormone secretion and action, Ca^{2+} supplements are lost in the urine), renal insufficiency (by PO_4^- retention and defective conversion of vitamin D), alkalosis (elevated pH increases the binding of Ca^{2+} to albumin and decreases the free level), pancreatitis, and massive citrate (blood) transfusion

       b. Findings — neuromuscular excitability (tetany, seizures, and hyperreflexia (Chvostek and Trousseau signs), and cardiovascular abnormalities (peripheral dilation, hypotension, prolonged QT segment, and left ventricular failure)

       c. Treatment — $CaCl_2$ or Ca^{2+} gluconate

   3. Hypercalcemia

       a. Causes — malignancies, sarcoid and hyperparathyroidism

       b. Findings (with levels >13) — hypotension (moans); fractures (bones); kidney stones (stones); ileus, pancreatitis, and ulcers (abdominal groans); and mental status changes (psychic undertones)

       c. Treatment — volume (NaCl infusion = urine volume every hour), furosemide (these patients are often volume depleted so use caution as furosemide may cause nephrocalcinosis), calcitonin 4 units/kg intramuscularly or subcutaneously every 12 hours, mithramycin, and dialysis if needed

E. Phosphorus

   1. Mostly intracellular with K^+ and Mg^{2+}, 60% is extracellular. It functions as a cofactor for glucose use. The normal serum level is 2.5–4.5 mEq/dL.

   2. Hypophosphatemia

       a. Causes — dextrose feedings (insulin pulls in PO_4^- with the glucose, especially in malnourished patients), respiratory alkalosis (elevated pH causes increased glycolysis with increased PO_4^- influx into cells), sepsis, diabetic ketoacidosis (PO_4 is lost in the urine and moves into the cells with insulin), antacids (aluminum binds PO_4^-), amphogel, and sucralfate

       b. Findings — rare, but include decreased cardiac contractility, hemolysis, decreased DPG (decreased tissue O_2 dissociation), and decreased ATP formation causing muscle weakness

       c. Treatment — 15 mg/kg Na^+ or K_4PO_4 over 4 hours. 1 mmol/L = 30 mg PO_4

   3. Hyperphosphatemia

       a. Causes — renal failure, cell necrosis, rhabdomyolysis, and diabetic ketoacidosis (serum levels may be elevated, but they will plummet with transcellular shift)

X. Nutrition

A. Respiratory quotient (CO_2 formed/O_2 used) — lipid = 0.7, protein = 0.8, carbohydrate = 1

B. Energy produced (kcal/g) — lipid = 9.1, protein = 4, carbohydrate = 3.75

C. Carbohydrates — comprise 60–90% of total dietary calories. Carbohydrate use is impaired in sepsis. Carbohydrates produce the most CO_2 molecules per energy produced, so one may attempt to reduce carbohydrate intake in patients with lung disease.

D. Lipids — should make up <30% of caloric intake. Linoleic acid is the only essential fatty acid provided in the diet. Deficiency causes rashes, neutropenia, and thrombocytopenia. Treat with oral or topical safflower oil.

E. Protein — diet should provide 0.8 g/kg/day. Demand is increased with catabolic states to 1.6 g/kg/day. The urine removes ⅔ of the nitrogen waste. Nitrogen balance (g) = (Protein intake/6.25) – (urinary nitrogen + 4). 1 g nitrogen = 6.25 g protein because protein is 16% nitrogen. The most successful way to improve protein balance is to supply enough nonprotein energy to avoid protein catabolism.

F. Vitamins

1. 12 essential vitamins: A, C, D, E, thiamine (B1), riboflavin (B2), pyridoxine (B6), B12, pantothenate, vitamin K, folate, and biotin. The most frequent deficiencies are A, C, E, folate, and thiamine.

2. Folate (1 mg/day) is required at increased doses with sepsis or postoperative stress. Deficiencies may cause thrombocytopenia and megaloblastic changes in the marrow.

3. Thiamine (100 mg/day) is needed as cofactor for glucose metabolism. Deficiencies cause beriberi heart disease, Wernicke encephalitis, peripheral neuropathy, and lactic acidosis.

G. Trace elements

1. There are seven essential trace elements: chromium, copper, iodine, iron, manganese, selenium, and zinc.

2. Chromium deficiency causes insulin resistance.

3. Zinc deficiency may increase the risk of infections.

4. Iron – 4.5 g of iron stored; bound to transferrin, hemoglobin, and ferritin

H. Enteral nutrition

1. Benefits include calories and trophic effects on the mucosal barrier. After a few days of bowel rest, there is atrophy of the mucosa and disruption causing refeeding diarrhea and bacterial translocation.

2. Avoid feedings with shock, bowel obstruction, or ischemia. Use low volumes if there is a partial obstruction or diarrhea. Gastric feedings are better than intestinal because they decrease ulcer formation, decrease diarrhea by lowering the osmolarity of gastric secretions, and increase trophic substances by distention.

3. Bolus feeding delays emptying. Continuous infusion is better tolerated and decreases aspiration and diarrhea. A slow or dilute start to feeding is only needed after long bowel rest, with high residuals or with jejunal feedings.

I. Caloric density of tube feedings

1. 1 kcal/mL — Osmolite (Abbott Laboratories, Abbott Park, IL), Isocal (Isocal Laboratories, Bloomfield, CT), and Ensure (Abbott Laboratories, Abbott Park, IL; isotonic so good for small bowel feedings)

2. 1.5 kcal/mL — Ensure plus

3. 2 kcal/mL — Isocal HCN and Osmolite HN (for gastric feedings or with fluid restriction)

J. Most tube feedings have proteins that provide < 20% of the calories (except Sustacal [Novartis, East Hanover, NJ] > 20%). Some formulas use peptides instead of protein for easier absorption with short gut, etc. Elemental formulas are even easier to absorb with amino acids for needle cannula jejunostomies. Fats in the form of long or medium chain triglycerides are easier to absorb.

K. Fiber is a carbohydrate not degradable by the normal routes. Fermentable (Kaopectate, Pfizer, New York, NY) fiber includes cellulose and pectin. These are metabolized by intestinal bacteria to produce short chain fatty acids for bowel mucosa energy. They delay gastric emptying and help decrease diarrhea. Nonfermentable fiber includes lignins (Metamucil, Procter & Gamble, Pharmaceuticals, Cincinnati, OH). They are nondegradable and their osmotic pull draws in H_2O to increase the stool bulk and prevent constipation. Jevity (Abbott Laboratories, Abbott Park, IL) and Enrich (Tate & Lyle PLC, London, UK) have both types of fiber.

L. Hepatic encephalopathy requires feedings with increased branched chain amino acids (leucine, isoleucine, and valine) to decrease the aromatic uptake across the blood–brain barrier (BBB; methionine, phenylalanine, tyrosine, and tryptophan).

M. Renal failure diet should avoid electrolytes and increase the essential amino acids because they produce less urea than nonessential amino acids do.

N. Respiratory failure diet should have fewer carbohydrates and more fats to decrease the CO_2 production. At least 50% of calories should come from lipids. A complication of this diet is steatorrhea.

O. Tube feeding complications

1. Diarrhea — occurs in 30% of patients who receive enteral feedings and is caused by osmotic forces and malabsorption

2. Aspiration — There is no increased risk in gastric feedings versus duodenal feedings.

P. Parenteral nutrition

1. Use if there is bowel obstruction or ischemia. Bowel sounds are made by air in the stomach or colon, rarely by air in the small intestine, although this is the first place to recover after stress or surgery.

2. There are three elemental nutrients: dextrose 10–70%, amino acids 3–10%, and fat 10–20% (from chylomicrons of safflower or soybean oil rich in linoleic acid). Add electrolytes and trace elements.

3. Daily caloric requirement is 25 kcal/kg/day (average 1750 kcal). The daily requirement of protein is 1.4 g/kg/day (average 100 g). Total parenteral nutrition formulation A10–D50 (actually provides amino acids 5% and dextrose 25%) provides 50 g of protein/L, so 2 L fulfills daily protein requirement (85 mL/hour). Dextrose provided is 475 g and daily calories from dextrose are 1615 kcal. Lipid requirement is 1750–1615 kcal = 135 kcal that is provided with 10% emulsion twice a week (500 mL infusion twice a week). Add standard electrolytes/L, daily multivitamins, and mineral pack.

4. When starting TPN, avoid glucose intolerance by starting at 2 mg dextrose/kg/minute for 12 hours then increasing to 5 mg/kg/minute. If the serum glucose is > 200 mg/dL, add insulin. Try to avoid insulin (it prevents lipoprotein lipase activity that draws fat from the adipose tissue). If needed, use less glucose and more fat. Use regular insulin 18 units/250 g glucose if the serum glucose is > 200 mg/dL.

5. Complications of TPN
   a. Carbohydrates — hyperglycemia and hyperosmolar coma. Chromium deficiency leads to glucose intolerance. Treat by decreasing the dextrose and increasing the lipids and adding insulin. PO_4^- may decrease because it is drawn into the cells with glucose. Fatty liver may develop because the glucose is converted to fatty acids in the liver when fat mobilization for energy is impaired. If the patient has pulmonary disease with CO_2 retention, increase the fat intake and lower the carbohydrates to keep the respiratory quotient < 0.95.
   b. Lipids — rarely adult respiratory distress syndrome due to damage to pulmonary capillaries by free fatty acids.
   c. Electrolytes — hyponatremia may develop because of increased free H_2O. Be sure to add PO_4^- and Mg^{++}.
   d. Bowel atrophy increases infections.
   e. Acalculous cholecystitis — the lack of lipid in the duodenum causes bile stasis.

XI. Endocrine

A. Adrenal gland

1. Responds to stress by secreting glucocorticoids, mineralocorticoids and catecholamines. They increase CO, vascular tone, plasma volume, and blood glucose. Levels increase up to 6 times with stress. There must be a loss of 90% of the adrenal tissue to produce a deficit.

2. Adrenal insufficiency — hypocorticolism
   a. Findings — lethargy, weight loss, anorexia, skin pigmentation (the precursor of adrenocorticotropic hormone (ACTH) also produces melanin-stimulating hormone), orthostatic hypotension, hyponatremia, and hyperkalemia. When very severe, there may be Addison syndrome with hypotension; decreased CO, PCWP, and SVR; oliguria; and hypoglycemia.
   b. Evaluation — ACTH stimulation test. 1 hour after administration of ACTH an incremental increase of serum cortisol < 7 µg/dL implies primary adrenal insufficiency.
   c. Treatment — dexamethasone 10 mg IV bolus followed by hydrocortisone 100 mg IV every 6 hours

3. Hypercortisolism (Cushing syndrome)
   a. Causes — iatrogenic, ACTH-secreting pituitary adenoma (Cushing disease, most frequent noniatrogenic cause, 65%), adrenal tumor (25%), and ectopic ACTH production (pulmonary oat cell tumors and carcinoids, 15%).
   b. Findings — hyperglycemia, hypertension, hypokalemia, hypercalciuria, osteoporosis, truncal obesity, moon facies, peripheral muscle wasting, lymphopenia, and increased infections
   c. Evaluation — serum cortisol, ACTH (decreased with adrenal tumor or iatrogenic causes and increased with ectopic ACTH or pituitary adenoma), 24-hour urine collection (poor patient compliance, also measure urine creatinine to determine result accuracy), low-dose dexamethasone suppression test (1 mg dexamethasone at midnight followed by morning cortisol), and high-dose dexamethasone suppression test (2 mg 4 times a day for 48 hours; suppression occurs with pituitary adenoma, but not with ectopic or adrenal disease)
   d. Treatment — Treat a pituitary adenoma with surgical resection.
   e. Complications of exogenous steroids include proximal myopathy, weight gain, diabetes, hypertension, infection, osteoporosis, and posterior subcapsular cataracts.

4. Hyperaldosteronism — characterized by hypernatremia, hypokalemia, metabolic alkalosis, hypertension, increased urine output, and lack of edema

B. Thyroid gland

1. Thyroxine (T_4) is the main hormone secreted and tri-iodothyronine (T_3) is the active form. Serum thyroid-stimulating hormone (TSH) concentration is useful to diagnose primary hypothyroidism if elevated, decreased TSH not as useful for diagnosis of hyperthyroidism. Serum T_3 and T_4 levels measure the total unbound and bound to thyroxine binding globulin. Free T_4 is better indication of thyroid function.

2. Hyperthyroidism
   a. Etiology — Grave disease most common cause from production of TSH receptor antibodies, which lead to stimulation of thyroid gland. Thyroiditis may initially present with hyperthyroidism. Toxic adenoma or multinodular goiter, TSH-producing pituitary adenomas or struma ovarii (functioning thyroid tissue in an ovarian malignancy) are all causes of hyperthyroidism.
   b. Findings — sinus tachycardia, atrial fibrillation, heat intolerance, and diarrhea. Thyroid storm is precipitated by surgery or illness and is characterized by fever, agitation, high output heart failure, hypotension, and possibly coma.

      c. Treatment — Propylthiouracil (inhibits thyroid hormone synthesis and conversion of T_4 to T_3), radioactive iodine, and lithium. Treat tachycardia with propranolol, 1 mg IV.

  3. Hypothyroidism

      a. Etiology — The most common cause is Hashimoto thyroiditis.

      b. Findings — bradycardia, mental impairment, hypoventilation, hypothermia, hyponatremia (by associated adrenal insufficiency), hypotension, constipation, hair loss, and myxedema coma

  4. Treatment — thyroxine (T_4)

C. Miscellaneous

  1. Multiple endocrine neoplasia 1 (MEN 1, Wermer syndrome) — autosomal dominant disorder associated with tumors of the parathyroid, pancreas, and pituitary gland.

  2. MEN IIa (Sipple syndrome) — autosomal dominant disorder characterized by parathyroid hyperplasia, medullary thyroid cancer and pheochromocytoma. Hypertension secondary to pheochromocytoma treated with phenoxybenzamine (Dibenzyline [GlaxoSmithKline, Brentford, London, UK], a blocker)

  3. MEN IIb — medullary thyroid cancer, pheochromocytoma, mucosal neuromas, intestinal ganglioneuromas; Marfanoid

XII. Infectious Diseases

A. Fever benefits include inhibition of viral replication, slowing bacterial growth, and temperatures > 40°C can kill pneumococcus and increase phagocytosis and lymphocyte transformation.

B. Postoperative day 1 fevers often due to atelectasis and do not need an extensive workup because they usually disappear without sequelae.

C. Etiology of fever — pneumonia, pulmonary embolus, acalculous cholecystitis, translocation enterocolitis, pancreatitis, urinary tract infection, wound infection, deep vein thrombosis, and drug reaction. Also consider a sinus infection when a nasogastric tube has been in place and line infection if there is an indwelling catheter.

D. Wound infections — usually occur on postoperative days 5–7. Necrotizing fascitis caused by Clostridia or β-hemolytic streptococcus may occur in the first 48 hours. Treatment is with penicillin and debridement. Mortality rate is 60%.

E. Pneumonia — community acquired is usually caused by *Pneumococcus, Hemophilus influenzae*, and *Mycoplasma pneumoniae*. Nosocomial is caused by gram-negative bacilli (*Pseudomonas, Klebsiella, Haemophilus influenzae*, and *Escherichia coli*) and *Staphylococcus*. The mechanism is mainly by oropharyngeal colonization that spreads to the lungs. Normal colonization is by streptococci and other anaerobes.

F. Urinary tract infections — 30% of nosocomial infections. Most commonly caused by *Escherichia coli, Enterococcus, Pseudomonas, Klebsiella,* or *Proteus*.

G. Meningitis — After basilar skull fractures, the most common pathogen is *Streptococcus pneumonia* and the infection usually occurs in 72 hours (although it may occur much later). Antibiotics with good CSF penetration include chloramphenicol, second- and third-generation cephalosporins, ciprofloxacin, metronidazole, rifampin, and sulfamethoxazole/trimethoprim. (see Chapter 3 section VII)

H. Ventriculoperitoneal shunt infections — usually caused by *Staphylococcus epidermidis*

I. Catheters — Infections caused by bacteria are brought in during placement or secondarily seed the catheter by means of the stopcock or tract. The most frequent pathogens are *Staphylococcus epidermidis* and *Staphylococcus aureus*.

J. Antibiotic side effects

  1. Aminoglycosides — nonoliguric ATN (appears in 5 to 7 days and is reversible), hearing loss (irreversible and conversational hearing is usually not affected), vestibular dysfunction and worsening of myasthenic syndrome (they decrease neurotransmitter release by decreasing Ca^{2+} influx at the nerve terminal).

  2. Amphotericin B — distal tubule RTA, anemia, hypomagnesemia, and hypokalemia

  3. Vancomycin — red man syndrome caused by histamine release after rapid infusion producing facial flushing, pruritus, and hypotension without a fever. It also is ototoxic and nephrotoxic.

K. Systemic inflammatory response syndrome — widespread inflammatory response to insult characterized by at least two of the following:

$$Temperature < 36 \text{ or } > 38°C$$
$$Heart\ rate > 10$$
$$Respiratory\ rate > 20 \text{ or } PaCO_2 < 32\ mm\ Hg$$
$$White\ blood\ cell\ count > 12 \text{ or } < 4$$

L. Multiple organ dysfunction syndrome — The inflammatory response includes activated neutrophils that adhere to endothelium and secrete proteolytic enzymes and oxygen metabolites that injure endothelium and impair organ function.

M. Sepsis – systemic inflammatory response syndrome where the insult is infection. Severe sepsis is when there is impaired perfusion that results in organ dysfunction.

N. Septic shock – The effects of hypoperfusion are more pronounced then severe sepsis and the patient is dependent on vasopressors. Septic encephalopathy has similar features to hepatic encephalopathy. Branched-chain amino acids are used for energy and decrease in number, causing a relative accumulation of aromatic amino acids. This causes the aromatic amino acids to cross the BBB and act as false neurotransmitters. Acute renal failure is caused by hypotension, endotoxin-mediated renal artery constriction, and drugs.

XIII. Anesthesia

A. Ketamine — increases cerebral blood flow (CBF) and cerebral metabolic rate for O_2 (CMRO$_2$). May elevate ICP but controversial. It causes dissociative anesthesia. Provides analgesia, amnesia, and sedation

B. Isoflurane — produces the least increase in CBF of inhalation anesthetics

C. Enflurane — lowers seizure threshold.

D. Thiopental—decreases CBF and CMRO$_2$. It is a cardiodepressant.

E. Etomidate — sedative-hypnotic agent, decreases CBF and cerebral metabolic oxygen demand, but preserves CPP. It suppresses the adrenocortical response to stress.

F. Fentanyl — decreases CBF and CMRO$_2$

G. All decrease CMRO$_2$ and cerebral metabolism except ketamine and nitrous oxide.

  1. Agents increasing CBF (in decreasing order) — halothane, ketamine, enflurane, isoflurane, and nitrous oxide

XIV. Miscellaneous

A. Wound healing

1. Inflammatory phase — 0–3 days characterized by histamine release; migration of polymorphonuclear leukocytes, which digest bacteria and necrotic tissue

2. Epithelialization — Basal cell proliferation and epithelial cell migration begins to occur in 12 hours.

3. Fibroplasia — Fibroblast proliferation begins 24 hours after injury and collagen synthesis (2 days–6 weeks) begins. Myofibroblasts are present by 5 days, which produce contractile proteins leading to wound contraction.

4. Maturation — collagen crosslinking, additional wound contraction. The plateau of the increased tensile strength of the wound is at 2 years.

B. Toxicology

1. Metal antidotes
    a. Lead — ethylenediaminetetraacetic acid (EDTA), 2,3-dimercaptopropanol (BAL), penicillamine
    b. Arsenic — BAL
    c. Mercury — penicillamine
    d. Iron — deferoxamine
    e. Gold — BAL and penicillamine

2. Organophosphate toxicity (increased anticholinesterase) — Use 2-pyridine aldoxime methochloride (PAM).

3. Tylenol overdose — metabolized in liver, which results in hepatotoxic reactive intermediate. Normally conjugated by glutathione pathway, but may get saturated. Hepatic injury may only become clinically apparent 72 hours after ingestion. Use *N*-acetylcysteine, which inactivates toxic metabolite.

4. Aspirin (acetylsalicylic acid) overdose — causes early respiratory alkalosis and late metabolic acidosis

5. Methanol and ethylene glycol intoxication — Use ethanol to saturate the alcohol dehydrogenase enzymes and prevent formation of formaldehyde.

6. Thallium intoxication — causes cardiac dysfunction, gastrointestinal disturbance, alopecia, lower limb joint pain, and peripheral neuropathy

7. Atropine toxicity — causes decreased sweating, tachycardia, dry mouth, decreased peristalsis, and blurred vision

8. Thiazide side effects — increased uric acid, glucose, and lipids; and decreased K^+

9. Dilantin levels — increased by cimetidine, warfarin, isoniazid, and sulfa drugs. They are decreased by carbamazepine.

10. Acute intermittent porphyria — causes abdominal pain, psychosis, hypertension, tachycardia, and polyneuropathy

11. Urine alkalization — increases the excretion of weak acids such as acetylsalicylic acid, tricyclic antidepressants, and phenobarbital. It does not help with amphetamines.

12. Benzodiazepines are the most common agent in drug overdose. Flumenazil antagonizes benzodiazepine effects.

13. Digitalis — Toxicity leads to lethargy, delirium, seizure disorder, and arrhythmias. Effects potentiated by hypokalemia.

14. Opioids — Naloxone is opioid antagonist.

15. Vincristine — may cause peripheral neuropathy

16. Baclofen (GABA agonist) — used to treat spasticity; may cause drowsiness, mental status changes, and seizures

List of Abbreviations

A

Aδ	A delta
ABCD1	ATP binding cassette, subfamily D (ALD), member 1 gene
ACA	anterior cerebral artery
ACAS	Asymptomatic Carotid Atherosclerosis Study
ACE	angiotensin converting enzyme
ACh	acetylcholine
ACh-R	acetylcholine receptor
ACST	Asymptomatic Carotid Surgery Trial
ACTH	adrenocorticotropic hormone
ADC	apparent diffusion coefficient
ADH	antidiuretic hormone
AFB	acid-fast bacillus
AFP	α-fetoprotein
AG	anion gap
AICA	anterior inferior cerebellar artery
AIDS	acquired immune deficiency syndrome
AIFA	anterior internal frontal artery
ALD	adrenoleukodystrophy
ALI	acute lung injury
ALL	acute lymphocytic leukemia; anterior longitudinal ligament
ALS	amyotrophic lateral sclerosis
AMPA	α-amino-3-hydroxy-5-methylisoxazole-4-propionic acid
AP	anteroposterior; action potential
APP	amyloid precursor protein
APUD	amine precursor uptake and decarboxylation
AR	autosomal recessive
ARAS	ascending reticular activating system
ARDS	acute respiratory distress syndrome
ASA	acetylsalicylic acid (aspirin)
ATN	acute tubular necrosis
ATP	adenosine triphosphate
ATPase	adenosine triphosphatase
AV	atrioventricular
AV-3V	anteroventral third ventricular
AVF	arteriovenous fistula
AVM	arteriovenous malformation

B

BAL	2,3-dimercaptopropanol
BBB	blood—brain barrier
BCNU	bischlorethylnitrosourea
BG	basal ganglia
BMR	basal metabolic rate
BP	blood pressure
BUN	blood urea nitrogen

C

cAMP	cyclic adenosine monophosphate
CBF	cerebral blood flow
CCA	common carotid artery
CCF	carotid cavernous fistula
CCK	cholecystokinin
CEA	carcinoembryonic antigen
cGMP	cyclic guanosine monophosphate
cGy	centigray
ChA	choroidal artery
CHF	congestive heart failure
CJD	Creutzfeldt–Jakob disease
CK	creatine kinase
CL	centralis lateralis; corpus luteum; cruciate ligament
CM	centromedial
$CMRO_2$	cerebral metabolic rate of oxygen
CMV	cytomegalovirus
CN	cranial nerve
CNS	central nervous system
CO	cardiac output
CoA	coenzyme A
COMT	catechol-O-methyl transferase
COPD	chronic obstructive pulmonary disease
CPA	cerebellopontine angle
CPAP	continuous positive airway pressure
CPM	central pontine myelinolysis
CPP	cerebral perfusion pressure
CPR	cardiopulmonary resuscitation
CSF	cerebrospinal fluid
CSW	cerebral salt wasting
CT	computed tomography

CTA	computed tomography angiography
CV	cardiovascular
CVP	central venous pressure
CVR	cortical venous reflux

D

D	diopter
DA	dopamine
DAG	diacylglycerol
DAI	diffuse axonal injury
DAVF	dural arteriovenous fistula
DBS	deep brain stimulation
DDAVP	desmopressin acetate
DDx	differential diagnosis
deoxyHb	deoxyhemoglobin
DI	diabetes insipidus
DISH	diffuse idiopathic skeletal hyperostosis
DM	dorsomedial
DNA	deoxyribonucleic acid
DNET	dysembryoplastic neuroepithelial tumor
DOPA	dihydroxyphenylalanine (methyldopa)
DPG	2,3-diphosphoglycerate
DREZ	dorsal root entry zone
DRG	dorsal root ganglion
DSA	digital subtraction angiography
DTR	deep tendon reflex
DWI	diffusion-weighted imaging

E

EBV	Epstein–Barr virus
ECA	external carotid artery
ECG	electrocardiogram
ECST	European Carotid Stenosis Trial
EDH	epidural hematoma
EDTA	ethylenediaminetetraacetic acid
EEG	electroencephalogram
ELISA	enzyme-linked immunosorbent assay
EMA	epithelial membrane antigen
EMG	electromyography
EML	external medullary lamina

EPI	epinephrine
EPSP	excitatory postsynaptic potential
ESR	erythrocyte sedimentation rate
ETOH	ethanol

F

F	female
FFH1	Forel's field H1 (thalamic fasciculus)
FFH2	Forel's field H2 (lenticular fasciculus)
FLAIR MRI	fluid-attenuated inversion-recovery magnetic resonance imaging
FMD	fibromuscular dysplasia
FSH	follicle-stimulating hormone

G

GABA	gamma-aminobutyric acid
GBM	glioblastoma multiforme
GCS	Glasgow Coma Scale
GDP	guanosine diphosphate
GFAP	glial fibrillary acidic protein
GH	growth hormone
GI	gastrointestinal
GP	globus pallidus
GPe	globus pallidus externa
GPi	globus pallidus interna
GPm	medial globus pallidus
GRE	gradient echo
GSA	general somatic afferent
GSE	general somatic efferent
GTP	guanosine triphosphate
GU	genitourinary
GVA	general visceral afferent
GVE	general visceral efferent
Gy	Gray

H

5-HT	5-hydroxytryptamine (serotonin)
H & E	hematoxylin and eosin
Hb	hemoglobin
HCG	human chorionic gonadotropin

HCP	hydrocephalus
HDL	high-density lipoprotein
HELLP	hemolysis, elevated liver enzymes, and low platelet count
HGPRT	hypoxanthine-guanine phosphoribosyltransferase
HHT	hereditary hemorrhagic telangiectasia
HIV	human immunodeficiency virus
HLA-DR2	human leukocyte antigen-DR2
HSM	hepatosplenomegaly
HSV	herpes simplex virus
HTLV	human T cell lymphotropic virus

I

IC	internal capsule
ICA	internal carotid artery
ICAM	intercellular adhesion molecule
ICH	intracranial hemorrhage
ICP	intracranial pressure
IgG	immunogobulin G
IJV	internal jugular vein
IML	internal medullary lamina
INO	internuclear ophthalmoplegia
IPH	intraparenchymal hemorrhage
IPSP	inhibitory postsynaptic potential
ISAT	International Subarachnoid Aneurysm Trial
IV	intravenous
IVH	intraventricular hemorrhage

L

LD	lateral dorsal
LE	lower extremity; lupus erythematosus
LGB	lateral geniculate body
LGP	lateral globus pallidus
LH	luteinizing hormone
LHRH	luteinizing hormone-releasing hormone
LL	lower limb
LMN	lower motor neuron
LOAF	lumbricals 1 and 2, opponens pollicis, and abductor and flexor pollicis brevis
LP	lateral posterior; lumbar puncture
LV	lateral ventricle

M

M	male
MAO	monoamine oxidase
MAP	mean arterial pressure
MBP	myelin basic protein
MCA	middle cerebral artery
MCP	metacarpophalangeal
MD	mediodorsal; muscular dystrophy
MELAS	myopathy, encephalopathy, lactic acidosis, and strokes
MEN	multiple endocrine neoplasia
MEP	motor evoked potential
MEPP	miniature end-plate potential
MERRF	myoclonus, epilepsy, and red-ragged fibers
MetHb	methemoglobin
MFB	medial forebrain bundle
MG	myasthenia gravis
MGB	medial geniculate body
MGMT	O^6-methylguanine-DNA methyltransferase gene
MGP	medial globus pallidus
MI	myocardial infarction
ML	medial lemniscus
MLF	medial longitudinal fasciculus
MMA	middle meningeal artery
MPS	mucopolysaccharides
MPTP	1-methyl-4-phenyl-1,2,3,6-tetrahydropyridine
MR	mental retardation
MRA	magnetic resonance angiography
MRI	magnetic resonance imaging
MRV	magnetic resonance venography
MS	multiple sclerosis

N

NAPA	*N*-acetylprocainamide
NASCET	North American Symptomatic Carotid Endarterectomy Trial
NCV	nerve conduction velocity
NE	norepinephrine
NF	neurofibromatosis
NMDA	*N*-methyl-D-aspartate
NMJ	neuromuscular junction
NO	nitric oxide

NPH	nucleus pulposus herniation; normal pressure hydrocephalus
NSAID	nonsteroidal antiinflammatory drug
NSol	nucleus solitarius

O

OFA	orbitofrontal artery
OPLL	ossified posterior longitudinal ligament
oxyHb	oxyhemoglobin

P

PAM	pyridine aldoxime methochloride
PAS	periodic acid– Schiff
PCA	posterior cerebral artery
PcommA	posterior communicating artery
PCR	polymerase chain reaction
PCV	procarbazine, CCNU (lomustine), vincristine
PCWP	pulmonary capillary wedge pressure
PEEP	positive end-expiratory pressure
PET	positron emission tomography
PF	parafasciculus
PICA	posterior inferior cerebellar artery
PLL	posterior longitudinal ligament
PLP	proteolipid protein
PML	progressive multifocal leukoencephalopathy
PMN	polymorphonuclear neutrophils
PNET	primitive neuroectodermal tumor
PNS	peripheral nervous system
POA	persistent otic artery
postop	postoperative
PPD	purified protein derivative
PPRF	paramedian pontine reticular formation
PRL	prolactin
preop	preoperative
PSA	persistent stapedial artery; prostate specific antigen
PT	prothrombin time
PTA	persistent trigeminal artery
PTAH	phosphotungstic acid hematoxylin
PTEN	phosphatase and tensin gene
PTT	partial thromboplastin time

R

RAS	reticular activating system
RBC	red blood cell
RCT	randomized controlled trial
REM	rapid eye movement
REZ	root entry zone
RF	radiofrequency
RiMLF	rostral interstitial nucleus of the MLF
RMP	resting membrane potential
RNA	ribonucleic acid
RQ	respiratory quotient
RTA	renal tubular acidosis

S

SA	special afferent; sinoatrial
SAH	subarachnoid hemorrhage
SBE	subacute bacterial endocarditis
SBP	systolic blood pressure
SCA	superior cerebellar artery
SCI	spinal cord injury
SDH	subdural hematoma
SI	substantia innominata; sacroiliac
SIADH	syndrome of inappropriate antidiuretic hormone (secretion)
SLE	systemic lupus erythematosus
SMA	spinal muscle atrophy
SN	substantia nigra
SNAP	sensory nerve action potential
SNpc	substantia nigra pars compacta
SNpr	substantia nigra pars reticulata
SPECT	single photon emission computed tomography
SR	sarcoplasmic reticulum
SSA	special somatic afferent
SSEP	somatosensory evoked potential
SSPE	subacute sclerosing panencephalitis
SSS	superior sagittal sinus
ST	subthalamus
STT	spinothalamic tract
SVA	special visceral afferent
SVE	special visceral efferent
SVR	systemic vascular resistance
SVT	supraventricular tachycardia

T

T_3	triiodothyronine
T_4	thyroxine
TB	tuberculosis
TENS	transcutaneous electrical nerve stimulation
TIA	transient ischemic attack
TOF	time-of-flight
tPA	tissue plasminogen activator
TPN	total parenteral nutrition
TRH	thyroid-releasing hormone
tRNA	transfer ribonucleic acid
TS	tuberous sclerosis
TSC	tuberous sclerosis complex
TSH	thyroid-stimulating hormone
t-SNARE	target synaptosome associated protein (SNAP) and *N*-ethylmaleimide-sensitive factor (NSF) attachment receptors

U

UE	upper extremity
UL	upper limb
UMN	upper motor neuron

V

VA	ventroanterior; visceral afferent
VApc	ventroanterior pars compacta
VAS	Veterans Administration Study
VEP	visual evoked potential
VHL	von Hippel--Lindau disease
Vim	ventrointermedius
VL	ventrolateral
VLm	ventrolateral medial
VLo	ventrolateral pars oralis
VP	ventriculoperitoneal
VPI	ventral posterior inferior
VPL	ventroposterolateral
VPLc	ventroposterolateral pars caudalis
VPLo	ventroposterolateral pars oralis
VPM	ventroposteromedial
VPMpc	ventroposteromedial pars compacta

v-SNAREs   vesicle synaptosome associated protein (SNAP) and *N*-ethylmaleimide-sensitive factor (NSF) attach-ment receptors
VT   ventricular tachycardia
vWF   von Willebrand factor

W

WBC   white blood cell
WHO   World Health Organization
WM   white matter

X

XR   x-linked recessive

Index

Note: Page numbers followed by *f* and *t* indicate figures and tables, respectively.

Aging, neurologic changes with, 286, 395
Agnosia, 400
  auditory, 401
  tactile, 438
  visual, 401
AICA. *See* Anterior inferior cerebellar artery
Aicardi syndrome, 190
AIDS. *See* Acquired immune deficiency
    syndrome
AIDS dementia complex, 217
Air embolism, 500
Akinetic mutism, 398, 403
Ala cinerea, 76f
Alar ligaments, 94, 95f–96f
Alar plate, 183
Albumin, 511
Alexander disease, 179, 286, 304t, 305
ALI. *See* Acute lung injury
Allergic angiitis, 323
Allergic encephalomyelitis, experimental,
    314
Allergic neuritis, experimental, 312, 382
Allocortex, 29, 397
Allodynia, 127
Alloesthesia, 438
Alpha-blockers, 163
Alpha-fetoprotein, with yolk sac tumors, 257
Alpha motor neuron, 90, 119f, 121
Alpha waves, 159–160, 159f
ALS. *See* Amyotrophic lateral sclerosis (ALS)
Aluminum toxicity, 178
Alveolar oxygen (O_2) pressure (P_AO_2), 502
Alveolar to arterial O_2 gradient ($P_AO_2 – P_aO_2$),
    502
Alzheimer disease, 56, 178–179, 306–307,
    396
  diagnosis, 307
  neurotransmitters in, 151
  pathology, 306, 307f
  positron emission tomography in, 182
  signs and symptoms, 306
  treatment, 307
  trisomy 21 and, 196
Amacrine cells, 129–130, 132
Amaurosis fugax, 419, 430
Ambulation, 438
Amiloride, 508
Amine precursor uptake and decarboxylation
    (APUD) cells, formation, 183
Amines, 117
Aminoacidopathy(ies), 300
Amino acids, as neurotransmitters, 117
Aminoglycosides
  adverse effects and side effects, 526
  effect on presynaptic ACh release, 387
Amiodarone, 499
Amitriptyline, 126
Ammon's horn, 53f
Amoebic meningoencephalitis, 208
Amorphosynthesis, 124–125
AMPA/quisqualate receptor, 118
Amphetamines, adverse effects and side
    effects, 295
Amphotericin B, adverse effects and side
    effects, 526
Ampulla (of semicircular canal), 145, 145f

Amygdala, 31f, 45, 53, 55–56, 64, 158, 403
  damage to, 155
  functions, 56
  inputs, 55–56
  lesions, 158
  outputs, 56
  stimulation, 56, 158
Amygdalocortical tract, 56
Amygdalofugal tract, ventral, 56
Amygdaloid complex, 54f
Amygdalostriate fibers, 46
Amygdalostriate tract, 56
Amyloid
  β peptides, 396
  effects on peripheral nerves, 379, 382
Amyloid angiopathy, 326–328, 327f, 396
Amyloidosis
  dural enhancement with, 283
  primary, 271
Amyloid precursor protein, 396
Amyotrophic lateral sclerosis (ALS), 179, 310,
    311f, 368, 403, 433
Anaerobes, epidural abscess, 454
Analeptics, adverse effects and side effects,
    295
Analgesia system, 126
Anaphylaxis, 509
Anatomic dead space, 502
Anencephaly, 184
Anesthesia, 526
Aneurysm(s), 328–340. *See also specific vessel*
  anterior circulation
    rupture, risk, 446t
    surgery for, 447–448
  carotid cavernous, rupture, risk, 446t
  Charcot-Bouchard, 325–326
  cranial
    clinical presentation, 446–447
    endovascular coiling for, 447–448
    epidemiology, 446
    Hunt and Hess clinical grading scale,
      446t
    natural history, 446–447
    rupture, risk, 446t
    surgery for, 446–448
    treatment, 447–448
    World Federation of Neurosurgical
      Societies clinical grading scale, 447t
  differential diagnosis, 279–280
  dissecting, 340, 447
  false, 340
  flow-related, 340
  fusiform, 339, 339f, 446
  infectious, 339, 340f, 447
  intrasellar, differential diagnosis, 280
  multiple, 329
  mycotic, 447
  oncotic, 340
  posterior circulation
    rupture, risk, 446t
    surgery for, 447–448
  risk factors for, 329
  rupture, 328–329, 446t
  saccular, 328–339, 446
  spinal, 362
  suprasellar, differential diagnosis, 280

traumatic, 340, 447
true, 340
Aneurysmal bone cyst, spinal, 356–357,
    357f, 481t
Angelman syndrome, 394
Angina, intractable, surgery for, 470–471
Angiofibroma(s), in Bourneville disease, 289
Angiography
  of arteriovenous malformation, 340, 341f
  in stroke patient, 317
Angiolipoma, spinal, 358
Angiomyolipoma, renal, in tuberous
    sclerosis, 289
Angiosarcoma, epidemiology, 463
Angiostrongylus cantonensis, 207
Angiotensin II, 156
Angular artery, 6f, 14f, 15
Angular gyrus, 30f, 152–153, 400, 402, 456
Anion gap, 516
Anion gap acidosis, 516
Anisocoria, 417
Ankylosing spondylitis, 368–370, 370f, 432,
    484–485
  epidemiology, 485
  presentation/natural history, 485
  treatment, 485
Anosmia, 423
Ansa cervicalis, 103, 104f
  inferior root, 103, 104f
  superior root, 103, 104f
Ansa lenticularis, 47
  features, 108
Anterior capsular artery, 9
Anterior caudate vein, 23f
Anterior cerebral artery, 12–13, 12f, 21, 44,
    45f
  aneurysm, 335f
  azygous, with callosal agenesis, 190
  distal segment (A3), 13
  postcommunicating segment (A2), 13
  precommunicating segment (A1), 12
  segments, 12
  stroke, 430
Anterior cerebral vein, 23f
Anterior chamber (of eye), defects, 420
Anterior choroidal artery, 10f, 11–12, 16f,
    18, 21, 44, 45f–46f
  aneurysms, 11, 322f
  cisternal segment, 11
  intraventricular segment, 11–12
  perforators arising from, 11
  stroke, 430
Anterior commissure, 31f, 52, 54f
  blood supply to, 12
  features, 108
  formation, 183
Anterior communicating artery, 12–13, 16f
  aneurysms, 13, 329, 334f–335f
    surgery for, 448
  perforators arising from, 12–13
Anterior cord syndrome, 376, 487t
Anterior ethmoidal artery, 10, 11f
Anterior ethmoidal nerve, 101f
Anterior femoral cutaneous nerve, 107
Anterior fontanelle, closure, 184
Anterior funiculus, 88

F

Fabry disease, 301, 301*t*, 390
　peripheral neuropathy in, 382
Facial artery, 6*f*, 7
Facial canal, 71*f*
Facial colliculus, 69, 76*f*
Facial muscles, innervation, 102
Facial nerve. *See* Cranial nerve(s), VII (facial)
Facial pain, atypical, 415
Facial pain syndromes, 415
Facioscapulohumeral dystrophy, 389
Factor VII
　deficiency, 515
　recombinant, 515
Factor VIII deficiency, 515
Factor IX deficiency, 515
Factor XII deficiency, 515
Factor XIII deficiency, 515
Fahr disease, 286, 308
Failed back syndrome, 374
Falciform ligament, 100
Familial myoclonic epilepsy, 310
Familial periodic paralysis, 391–392
Farsightedness. *See* Presbyopia
Fascicles, *to memorize,* 108–109
Fasciculus cuneatus, 76*f*, 78*f*, 85*f*, 89, 123
　lateral, 78*f*
Fasciculus cuneatus (spinal cord), 91*f*
Fasciculus gracilis, 76*f*, 78*f*, 85*f*, 89
　medial, 78*f*
Fasciculus gracilis (spinal cord), 91*f*
Fasciculus retroflexus, 44
　features, 108
Fasciolar gyrus, 54*f*
Fastigial nucleus, 61–62, 148
Fastigium, 59*f*
Fatal familial insomnia, 216
Fatigue, synaptic, 116, 122
Fear, 157, 403
Febrile seizures, 405
Feeding, 173
　regulation, 157
Feeding center, 51
Felbamate, 409
Femoral nerve, 106*f*
　muscles innervated by, 107
Fencing posture, 394
Fentanyl, 526
Ferrugination, 178
Festinating gait, 439
Fetal alcohol syndrome, 193, 293
Fever, 175
　benefits, 525
　etiology, 175, 525
　postoperative, 525
　treatment, 175
FFH1 (Forel's field H1). *See* Thalamic fasciculus
FFH2 (Forel's field H2). *See* Lenticular fasciculus
FFP. *See* Fresh-frozen plasma (FFP)
Fiber
　dietary, 522
　fermentable, 522

　nonfermentable, 522
Fibrinogen deficiency, 515
Fibrolipoma, of filum terminale, 353
Fibromuscular disease, 321
　aneurysm risk with, 329
Fibronectin, 511
Fibrosarcoma, 221
　epidemiology, 463
　spinal, 357
Fibrous dysplasia
　monostotic, 282, 352
　polyostotic, 282, 352
　of skull, 352
　of skull base, 281–282, 282*f*
Filum terminale, 1, 87
　fibrolipoma, 353
Fimbria, 54*f*
FiO₂, 501
Flaccidity, 437
FLAIR. *See* Fluid-attenuated inversion-recovery (FLAIR)
Flatworms. *See* Platyhelminths
Flavivirus, 209–211
Flexner-Wintersteiner rosettes, 245, 246*f*
Flexor carpi radialis muscle, innervation, 105
Flexor carpi ulnaris muscle, innervation, 105
Flexor digiti minimi muscle, innervation, 105, 107
Flexor digitorum brevis muscle, innervation, 107
Flexor digitorum longus muscle, innervation, 107
Flexor digitorum profundus muscle, innervation, 105
Flexor digitorum superficialis muscle, innervation, 105
Flexor hallucis brevis muscle, innervation, 107
Flexor hallucis longus muscle, innervation, 107
Flexor pollicis brevis muscle, innervation, 105
Flexor pollicis longus muscle, innervation, 105
Flexor (withdrawal) reflex, 141
Flocculonodular lobe, 147–148, 416
Flocculus, 30*f*, 57, 58*f*
　lesions, functional deficits caused by, 63
　peduncle, 58*f*
Floppy infant syndrome, 310
Flow, 510–511
Fluid-attenuated inversion-recovery (FLAIR), 181
Fluid replacement, 510–511
Flukes, 207
Flumazenil, 527
Fluorophosphate, 167
FMD. *See* Fibromuscular disease
FMR1 gene, 197
fMRI. *See* Magnetic resonance imaging (MRI), functional (fMRI)
Focal length (f), 128
Focal response (sympathetic), 163
Foix-Alajouanine syndrome, 363
Folate
　deficiency, 522

　requirements, 522
Folia, 57
Folium of vermis, 57, 58*f*–59*f*
Follicle-stimulating hormone (FSH), 176
Fontanelle(s), closure, 184
Foot, innervation, 107
Foramen cecum, 97
Foramen lacerum, 97, 99*f*
Foramen magnum, 97, 99*f*
　lesions, 352
　tumors, differential diagnosis, 280
Foramen of Monro, anatomy, 455, 455*f*
Foramen ovale, 97, 99*f*
Foramen rotundum, 97, 99*f*
Foramen spinosum, 97, 99*f*
Forearm, innervation, 105, 106*f*
Forel's field H1. *See* Thalamic fasciculus
Forel's field H2. *See* Lenticular fasciculus
Fornix (pl., fornices), 31*f*, 40*f*, 41, 43*f*, 49*f*, 50, 53, 53*f*–54*f*
　body, 31*f*
　components, 55
　features, 108
　formation, 183
　pillars, blood supply to, 12
　postcommissural, 55
　precommissural, 55
Foster-Kennedy syndrome, 249, 250*f*
Fourth ventricle, 31*f*, 58*f*, 76*f*
　floor, 84
　formation, 183
　lateral recess, 76*f*
　neoplasia in, surgical approach for, 455
　rosette-forming glioneuronal tumor
　　epidemiology, 459
　　presentation/natural history, 459
　　treatment, 459
　tenia, 76*f*
　tumors, differential diagnosis, 279
Fovea, 129
Fovea centralis, 133*f*, 419
Fractional excretion, 506
Fracture(s)
　basilar, 347, 348*f*
　burst, 379, 381*f*, 490
　clay shoveler's, 379, 381*f*, 490
　comminuted, 347
　compound (open), 347
　definition, 347
　depressed, 347, 347*f*
　　epidemiology, 474
　　presentation/natural history, 474
　　treatment, 474
　diastatic, 347
　hangman's, 378, 379*f*, 489
　Jefferson, 377, 377*f*, 488
　linear, 347
　nonaccidental, 347
　occipital condyle, 488
　odontoid, 377–378, 378*f*, 488–489
　spinal, 376
Fragile X syndrome, 196–197
Free nerve endings, 122
Fresh-frozen plasma (FFP), 511, 515
F response, 435

Pseudoaneurysm(s), 340
Pseudobulbar palsy, 399
  with frontal lobe lesion, 398
Pseudodementia, 396
Pseudolaminar cortical necrosis, 317
Pseudomembranous colitis, 508
Pseudorosettes
  in ependymoma, 235, 236f
  in PNETs, 244
Pseudoseizures, 407
Pseudotumor cerebri, 427
  epidemiology, 472
  presentation/natural history, 472
  treatment, 472
Psoas muscle, innervation, 107
Psychic blindness, 401
PT. *See* Prothrombin time (PT)
Pterion, 455
Pterygoid canal, 98
Pterygopalatine fossa, 98
Pterygopalatine ganglion, 67f, 70, 70f, 101f
  features, 109
Pterygopalatine nerve, 68
Ptosis, 418
PTT. *See* Partial thromboplastin time (PTT)
Pudendal nerve, 106f
  function, 110
  muscles innervated by, 107
Pulmonary disorders, 502–503
Pulmonary edema, cardiogenic, 502–503,
    503t
Pulmonary embolism, ECG findings with, 499
Pulse oximetry, 501
Pulvinar, 40f, 41, 43f, 76f
Punishment centers, 157
Pupil(s), 129, 417–419
  in comatose patient, 426–427
  dilated, in comatose patient, 426–427
  fixed and dilated, 417
  midsized fixed, in comatose patient, 427
  pinpoint, 418
    in comatose patient, 427
Pure word blindness, 403
Pure word deafness, 401, 403
Purkinje cells, 57, 60, 148–149, 416
Putamen, 31f
  damage to, 150
  formation, 183
Putamen circuit, 48, 149
P waves, 497, 497t
Pyramid(s), 30f, 76f–77f, 399
  decussation, 77f, 85f
Pyramidal cells, 152, 397
Pyramidal tract, 79f, 85f, 143
Pyramid of vermis, 57, 58f–59f
Pyramis. *See* Pyramid of vermis
Pyrexia, in trauma, 496
Pyridostigmine, 163
Pyridoxine deficiency, 298
Pyriform cortex, 64

Q

Quadriceps femoris muscles, innervation,
    107

Quinidine, 499
  toxicity, ECG findings with, 499

R

Rabies, 179, 209–210, 213, 213f
Raccoon eyes, 347
Radial nerve, 105, 106f
  entrapments, 493–494
Radiation, vertebral body changes caused
    by, 224f
Radiation myelopathy, 223, 367–368, 368f
Radiation necrosis, 223, 224f
Radiation therapy
  for single-level spinal cord compression,
      comparison to surgery, 481, 482t
  standard doses, 223
Radiation vasculopathy, 321
Radicular artery(ies), 24, 25f, 26
Radicular pain, spinal disorders and, 432
Raeder syndrome, 323, 415
Rage, 157
RAH. *See* Recurrent artery of Heubner
Ramsay Hunt syndrome, 213, 386, 415
Ramsay-Hunt zoster otitis, differential
    diagnosis, 280
Ranawat scale, for neurologic symptoms
    from rheumatoid arthritis, 484,
    484t
Raphe nucleus, 46, 56, 61, 84, 156, 159
Rapid eye movements (REM), 158–160,
    439–440
Rasmussen chronic encephalitis, 218
Rathke cleft cyst, 261, 261f, 467
  differential diagnosis, 280
Raynaud disease, surgery for, 470–471
Raynaud syndrome, 443
Rebound, 149
Receptive fields, of nerve fibers, 119f, 121
Receptor potential, 120
Reciprocal inhibitory circuit, 121
Rectus capitis anterior muscle, innervation,
    103, 104f
Rectus capitis lateralis muscle, innervation,
    103, 104f
Rectus capitis posterior muscle(s), major and
    minor, innervation, 103
Recurrent artery of Heubner, 12–13, 21,
    45f–46f
Recurrent laryngeal nerve, 75
  muscles innervated by, 102
Recurrent meningeal artery, 10
Red nucleus, 61, 77f, 78, 79f, 81–82, 143
Reentrant tachycardia, 497, 497t
Referred pain, spinal disorders and, 432
Reflex(es)
  autonomic, 142, 162–163
  gastrointestinal, 172
  hung-up, 411
  muscle spindle-related, 141
  pendular, 411
  primitive, 394
  programmed in spinal cord, 141–142
Reflex epilepsy, 407
Reflexive learning, 155

Reflex sympathetic dystrophy, 127, 386
  facial, 415
Refraction, 128–129
Refractive power, 128
Refractory period, 114–115
  absolute, 114
  relative, 115
Refsum disease, 304t, 305, 312, 383
Reinnervation, 166, 436
Reissner membrane, 135f–136f, 137
Reiter syndrome, 432
REM. *See* Rapid eye movements (REM)
REM sleep behavior disorder, 441
Renal cell carcinoma
  metastases
    cerebral, epidemiology, 467t
    hemorrhage with, 328
    spinal, 481
  in von Hippel-Lindau disease, 289–290
Renal critical care, 506–508
Renal failure
  acute
    approach to, 507
    drug adjustments in, 507
    impaired platelet adhesion in, 513–514
    nutrition in, 523
    prerenal causes, 506, 507t
    renal causes, 506, 507t
Renal tubular acidosis, 507–508
Rendu-Osler-Weber disease, 201
Renshaw cells, 140
Reovirus, 210–211
Repolarization, and action potential, 113
Reserpine, 163
Respiration
  control, 171–172
  physiology, 171–172
Respiratory acidosis, 517
  acute, 516
  chronic, 516
Respiratory alkalosis, 517
  acute, 516
  chronic, 516
Respiratory center, 171
Respiratory critical care, 501–506
Respiratory failure, nutrition in, 523
Respiratory medications, 503–504
Respiratory quotient, 502, 521
Restiform body, 61, 147
  features, 109
Resting membrane potential, 112–113
  in cardiac cells, 169
Restless leg syndrome, 440
Restlessness, 157
Reticular activating system, 155–156
Reticular formation, 79f, 85f, 86
  inhibitory, 155
Reticular formation zones, 82
Reticular nucleus, 41
Reticulocerebellar tract, 60, 147
Reticulospinal tract, 91f, 143–144
  lateral (medullary), 93–94
  medial (pontine), 93–94
Reticulotegmental tract, 61
Retina, 419
  blood supply to, 129

drug interactions with, 408
indications for, 409
pharmacology, 408
Vancomycin, adverse effects and side effects, 526
Varicella-zoster virus (VZV), 209, 213
detection, 210
in HIV-infected (AIDS) patients, 218
peripheral neuropathy, 383
Vascular dementia, 396
Vascular disease(s), 315–347
cranial, surgery for, 446–452
extrinsic compressive lesions and, 322
spinal, 362–364
surgery for, 476–477
Vascular lesion(s), differential diagnosis, 280
Vascular malformations, 183, 340–347.
See also Arteriovenous fistula;
Arteriovenous malformation
differential diagnosis, 278
Vascular steal, 341
Vasculitis, 323–324
cell-mediated, 323–324
chemical, 324
immune complex, 323
infectious, 323
lupus, 323, 323f
mononeuropathy multiplex in, 385
tuberculous, 323
Vasculopathy, 323–324. See also Vascular disease(s)
Vasoconstrictor area, 170
Vasocorona, of spinal arteries, 25f
Vasodepressor (vasovagal) syncope, 425
Vasodilator area, 170
Vasomotor center, 170
Vasopressin, 499
Vater-Pacini corpuscle, 119f. See also Pacinian corpuscle
Vecuronium, 504
Vein of Galen, 23f, 24
aneurysm/malformation, 342, 342f
Venezuelan equine encephalitis (VEE) virus, 210
Venous angle, 23f
Venous lakes, 283
Venous malformations, 344, 346f
spinal, 364
Venous sinus thrombosis, 318, 318f
Venous varix, 344
Ventilation, 502
Ventral induction, 183
Ventral median fissure, 77f
Ventral tegmental nucleus, 81
Ventricular system (cerebral), 3, 3f
Ventricular tachycardia, 497t, 498
Ventriculoperitoneal shunt infection, 525
Ventrobasal complex, 123
Ventrolateral sulcus, 76f–77f
Ventroposterolateral thalamic nuclei, 40f, 42, 123, 124f
Ventroposteromedial thalamic nuclei, 40f, 42, 123, 124f
VEP. See Visual evoked potentials (VEP)
Verbal apraxia, 399

Vermis of cerebellum, 31f, 58f–59f, 147–148, 416
lobules, 57
posterior, lesions, functional deficits caused by, 63
Verocay bodies, 274, 274f
Vertebrae
age-related changes in, 431–432
body, 95f
inflammatory diseases, 368–370
osteomyelitis
epidemiology, 478
presentation/natural history, 478
treatment, 478
postradiation changes in, 368
Vertebrae plana, 357
Vertebral arch, 95f
Vertebral artery, 5, 6f, 19–20, 19f, 21, 87f
branches, 19–20
dissection, 322, 323f, 350
hypoplastic, 5
meningeal branches, 19f
stroke, 431
Vertebral artery(ies) (spinal), 24
Vertebral veins, 87f
Vertebrobasilar junction, aneurysm, 329, 336f
Vertebrobasilar system, atherosclerosis, 426
Vertigo
benign positional, 424
definition, 424
Vestibula (ear), 71f
Vestibular area, 76f
Vestibular cortex, 37, 401
Vestibular ganglion, 71f
Vestibular nerve, 71f, 145
Vestibular neuroma, unilateral, 288
Vestibular neuronitis, 424
Vestibular nucleus (pl., nuclei), 72, 144
inferior, 146
lateral, 146
medial, 146
superior, 146
Vestibular schwannoma(s), 221, 273, 274f–275f
bilateral, 288
differential diagnosis, 279–280
hearing loss caused by, 424
radiation sensitivity, 223
Vestibular system, 144–146
anatomy, 144–146, 145f
Vestibulocerebellar tract, 60, 147
Vestibulocerebellum, 416
Vestibulocochlear nerve. See Cranial nerve(s), VIII (vestibulocochlear)
Vestibulospinal tract(s), 91f, 93, 143–144
lateral, 94
medial, 72, 94
VHL. See von Hippel-Lindau disease
Vibration sense, 122
Vidian artery, 8
Vidian canal, 98
Vidian nerve of pterygoid canal, 70, 70f
Vinblastine, adverse effects and side effects, 380

Vincristine, adverse effects and side effects, 296, 380, 528
Viral infection(s), 209–219
access to CNS, 209
acute disseminated encephalomyelitis after, 218–219
encephalitis caused by, 210
meningitis caused by, 210
transmission, 209
Viral myositis, 391
Virchow-Robin spaces, 1, 283
Virus(es), 209
detection, 210
DNA, 210
neurotropic, 209
RNA, 210
neurotropic, 209
Viscosity, 510
Vision, 128–135, 417–422
central pathways, 65–66
disorders, 130–131
physics, 128–129
Visual agnosia, 401
Visual cortex, 134
layers, 134
primary, 36, 134
secondary, 36
Visual deficits
parietal lobe lesions and, 400
temporal lobe lesions and, 401
Visual evoked potentials (VEP), 434
Visual fields, 133f, 420–421
chiasmatic lesion deficits, 420–421
concentric constriction, 420
"pie in the sky" deficit, 421
prechiasmatic lesion deficits, 420
retrochiasmatic lesion deficits, 421
Visual loss
episodic, 420
of glaucoma, 420
neurologic causes, 419–420
nonneurologic causes, 420
sudden painless, 419
Visual pathway(s), 132–134, 133f
Visual pursuit movements, 134
Visual system, blood supply to, 11
Visuotopic thalamocortical pathways, 41
Vitamin(s), 521–522
deficiency(ies), 297–298, 522
and optic neuropathy, 420
peripheral neuropathy in, 382
requirements, 522
Vitamin A
deficiency, 131, 298, 522
in photochemistry, 131
Vitamin B$_6$. See Pyridoxine
Vitamin B$_{12}$ deficiency, 297–298, 298f
Vitamin C deficiency, 522
Vitamin D deficiency, 298
Vitamin E deficiency, 298, 522
Vitamin K-dependent factors, 514
Vitreous humor, 129
defects, 420
V$_m$. See Membrane potential
Voltage-gated channels, 111
von Hippel-Lindau disease, 252, 289–290, 291f